Emerging Perspectives in Health Communication

This collection highlights the changing landscape of health communication scholarship through its coverage of interpretive, cultural, and critical approaches to health communication research and practice. It introduces theoretical perspectives, methodological questions, and empirical evidence to demonstrate the importance of meaning construction, culture, power, inequality, participation and voice to our understanding of health discourse and everyday experience. Contributors actively engage with health problems in local, national and transnational contexts.

This distinctive volume serves as a catalyst for future study, presenting the latest research by top scholars in health and popular discourse; culturally-based health promotion; medical communication; and health policy. It provides a rich foundation for scholars who seek to use interpretive, critical or cultural frameworks in academic and applied health communication settings. It will be a key resource for health communication scholars, researchers, and students as well as interpretive, cultural, and critical communication scholars and graduate students. It will also appeal to scholars and practitioners in the allied health areas.

Heather M. Zoller (Ph.D., Purdue University) is an Associate Professor in the Department of Communication at the University of Cincinnati. Her research in health and organizational communication focuses on the politics of public health, including corporate issue management and occupational health, community organizing/public participation, and health activism.

Mohan J. Dutta (Ph.D., University of Minnesota) is Associate Professor of health communication, public relations and mass media and Director of Graduate Studies in the Department of Communication at Purdue University. Professor Dutta is the 2006 Lewis Donohew Outstanding Scholar in Health Communication and has received multiple research and teaching awards for his scholarly contributions. His research in health communication focuses on the culture-centered approach to health communication, politics of resistance in health, subaltern studies and postcolonial theories, and performance-based strategies of social change.

LEA's communication series
Jennings Bryant/Dolf Zillmann, General Editors

Selected titles in Applied Communication
(Teresa L. Thompson, Advisory Editor) include:

Communication Perspectives on HIV/AIDS for the 21st Century
Edgar/Noar/Freimuth

Privacy and Disclosure of HIV in Interpersonal Relationships
A sourcebook for researchers and practitioners
Greene/Derlega/Yep/Petronio

Narratives, Health, and Healing
Communication theory, research, and practice
Harter/Japp/Beck

Aging, Communication, and Health
Linking research and practice for successful aging
Hummert/Nussbaum

Handbook of Communication and Aging Research, Second Edition
Nussbaum/Coupland

Lifespan Communication
Pecchioni/Wright/Nussbaum

Health Communication in Practice
A case study approach
Ray

Family Communication
Segrin/Flora

Handbook of Health Communication
Thompson/Dorsey/Miller/Parrott

Handbook of Family Communication
Vangelisti

Emerging Perspectives in Health Communication

Meaning, Culture, and Power

Edited by
Heather M. Zoller and
Mohan J. Dutta

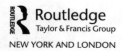

Routledge
Taylor & Francis Group

NEW YORK AND LONDON

First published 2008
by Routledge
270 Madison Ave, New York, NY 10016

Simultaneously published in the UK
by Routledge
2 Park Square, Milton Park, Abingdon, Oxon OX14 4RN

Routledge is an imprint of the Taylor & Francis Group, an informa business

© 2008 Taylor & Francis

Typeset in Goudy and Gill Sans by
Keystroke, 28 High Street, Tettenhall, Wolverhampton
Printed and bound in the United States of America on acid-free paper by
Edwards Brothers, Inc

Library of Congress Cataloging in Publication Data
Emerging perspectives in health communication : meaning, culture, and power /
[edited] by Heather M. Zoller and Mohan J. Dutta.
p. ; cm.
Includes bibliographical references.
ISBN 978-0-8058-6195-2 (alk. paper) – ISBN 978-1-4106-1550-3 (alk. paper)
1. Communication in public health. 2. Health promotion. I. Zoller, Heather M.
II. Dutta, Mohan J.
[DNLM: 1. Delivery of Health Care. 2. Communication. 3. Health Promotion.
W 84.1 E53 2008]
RA423.2.E44 2008
362.101'4—dc22
2007038207

ISBN10: 0–8058–6195–5 HB
ISBN10: 0–8058–6196–3 PB
ISBN10: 1–4106–1550–2 EB

ISBN13: 978–0–8058–6195–2 HB
ISBN13: 978–0–8058–6196–9 PB
ISBN13: 978–1–4106–1550–3 EB

Contents

List of illustrations   ix

1 Theoretical foundations: interpretive, critical, and cultural
  approaches to health communication   1
  MOHAN J. DUTTA AND HEATHER M. ZOLLER

PART I
Popular discourse and constructions of
health and healing   **29**

  Introduction   30
  MOHAN J. DUTTA AND HEATHER M. ZOLLER

2 Let me tell you a story: narratives and narration in health
  communication research   39
  CECILIA BOSTICCO AND TERESA L. THOMPSON

3 Supporting breastfeeding(?): nursing mothers' resistance to
  and accommodation of medical and social discourses   63
  EMILY T. CRIPE

4 Communicating healing holistically   85
  PATRICIA GEIST-MARTIN, BARBARA SHARF, AND NATALIE JEHA

5 'You feel so responsible': Australian mothers' concepts and
  experiences related to promoting the health and development
  of their young children   113
  DEBORAH LUPTON

6 Destigmatizing leprosy: implications for communication
   theory and practice   129
   SRINIVAS R. MELKOTE, PRADEEP KRISHNATRAY, AND SANGEETA
   KRISHNATRAY

PART II
Culture in health communication   147

   Introduction
   MOHAN J. DUTTA AND HEATHER M. ZOLLER

7 Teach-with-stories method for prenatal education: using
   photonovels and a participatory approach with Latinos   155
   SUSAN J. AUGER, MARY E. DECOSTER, AND MELIDA D. COLINDRES

8 Ethical paradoxes in community-based participatory research 182
   VIRGINIA M. MCDERMOTT, JOHN G. OETZEL, AND KALVIN WHITE

9 *Voces de Las Colonias*: dialectical tensions about control
   and cultural identification in Latinas' communication
   about cancer   203
   MELINDA VILLAGRAN, DOROTHY COLLINS, AND SARA GARCIA

10 *El Poder y la Fuerza de la Pasión*: toward a model of
   HIV/AIDS education and service delivery from the
   "bottom-up"   224
   ARIANA OCHOA CAMACHO, GUST A. YEP, PRADO Y. GOMEZ,
   AND ELISSA VELEZ

11 Interrogating the Radio Communication Project in Nepal:
   the participatory framing of colonization   247
   MOHAN J. DUTTA AND ICCHA BASNYAT

PART III
Medical communication   **267**

Introduction
HEATHER M. ZOLLER AND MOHAN J. DUTTA

12 Contested streams of action: power and deference in
emergency medicine   275
ALEXANDRA G. MURPHY, ERIC M. EISENBERG, ROBERT WEARS,
AND SHAWNA J. PERRY

13 Changing realities and entrenched norms in dialysis: a case
study of power, knowledge, and communication in
health-care delivery   293
LAURA L. ELLINGSON

14 Changing lanes and changing lives: the *shifting scenes*
and *continuity* of care of a mobile health clinic   313
LYNN M. HARTER, KAREN DEARDORFF, PAMELA KENNISTON,
HEATHER CARMACK, AND ELIZABETH RATTINE-FLAHERTY

15 The paradox of pharmaceutical empowerment: Healthology
and online health public relations   335
ASHLI QUESINBERRY STOKES

PART IV
Communication and health policy   **357**

Introduction
HEATHER M. ZOLLER AND MOHAN J. DUTTA

16 Dealing drugs on the border: power and policy in
pharmaceutical reimportation debates   365
CHARLES CONRAD AND DENISE JODLOWSKI

17 Technologies of neoliberal governmentality: the discursive
influence of global economic policies on public health   390
HEATHER M. ZOLLER

18 The paradox of "fair trade": the influence of neoliberal
trade agreements on food security and health   411
REBECCA DESOUZA, AMBAR BASU, INDUK KIM, ICCHA BASNYAT,
AND MOHAN J. DUTTA

19 Globalization, social justice movements, and the human
genome diversity debates: a case study in health activism   431
RULON WOOD, DAMON M. HALL, AND MAROUF HASIAN, JR.

PART V
Afterword   **447**

20 Emerging agendas in health communication and the
challenge of multiple perspectives   449
HEATHER M. ZOLLER AND MOHAN J. DUTTA

List of contributors   464
Index   472

Illustrations

Tables

6.1 Differences in perception of leprosy between the state
   health agencies and the local community   134
6.2 Comparison of the Diffusion of Innovations and Participatory
   Communication Models in leprosy communication, cure, and
   its desigmatization   136
6.3 Comparison of development communication theories and
   approaches in the modernization and empowerment
   frameworks   140
7.1 Summary of PDSA cycles   164
7.2 Definitions of common Latino cultural values and norms   167
9.1 Research participant demographics   211
9.2 Interview guide   213

Figures

6.1 Relevant actors in leprosy cure and its destigmatization   144
7.1 De Madre a Madre prenatal education: six steps in the
   Teach-With-Stories Method™   160
11.1 A culture-centered model of health communication   248

Chapter 1

Theoretical foundations

Interpretive, critical, and cultural approaches to health communication

Mohan J. Dutta and Heather M. Zoller

In some ways, the field of "health communication" may appear to address a relatively straightforward set of goals and concerns. For example, health provider communication may be studied to improve patient compliance with health directives, such as completing prescriptions or reducing cholesterol intake. Public health communication interventions may be designed to bring about some desired health improvement goal in a target audience, and the results measured in terms of their effectiveness in achieving change. Certainly, these health initiatives are ubiquitous: African Americans in the rural South are encouraged to take five or more servings of fruits and vegetables to reduce their cancer risks, people are encouraged not to smoke, workplaces cajole employees to exercise so as to lower absenteeism and reduce insurance rates. In these efforts, communication involves methods of persuasion (such as motivation, fear, encouragement) that can be measured in terms of effectiveness.

Of course, achieving these goals is not straightforward. Health communication research shows us that communication is not a "magic bullet" that can create change. Health messages, whether mass mediated or interpersonal, must engage with the complexities of human needs, motivations, and priorities. Indeed, health communicators are working to create interventions more sensitive to these issues (Edgar et al., 2003).

However, there are still more complexities in the communicative endeavors described above beyond the challenge of effective behavior change. Each of these goals relies on a particular approach to the meaning of health, making assumptions about how health can be achieved and who has the authority to instruct others. The ways in which intervention objectives are determined and evaluative criteria are configured are predicated upon certain assumptions that are taken for granted about what it means to be healthy and what constitutes health (Dutta, in press; Dutta & Basu, 2007; Dutta-Bergman, 2004b). The projects themselves may come into question when contextually embedded in social and political systems. What counts as illness, whose therapies are recommended, and who has the means to pay for prescriptions? Why is fruit and vegetable consumption addressed as the predominant means for preventing cancer? Why does management promote exercise when their companies have high rates of occupational illness and accidents? Each of these questions involves broadening our conception of communication to address the social construction of health and illness and the underlying dimensions of power that are central to health communication. In this book, we would like to add multiple layers of complexity to our understanding of relationships between health and meaning. By highlighting the emergence of interpretive, critical, and cultural research perspectives, chapters in this book will demonstrate the utility of asking an array of questions about health communication, including: what meanings of health are operating in a particular circumstance, how have those meanings been culturally constructed, whose meanings are circulating, and with what material and symbolic consequences?

In organizing this introductory chapter to the book, we decided to begin by examining what it means to study health communication. What is health communication? What unites the different approaches to the study of health communication? What are some of the common threads that join these different approaches? After setting up the scope of health communication as a field of inquiry, we shift our attention to theory. What constitutes a theory and what are the different approaches to theory building? What criteria shall we as students and scholars of health communication use in evaluating these different theories, and how do these criteria vary based on the approach we take toward the study of health communication? Our introductory discussion of theory will lay out the foundations for discussing the post-positivistic, interpretive, critical, and cultural approaches to health communication. After setting up each of these approaches, we compare and contrast them and provide exemplars of each in the study of health communication. Following the framework proposed by Babrow and Mattson (2003), we lay out the dialectical tensions that are inherent in the different approaches. We conclude our chapter by discussing the contributions of interpretive, critical, and cultural approaches and previewing the chapters to follow.

The discipline

In the introduction to the *Handbook of Health Communication*, Teresa Thompson (2003) points out that the field of health communication has grown dramatically in the last twenty-five years. As she notes, the field started with the creation of the Health Communication Division of the International Communication Association in 1975, and subsequently became a division under the same name at the National Communication Association in 1985. The flagship journal of the field, *Health Communication*, was started in 1989, devoted specifically to the coverage of research focused on the study of communication in health care. In her review of the field, Thompson notes that the field has grown substantively from its early years not only in terms of the amount of research being conducted, but also in the growth of its scope. Whereas the early years of health communication scholarship focused on the interpersonal aspects of health communication, current research in health communication encompasses (a) organizational issues in health communication, (b) community-based aspects of health communication, and (c) popular media issues and campaigns in the context of public health and medicine. We also are beginning to see greater attention to cultural and policy levels of analysis.

Furthermore, we are seeing a growth in the variety of perspectives applied in health communication research. Whereas most of the early research approached the field from a post-positivistic lens, an increasing body of research has started addressing interpretive, critical, and cultural issues in health communication scholarship (Zoller & Kline, 2008). The popularity of these alternative approaches to the study of health communication is witnessed in the growing number of articles in field journals such as *Health Communication*, *Journal of Applied Communication Research*, and *Journal of Health Communication* that approach the study of health communication from these perspectives. One of the goals of this book is to highlight and showcase this increasingly important body of scholarship. As we do so, we hope to provide a launching pad for the student and the scholar in health communication who is interested in exploring these perspectives, as well as to demonstrate their utility to health scholars in disciplines such as sociology, psychology, and anthropology. This book features the works of scholars who embrace the interpretive, critical, and cultural frameworks as ways of understanding, explaining, and engaging with health communication processes and phenomena.

Whereas some of these approaches presented in the book emphasize in-depth understanding of health constructions, others explicitly focus on raising questions of social change. Most of the contributors employ qualitative methods, reflecting current trends in interpretive, cultural, and critical work in the field. Indeed, this predominance of qualitative methods may suggest the need for developing more quantitative approaches to health communication that ask critical questions and seek to engage in transformative politics.

What does it mean to study health communication?

Health communication refers to the array of communication processes and messages that are constituted around health issues. Scholarship in the field may be categorized into two broad categories based on its emphasis: the process-based perspective and the message-based perspective. The process-based approach to health communication explores the ways in which health meanings are constituted, interpreted, and circulated, investigating processes of symbolic interaction and structuration as they relate to health. The message-based perspective is concerned with the creation of effective messages about health, and it attempts to address strategies for creating effective communication that would accomplish the goals of the involved stakeholders. Of course, all of this begs the question of what constitutes health, but we would argue that this foundational question is one that must be situated in light of particular contexts.

Elements of health communication scholarship

Despite the wide variety of paradigmatic approaches to the study of health communication that we will discuss, there are certain underlying principles that run through the various areas and levels of health communication scholarship. One of the salient features of this communication research is its commitment to praxis. Praxis encompasses the ways in which health communication scholarship comes to be enacted in the world. In this sense, health communication researchers examine the practice of health communication, and are concerned with the applications through which the study of health messages, meanings, and processes can inform the practice of health communication (Thompson, 2003). Studies in the field explore the possibilities of developing meaningful applications that are humane, effective, and responsive to the health needs of individuals, groups, and communities. Although scholars might disagree on what comes to constitute humane, effective, and meaningful communication, the field nevertheless is committed to the possibilities of developing meaningful applications.

The commitment to the examination of communication messages and processes in health settings also suggests that health communication scholars "get dirty" and immerse themselves in the field. Therefore, most health communication scholarship takes place in the context of physician–patient interactions, workplace health interventions, media outlets, community coalition building to create health infrastructures, and other applied situations. Sub-disciplinary journals such as *Health Communication* and the *Journal of Health Communication* attest to the engagement of health communication scholarship in "real world" settings, exemplifying research that typically takes place outside the realm of the typical convenience sample of classroom subjects that are overrepresented in much communication scholarship.

Yet another common feature of health communication scholarship is its interdisciplinary nature. The complex nature of health communication problems calls for the need to engage with theories and methods spanning across (a) various sub-disciplines of communication, and (b) various other disciplines beyond communication. For instance, scholars studying communication patterns in the physician–patient relationship not only need to engage interpersonal communication scholarship, but also need to interact with bodies of knowledge from medicine, nursing, medical anthropology, and medical sociology that engage with the question of the physician–patient relationship. Similarly, scholars examining the role of health policies in creating certain communication outcomes ought to engage with economists, sociologists, and others in order to develop a sophisticated understanding of health communication phenomena.

Finally, the field of health communication is dynamic, thus calling for continuous movement in the theories and methodologies that are applied in studying the health communication messages and processes. The continuously shifting terrain of health care today calls for constant updating of the ways in which we come to understand and study health communication phenomena. For example, present-day health communication scholars ought to understand the existence of health communication at the intersections of technology and globalization, two key trends in the current social configuration of the world that continue to profoundly influence our understanding of health and the ways in which it has come to be constituted in the world. Health communication theorizing is in a state of continual flux, necessitating that we revisit old theories, offer new ones, and continually revise the knowledge that has come to constitute the field.

Theoretical perspectives in health communication: dominant and emerging perspectives

Broadly speaking, the study of health communication may be grouped into one of the four following approaches: post-positivistic, interpretive, critical, or cultural studies. The dominant approach in health communication is the post-positivistic, with an emphasis on improving a variety of health outcomes as outlined by the biomedical model (Dutta, in press). The field, however, has witnessed an increasing trend toward the incorporation of interpretive approaches that emphasize health meanings and narratives, critical approaches that raise questions of power and control, and cultural studies that situate critical questions in cultural contexts (Zoller & Kline, 2008). It is worth pointing out at the onset that although this categorization scheme is offered as a way of labeling and understanding the different approaches to heath communication, it surely is not our goal to limit the scope of current health communication scholarship within these distinctly defined categories.

The post-positivistic approach is concerned with explaining, controlling, and predicting various levels of health outcomes by investigating the roles of communicative, social, and psychological variables. This line of research has typically been concerned with the identification of constructs, operationalization, measurement, and prediction of health-related communication constructs. For instance, the post-positivistic line of research on communication competence in health settings operationalizes what it means to be a competent communicator, measures communication competence, examines the effects of competence on heath outcomes and suggests communication skills for improving the communication competence in the population (Makoul et al., 1995). Similarly, the post-positivistic research on health campaigns focuses on identifying variables such as perceived benefits and barriers to action in order to develop effective health interventions. Ultimately, the goal of this line of scholarship is to create effective health communication solutions to tackle problems addressed typically at the individual level (Murray-Johnson & Witte, 2003).

Much of the extant health communication research may be categorized under the post-positivistic paradigm, and has primarily focused on the roles of effective messaging strategies in health communication settings (social support systems, provider–patient interactions, health campaigns, health organizations, and media systems). This research focuses on identifying communication variables that influence health outcomes.

Interpretive, critical, and cultural studies approaches to health communication tend to be thought of as "alternative" because of the dominance of post-positivistic approaches (Zoller & Kline, 2008). In using the term "alternative," we realize that what is alternative can become dominant as discursive spaces of scholarship shift terrains and as the power structures within and across institutional systems change. The publication of this book and the increasing popularity of interpretive, critical, and cultural studies in health communication attest to the shifting mood in the field (Beck et al., 2004).

The interpretive approach to health communication emphasizes the construction of meanings related to health and medicine. Drawing from the theoretical traditions of hermeneutics, phenomenology, ethnomethodology, and symbolic interactionism among others (Lindlof & Taylor, 2002), interpretive theorists seek to understand how meaning is constituted and contested through interaction. Scholars applying the interpretive approach to health communication typically engage in documenting detailed descriptions of health meanings and the processes through which they are constructed and enacted, using a variety of techniques such as in-depth interviews, focus groups, participant observations, textual and rhetorical analysis, and ethnographies (Sharf & Vandeford, 2003; Geist & Dreyer, 1993; Ellingson, 2005). Most of these approaches are qualitative in nature, and emphasize contextually located accounts rather than generalizable explanations that predict health behaviors and outcomes. This qualitative approach allows for understanding the embodied performance of health and illness, as well as issues of textual style and artistry that are difficult to capture quantitatively. Increasingly, health communication scholars are adopting narrative perspectives, focusing on the role of stories in narrating health and illness experiences. The growth of this perspective is evident in the publishing of the edited book, *Narratives, Health, and Healing: Communication Theory, Research, and Practice* (Harter et al., 2005), which investigates the "murky, cluttered, and complicated interrelationships" addressed by narrative (p. 8).

Critical approaches emphasize understanding the role of health communication in constructing and reinforcing dominant power relationships, and in simultaneously marginalizing certain sectors of society. How do communication practices in health settings serve the status quo? How are the interests of the underprivileged sectors of social systems represented in the discursive space of health communication theories and applications? Critical theorists in communication may be influenced by the same hermeneutic, phenomenological, and rhetorical perspectives as interpretive scholars, but also draw critical concepts from a number of sources. These sources include the neo-Marxist perspectives of the Frankfurt School, Antonio Gramsci, and Stuart Hall (Mumby, 1988), as well as what may be considered postmodern research derived from scholars such as Foucault and Derrida (Lupton, 1994; Waitzkin, 1991). Other branches include postcolonial theory (Spivak, 1999), feminist studies (Dow & Condit, 2005) and queer theory (Yep et al., 2003). Because of their explicit interest in issues of social justice, critical scholars studying health communication campaigns, for example, suggest that such campaigns contribute to the marginalization of the lower socioeconomic segments of society by shifting the responsibility of health on the individual, and obscuring issues of structural change that would address health inequities and disparities (Dutta-Bergman, 2005; Lupton, 1995; McKnight, 1988; Zoller, 2003a). Furthermore, the critical approach draws our attention to ideologies, "the interlocking set of ideas and doctrines that form the distinctive perspective of a social group" (Waitzkin, 1991, p. 12), which justify and reinforce capitalist relations as well as racial and gender inequalities related to health and health outcomes (Ellingson & Buzzanell, 1999; Gillespie, 2001; Waitzkin, 1991). Some critical scholars explore the intersections of health care and market forces with the goal of understanding the ways in which market logic undermines possibilities of structural health programs that would benefit marginalized communities (Conrad & McIntush, 2003; Gillespie, 2001; Waitzkin, 1983). Scholars investigating the constitution of health in the realm of national and global policies may interrogate health-care policies, and draw the interconnections between such policies and the material conditions of marginalization in the underserved sectors of the globe (Melkote et al., 2000). Critical perspectives are interested in hegemony as a relationship of consent between dominant and subordinate groups. However, hegemony is understood as a dialectical relationship of control and resistance (Gramsci, 1971; Mumby, 1997), so that critical perspectives also give attention to agency among marginalized groups by investigating the potential for nonconformity, resistance, and transformation (Lupton, 1995; Sharf, 1997; Zoller, 2005a).

The cultural studies approach emphasizes the culturally situated nature of health communication interactions and processes, and locates culture in the realm of structure and power (Dutta-Bergman, 2004a). In exploring the culturally constituted nature of health and in connecting the discussions of culture with issues of structure and power, the cultural studies approach provides a bridge between the interpretive and critical approaches. On one hand, it demonstrates commitment to the interpretive paradigm by emphasizing the local contexts within which health meanings are constituted; on the other hand, it shares commonalities with the critical tradition by emphasizing questions of power and the ways in which such questions of power shape the socially constructed nature of discourse (Airhihenbuwa et al., 2000). Cultural studies emphasize "deconstructing the apparent 'naturalness' of the way culture is understood" (Lupton, 1994, p. 16). Often focused on how mass media influence society through the production of knowledge, the cultural studies approach also draws attention to the way that social structures are constituted at macro and micro levels. Furthermore, it creates openings for examining the ways in which agency is played out within the locally situated contexts (Dutta-Bergman 2004a). Culture here is dynamic and transformative, constituted through the locally situated meanings that are co-constructed in the realm of social structures (Airhihenbuwa, 1995; Dutta, in press).

The rise in interpretive, critical, and cultural approaches in the field necessitates additional platforms for academic exchanges, debates, and collaborations that involve these emerging approaches to the study of health communication. We embarked on this project of putting together a book that would highlight some of the best scholarship in these areas with the goal of providing a theoretical and methodological framework for scholars interested in these approaches, and documenting exemplars that illustrate how health communication scholars can engage in interpretive, critical, and cultural studies projects. We believe that the proliferation of these approaches to the study of health communication is a sign of healthy growth of the discipline, which opens up avenues for building the study of health communication processes and messages in ways that have hitherto been unexplored. In the next section, we situate this growth within the historical development of the field.

Historical developments

The early studies of health communication examined interpersonal issues such as physician–patient relationship and sought to measure outcomes with the goal of identifying skills-building exercises to train physicians and patients (Cegala & Broz, 2003). This line of work was complemented by a growth in health communication studies that sought to measure and examine the effectiveness of health prevention messages (Witte, 1994). What was common to both of these areas of study in health communication was the emphasis on understanding universal characteristics that might be generalized to the population, and the development of predictions based on systematic observations of certain health communication phenomena.

Post-positivism employs mostly quantitative research. This research focused on behavior change in both doctor–patient communication and health campaign research. Indeed, Burgoon (1995) went so far as to suggest that in the medical context, "The only models (statistical) that make any sense are probit or logistical regression procedures with 'Dead/Not Dead' as the prime dependent measurement" (p. 3). In campaign research, scholars emphasized the goal of gaining compliance from "targets" (Burgoon, 1995; Freimuth et al., 1993; Rogers, 1996). For instance, Scherer and Juanillo (1992) described the responsibilities of public health communicators as informing the public of risk, training them with skills for "more healthful lifestyles" and persuading them to "assume more effective responsibility for maintaining their own health" (p. 313).

Witte (1994) argued unapologetically that health communication involves manipulating the public into behavior change. "Manipulation is not a popular word, yet it is really a major part of what health promotion and disease prevention is all about. Broadly defined, to manipulate or persuade means to influence people into doing what we want them to do" (p. 285). The focus on creating behavior change rests upon a relatively linear notion of communication that gives less attention to the role of the audience in giving meaning and embodiment to health messages. These models left little room for investigating the cultural and political implications of discourse such as HIV or substance abuse prevention.

The idea of manipulation invokes paternalistic attitudes. Rogers (1996) claimed that "The main independent variables of study in health communication research are usually of unquestioned good" and these include "HIV/ AIDS prevention, substance abuse prevention and early treatment" (p. 18). Although reducing and preventing illness is generally positive, researchers should be careful not to assume that they know what is best for people. Paternalistic attitudes deflect the potential for critique of the researcher's goals and methods, which is important given the constantly changing landscape of medical and health-related knowledge and the complexity of experience.

Scholars began to comment on the limitations of this orthodoxy in the late 1980s and early 1990s, starting a conversation that would introduce alternative approaches to the study of health communication. These approaches were more meaning-focused, including interpretive, critical, and cultural perspectives. For example, McKnight (1988) questioned the emphasis on medical communication as a primary source of good health, and argued that health communication scholars should work toward empowering the disenfranchised as the key to improving health. Sharf (1990) introduced a rhetorical perspective for understanding physician–patient communication. Geist and Dreyer (1993) critiqued dominant approaches to doctor–patient communication, introducing dialogue as a theoretical lens for re-conceptualizing medical communication. Zook (1994) described a more holistic approach to defining health, calling for attention to the embodied experience of health.

Deborah Lupton (1994) called for work that focuses "attention on discourse and the ways that the use of language in the medical setting acts to perpetuate the interests of some groups over others" (p. 60). Lupton's book *The Imperative of Health* (1995) applied a critical perspective to the study of health campaigns, interrogating how dominant values are encoded in health messages with important implications for health, social identity, and material resources. During this time period, Airhihenbuwa (1995) also introduced a cultural perspective and critiqued the Western paradigm that guides health interventions. Ray's (1996) volume on disenfranchisement brought attention to the role of marginalization in health status. As a result of this early work, interest in issues of meaning, culture, and even power are becoming more central to health communication research.

We are now seeing exciting growth in the development of interpretive, critical, and cultural perspectives in health communication (for instance Ellingson, 2005; Geist-Martin, Ray, & Sharf, 2003; Harter, Japp & Beck, 2005; Kline, 1999). We believe the growth and development of these perspectives represents a positive trend for the field. Indeed, we see this book as a celebration of the growth of this scholarship in health communication and as a way to share its theoretical and practical value with scholars working in the communication and health disciplines. We also see the need to evaluate existing research and theory in the area in order to help chart new territory that can foster and shape research agendas over the coming years. Thus this book presents the state of existing research and, we hope, offers insights into the potential of interpretive, critical, and cultural research to contribute to both the research and the practice of health communication. Ultimately, we hope that this book will provide not only a theoretical entry point for scholars interested in the study of health communication, but also a pragmatic point of entry into the practice of health communication.

Defining health communication theory

In order to describe theoretical contributions of "alternative" approaches, we must first revisit how theory building itself is seen differently by various research perspectives, and explain how we conceptualize the intellectual commitments of what we call interpretive, critical, and cultural perspectives. In the next few sections, we describe how theories are built in each of these domains. As we describe the theoretical underpinnings of various research traditions in health communication, we want to avoid making overly rigid distinctions that would fail to note how these traditions may overlap and complement each other, and avoid underplaying significant areas of conflict and difference. As outlined earlier, each of these approaches are founded upon certain tensions with the other approaches to the study of health communication. Although these tensions at times indicate opposite ends of a spectrum, it is also worthwhile pointing out that they exist on a continuum.

Research in communication is often divided into "Worldview I" and "Worldview II" perspectives, referring to scientific/positivistic/post-positivistic research, and interpretive/humanistic research respectively. Consistent with the discussions of Craig (1999) and Babrow & Mattson (2003), we suggest that the different approaches to health communication are founded upon the dialectical tensions of materiality/social construction, universal/specific, and social change/status quo. The dialectical tension of materiality versus social construction focuses on the ways in which health communication scholarship conceptualizes the nature of communication. Whereas perspectives drawing upon materiality emphasize the material basis of communicative phenomena, the social construction approach focuses on the ways in which communicative meanings are constituted through interactions and exchanges. The tension between the universal and specific aspects of health communication processes touches upon the scope of health communication theorizing, and the degree to which the goals of research are to generalize findings across cases or to understand the role of the local context. The social change–status quo tension in health communication scholarship is built around the goals and objectives of the scholarly enterprise, based on the degree to which research seeks to understand and reinforce the status quo or seeks to understand and bring about changes in the status quo. We also find that Deetz (2001) provides a key dimension by which we can contrast research as he asks whose concepts are used in research. "Elite, a priori" approaches to communication privilege the questions and concepts of the researcher, and tend to define or operationalize research terms prior to the study. "Local, emergent" research, on the other hand, privileges local questions and concepts, defining the issues of interest and the meaning of important terms during the study itself. In the next section, we describe the three research perspectives in terms of their orientation toward these issues as we discuss their views of theory.

Scientific discourses: defining and judging theory

Scientific perspectives in health communication generally orient toward the universal, as they are driven by the goals of prediction, control, and generalization. Theories are judged on the basis of their ability to explain phenomena and to predict relational patterns among message and process variables identified by the health communication scholar (Chafee & Berger, 1987; Dutta-Bergman, 2005). The goal is to identify broader patterns in health communication that apply across contexts, and hold true above and beyond the contextual limits. Given these goals, theories such as the Health Belief Model, Theory of Reasoned Action and the Extended Parallel Process model seek to explain human behavior in universal terms, based on certain primary characteristics of communication phenomena. Post-positivist research may orient either toward a material or a social constructionist view of reality, but the research itself is generally judged with theories of validity that suggest a correspondence model of truth. Post-positivist research is generally associated with the status quo; quantitative measurements often study *what is* rather than *what could be*, so that existing social arrangements are taken as a given (Bochner, 1985). However, because health communication research tends to be interventionist, this research does orient toward some level of change, albeit in the realm of individual behaviors and lifestyles, leaving dominant social arrangements intact. For example, scholarship focused on improving the quality of physician–patient interaction rarely proposes altering the structural barriers to care or even the biomedical model itself.

Post-positivist research describes theory testing and theory building as an "objective" process in which values and biases are counteracted by the scientific method. Yet, as we have articulated in this chapter, this presumed objectivity hides a number of values in the dominant approach to health communication. These include assumptions of the universality of the biomedical model and endorsement of theories of health that emphasize lifestyle factors as the root of health problems (Lupton, 1994). Campaigns that predict individual level behaviors such as healthy eating and exercising, and develop messages to alter the underlying beliefs and barriers associated with these behaviors, tend to privilege the a priori concepts and issues behind those theories and give less attention to the sociocultural and environmental factors that are integral to the health experiences of individuals, groups, and communities. Much of this research on campaigns assumes the superiority of the health solution being proposed, without interrogating the contexts within which health and illness are situated. Promoting five servings of fruits and vegetables to reduce cancer risk appears to be a value neutral approach, but we note that the lifestyle approach does not address material barriers to compliance and it obscures the environmental, sociocultural, and economic risks of cancer. The emphasis on the individual not only reflects a eurocentric cultural bias, but also serves the political role of determining the key topics in policy agenda, and shifts attention away from the need for structural changes in social systems that promote unhealthy conditions (Dutta, 2007).

Interpretive and critical scholars have developed alternative theoretical approaches that adopt an explicit value-orientation. The interpretive framework is often thought of as an alternative to this dominant scholarship in health communication, exploring issues of local meaning rather than universal generalizations.

Interpretive discourses: defining and judging theory

In an interpretive framework, health communication theorists provide descriptions of health communication processes, orienting toward a concern with the specific. In other words, the role of theory under this framework is to provide a detailed account of the processes and phenomena that are enacted in health settings. Theories within the interpretive paradigm are committed to the local contexts within which health meanings are constituted, health-care relationships are negotiated, and health practices are enacted. Rather than test concepts defined by researchers, in interpretive research, the concepts and issues studied emerge through the research process itself (Anderson, 1987; Charmaz, 2002).

Following its hermeneutic and phenomenological roots, this perspective focuses on how reality is socially constructed. Instead of questions of validity, which assume that findings can be compared against objective reality (or at least triangulated), interpretive theories are evaluated in terms of the richness of the accounts they provide of health communication processes, and the extent to which they equip us with an understanding of the health experiences of the participants. Insight, utility, and the ethics of the research process itself are important criteria for judging interpretive research (Bochner, 1985; Patton, 2002).

The universal–specific relationship is dialectical, however, and this is a frequent point of misunderstanding across perspectives. Geertz (1973) describes how interpretive theories of culture differ from the aims of prediction, control, and generalization, noting that interpretive theories should "stay rather closer to the ground" (p. 55). Yet interpretive researchers do not completely ignore the "universal" that exists in tension with the "specific." Whereas Geertz states that "the essential task of theory building here is not to codify abstract regularities but to make thick description possible, not to generalize across cases but to generalize within them" (p. 56), he also notes that theory building is a dialectic between local and more generalized knowledge. Theory building occurs "between setting down the meaning particular social actions have for the actors whose actions they are, and stating, as explicitly as we can manage, what the knowledge thus attained demonstrates about the society in which it is found and, beyond that, about social life as such" (p. 57).

Focusing on description, interpretive research allows research concepts and concerns to emerge from the study itself (local emergent). This focus on description often leads interpretive scholars to orient toward understanding social consensus rather than critiquing that consensus or seeking transformation (Deetz, 2001). This orientation can be contrasted with critical perspectives.

Critical discourses: defining and judging theory

Whereas interpretive approaches to the study of health communication emphasize the descriptive act, critical discourses add explicit focus on the critique of social relations and social change (Waitzkin, 1991). Critical studies evaluate theory in terms of the degree to which it opens closed systems of meaning for assessment and provides for the possibility of changing the status quo related to health and health outcomes. One of the goals of critical theory is to understand the communicative processes and meaning constructions in the realm of power, thus exploring the ways in which communication is constituted within structural realms, and the processes through which the discursive constructions of health reflect and reinforce dominant power structures (Lupton, 1994; Mokros & Deetz, 1996). Simultaneously, critical studies also provide entry points for looking at the ways in which human agency is enacted as social actors resist power relationships through various communicative acts.

Critical scholars may take multiple approaches toward the materiality/social construction dialectic. Because of the commitment to social change, critical research generally explores the connections between discourse (as both talk in interaction and in the Foucauldian (1980a) sense of systems of thought, ideas, assumptions, and practices that constitute power/knowledge configurations) and the material conditions surrounding the production of discourse. While some in the Marxist tradition emphasize the relationship between communication and pre-existing material realities (Dutta & Basu, 2007), critical–interpretive and critical postmodern perspectives emphasize the relationship between constructed views of reality and power relations, positioning materiality in a mediating role (Lupton, 1995; Waitzkin, 1991). Theoretical commitments to issues of power and inequality mean that critical scholars may seek understanding at the local emergent level in data gathering, and then introduce what can be considered elite, a priori concepts such as ideology and hegemony in terms of analysis.

We can evaluate critical theories in terms of their contributions to our understanding of relationships between discursive meanings and material realities, and the ways in which these meanings reflect and reinforce dominant interests. Critical theories are concerned with praxis, so we also judge critical theories in terms of their emancipatory potential. This emancipatory potential may be achieved through ideology critique in the Frankfurt school tradition, reclaiming conflict from apparent consensus with the goal of overcoming false consciousness to allow actors to represent their own social interests (Deetz, 2001). Deetz (2005) also describes "communicative action" (Habermas, 1984) as an alternative approach to ideology critique. Here, critical scholars focus less on the substance of value conflicts and more on the possibility for symmetrical communication processes based on procedural ideals. This work can be judged in terms of its ability to facilitate more open and inclusive dialogue.

Cultural studies: defining and judging theory

Cultural studies scholarship examines the intersections of critical and interpretive frameworks by locating discourse in the realm of culture and by connecting the exploration of discourse to the structures that surround the discursive spaces. The locally situated narratives, identities, and relationships of cultural participants are constituted within the broader framework of the culture, and are negotiated in the realm of social structures that define the possibilities of discourse (Dutta, in press; Dutta & Basu, 2007). The cultural studies approach explores the ways in which the stories of cultures perpetuate hegemonic configurations, and thereby serve the status quo. In this sense, the cultural studies approach judges research in terms of its ability to connect issues of meaning, culture, and power. Culture, as conceptualized in cultural studies, is dynamic and constitutive rather than being conceptualized in terms of a stable set of characteristics as articulated in the cultural differences approach of post-positivism. By examining the interplay of hegemony and ideology in the constitution of health discourse, critical–cultural studies draw our attention to the marginalizing practices of the dominant frameworks of health communication, and the possibilities of social change through the rupture of these dominant frameworks (Basu & Dutta, 2007).

Methodological issues in health communication theory

The paradigms within which health communication theories are proposed are also tied to the methodological approaches that inform health communication scholarship. In other words, methodological choices are deeply embedded within the paradigms that provide the overarching frameworks for health communication scholarship.

Because post-positivism emphasizes prediction and generalizability, the relevant methodologies tend to be quantitative because they facilitate testing and replication. For instance, physician–patient researchers survey patients to measure relationships between communication (such as satisfaction) and health outcomes, or observe physician–patient interactions and content analyze them based on their communicative features (Street, 2003). Similarly, researchers may study health communication campaigns by measuring self-reports of attitudes, beliefs, and behavioral intentions before and after the campaign (Murray-Johnson & Witte, 2003). When post-positivist researchers use qualitative research, they often treat it as preliminary to quantitative testing (Brashers et al., 2000).

In contrast, interpretive scholarship typically uses qualitative methodologies in order to provide thick descriptions of texts, phenomena, and processes in health settings. Rhetorical scholars provide unique interpretations of texts, helping us to understand how they invite certain meanings in audiences (Perez & Dionisopoulos, 1995; Solomon, 1985; Zoller & Kline, in press). Methods such as focus groups offer descriptions of health phenomena through the group's participation in the constitution of discourse, whereas in-depth interviews are built upon one-on-one face-to-face interviews with participants that dig deeper into the "meanings of things" (Sharf et al., 1996). Ethnographic projects are typically longitudinal in nature and often involve combinations of participant observations and in-depth interviews (Ellingson, 2003). Scholars using ethnographies immerse themselves in the field in order to provide thick descriptions of the health communication phenomena they are studying.

Critical theory is heavily influenced by interpretive perspectives in the communication field. Therefore, this research uses the same array of methodological tools. Analysis typically differs because of the explicit commitment to recovering hidden conflict and challenging dominant power relationships. For instance, critical theorists examining health discourse may use discourse analysis or thematic analysis to understand the ways in which such discourses reflect the dominant positions of power, and are imbedded within ideological and hegemonic configurations (Lupton, 1995; Zoller, 2005b). From this standpoint, the goal of the critical theorist is to bring out the taken-for-granted assumptions in discourse that reify dominant perspectives and guide practice. By doing so, critical research encourages attention to the conditions for more open and equitable participation in health discourse and practice, and for change in problematic social structures and relationships of power. Similarly, cultural studies emphasize the socially constituted nature of health and locate such social constructions in the realm of power; therefore, such studies typically use in-depth interviews, ethnographies, and discourse analyses to explore the interactions among culture, structure, and agency, with a particular emphasis on hearing the voices of the marginalized (Dutta-Bergman, 2004a, 2004b).

Although critical theorists in health communication generally adopt qualitative methods that allow research participants to help define problems and issues, this does not rule out quantitative methodology. Critical scholars who investigate the health outcomes associated with the macro-level disparities in infrastructures may rely on or produce quantitative methods such as survey-based observations to locate health outcomes in the realm of material disparities (Waitzkin, 1983).

Contributions

The preceding discussion notes the common threads and tensions among interpretive, critical, and cultural perspectives in terms of theory and methodology. Taken together, this research can act in complementary ways to build systematic knowledge. The goals of prediction, description, and critique may operate within a particular study or across research projects to elucidate health communication. Here we provide an initial discussion of the theoretical and practical contributions of interpretive, critical, and cultural research (see also Zoller & Kline, 2008).

Interpretive research informs us about the social construction of health meanings in everyday contexts (DeSantis, 2002; Ellingson & Buzzanell, 1999; Japp & Japp, 2005). Common theoretical concerns include how various groups define the basic concepts of health and illness, including attention to the body, mind, and spirit as well as material dimensions. Interpretive media studies investigate the mediated construction of health and illness (Kline, 2003), such as Barbara Sharf and Vicky Freimuth's (1993) rhetorical analysis of how the televised program *Thirtysomething* depicted the illness experiences of a woman with cancer. From a critical perspective, Zoller (2003b) investigated the political implications of how an auto manufacturer defined health in worksite promotion campaigns, finding that they emphasized individual efforts over attention to the role of occupational health practices, and that employees adopted much of this discourse. Dutta-Bergman (2004a) used a cultural approach to understand how the Santali community in India conceptualizes health, noting the tensions between adopting the views of dominant groups versus maintaining their own traditions.

Researchers from alternative perspectives have investigated the ways in which issues of identity are central to our understanding of health communication (Elwood, Dayton, & Richard, 1996; Kirkwood & Brown, 1995; Zoller, 2003a). Scholars have investigated the influence of illness on one's sense of self and the influence of group identity on health communication. For example, Harter et al. (2005) critically assessed the degree to which dominant assumptions about age-related infertility discourse about women reflect gendered stereotypes. These perspectives also often focus on the recursive role of culture in constituting and shaping individual understanding of health and illness (Airhihenbuwa, 1995; Dutta-Bergman, 2004a). Culture-centered approaches situate individual identities of health within a continuously shifting terrain of culture that offers the script for understanding and interpreting illness and disease, and for choosing courses of action in response to disease and illness. For instance, Dutta-Bergman's (2004a) narrative co-construction with the Santalis of rural Bengal suggests that the individual choices of healing and curing are based on a polymorphic worldview that celebrates multiple approaches to knowing and places them in complementary spaces that create openings for synergistic co-existence of seemingly contradictory or opposing approaches.

Interpretive, critical, and cultural perspectives also have introduced previously marginalized voices into health communication theorizing, including women, ethnic minorities, and low-income groups (Johnson, Bottorff, & Browne, 2004; Nadesan & Sotirin, 1998; Yep et al., 2003). For instance, in their work on the culture-centered approach to health communication, Airhihenbuwa (1995) and Dutta (in press) emphasize the relevance of exploring the intersections of culture, structure, and power among marginalized cultural groups. Dutta-Bergman (2004a) suggests that meanings of health are constituted at the intersections of culture and structure; the privileging and silencing of different culturally situated approaches, and the rational universalization of certain approaches over others are predicated upon the knowledge structures and power differentials that underlie these cultural spaces. Drawing upon the transformative politics of postcolonial and subaltern studies theories, the culture-centered approach then seeks to interrupt the dominant logics of health communication by noting the violent erasures of alternative epistemologies achieved through the rational scientific enterprise of modernity, and co-constructs alternative epistemologies of health through relationships of solidarity with marginalized groups that have otherwise been silenced in the dominant spaces.

It is this commitment to transformative politics that is evident in the works of health communication scholars studying the ways in which health-care policies are discursively constructed, implemented, and circulated (Conrad & McIntush, 2003; Melkote et al., 2000). Scholars are coming to explore the role of health activism in challenging the unhealthy structures of health and bringing about changes in global health-care policies that create and sustain health inequities across the globe (Christiansen & Hanson, 1996; Fabj & Sobnosky, 1995; Sobnosky & Hauser, 1999; Zoller, 2005a). Researchers are building our understanding of community-based approaches to health promotion focused on local empowerment (Ford & Yep, 2003; McLean, 1997; Minkler, 1997).

This discussion of contributions is preliminary. The chapters in this book will describe a number of other theoretical and practical contributions of these "alternate" perspectives that address issues of meaning, culture, and power. In the next section, we explain how the book is organized and provide an overview of the major sections and their chapters.

Organization of the book

The book is divided into four parts based on topical similarities. Part I, "Popular discourse and constructions of health and healing," focuses on the emerging interest in discourse, including linkages among textuality, talk-in-interaction, and larger knowledge formations in constructing everyday beliefs about health and illness. After an introduction that situates the chapters within discursive approaches to health communication, Chapter 2 by Cecilia Bosticco and Teresa L. Thompson describes the richness that narrative perspectives contribute to our understanding of health and healing in their chapter "Let me tell you a story: narratives and narration in health communication research." In Chapter 3, "Supporting breastfeeding(?): nursing mothers' resistance to and accommodation of medical and social discourses," Emily Cripe uses ethnography to understand women's discourse about breastfeeding in a support group, and links their communication to larger medical and gendered discourses. Patricia Geist-Martin, Barbara Sharf, and Natalie Jeha's chapter, "Communicating healing holistically," describes the role of communication in holistic healing practices, providing a contrast to the role of communication in biomedical interactions. In Chapter 5, "'You feel so responsible': Australian mothers' concepts and experiences related to promoting the health and development of their young children," Deborah Lupton interviews women to understand how mothers talk about promoting the health of their children, connecting their views to larger social constructions of responsibility, health, and motherhood. Finally in Chapter 6, "Destigmatizing leprosy: implications for communication theory and practice," Srinivas R. Melkote, Pradeep Krishnatray, and Sangeeta Krishnatray discuss the role of stigma in health care, situating the care of leprosy within neoliberal models of health and development, and suggesting the relevance of participatory processes in creating community-based health communication efforts. These chapters draw our attention to the selective nature of discourse; just as certain dominant understandings are selected and foregrounded, other understandings are omitted and backgrounded in the discursive space. The emphasis is on understanding the discursive formations within which health comes to be constructed and codified; it is, after all, within these discourses that (im)possibilities of health practices are imagined.

Part II draws our attention to alternative approaches to health campaign scholarship that sensitize us to the cultural rootedness of health promotion efforts. The section introduction describes the development of research in culturally based participatory health promotion. In their chapter titled "Teach-with-stories method for prenatal education: using photonovels and a participatory approach with Latinos", Susan Auger, Mary DeCoster and Melinda Colindres describe how photonovels can be used to make prenatal education more culturally appropriate through the sharing of stories. Story-telling encourages active participation among women in the education process. The theme of culturally based participatory communication is also articulated in Chapter 8, "Ethical paradoxes in community-based participatory research," by Virginia McDermott, John Oetzel and Kalvin White, which discusses the ethical paradoxes in community-based participatory research. The chapter brings out the various tensions that are inherent in community-based parti-cipatory research processes as researchers engage with community members in the production of knowledge. In Chapter 9, *Voces de Las Colonias*: dialectical tensions about control and cultural identification in Latinas' communication about cancer, Melinda Villagran, Dorothy Collins, and Sara Garcia participate in co-constructive meaning making with Latina community members to explore these residents' interpretations and explanations of health and illness around cancer. Through this co-constructive journey, the authors elucidate the tensions around control and cultural identification that circulate in this cultural community. Chapter 10, *El Poder y La Fuerza de la Pasión: toward a model of HIV/AIDS education and service delivery from the bottom-up*, presents the concepts of critical health communication praxis, "third-order" research, and collaborative community dialogue to describe the communicative strategies utilized by the organization Proyecto ContraSIDA Por Vida (PCPV) in Latino communities in San Francisco, California. Finally, Chapter 11, "Interrogating the Radio Communication Project in Nepal: the participatory framing of colonization," concludes Part II by utilizing the basic tenets of the culture-centered approach (Dutta-Bergman, 2004a) to interrogate the participatory claims of the Radio Communication project in Nepal; the chapter details the ways in which participatory avenues might be co-opted to serve the goals of planners in top-down hegemonic agendas. Each of the chapters in this section elucidates the tenets and tensions invoked by the culture-centered approach to health communication, drawing out the interactions among culture, structure, and agency in the realm of health meanings and health com-munication processes. The chapters engage with the contextually embedded nature of culture that is simultaneously regenerative and transformative; therefore, each of these chapters suggest openings for transformative politics in the realm of how we think about health communication and the ways in which health communication practices might be mobilized in solidarity with cultural members.

Part III focuses on communication in medical settings. The section introduction describes the growth of interpretive, critical, and cultural research into communication that constitutes and supports biomedical approaches to health care. The following chapters represent emerging interest in medical settings outside the standard physician–patient interaction as well as issues of power in medical communication. In Chapter 12, "Contested streams of action: power and deference in emergency medicine," Alexandra Murphy, Eric Eisenberg, Robert Wears, and Shawna J. Perry investigate the role of power and authority in sense-making processes in an emergency department, describing the influence of systems of authority on patient care through extended examples from their extensive observations. In Chapter 13, "Changing realities and entrenched norms in dialysis: a case study of power, knowledge, and communication in health-care delivery," Laura Ellingson provides in-depth understanding of how macro-level issues, including acute care models of health and professional hierarchies, influence everyday interaction in a dialysis care clinic where paraprofessionals must deal with chronic illness. Chapter 14, "Changing lanes and changing lives: the *shifting* scenes and *continuity* of care of a mobile health clinic," by Lynn Harter, Karen Deardorff, Pamela Kenniston, Heather Carmack, and Elizabeth Rattine-Flaherty, is an ethnography of a mobile health clinic. The authors focus on how health-care workers improvise to manage the physical and material barriers to care they face in this mobile unit. Finally, in Chapter 15, "The paradox of pharmaceutical empowerment: Healthology and online health public relations", Ashli Quesinberry Stokes takes us out of the clinic and onto the web, where she examines the contradictions of pharmaceutical rhetoric on the site "Healthology." She describes the paradox of "empowerment" discourse and its influence on audience identity. This section illustrates how the emergence of qualitative research such as ethnography, observation, and textual analysis expands the existing literature by focusing on issues of meaning, culture, and power in medical communication. As such, these chapters are excellent models of research that is both theoretically and practically grounded, with clear implications for the revision of dominant medical scripts.

Part IV represents what is in some ways the most newly emergent trend in health communication by focusing on health policy. As we describe in the section introduction, we see this area of the book drawing together the previous chapters that address popular discourses of health, community and culturally based health promotion, and medical communication, because it investigates how formal and informal political processes structure the experience of health at these other levels. This section also represents newly emerging attention in the field to issues of globalization. The chapters address the influence of transnational trade policies on pharmaceutical pricing and access, public health protections, food security, and genetic research. It begins with Chapter 16, "Dealing drugs on the border: power and policy in pharmaceutical reimportation debates," by Charles Conrad and Denise Jodlowski. These authors engage in a rhetorical analysis of the interrelation of U.S. and Canadian pharmaceutical policy making, describing the processes through which elites may outflank public groups through overt and hidden forms of influence. In Chapter 17, "Technologies of neoliberal governmentality: the discursive influence of global economic policies on public health," Heather M. Zoller broadens the definition of health policy to examine critically the governmental discourse of neoliberal trade mechanisms from the perspective of public health. The chapter encourages attention to multisectoral policy activism and advocacy as a form of health promotion. Chapter 18, "The paradox of 'Fair Trade': the influence of neoliberal trade agreements on food security and health," by Rebecca DeSouza, Ambar Basu, Induk Kim, Iccha Basnyat, and Mohan Dutta focuses on the impact of neoliberal trade policies on one of the most important elements of public health—access to adequate and safe food and water. Finally, in Chapter 19, "Globalization, social justice movements, and the human genome diversity debates: a case study in health activism," Rulon Wood, Damon Hall, and Marouf Hasian describe the politicization of the Human Genome Diversity Project (HGDP), an attempt to accrue diverse genetic samples ostensibly to create a more complete genetic map. The chapter traces the development of activism among subaltern groups as alliances form to contest the perceived colonialist assumptions of the project, and describes how the leaders of the project responded to this activism. We believe that these chapters provide a foundation for continued research into communication and health policy making that addresses a broad array of policies that influence the health contexts we study.

In the Afterword, the editors discuss the overarching contributions to health communication research made by the chapter authors. We describe how the interpretive, critical, and cultural perspectives in this book contribute to health communication theory and practice. We also discuss how we can expand on these through our future research agendas. Finally, given the growth of multiple theoretical and methodological perspectives in health communication, we talk about how the field can maintain productive dialogue across different philosophical and methodological commitments.

Conclusion

In conclusion, this chapter laid out the foundation for examining the different ways in which theory is conceptualized in health communication scholarship. The evaluative criteria that are applied in order to examine various health communication theories vary with the specific paradigms within which these theories are located. Also, our discussions pointed out the different methodological commitments that align themselves with the different approaches to theory building, suggesting that methodological questions emerge from the broader theoretical net that is cast on a specific health communication problem. Interpretive, critical, and cultural studies offer new ground for health communication scholars in conceptualizing communicative phenomena around health, studying these phenomena, and implementing them in practice.

As we pointed out here, whereas much of the existing scholarship in health communication falls under the rubric of the post-positivistic approach, recent trends demonstrate an increase in the number of articles that study health communication processes from interpretive, critical, and cultural approaches (Beck et al., 2004). This trend warrants discussion about avenues for engaging in and presenting such scholarship, as well as useful directions for building theory and practice. The chapters in this book provide valuable exemplars of how the study of health communication phenomena may be approached from interpretive, critical, and cultural perspectives.

Note: The authors wish to thank Kim Kline for helpful comments on this chapter.

References

Airhihenbuwa, C. (1995). *Health and Culture: Beyond the Western Paradigm*. Thousand Oaks, CA: Sage.

Airhihenbuwa, C., Makinwa, B., & Obregon, R. (2000). Towards a new communications framework for HIV/AIDS. *Journal of Health Communication*, 5(1), 101–111.

Anderson, J.A. (1987). *Communication Research: Issues and Methods*. New York: McGraw-Hill.

Babrow, A., & Mattson, M. (2003). Theorizing about health communication. In T.L. Thompson, A.M. Dorsey, K.I. Miller, & R. Parrot (eds), *Handbook of Health Communication*. Mahwah, NJ: Lawrence Erlbaum Associates, pp. 35–62.

Basu, A., & Dutta, M. (2007). Centralizing context and culture in the co-construction of health: localizing and vocalizing health messages in rural India. *Health Communication*, 21, 187–196.

Beck, C., Benitez, J.L., Edwards, A., Olson, A., Pai, A., & Torres, M.B. (2004). Enacting "Health Communication": The field of health communication as constructed through publication in scholarly journals. *Health Communication*, 16(4), 475–492.

Bochner, A.P. (1985). Perspectives on inquiry: Representation, conversation and reflection. In M.L. Knapp & G.R. Miller (eds., *Handbook of Interpersonal Communication*. Beverly Hills: Sage, pp. 27–58.

Brashers, D.E., Neidig, J.L., Haas, S.M., Dobbs, L.K., Cardillo, L.W., & Russell, J.A. (2000). Communication in the management of uncertainty: the case of persons living with HIV or AIDS. *Communication Monographs*, 67, 63–84.

Burgoon, M. (1995). Navigating the treacherous waters of health communication: dawning of the age of aquarius or the rule of proteus? Paper presented at the SCA summer conference on Communication and Health, Washington, DC.

Cegala, D.J., & Broz, S.L. (2003). Provider and patient communication skills training. In T.L. Thompson, A.M. Dorsey, K.I. Miller, & R. Parrot (eds), *Handbook of Health Communication*. Mahwah, NJ: Lawrence Erlbaum Associates, pp. 95–120.

Chafee, S. & Berger, C. (1987). What communication scientists do. In Berger, C. and Chaffee, S. (eds), *Handbook of Communication Science*. Sage: London, pp. 99–123.

Charmaz, K. (2002). Qualitative interviewing and grounded theory analysis. In J.F. Gubrium & J.A. Holstein (eds), *Handbook of Interview Research*. London: Sage, pp. 675–694.

Christiansen, A., & Hanson, J. (1996). Comedy as cure for tragedy: ACT UP! and the rhetoric of AIDS. *Quarterly Journal of Speech*, 82, 157–170.

Conrad, C., & McIntush, H.G. (2003). Organizational rhetoric and healthcare policymaking. In T.L. Thompson, A.M. Dorsey, K.I. Miller, & R. Parrott (eds), *Handbook of Health Communication*. Mahwah, NJ: Lawrence Erlbaum Associates, pp. 403–422.

Craig, R.T. (1999). Communication theory as a field. *Communication Theory*, 9, 119–161.

Deetz, S.A. (2001). Conceptual foundations. In F.M. Jablin & L.L. Putnam (eds), *The New Handbook of Organizational Communication*. Thousand Oaks, CA: Sage, pp. 3–47.

Deetz, S.A. (2005). Critical theory. In S. May & D.K. Mumby (eds), *Engaging Organizational Communication Theory and Research: Multiple Perspectives*. Thousand Oaks, CA: Sage, pp. 85–112.

DeSantis, A. (2002). Smoke screen: An ethnographic study of a cigar shop's collective rationalization. *Health Communication*, 14(2), 167–198.

Dow, B.J., & Condit, C.M. (2005). The state of the art in feminist scholarship in communication. *Journal of Communication*, 55, 448–478.

Dutta, M.J. (2007). Communicating about culture and health: Theorizing culture-centered and cultural sensitivity approaches. *Communication Theory*, 17, 304–328.

Dutta, M.J. (in press). *Communicating Health: A Culture-centered Perspective*. London: Polity.

Dutta, M.J., & Basu, A. (2007). Health among men in rural Bengal: exploring meanings through a culture-centered approach. *Qualitative Health Research*, 17(1), 38–48.

Dutta-Bergman, M. (2004a). Poverty, structural barriers, and health: A Santali narrative of health communication. *Qualitative Health Research*, 14(8), 1107–1123.

Dutta-Bergman, M. (2004b). The unheard voices of Santalis: Communicating about health from the margins of India. *Communication Theory*, 14, 237–263.

Dutta-Bergman, M. (2005). Theory and practice in health communication campaigns: A critical interrogation. *Health Communication*, 18(2), 103–122.

Edgar, T., Freimuth, V.S., & Hammond, S. (2003). Lessons learned from the field on prevention and health campaigns. In T.L. Thompson, A.M. Dorsey, K.I. Miller, & R. Parrot (eds), *Handbook of Health Communication*. Mahwah, NJ: Erlbaum Associates, pp. 625–636.

Ellingson, L. (2003). Interdisciplinary health care teamwork in the clinic backstage. *Journal of Applied Communication Research*, 31(2), 93–117.

Ellingson, L. (2005). *Communicating in the Clinic: Negotiating Frontstage and Backstage Teamwork.* Cresskill, NJ: Hampton Press.

Ellingson, L.L., & Buzzanell, P.M. (1999). Listening to women's narratives of breast cancer treatment: a feminist approach to patient communication. *Health Communication, 11*(2).

Elwood, W.L., Dayton, C., & Richard, A. (1996). Ethnography and illegal drug users: the efficacy of outreach as HIV prevention. *Communication Studies, 46*(3–4), 261–275.

Fabj, V., & Sobnosky, M.J. (1995). AIDS activism and the rejuvenation of the public sphere. *Argumentation & Advocacy, 31*(Spring), 163–184.

Ford, L.A., & Yep, G.A. (2003). Working along the margins: Developing community-based strategies for communicating about health within marginalized groups. In T.L. Thompson, A. M. Dorsey, K. I. Miller, & R. Parrott (eds), *Handbook of Health Communication.* Mahwah, NJ: Lawrence Erlbaum Associates, pp. 241–262.

Foucault, M. (1980a). *Power/knowledge: Selected Interviews and Other Writings 1972–1977* (C. Gordon, L. Marshal, J. Mepham, & K. Soper, trans.). New York: Pantheon.

Freimuth, V.S., Edgar, T., & Fitzpatrick, M.A. (1993). Introduction: The role of communication in health promotion. *Communication Research, 20*(4), 509–516.

Geertz, C. (1973). *The Interpretation of Cultures.* New York: Basic Books.

Geist, P., & Dreyer, J. (1993). The demise of dialogue: a critique of medical encounter ideology. *Western Journal of Communication, 57*(Spring), 233–246.

Geist-Martin, P., Ray, E.B., & Sharf, B.F. (2003). *Communicating Health: Personal, Cultural, and Political Complexities.* Belmont, CA: Thomson/Wadsworth.

Gillespie, S.R. (2001). The politics of breathing: asthmatic Medicaid patients under managed care. *Journal of Applied Communication Research, 29*(2), 97–116.

Gramsci, A. (1971). *Selections from the Prison Notebooks* (Q. Hoare & G.N. Smith, trans.). New York: International Publishers.

Habermas, J. (1984). *The Theory of Communicative Action: Reason and the Rationalization of Society* (T. McCarthy, trans. Vol. 1). Boston: Beacon Press.

Harter, L.M., Japp, P.M., & Beck, C. (2005). *Narratives, Health, and Healing.* Mahwah, NJ: Lawrence Erlbaum Associates.

Harter, L.M., Kirby, E., Edwards, A., & McClanahan, A. (2005). Time, technology and meritocracy: The disciplining of women's bodies in narratives constructions of age-related infertility. In L.M. Harte, & P.M. Japp & C. Beck (eds), *Narratives, Health, and Healing.* Mahwah, NJ: Lawrence Erlbaum Associates, pp. 83–106.

Japp, P., & Japp, D. (2005). Desperately seeking legitimacy: narratives of a biomedically invisible disease. In L.M. Harter, P.M. Japp, & C. Beck (eds), *Narratives, Health, and Healing.* Mahwah, NJ: Lawrence Erlbaum Associates, pp. 107–130.

Johnson, J., Bottorff, J., & Browne, A. (2004). Othering and being othered in the context of health care services. *Health Communication, 16*(2), 253–271.

Kirkwood, W.G., & Brown, D. (1995). Public communication about the causes of disease: The rhetoric of responsibility. *Journal of Communication, 45*(1), 55–76.

Kline, K.N. (1999). Reading and re-forming breast self-examination discourse: Claiming missed opportunities for empowerment. *Journal of Health Communication, 4,* 119–141.

Kline, K.N. (2003). Popular media and health: images, effects, and institutions. In T.L. Thompson, A.M. Dorsey, K.I. Miller, & R. Parrott (eds), *Handbook of Health Communication*. Mahwah, NJ: Lawrence Erlbaum Associates, pp. 557–581.

Lindlof, T. & Taylor, B. (2002). *Qualitative Communication Research Methods*, 2nd edn. Thousand Oaks, CA: Sage Publications.

Lupton, D. (1994). Toward the development of critical health communication praxis. *Health Communication*, 6, 55–67.

Lupton, D. (1995). *The Imperative of Health: Public Health and the Regulated Body*. London: Sage Publications.

Makoul, G., Arntson, P., & Schofield, T. (1995). Health promotion in primary care: Physician–patient communication and decision making about prescription medications. *Social Science and Medicine*, 41, 1241–1254.

McKnight, J. (1988). Where can health communication be found? *Journal of Applied Communication Research*, 16(1), 39–43.

McLean, S. (1997). A communication analysis of community mobilization on the Warm Springs Indian Reservation. *Journal of Health Communication*, 2, 113–125.

Melkote, S., Muppidi, S., & Goswami, D. (2000). Social and economic factors in an integrated behavioral and societal approach to communications in HIV/AIDS. *Journal of Health Communication*, 5(3), 17–27.

Minkler, M. (ed.) (1997). *Community Organizing and Community Building for Health*. New Brunswick, NJ: Rutgers University Press.

Mokros, H.B. & Deetz, S. (1996). What counts as real? A constitutive view of communication and the disenfranchised in the context of health. In E.B. Ray (ed.), *Communication and the Disenfranchised: Social Health Issues and Implications*. Hillsdale, NJ: Erlbaum, pp. 29–44.

Mumby, D.K. (1997). The problem of hegemony: Re-reading Gramsci for organizational studies. *Western Journal of Communication*, 61, 343–375.

Mumby, D.K. (1988). *Communication and Power in Organizations: Discourse, Ideology and Domination*. New Jersey: Ablex Publishing Corporation.

Murray-Johnson, L., & Witte, K. (2003). Looking toward the future: Health message design strategies. In T.L. Thompson, A.M. Dorsey, K.I. Miller, & R. Parrot (eds), *Handbook of Health Communication*. Mahwah, N.J.: Lawrence Erlbaum Associates, pp. 473–497.

Nadesan, M.H., & Sotirin, P. (1998). The romance and science of "Breast is Best": Discursive contradictions and contexts of breast-feeding choices. *Text and Performance Quarterly*, 18, 217–232.

Patton, M.Q. (2002). *Qualitative Research & Evaluation Methods*. Thousand Oaks, CA: Sage.

Perez, T.L., & Dionisopoulos, G.N. (1995). Presidential silence, C. Everett Koop, and the Surgeon General's Report on AIDS. *Communication Studies*, 46, 1–2.

Ray, E.B. (ed.) (1996). *Communication and Disenfranchisement: Social Health Issues and Implications*. Mahweh, NJ: Lawrence Erlbaum Associates.

Rogers, E.M. (1996). The field of health communication today: An up-to-date report. *Journal of Health Communication*, 1, 25–41.

Scherer, C.W., & Juanillo, N.K. (1992). Bridging theory and praxis: Re-examining public health communication. In S. Deetz (ed.), *Communication Yearbook 15*. Newbury Park, CA: Sage.

Sharf, B.F. (1990). Physician–patient communication as interpersonal rhetoric: A narrative approach. *Health Communication*, 2(4), 217–231.

Sharf, B.F. (1997). Communicating breast cancer on-line: Support and empowerment on the Internet. *Women & Health*, 26(1), 65–84.

Sharf, B.F., & Freimuth, V.S. (1993). The construction of illness on entertainment television. *Health Communication*, 5(3), 141–160.

Sharf, B.F., Freimuth, V.S., Greenspon, P., & Plotnick, C. (1996). Confronting cancer on *Thirtysomething*: audience response to health content on entertainment television. *Journal of Health Communication*, 1(2), 157–172.

Sharf, B.F., & Vandeford, M. (2003). Illness narratives and the social construction of health. In T.L. Thompson, A.M. Dorsey, K.I. Miller, & R. Parrott (eds), *Handbook of Health Communication*. Mahwah, NJ: Lawrence Erlbaum, pp. 9–34.

Sobnosky, M.J., & Hauser, E. (1999). Initiating or avoiding activism: Red ribbons, pink triangles, and public argument about AIDS. In W.N. Elwood (ed.), *Power in the Blood: A Handbook on AIDS, Politics, and Communication*. Mahwah, NJ: Lawrence Erlbaum Associates, pp. 25–38.

Solomon, M. (1985). The rhetoric of dehuminization: An analysis of medical reports of the Tuskegee Syphilis Project. *Western Journal of Speech Communication*, 49, 233–247.

Spivak, G. (1999). *A Critique of Postcolonial Reason: Towards History of the Vanishing Present*. Cambridge: Harvard University Press.

Street, R.L. (2003). Communication in medical encounters: An ecological perspective. In T.L. Thompson, A.M. Dorsey, K.I. Miller, & R. Parrott (eds), *Handbook of Health Communication*. Mahwah, NJ: Lawrence Erlbaum Associates, pp. 63–89.

Thompson, T.L. (2003). Introduction. In T.L. Thompson, A.M. Dorsey, K.I. Miller, & R. Parrott (eds), *Handbook of Health Communication*. Mahwah, NJ: Lawrence Erlbaum Associates, pp. 1–8.

Waitzkin, H. (1983). *The Second Sickness*. New York: The Free Press.

Waitzkin, H. (1991). *The Politics of Medical Encounters*. New Haven: Yale University Press.

Witte, K. (1994). The manipulative nature of health communication research: Ethical issues and guidelines. *American Behavioral Scientist*, 38, 285–293.

Yep, G.A., Lovaas, K., & Elia, J.P. (eds) (2003). *Queer Theory and Communication: From Disciplining Queers to Queering the Discipline*. Bingharton, NY: Harrington Park Press.

Yep, G.A., Reece, S., & Negron, E. (2003). Culture and stigma in a bona fide group: Boundaries and context in a 'closed' support group for 'Asian Americans' living with HIV infection. In L. Frey (ed.), *Group Communication in Context: Studies of Bona-fide Groups*. Mahwah, NJ: Lawrence Erlbaum Associates, pp. 157–180.

Zoller, H.M. (2003a). Health on the line: Identity and disciplinary control in employee occupational health and safety discourse. *Journal of Applied Communication Research*, 31(2), 118–139.

Zoller, H.M. (2003b). Working out: Managerialism in workplace health promotion. *Management Communication Quarterly*, 17(2), 171–205.

Zoller, H.M. (2005a). Health activism: Communication theory and action for social change. *Communication Theory*, 15(4), 341–364.

Zoller, H.M. (2005b). Women caught in the multicausal web: A gendered analysis of *Healthy People 2010*. *Communication Studies*.

Zoller, H.M., & Kline, K.N. (2008). Theoretical contributions of interpretive and critical research in Health Communication. *Communication Yearbook*, 32.

Zook, E.G. (1994). Embodied health and constitutive communication: Toward an authentic conceptualization of health communication. In S.A. Deetz (ed.), *Communication Yearbook*. Thousand Oaks, CA: Sage, Vol. 17, pp. 378–387.

Part I

Popular discourse and constructions of health and healing

Introduction

Mohan J. Dutta and Heather M. Zoller

Emerging scholarship in health communication attends to the discursive nature of health-care processes and messages (Lupton, 2003). Lupton defines discourse as a "patterned system of texts, messages, talk, dialogue or conversation which can both be identified in and located in social structures" (p. 142). Inherent in this description of discourse is the recognition of a patterned configuration that is rendered meaningful through a certain structural arrangement of statements. Thus, we can understand relationships between micro-level discourses as talk-in-interaction, and macro-level social discourses. Worth noting here is that discourse both constructs and is constructed by the contexts in which it is articulated. Building on this contextually situated nature of discourse, Foucault (1979, 1990) emphasizes that discourse is historic, and suggests that a *discourse* is a cluster of statements that define and simultaneously constrain the ways in which a particular phenomenon gets talked about, interpreted, and circulated at a particular historical moment. It is by attending to this historical moment that we come to understand the organizing role of discourse that puts forth a dominant set of meaning configurations that are aligned with the specific context. The historically situated nature of discourse was eloquently articulated in the writing of Foucault in classics such as *Madness and Civilization* (1967), *The Birth of the Clinic* (1975), and *The History of Sexuality* Volumes 1–3 (1979, 1986, 1988) that pointed out the ways in which historically situated networks of power constituted medical knowledges, practices, and experiences.

Foucault's (1967, 1975, 1979, 1986, 1988) work drew attention to the connections among discourse, knowledge, and social practices. Therefore, discourse is not only linguistic but also constituted through social practices because these practices both define and limit the production of all forms of knowledge just as they are defined, produced, and constrained by knowledge configurations. In other words, discourse is intertwined with practices as it defines and constrains the scope of such social practices; it is also in the realm of social practices that discourse opens up the possibilities for transformative politics by suggesting new knowledge configurations through which social phenomena come to be understood. Health communication scholars note that discourse is intrinsically connected with the practice of health care as it sets the parameters, norms, and guidelines for expectations, choices, and actions in the domain of health. For instance, discourses of medical authority legitimize the power and control held by experts trained in institutionally accepted medical practices (Foucault, 1973). Similarly, the *professionalization* discourse of health-care privileges a certain set of practices located within the biomedical paradigm, simultaneously discarding and/or undermining other ways of approaching and understanding health (Freidson, 1970; Illich, 1976; Zola, 1981). For these critics, the institutionalization of medicine has led to the increasing scope of jurisdiction of the medical profession, the increasing allocation of social resources toward illness, and the increasingly uncontested power and control of the medical profession in the twentieth century.

The *professionalization* discourse demonstrates the selection function served by discourse. Just as the magical power of the medical profession is foregrounded under the biomedical paradigm, the social, political, and economic conditions underlying ill health are obscured (Illich, 1976). Discourse simultaneously selects and foregrounds certain meaning configurations just as it omits and backgrounds other meaning configurations. This selectivity of discursive configurations is also well articulated in Lupton's work on the metaphoric nature of health discourse that suggests that metaphors provide a way for understanding and interpreting health and illness. They provide a conceptual map, provide the bases for deriving notions of reality, and construct human subjectivity (Clatts & Mutchler, 1989; Lakoff & Johnson, 1981; Lupton, 1994, 2003). Lupton draws our attention to metaphors such as the *machinery* metaphor defining the body as a "workshop full of instruments and tools" (Lupton, 2003, p. 62) that circulate in elite, popular, and lay discourses of health.

Going back to the interconnectedness between discourse and social practice, such metaphors as the *"body as machine"* validate a set of social practices such as dissection, the emphasis on medical technology, medical techniques, and surgery that focus on locating and identifying a specific problem in a part of the body and only treating that part (Helman, 1986). Just as this selectivity of discourse foregrounds the role of medical technology in disease and illness, it simultaneously undermines the interconnectedness of the mind and the body, and the role of healing relationships that draw from spirituality, mutual trust, interpersonal intimacy, and community ties (Helman, 1986; Stein, 1990). On a similar note, connecting the broader social–cultural embeddedness of discourse, Sontag (1988) posits that the *military* discourse in health circulates widely because it resonates with the broader culture's emphasis on mobilizing resources to counter the threats imposed by an emergency.

Discourses also function as narratives; in other words, they constitute certain meaning configurations through the stories they narrate. Individuals come to constitute their identities discursively through the construction and re-construction of certain narratives of health and illness. It is also in the realm of narratives that health-care relationships are constituted. Narratives serve as entry points for articulating structures through relationships of power, and they also create transformative openings through the opportunities they offer for new ways of sharing and constituting stories.

Just as discourse is constraining and limiting, it is also productive and enabling (Armstrong, 1982). Agency is enacted in the realm of discursive constitutions and is constituted in a certain community of social practices. Drawing upon the work of Foucault, poststructuralists point out that power operates through discourse not in a monolithic top-down manner, but rather within a set of strategic relationships that are diffuse and invisible. By producing subjectivities and realms of knowledge, power often retains social order and conformity through voluntary means; in medical encounters, it is continuously negotiated and renegotiated among the interactants as they define their identities. Health communication scholars exploring the role of discourse attend to both the constraining and the enabling roles of discourse (Kline, 2003; Lupton, 1995). This line of work on discursive constructions of health suggests that health is constituted and negotiated through discourse. It is in the realm of discourse that meanings of health are articulated and realms of possibilities are imagined; it is also in the realm of discourse that new openings are created for transformative action.

Much of the health communication scholarship exploring public discourses of health draws from both interpretive and critical lines of scholarship to investigate both the meanings of health in discursive spaces and the ways in which transformations in these meanings can create new openings for imagining health-care processes that resist the dominant structures of health. Public discourses of health circulate in a variety of spaces ranging from the media to the community to the physician–patient relationship to individual identity and play out ultimately in the ways in which the individual comes to understand health and illness, constructs and negotiates his/her identity in the realm of health-care processes, and goes about making her/his everyday health choices.

Also, meanings of health are continually constituted in everyday discursive practices, drawing our attention to the ways in which discourse constrains and enables possibilities for everyday practices. Suggesting the relevance of discourse analysis in health communication scholarship, sociologist Deborah Lupton (1994a) noted that "discourse analysis centers its attention upon the rhetorical devices and linguistic structure, the 'style' as well as the subject matter of verbal communications, and the manner in which ideology is reproduced in them" (p. 145). Lupton studied the mediated construction of health issues such as HIV/AIDS (Lupton, 1994a), cholesterol (Lupton, 1994b), and condom use (Lupton, 1994a) in Australian newspapers, demonstrating how the discourse defines problems and presents a range of potential responses. Similarly, Sharf and Freimuth (1993) demonstrated the value of a more interpretive approach in their analysis of the ongoing storyline in the television show *Thirtysomething*, wherein a major character suffers from ovarian cancer.

The authors "construct [their] own reading of this text in the context of contemporary biomedical and cultural information regarding ovarian cancer" (p. 145). Here, they point out the ways in which mediated representations addressed various issues of information seeking choices, self-image, sexuality, relationships with family and friends, relationships with doctors, and spirituality, also noting throughout missed opportunities for presenting additional information and perspectives that might be useful to a diverse audience. In her review of mediated health discourse analyses, Kline (2003) outlines the rhetorical manipulations that have undermined the informational value of media representations (e.g., over- or underreporting relevant information and the depiction of characters engaging in unhealthy behaviors) and fostered medical establishment hegemony (e.g., framing medical knowledge as authoritative and definitive while disregarding folk remedies, negative stereotyping, selective use of personal narratives and lay commentary in support of medicalization, and emphasizing risk factors presumably controlled by the individual which effectively deflect attention from systemic social, political and economic influences). In a later piece, Kline (2006) further notes that research related to challenges to bodily health (acute illness, chronic conditions, at-risk lifestyles, wellness) "tacitly assumed that some form of consensus could be reached about the 'right' way to represent health issues" (p. 49), whereas research related to politics and sociocultural context (public policy, controversies, health scares, ideologies) "suggested that the issues discussed are contested and that competing groups are making claims on the system" (p. 49). The discursive turn is also elucidated in the culture-centered approach to health campaigns (Dutta & Basnyat, in press; Dutta-Bergman, 2005) where scholars have noted the relevance of interrogating the discursive constructions of health campaigns and the ways in which these turns hide the hegemonic configurations of campaigns. Ultimately then, discourse influences the realms of possibilities by constituting the range of interpretations of health issues and problems.

This capacity to articulate and constrain individual understanding led Foucault (1990) to argue that social discourses are productive in that they produce the vocabularies and practices within which individuals come to know themselves. Public discourse also shapes and constrains the possibilities for transformative action in the realm of the politics of health care, and the structural access to health resources. Inherent in discourses are the social structures within which they are constituted. For instance, the ways in which health is constituted in the realm of work and productivity ties in to the social structures of capitalism where health is seen as a resource for productive management of workers (Waitzkin, 1981, 1983, 1991). Similarly, the discursive constructions of new-age corporate spiritualism in the workplace serves the interests of postindustrial Western capitalism by seeking to address the symptoms rather than causes of employee distress in current work conditions. Instead of locating growing work pressures, the number of hours spent at work, and the decreasing levels of community and family time available to employees, the discourse of corporate spiritualism foregrounds the importance of change of attitude with respect to work, achieved through inward reflection and spiritual journey. Also, disease and illness are often represented in military discourse, thus legitimizing the power and control held by the biomedical community in defining, detecting and treating disease and illness (Sontag, 1977).

For critical theorists, discourses of health are embedded in relationships of power. Powerful social actors with access to dominant spaces in the public sphere shape the nature of health discourses, and thus dictate the possibilities within which health choices are negotiated. Through their access to the sources of meaning making, powerful social actors define and constrain the realm of possibilities for how health is conceptualized, and the ways in which health and illness are understood. It is by challenging these dominant structures within which health discourses are located that critical theorists create openings for social change. For example, Dutta and Basnyat (in press) deconstruct the participatory claims made by entertainment education programming in Nepal, suggesting that such participatory claims serve as rhetorical strategies for positioning the campaigns as dialogic, hiding the fundamentally top-down nature of such campaigns.

In Chapter 2, "Let me tell you a story: narratives and narration in health communication research," Bosticco and Thompson provide an excellent overview of the ways in which narration serves as a fulcrum that facilitates understanding of the self in the context of health and illness, the meaning of health and illness, and the possibilities of human action constituted in the realm of health and illness. Furthermore, the chapter explores the role of narration in the context of healing and coping, and the effect of narration on healing. The authors cogently articulate the different functions of narration such as sense-making, asserting control and coping, transforming identity, creating community, and reinforcing and challenging dominant ideologies. These functions navigate from the micro to the macro, suggesting ways of understanding the role of communication in the realm of health and health-care delivery. The authors suggest that communication scholars can uniquely contribute to our understanding of health by exploring the use of language and the structure of discourse in the realm of health narratives. They conclude their discussion of narratives by suggesting possibilities for combining the critical and cultural approaches with the narrative approach that explores the intersections of power, control, and resistance in the realm of the stories of health that circulate in cultures.

Emily Cripe addresses this intersection of power, control and resistance in the context of narratives of breastfeeding in Chapter 3, "Supporting breastfeeding(?): nursing mothers' resistance to and accommodation of medical and social discourses." In her study of a breastfeeding support group held at a suburban hospital in a large southwestern city, the author explores the *medicalization* of breastfeeding, the micro and macro level dialectical tensions that are inherent in breastfeeding discourses, and the ways in which these dialectical tensions are connected with the practice of breastfeeding. Noting the contradictions inherent in breastfeeding discourses, Cripe observes that reinforcements of and resistance to such contradictory discourses are contextually situated and are tied to the sources of these contradictions. In the narratives of the women, whereas societal norms were often reinforced discursively, contradictory and ambiguous advice originating from medical expertise was resisted through a variety of tactics such as noncompliance and verbal criticism of physician advice. The author uses her analysis to suggest the importance of problematizing monolithic medical advice such as "breast is best." Instead, she suggests the need for narrative scholarship that engages with women's own experiences, and acknowledges the tensions and contradictions in narratives of health, thus creating alternative entry points for discourses of health.

The emphasis on alternative discourses is further reiterated in Chapter 4, "Communicating healing holistically," written by Patricia Geist-Martin, Barbara Sharf, and Natalie Jeha. In this chapter, the authors look beyond the biomedical model to articulate the role of communication in the holistic healing practices, the epistemology guiding the work of holistic practitioners, and the ways in which this epistemology is communicated in healing practices. Through two case studies that draw upon interviews conducted with practitioners of holistic healing, the authors suggest alternative entry points for health and healing that are epistemologically located in the realm of the divine, connecting the mind, body, and soul. Noting the role of communication in holistic healing, the authors point out that in addition to using communication tools such as listening that has been discussed in the health communication literature, holistic healers also use tools such as acute sensory observation, and environmental, tactile and other forms of nonverbal communication. The interviews further articulate the restrictions on holistic healing within the U.S. that are structurally situated within the biomedical model and the economic incentives tied to the model. Ultimately, through their elucidation of epistemologies and communicative practices around health and healing among holistic healing practitioners, the authors draw our attention to the dialectical tensions that circulate in discourses of health, and the networks of power that legitimize technologies of biomedicine and simultaneously delegitimize alternative ways of healing.

The role of networks of power in discourses of health is eloquently brought out in Deborah Lupton's Chapter 5, "Australian mothers' concepts and experiences related to promoting the health and development of their young children." Based on in-depth, semi-structured interviews with ninety mothers who were caring for at least one young child between 0 and 5 years of age in Australia, Lupton elucidates the ways in which discourses of child care center around the responsibility of the mother, suggesting that children's health requires constant monitoring and vigilance from their mothers. Drawing upon

Foucault's work, Lupton argues that in the context of the apparatuses of biopolitics in neoliberal societies, discourses of *responsible motherhood* serve as instruments of governmentality and biopower. Lupton summarizes her chapter by noting that "women as the mothers of young children, are positioned, and, importantly, position themselves and other mothers as responsible for the health of their children through a complex and intersecting network of discourse, practice, and power relations" (p. 126). These largely invisible power relations are embedded within the larger social structures surrounding discourses of health.

In the final chapter in this section, "Destigmatizing leprosy: implications for communication theory and practice," Srinivas R. Melkote, Pradeep Krishnatray, and Sangeeta Krishnatray criticize the dominant diffusion of innovation approach to leprosy destigmatization employed by health agencies in Madhya Pradesh, India. Instead, they suggest the relevance of more participatory strategies in health communication that are aligned with the basic tenets of the culture-centered approach to health communication discussed in Section II of the book. Through dialogue with local community members, they find dialectical tensions and contradictions in discourses of leprosy. The authors posit the importance of community capacity building and collective organizing as strategies for improving health. Through organizing at the local level, communities are able to address structures of health, and secure access to resources and relevant authorities outside the community that are crucial to solving their problems.

In summary, the chapters in this section of the book all draw attention to the contested nature of discourses as sites of meaning making. As they demonstrate the hegemonic nature of discursive constructions in articulating and circulating certain meanings and interpretations of health and illness, they also suggest entry points for change by noting the resistive capacity of discourse. This resistive capacity is noted both in the realm of everyday language practices and narrative constructions and in the realm of larger societal level changes in attitudes toward health and illness. The chapters provide openings for future health communication work that situates discourses of health in the realm of material structures, and engages with the continuing linkages between the material and symbolic realms of power and control. What are the ways in which discourses reflect material inequities and continue to circulate them? What material functions do discourses serve? Also, the chapters suggest possibilities for additional health communication scholarship that explores the transformative capacity of discourse. What are the ways in which discourses are mobilized for health communication activism that seeks to bring about changes in unhealthy social structures? What are the discursive practices that imagine new possibilities for health and health care that is accessible, equitable, and meaningful to those communities that are typically marginalized by mainstream health communication practices?

References

Armstrong, D. (1982). The doctor-patient relationship: 1930–80. In P. Wright, & A. Treacher (Eds), *The Problem of Medical Knowledge: Examining the Social Construction of Medicine*. Edinburgh: Edinburgh University Press, pp. 109–122.

Clatts, M., & Mutchler, K. (1989). AIDS and the dangerous other: Metaphors of sex and deviance in the representation of disease. *Medical Anthropology, 10*, 105–114.

Dutta-Bergman, M. (2005). Theory and practice in health communication campaigns: A critical interrogation. *Health Communication, 18*(2), 103–122.

Dutta, M., & Basnyat, I. (in press). The Radio Communication Project in Nepal: A critical analysis. *Health Education and Behavior*.

Foucault, M. (1967). *Madness and Civilization: A History of Insanity in the Age of Reason*. London: Tavistock.

Foucault, M. (1973). *The Order of Things: An Archaeology of the Human Sciences*. New York: Vintage.

Foucault, M. (1975). *The Birth of the Clinic: An Archaeology of Medical Perception*. New York, NY: Vintage Books.

Foucault, M. (1979). *The History of Sexuality, Volume One: An Introduction*. London: Penguin.

Foucault, M. (1986). *The Use of Pleasure: The History of Sexuality, Volume Two*. London: Viking.

Foucault, M. (1988). *The Care of the Self: The History of Sexuality, Volume Three*. London: Allen Lane/Penguin.

Foucault, M. (1990). *The History of Sexuality, Volume 3*. New York: Vintage.

Freidson, E. (1970). *Professional Dominance: The Social Structure of Medical Care*. Chicago, IL: Aldine.

Helman, C. (1986). *Culture, Health and Illness*. Bristol, England: Wright.

Illich, I. (1976). *Limits to Medicine: Medical Nemesis: The Expropriation of Health*. London: Marion Boyars.

Kline, K.N. (2003). Popular media and health: Images, effects, and institutions. In T.L. Thompson, A.M. Dorsey, K.I. Miller, & R. Parrott (eds), *Handbook of Health Communication*. Mahwah, NJ: Erlbaum, pp. 557–581.

Kline, K. N. (2006). A decade of research on health content in the media: The focus on health challenges and sociocultural context and attendant informational and ideological problems. *Journal of Health Communication, 11*, 43–59.

Lakoff, G., & Johnson, M. (1981). *Metaphors We Live By*. Chicago, IL: University of Chicago Press.

Lupton, D. (1994a). *Medicine as Culture: Illness, Disease and the Body in Western Societies*. London: Sage.

Lupton, D. (1994b). Toward the development of critical health communication praxis. *Health Communication, 6*, 55–67.

Lupton, D. (1995). *The imperative of health: Public health and the regulated body*. London: Sage Publications.

Lupton, D. (2003). *Medicine as culture*, 1st edn. Thousand Oaks, CA: Sage.

Sharf, B.F., & Freimuth, V.S. (1993). The construction of illness on entertainment television. *Health Communication, 5*(3), 141–160.

Sontag, S. (1977). *Illness as metaphor*. New York: Vintage.

Sontag, S. (1988). *AIDS and Its Metaphors*. New York: Farrar Straius Giroux.

Stein, H. (1990). *American Medicine as Culture*. Boulder, CO: Westview Press.

Waitzkin, H. (1981). The social origins of illness: A neglected history. *International Journal of Health Services*, 11, 77–103.

Waitzkin, H. (1983). *The Second Sickness: Contradictions of Capitalist Health Care*. New York: Free Press.

Waitzkin, H. (1991). *The Politics of Medical Encounters: How Patients and Doctors Deal With Social Problems*. New Haven, CT: Yale University Press.

Zola, I. (1981). Medicine as an institution of social control. In P. Conrad, & R. Kerns (ed.), *The Sociology of Health and Illness: Critical Perspectives*. New York, NY: St. Martin's Press, pp. 511–527.

Chapter 2

Let me tell you a story

Narratives and narration in health communication research

Cecilia Bosticco and Teresa L. Thompson

The area of study known as health communication has traditionally been a very empirical, social scientific field of research. In the last fifteen years, however, researchers have begun expanding the horizons of health communication by employing and legitimizing alternative approaches to the understanding of communicative processes as they relate to health and illness and to the delivery of health care. Notable amongst those approaches is an application of narrative theory and an examination of the role of narratives and stories in the health, healing, coping, and dying processes. This chapter will provide an overview of how this approach has come to be applied within the area of health communication. It will begin with a conceptualization of narrative and the process of narration. The overarching social functions of narration will be discussed, followed by an exploration of varying perspectives on narrative and narration. The focus will then move to a more specific application of the concepts of narrative and narration to health, healing, illness, and coping. Discussion will focus on narration as it functions to facilitate understanding of patients and health conditions, on narration in the self-identify process and how that relates to coping and healing, the broader roles of narration in coping and healing (beyond identity concerns), narration as it helps us understand the nature of health and illness, narration as it impacts healing, and narration as it helps tell us how to live. Particularly interesting and insightful examples of the application of narrative theory and the examination of health/illness/coping narratives will be highlighted.

What is a story?

The basic elements of a story consist of an individual (or individuals) and movement through a series of developments over time (Brockmeier & Harré, 1997). The emphasis in this definition is on change over time based on some type of action by or directed at the characters. Stein and Policastro's (1984) review of story definitions includes this type, based on change over time. They also mention definitions based on goals and some that are even more complex. However, they hypothesize that people may hold a perfect model of a story, yet also recognize as stories some passages that differ from the ideal. They propose that the definition of a story may change for individuals as they gain life experience. Their research among second graders and teachers appeared to confirm their hypotheses and to support goal-directed story definitions as the most precise.

Why do people tell stories?

People tell stories to help them understand the world, and, more specifically, what is happening to them in their daily experiences (Lule, 1990; Weick, 1995). The structure of a story imposes order on what might otherwise seem to be disorder in their lives and makes connections between themselves, others, and reality in general (Tannen, 1988). Stories coordinate unrelated events, developing a logical progression of events (McAdams, 1990). Stories combine facts with possibilities, thus allowing for explanation of events through the development of probable and plausible causal relationships (Robinson & Hawpe, 1986). A story is never an exact representation of an individual's experience, according to Weick (1995), because only certain elements of that experience can be used to create a believable story. Storytelling combines details of an experience into a particular relationship that remains together in distinct memory fragments over time (Schrank, 1990).

Stories are an instinctively human way of passing on intentionality and understanding of experience. They discover causes for the actions of individuals, while taking their order from those action causes (McAdams, 1990). Storytellers consciously create meaning-carrying patterns in their stories. While stories arrange events in coherent ways, they also allow for tellers to reorganize those elements as new events or perceptions arise. Stories generate analogies between unexplained everyday happenings and well-known narrative structures (Brockmeier & Harré, 1997). These structures are familiar groupings into which experiences can be sorted, highlighting consistency in everyday situations (Robinson & Hawpe, 1986).

Stories have the ability to secure emotional experiences, allowing people to gain control of them. They provide an opportunity for catharsis and tension release. Stories can provide a vehicle for linking the experiences of different individuals to a central event (Sedney et al., 1994; Downs, 1993). In fact, Weick (1995) asserts, stories slow the build-up of tension and facilitate future actions. Stories allow people to consider other possible viewpoints that might rationalize and shed light on their experiences (Brockmeier & Harré, 1997). They provide a way to try out possible scenarios and test problem solutions (Weick, 1995).

Storytelling is the essence of intelligence, according to Schrank (1990). The ability to distinguish relationships among events, to recognize likenesses and differences between others' stories and one's own, and to convey a suitable story at the correct time is significant. The talent of relating current happenings to similar preceding events helps create understanding and facilitates sense-making (Schrank, 1990).

The functions of narration

Building on the early writing on narrative by Walter Fisher (1985, 1987), Barbara Sharf and Marsha Vanderford (2003) provide a useful overview of the application of the narrative approach to the social construction of health in their chapter in the *Handbook of Health Communication*. They outline several key functions for health narratives, which include sense making, asserting control, transforming identity, and building community. As much of the recent writing on narratives in health and illness falls nicely into one of these categories, we organize the earlier part of our review around them. Additionally, however, several more specific functions of narrative or ways of using narrative are evident in the scholarly writing on the topic, so our review will then turn to such topics as the structure of narratives, the roles of narrative in health and healing and in diagnosis, narratives as they relate to particular health problems or populations, narratives and health interventions, narratives of caregivers, and narrative competence.

Sense making

People tell stories to make sense of or find meaning in things that happen to them. Murphy and Johnson (2003) conducted a longitudinal study in which 167 parents who had lost children to sudden, violent events were interviewed at four, twelve, twenty-four and sixty months post-death. They measured five parent outcomes to determine whether finding meaning in the deaths of their children (or not) influenced the general health and well-being of the parents. A dual measure for meaning making was used: being able to understand and coming to a new sense of what is important. They found that at four months, no parents reported having come to the second kind of meaning, while at sixty months, 57 percent of the parents had been able to do so. The remaining 43 percent could not come to the second type of meaning. One such parent stated, "Suicide seems a bottomless pit without any real answers" (p. 396). Results show that those who were able to find meaning in the deaths of their children recounted less mental distress and more marital satisfaction than those who were not able to do so.

Many studies use self-narratives of sufferers/survivors to develop new understandings of ailments or conditions that often contrast with established medically, psychologically, or socially accepted perceptions. Squier (1999) presents one particularly interesting example in which views contained in narratives of three people with disabilities are compared to attitudes reflected in the 1999 Supreme Court rulings on the ADA. One narrator wrote:

> When it was all over, my doctor named my disorder "macular degenera-
> tion," defined my level of impairment as legally blind, and told me that
> there was no treatment or cure, and no chance of improvement. And that
> was all. Like many ophthalmologists then and perhaps now, he did not feel
> that it was his responsibility to recommend special education or training.
>
> (Squier, 1999, p. 155)

Other researchers investigate therapeutic uses for narrative in which patients
are helped by health-care providers to develop stories that support wellness and
healing attitudes. For example, Arnstein (2003) reports on efforts to help
patients challenge their own emotional responses that escalate perceptions of
pain while developing more positive stories about their lives despite the pain.
He reports patients saying such things as "I just want someone to make the pain
go away" and "my life is ruined; I'll never be a good parent because of my pain"
(p. 406).

Asserting control and coping

Our own writing on narratives came out of a focus on the role of narratives in
the coping process. This work was prompted by the death of Cecilia's daughter
during Cecilia's graduate school years and her experiences with the role of
narratives in bereavement (Bosticco & Thompson, 2005). An examination of
the writing on narratives makes evident the functional role of storytelling in
the grieving process (Fletcher, 2002). As articulated by one of Bosticco and
Thompson's (2005) interviewees: "we didn't really get the details of everything
until the guys came down and we spoke to them and on the side. . . . They told
us the stories . . . and it was wonderful for us" (p. 397). The interviews of
parents who have lost a child reported by Bosticco and Thompson make clear
that this is just one of the many ways that narrative helps one assert control
over one's life.

The scholars who have written about the role of narrative in grief and
coping have focused upon such issues as using stories to challenge fear, analyzed
through an examination of eight caregiver narratives (Penson et al., 2005),
stories to appear strong and hide feelings of grief and anger (McCreight, 2004),
stories of living with terminal illness (Ogle et al., 2003), integrating a sibling's
illness experience into one's own story (DiGallo et al., 2003), reauthoring life
narratives to facilitate grieving and meaning reconstruction (Neimeyer, 2001),
coping with a lost childhood through narrative (Dasberg et al., 2001),
uncertainty and revival in persons living with HIV or AIDS (Brashers et al.,
1999), the positive symbolic functions of stories of suicidality in coping with
HIV (Siegel & Meyer, 1999), the experience of coping with traumatic brain
injury (Nochi, 2000), the function of narrative for children with HIV to
integrate the fragmented portions of their family lives (Gewirtz & Gossart-
Walker, 2000), coping with mother-loss by recreating the relationship

(Dietrich et al., 1999), coping with the mental illness of a family members (Jones, 2004), grieving following youth suicide (Kalischuk & Hayes, 2003–2004), narrative in complicated grief (Lichtenthal et al., 2004), coming to grips with loss and enhancing quality of life (Gullickson & Ramser, 1996), and facing acute illness or invasive procedures (Rybarczyk & Bellg, 1997).

Sharf's (2005) narrative of firing her doctor describes a regaining of control, as narrative makes meaning. She writes: "This story illustrates how the communicative road toward patient autonomy and clinical partnership became detoured by the pain, fatigue, and stress of illness, then was blockaded by significant differences in expectations and styles between me and my doctor" (p. 325). We know that stories can help patients/clients discover competencies, talents, and resources within themselves to create hope (Monk et al., 1997) and that the story brought to the patient by the care provider helps determine coping with terminality (Hallberg, 2001), as does the story created in therapy (Hoyt, 2000). Hoyt's analysis was based on interviews with twenty-one patients who had been treated for mental illness. Facing the life-limiting illness of a child appears in father's narratives as "living in a dragon's shadow" (Davies et al., 2004, p. 111), while analysis of narratives of loss show the exploration of misunderstanding, tension, conflict, rage, fear, abandonment, and ambivalence (Lurier, 2004). Research talks about narrative hunger as we face terminality (Balber, 2003).

Even writing a narrative about the death of another helps create more realistic considerations of death (Evans, Walters, & Hatch-Woodruff, 1999). On a very foundational level, narrative can help create more empathic and compassionate care of the dying by showing that every death is a story waiting to be told (Fins et al., 2000).

Transforming identity

Ungar (2000, 2001) discusses therapeutic attempts to create positive self-narratives in regard to health behavior in adolescents. Androutsopoulou (2001) presents another example of narrative therapy in work based on self-characterization in individual and family analysis. Reporting on the use of Video Intervention/Prevention Assessment (which allows patients to create a video narrative about their diseases and the impact on their lives), Rich et al. (2000) point to increased understanding on the part of the therapist as well as enhanced coping ability in the teens who used the technology.

Williams, Labonte and O'Brien (2003) describe a social action program that used cultural and identity stories to encourage native women in New Zealand to claim their health status rights. In a creative use of narrative analysis, Arvay et al. (1999) make use of personal experiences of self to advance theory and practice among health-care providers.

Two other studies look at the reflection of self in stories by subjects experiencing chronic conditions. Hellstrom et al.'s (1999) interviews with eighteen patients discovered that sufferers of fibromyalgia struggled so much to have their status as people with an illness confirmed that they often had trouble coping with their symptoms. On the other hand, Scherman et al. (2002) found that asthma/allergy patients moved away from medically related self-perceptions toward more normal health perspectives over time. A common observation from these two studies is that health-care providers need to be aware of their influence on the identity narratives of patients.

While the preceding works chronicle the direct use of narrative to accomplish a result, the following works make use of analysis of the stories and interviews of the subjects. Bauer and Bonanno (2001) accurately predicted outcomes of the grieving process based on self-narratives of abilities, behaviors, and characteristics. Pals (2001) reports that self-narratives of the women in his study both reflect and impact their identity and are associated with predictable health outcomes. Based on personal stories, Nilsson et al. (2000) identified transition periods in people 85–96 years old by observing the subjects' perceptions of their own agedness.

Kirkman (2003) looked at the intentions of parents of offspring conceived by donor-assisted methods to divulge that fact to them and at what point. The researcher reported on interviews with fifty-five recipient parents and twelve offspring. Although the intentions of the parents to tell their children about their origins fell along a continuum, the researcher placed them into three broad categories: those who will not tell, those who are questioning or confused about telling, and those who have already told or plan to tell their offspring about having a possible donor as one of their parents. Most parents fell into the middle category. Some parents who do not plan to tell or who are not sure report that they must first consider their own narrative relating to conception problems before they can consider the impact on their children. Many wonder how to go about disclosing the information to their children, "What do you say?" (p. 2234). One way some parents use to inform their children is to create a book that may include images of the child as a few cells, photos of the parents during pregnancy and a simple clear narrative about why the family wanted a child, how things usually work, and the role of the doctor in the conception. The study also includes comments from people conceived through donor assistance. One woman said, "I would say that being told at a young age and being raised in openness has contributed to me having a stable sense of self" (p. 2239). A man who was told at age 35 a few days after his father's death was depressed and angry, "As a human being, I should have a right to the truth about my own identity and history . . . It was so painful to find out my dad had lied to me our whole life together about our true relationship, and that he felt it was none of my business" (p. 2229). Based in part on the experiences of children of donor-assisted conception and in part on human rights issues, the increasing importance of genetic information and studies of identity development, the researcher encourages families to plan and execute early disclosure to their children.

Several studies analyze narratives related to the sense of self of the subjects. Kameny and Bearison (1999) explore the development and description of a sense of self among adolescents with cancer by examining the interview-elicited narratives of seventy-five children. Belknap (2002) looks at relationship, connection, and moral development among women who have been in abusive situations. Murdoch (1999) investigates the effect of employment on the development of user and nonuser identities among drug addicts. In a re-analysis of the stories of two men with multiple sclerosis, Riessman (2003) explores gender, disability, and ability to perform as they impact self-identity. Copeland (2004) reports that, for hepatitis C antibody positive drug users, the hepatitis C status is engulfed by the problem drug user identity of those interviewed.

These studies are representative of many others in which new attitudes are developed by patients related to self-image via narrative or new concepts about health and healing are revealed by analysis of the self-narratives of patients.

Community

Sharf and Vanderford (2003) also focus upon the role of narratives in building community. This function is evident on many levels, including building a sense of community amongst members of an illness group, amongst care providers, and amongst family caregivers. This perspective is elaborated in Morgan-Witte's (2005) analysis of stories from the nurses' station and their role in the framing of patients, in dealing with the stress of care provision, and in coping with the treatment of nurses by doctors and family members. One story focused on a patient who had tried to remove a pimple from a testicle with a knife. The nurse told the story of the wife casually doing a crossword puzzle and exhorting her husband to "go ahead, tell her [the triage nurse] what you did. Go ahead, tell her why you did it. Go ahead, tell her what you used to do it!" (p. 223). Morgan-Witte also identifies story chains and discusses the potential negative ramifications on care of the framing of some patients. Similarly, Sunwolf et al.'s (2005) examination of the healing effects of storytelling reminds us of its role in connecting others, as does Callister's (2004) report of the sharing of women's birth narratives. Tardy and Hale's (1998) observational study of mothers' discussions of health-related issues in informal, interpersonal networks echoes some of the themes noted in Callister's work, but extends it to a focus on the role of such communities in health decision making.

Several narrative analysts discuss the process of making the private public through storytelling. It has been argued, for instance, that personal narratives energize public narratives (Japp et al., 2005), that personal stories are co-constructed and negotiated in public dialogues (Beck, 2005), and that public discourses of health and healing are narratively constructed (Harter et al., 2005). The relational nature of narrative construction is made evident in such analyses (Babrow et al., 2005; Beck, 2005). Much writing by scholars also emphasizes this co-construction and its value in confirming self-stories (Gaydos,

2005) and in influencing both forgiveness and physiological measures (Porter, 2004). Beck thoughtfully traces the manner in which "my" story becomes "our" story in public discourse, prompting public decision making. Rawlins (2005) shows how the family physician becomes a trusted co-author of individual narrative, making him or her a better care provider. Rawlins quotes the physician, "I felt I was part of the family. And in many cases, I've still been considered that way. This is a rare privilege to be in people's lives and be involved *with* them and be considered part of the family" (p. 206). Co-construction is also evident in Morgan-Witte's (2005) story of nurses, noted above, in our earlier analysis of narratives in bereavement (Bosticco & Thompson, 2005), and in Hess's (2003) discussion of co-construction to create a sought "good." Similarly, Jordens et al. (2001), drawing on sociolinguistic analyses of ten cancer patients, note the work that illness narratives do for both listener and narrator, and Harden (2000) describes the value of narratives in sharing "otherness." Positional differences as they impact co-construction have also been discussed (Murray, 2000).

Understanding the role of narrative in building community within groups of individuals concerned with a particular health focus is made evident in Martins et al.'s (2004) study of communication about genetic diseases, research on cancer patients (Bertero, 1999; Gray et al., 2005), Milton's (2004) analysis of nursing ethics, and Romyn's (2003) examination of nurse practitioners entering into relational dialogue. Brown et al. (1996) build on the theme of co-construction as they remind therapists that they do not merely reflect client's narratives—they help construct them.

The emphasis on care providers' narratives is an important in this body of work. Health communication scholars have written about the need for mindfulness in this regard (Connelly, 2005), emergency medicine narratives (Hawkins, 2004; Nairn, 2004), the need to place narratives in a structure practice context (Nelson & McGillion, 2004), nurse managers' narratives (Sorlie et al., 2004), and death stories told by internists (DelVecchio Good et al., 2004).

Dominant ideology

As narratives create a sense of community, they also function to reinforce or to challenge dominant ideologies. This notion is clarified in Japp's (2005) assertion that any narrative ultimately silences other narratives, frequently reinforcing a dominant ideology. Workman (2005) builds on this point as he outlines how the use of the death story as the "representative anecdote" (p. 131) in discussions of college drinking serves to focus attention on only that aspect of the college drinking problem. Such a story is not seen as relevant to most college-age drinkers, but other, more relevant stories are silenced by the focus on death stories. Looking cross-culturally, Singhal et al. (2005) demonstrate the narrative transparency or lack thereof in safe-sex episodes of the American television series, *Friends*. They note that their analysis enabled them to "gain theoretically rich insights on how Hollywood weaves its global web of transparent mass mediated narratives" (p. 187).

Buzzanell and Ellingson (2005) address this issue of dominant ideologies and contesting narratives most explicitly in their insightful analysis of the story of Tara, a pregnant photo technician for a national retailer. Tara's stories of her struggle through a difficult pregnancy vividly demonstrate the dominant corporate view of pregnancy as a negative medical condition—a disability. However, it is not an ADA (Americans with Disabilities Act) disability, so does not require accommodation. Tara has no power—the corporation has all of the power. Tara's story makes clear the role of narratives in maintaining social control. We hear Tara say,

> I thought that [my supervisors] would more or less help [when I was pregnant] and not really so much [give] special privileges, but they would be a little bit more understanding; but instead it was like they were out to get you.
>
> (Buzzanell & Ellingson, 2005, p. 277)

Similarly, Courtial and LeDreff (2004) analyze pregnancy narratives to understand a "normative conditioning toward medical norms" (p. 105). Focusing on the not-yet-pregnant, Kirkman (2001) identifies women's resentment at having to construct a narrative that publicly justifies the desire to become a mother while simultaneously explaining why they are not yet mothers.

Competing ideologies are also addressed in Coker's (2003) examination of the narratives found in patient medical charts in Egypt. Coker argues that these narratives are cultural negotiations in which the world views of Western biomedicine and traditional Egyptian culture must be reconciled. In a related conceptualization, Skultans's (2003) critical analysis looks at the construction of depression in Latvia to understand how patient narratives are suppressed during psychiatric consultations.

Related narratives may be used to reinforce different dominant ideologies during difficult social eras, as is demonstrated by the different narratives told about Franklin Roosevelt during times of conformity/homogeneity (such as the 1940s and 1950s, when narratives about him emphasized recovery), as compared to times of unrest (the 1960s, when narratives about him focused upon the reality of living with a chronic disability; Fairchild, 2001). Sakalys (2000) points out how the analysis of illness narratives highlights the ideological differences between patient and health-care cultures and shows the dominance of the health-care ideologies. Similar politicalization is noted in Harter et al.'s (2005) study of narrative constructions of age-related infertility.

Narrative structure

Thomas-MacLean (2004) has noted that, although health narratives are prevalent in all cultures, few researchers have explored the structure of them. Commonly discussed structures of narratives include restitution, quest, and chaos narratives (Frank, 1995). Restitution stories show an instance of health being restored—a happy ending. Quest narratives demonstrate how everyone involved in a story has grown through the task of dealing with troubles and adversity—they meet suffering head on, accepting illness and using it (Frank, 1995). Sharf (2005) makes clear the use to which a quest narrative can be put when she writes, "I have an appreciation for [her doctor's] candor, which ultimately contributed to reshaping the conclusion to my story" (p. 339). A chaos narrative, by contrast, presents a series of events that are not well connected to each other—closure is not obtained and uncertainty continues.

How a narrative is structured relates to its function and use. For instance, Myers (2002) writes about how emphasis on the restitution narrative prevents terminally ill patients from shifting their emphasis from a hope for cure to quality to life issues. As a result, hospice options are frequently underused by patients who could benefit from them. Also writing about restitution narratives, Stern et al. (1999) discuss the impact of stories on the abilities of family caregivers to transform the experience of caregiving into something that has meaning and occupies a place in their lives. By contrast, what they call chaotic or frozen narratives leave the illness as a series of random events, making coping more difficult.

The relationship of narrative structure to coping also underlies work that focuses upon the assimilation of problematic experiences. Stiles, Honos-Webb, and Lani (1999) uncovered four such narrative structures in their examination of narratives in psychotherapy: those that avoid encounters with threatening material, those that approach such material indirectly and symbolically, those through which individuals re-experience trauma, and those that help construct a mature understanding.

Different "players" in health care also structure their narratives differently. Little et al. (2003) note that patients tend to speak of their illness experiences in ways that identify them as victims of circumstance, policy makers narrate them as opportunities to be taken, and health-care workers take a perspective that alternately focuses on themselves as both victims and opportunists, depending on the context. The narratives of health science are also analyzed in Abma's (2002) assessment of health science, which focuses on narrative plotting, author's stance, character building, voices, and rhetorical tropes.

The structure of narratives also varies between somatizing and nonsomatizing patients (Elderkin-Thompson, 1997). Somatizing patients use well-structured narratives, but amplify the seriousness of symptoms. Those somatizers with a history of depression present narratives that are less well-structured, focus on their mental illness histories, and demonstrate more digression, equivocation, and ignoring of physician requests.

Health, healing, and intervention

Of great interest in the narrative literature is the relationship between storytelling and health and healing. This connection is articulated by Sunwolf, Frey, and Keranen (2005), as they describe healing by offering examples of success, healing by reducing unhealthy anxieties, cohealing of both the teller and the listener, healing the practitioner, and healing the community. Other work looks at narrative therapy regarding final conversation narratives (Keeley & Koenig Kellas, 2005), telling such stories as "But, I think because I was nonjudgmental and respected, you know, and just listened openly, I think it gave him a sense of belonging and being respected. . . . I was honored that he opened up and shared with me" (p. 373), or the role of transforming narratives in recovery from schizophrenia (Lysaker et al., 2003). Lysaker et al. examined the narratives elicited from twenty-five participants with schizophrenia spectrum disorders and a comparison group of eight legally blind participants and four with major depressive disorders. Flexibility of abstract thought and positive, negative, and emotional discomfort symptoms were assessed.

We also know that sharing a traumatic narrative is related to frequency of doctor visits, immune function, reports of symptoms, depression, anxiety, and well-being (Horn & Mehl, 2004). Horn and Mehl conclude that developing a coherent narrative enables an event to be stored in memory and then forgotten more easily. Even adolescents respond positively to narrative therapy (Kaptain, 2004). Research on the caregivers of children and adolescents has reported that sharing narratives decreases negative emotion, increases cognitive functioning, and leads to beneficial effects on health-related quality of life (Schwartz & Drotar, 2004). Another way in which reliance on sharing narratives improves health is by leading to greater social interaction (Pennebaker, 2003). Narratives help individuals integrate illness experiences into their personal biographies, facilitating health and coping (DiGallo et al., 2003). DiGallo et al. asked thirty-three adult siblings of former childhood cancer patients how they had experienced illness and treatment of their brother or sister.

Other research, too, has reported decrements in health in those who do not share narratives (Klein, 2002; Park & Blumberg, 2002). Smyth and True (2001) found positive health effects of sharing a structured narrative, but not for the random or fragmented sharing of traumatic events. Structured narration is even related to more successful rehabilitation (Krieshok et al., 1999). The impact of narrative is so strong that Jerome Bruner (1999) argued that willingness to story is tantamount to desire to live.

Diagnosis

The value of understanding narrative to facilitate diagnosis is also a frequent theme in the literature. Ragan, Mindt, and Wittenberg-Lyles (2005) remind us that understanding the patient's story is the key to diagnosis (see also Olesen, 2003). Ragan et al. share the story of a prostate cancer sufferer who notes, "My initial experience of illness was as a series of disconnected shocks, and my first instinct was to try to bring it under control by turning it into a narrative" (p. 259). Young and Flower (2002) describe using narratives to build a complete and coherent diagnostic story, and Roth and Nelson (1997) examined narratives to assess problems with the communication of a diagnosis. Even diagnosis of schizophrenia (Lysaker et al., 2002; Lysaker et al., 2005), personality avoidant disorders (Meyer & Carver, 2000), childhood anxiety (Warren et al., 2000), and attachment and behavior problems (Ramos-Marcuse & Arsenio, 2001) have been linked to an examination of narratives. Looking at stories helps us more fully understand medical mistakes (Woolf et al., 2004) and cancer diagnostic difficulties (Dixon-Woods et al., 2001). Dixon-Woods et al. conducted semistructured interviews with twenty parents whose children (aged 4–18 years) had a confirmed diagnosis of cancer or brain tumor in their examination of diagnostic difficulties.

Narratives and particular health problems or populations

Yet another role of narrative in health communication is to provide information to health practitioners about the experience of a particular health problem or illness population. Examples of such writing are too numerous to itemize, but we do want to draw the reader's attention to this function of narrative as we move forward in our discussion. For examples one might look at Elofsson and Ohlen's (2004) report on chronic obstructive pulmonary disease or Broussard's (2005) examination of bulimia narratives. Broussard's phenomenological analysis of the narratives of thirteen actively bulimic women identified four themes: isolation (as the practices of bulimic women are carried out in secret), living in fear (because the behaviors of binge eating and purging are regarded as abnormal, and the women were scared of others finding out about them), being at war with the mind (an internal struggle between the guilt of bingeing then purging conflicts with the guilt it causes), and pacifying the inner voice (by feeding the compulsion to eat but then erasing guilt by self-induced vomiting). Capturing such feelings, one participant said, "I think that if anything I was relieved as I usually am after I throw up even though I know what I'm doing isn't good for me. I've found a way to continue my food obsession and not have to suffer the consequences of gaining weight" (Broussard, 2005, p. 48).

Learning from narratives for intervention

Yet other narrative researchers have examined stories in order to attempt to understand how to persuade audience members about certain health issues. For instance, Workman's (2005) examination of binge-drinking narratives provides insight that can be used to design more effective campaigns for the prevention of alcohol abuse and the work of Johnson et al. (2003) on smoking narratives can facilitate the development of useful anti-smoking messages. Johnson et al. conducted in-depth interviews with a purposeful sample of thirty-five youths aged 14–18 years with a variety of smoking histories (all had tried smoking). One story shared by Workman (2005), for instance, includes such issues as "That night, however, something had gone terribly wrong. . . . Scott Krueger . . . remained in a coma until he died late Monday" (p. 131). Workman's argument, however, is that reliance on such drastic anecdotes as Scott Krueger's enables students to discard any similarity between his experience and their own. He argues, quite convincingly, that this is not the most effective approach. Numerous other examples of such reliance on narrative for more effective intervention also abound.

Narratives of caregivers

The stress of providing ongoing care for an ill family member has prompted many narrative scholars to turn their attention to the narratives told by these caregivers. Again, we mention only a few of many such examples. Kirsi et al.'s (2004) examination of the narratives of husbands caring for demented wives indicates a feeling of being "always one step behind" (p. 159), a passive voice, and an emphasis on duty and responsive agency, while Meeker's (2004) study of caregiver narratives at the end of the patient's life help us understand the surrogate decision-making roles required of these caregivers. Ayres (2000) identified four story types in the narratives of family caregivers, and themes of stress, appraisal and coping emerge in an assessment of care-giving of Aphasic stroke survivors (Biggins, 2003). Much other research focuses on narratives of professional health-care providers about the caring process (Bertero, 1999; Fins et al., 2000; Fosgarde et al., 2002; Gattuso & Bevan, 2000; Jaye & Wilson, 2003; Loftus & McDowell, 2000; Mahera & Souter, 2002; Olofsson & Norberg, 2001; Rabin et al., 1999; Skhorshammer, 2002; Skovdahl et al., 2003; Sorlie et al., 2003; Sorlie et al., 2000; Svedlund et al., 1999; Valente & Saunders, 2000; Vegni et al., 2001; Wear, 2002; Zerwekh, 2000).

Narrative competence

Taking a very different approach to the study of narratives, some scholars study narrative competence or the lack thereof as they attempt to understand why some people are very good at narration and, thus, more likely to reap the benefits described above. Narrative competence is not defined in a consistent way across researchers, but typically focuses upon being good at storytelling, good at eliciting stories from others, or good at interpreting and learning from the stories of others (Montello, 1997). Narrative skills include interpretation, empathy, and reflection (Ragan et al., 2005) and narrative competence is the ability to effectively exercise those skills and respond to the plight of others.

Montello (1997) relates narrative competence in providers to ethics and the ability to learn about moral issues from stories. She notes that "the ability to make sound moral choices involves facility with comprehending the motivations and consequences of behaviors and choices" (p. 190) and that narrative competence relates directly to negotiating the balance between involvement and detachment.

Other researchers look at the characteristics of stories to determine competence, rather than storytellers. For instance, Connelly (2005) writes about how doctors may be able to "help the patient tell the story that is most important, meaningful, and descriptive" (p. 84). Dimaggio et al. (2003) wrote about "impoverished narratives" (p. 385) that lack description of inner states, the perspective of others, and information about the action scenario, and thus hamper the narrator's ability to relate to others. Dimaggio et al. illustrate this narrative deficit with a psychotherapy case study and provide suggestions about the way a therapist ought to operate in order to tackle the deficit.

Narrative competence is a developmental ability (Shiro, 2003) and is also affected by some illnesses, disabilities, and treatments (Hemphill et al., 2002). Narrative competence, however, can also be taught (Kaufert & Koch, 2003; Marchand & Kushner, 2004; Yamada et al., 2003) and encouraging the telling of narratives facilitates the development of empathy (DasGupta & Charon, 2004). Those medical students who are encouraged to tell their own illness narratives become more empathic toward patients.

Conclusion

The value and potential of narrative is powerful. It is hoped that this review has made clear the many ways in which an understanding of narrative can facilitate work and intervention in health communication and that such work will continue to enrich our understanding of communication as it relates to health and health-care delivery. Communication scholars, with our focus on messages, are uniquely poised to contribute to an understanding of narrative processes both in terms of the language used in narratives and in terms of the functions of narratives. Contrast this, for instance, with a more sociological perspective on narrative (see, for instance, Elliott, 2005). Whereas Elliott's examples of narrative approaches focus on the role of narrative in understanding identity or an analysis of demographics in constructing a narrative, little insight is provided into the functions served by various narratives. Although each approach has value, an understanding of narrative that does not look at the language of stories or how the stories function to enable coping, diagnosis, healing, etc. would be inherently incomplete. Communication scholars stand at the brink of unique contributions in this regard.

Similarly, communication scholars are distinctively positioned to combine a narrative approach with a critical or cultural approach to health communication. The import and value of critical and cultural approaches to health communication are made clear throughout this book. Examples of research combining narrative with critical and cultural approaches may already be seen in such literature as the work of Harter et al. (2005) examining how narratives of age-related infertility structure women's lives and bodies. Their critique of this body of work provides a promising example of the kind of contribution that communication scholars can make as we move ahead in our applications of narrative, cultural, and critical health communication research.

References

Abma, T.A. (2002). Emerging narrative forms of knowledge representation in the health sciences: Two texts in a postmodern context. *Qualitative Health Research, 12,* 5–27.

Androutsopoulou, A. (2001). Self-characterization as a narrative tool: Applications in therapy with individuals and families. *Family Process, 40,* 79–94.

Arnstein, P. (2003). Comprehensive analysis and management of chronic pain. *Nursing Clinics of North America, 38,* 403–417.

Arvay, M., Banister, E., Hoskins, M., & Snell, A. (1999). Women's lived experience of conceptualizing the self: Implications for health care practice. *Health Care for Women International, 20,* 363–380.

Ayres, L. (2000). Narratives of family caregiving: Four story types. *Research in Nursing & Health, 23,* 359–371.

Babrow, A.S., Kline, K.N., & Rawlins, W.K. (2005). Narrative problems and problematizing narratives: Linking problematic integration and narrative theory in telling stories about our health. In L.M. Harter, P.M. Japp, & C.S. Beck (eds), *Narratives, Health, and Healing: Communication Theory, Research, and Practice.* Mahwah, NJ: Erlbaum, pp. 31–52.

Balber, P.G. (2003). Stories of the living dying: The Hermes listener. In I. Corless & B.B. Germino (ed.), *Dying, Death, and Bereavement: A Challenge for Living,* 2nd edn. New York: Springer, pp. 117–143.

Bauer, J.J. & Bonanno, G.A. (2001). I can, I do, I am: The narrative differentiation of self-efficacy and other self-evaluations while adapting to bereavement. *Journal of Research in Personality, 35,* 424–448.

Beck, C.S. (2005). Becoming the story: Narratives as collaborative, social enactments of individual, relational, and public identities. In L.M. Harter, P.M. Japp, & C.S. Beck (eds), *Narratives, Health, and Healing: Communication Theory, Research, and Practice.* Mahwah, NJ: Erlbaum, pp. 61–82.

Belknap, R.A. (2002). Sense of self: Voices of separation and connection in women who have experienced abuse. *Canadian Journal of Nursing Research, 33,* 139–153.

Bertero, C. (1999). Caring for and about cancer patients: Identifying the meaning of the phenomenon "caring" through narratives. *Cancer Nursing, 22,* 414–420.

Biggins, N.A. (2003). Long-term caregiving of Aphasic stroke survivors: The lived experience. *Dissertation Abstracts, 63*(12-B), 5796.

Bosticco, C., & Thompson, T.L. (2005). An examination of the role of narratives and storytelling in bereavement. In L.M. Harter, P.M. Japp, & C.S. Beck (eds), *Narratives, Health, and Healing: Communication Theory, Research, and Practice.* Mahwah, NJ: Erlbaum, pp. 391–412.

Brashers, D.E., Neidig, J.L, Cardillo, L.W., Dobbs, L.K., Russell, J.A., & Haas, S.M. (1999). "In an important way, I did die": Uncertainty and revival in persons living with HIV or AIDS. *AIDS Care, 11*, 201–219.

Brockmeier, J. & Harré, R. (1997). Narrative: Problems and promises of an alternative paradigm. *Research on Language and Social Interaction, 30*, 263–283.

Broussard, B.B. (2005). Women's experiences of bulimia nervosa. *Journal of Advanced Nursing, 49*, 43–50.

Brown, B., Nolan, P., Crawford, P., & Lewis, A. (1996). Interaction, language, and the "narrative turn" in psychotherapy and psychiatry. *Social Science & Medicine, 43*, 1569–1578.

Bruner, J. (1999). Narratives of aging. *Journal of Aging Studies, 13*, 7–9.

Buzzanell, P.M., & Ellingson, L.L. (2005). Contesting narratives of workplace maternity. In L.M. Harter, P.M. Japp, & C.S. Beck (eds), *Narratives, Health, and Healing: Communication Theory, Research, and Practice*. Mahwah, NJ: Erlbaum, pp. 277–294.

Callister, L.C. (2004). Making meaning: Women's birth narratives. *Journal of Obstetric, Gynecologic, and Neonatal Nursing, 33*, 508–518.

Coker, E.M. (2003). Narrative strategies in medical discourse: Constructing the psychiatric "case" in a non-western setting. *Social Science & Medicine, 57*, 905–916.

Connelly, J.E. (2005). Narrative possibilities: Using mindfulness in clinical practice. *Perspectives in Biology and Medicine, 48*, 84–94.

Copeland, L. (2004). Drug user's identity and how it relates to being hepatitis C antibody positive: A qualitative study. *Drugs: Education, Prevention & Policy, 2*, 129–147.

Courtial, J.P., & Le Dreff, G. (2004). Analysis of pregnant women's narratives. *Sante Publique, 16*, 105–121.

Dasberg, H., Bartura, J., & Amit, Y. (2001). Narrative group therapy with aging child survivors of the Holocaust. *The Israel Journal of Psychiatry & Related Sciences, 38*, 27–35.

DasGupta, S., & Charon, R. (2004). Personal illness narratives: Using reflective writing to teach empathy. *Academic Medicine, 79*, 351–356.

Davies, B., Gudmundsdottir, M., Worden, B., Orloff, S., & Brenner, P. (2004). "Living in the dragon's shadow": Fathers' experiences of a child's life-limiting illness. *Death Studies, 28*, 111–135.

DelVeccio Good, M.J., Gadmer, N.M., Ruopp, P., Lakoma, M., Sullivan, A.M., Redinbaugh, E., Arnold, R.M., & Block, S.D. (2004). Narrative nuances on good and bad deaths: Internists' tales from high-technology work places. *Social Science & Medicine, 58*, 939–953.

Dietrich, P.J., McWilliam, C.L., Ralyea, S.F., & Schweitzer, A.T. (1999). Mother-loss: Recreating relationship and meaning. *The Canadian Journal of Nursing Research, 31*, 77–101.

DiGallo, A., Gwerder, C., Amslwer, A., & Burgin, D. (2003). Siblings of children with cancer: Integration of the illness experiences into personal biography. *Praxis der Kinderpsychologie und Kinderpsychiatrie, 52*, 141–155.

Dimaggio, G., Salvatore, G., Azzara, C., Catania, D., Samerari, A., & Herman, H.J.M. (2003). Dialogical relationships in impoverished narratives: From theory to clinical practice. *Psychology and Psychotherapy, 76*, 385–409.

Dixon-Woods, M., Findlay, M., Young, B., Cox, H., & Heney, D. (2001). Parents' accounts of obtaining a diagnosis of childhood cancer. *Lancet, 357,* 670–674.

Downs, B. (1993). Lessons in loss and grief. *Communication Education, 42,* 300–303.

Elderkin-Thompson, V.D. (1997). Narrative and nonverbal communication of somatizing and nonsomatizing patients in a primary care setting. *Dissertation Abstracts, 57*(10-B), 6568.

Elliott, J. (2005). *Using Narrative in Social Research: Qualitative and Quantitative Approaches.* Thousand Oaks, CA: Sage.

Elofsson, L.C., & Ohlen, J. (2004). Meanings of being old and living with chronic obstructive pulmonary disease. *Palliative Medicine, 18,* 611–618.

Evans, J.W., Walters, A.S., & Hatch-Woodruff, M.L. (1999). Deathbed scene narratives: A construct and linguistic analysis. *Death Studies, 23,* 715–733.

Fairchild, A.L. (2001). The polio narratives: Dialogues with FDR. *Bulletin of the History of Medicine, 75,* 488–534.

Fins, J.J., Schwager Guest, R., & Acres, C.A. (2000). Gaining insight into the care of hospitalized dying patients: An interpretive narrative analysis. *Journal of Pain & Symptom Management, 20,* 399–407.

Fisher, W.R. (1985). The narrative paradigm: In the beginning. *Journal of Communication, 35*(4), 74–89.

Fisher, W.R. (1987). *Human Communication as Narration: Toward a Philosophy of Reason, Value, and Action.* Columbia, SC: University of South Carolina Press.

Fletcher, P.N. (2002). Experiences in family bereavement. *Family & Community Health, 25,* 57–70.

Forsgarde, M., Westman, B., & Jansson, L. (2002). Professional carers' struggle to be confirmed: Narratives within the care of the elderly and disabled. *Scandinavian Journal of Caring Sciences, 16,* 12–18.

Frank, A.W. (1995). *The Wounded Storyteller: Body, Illness, and Ethics.* Chicago: University of Chicago.

Gattuso, S., & Bevan, C. (2000). Mother, daughter, patient, nurse: Women's emotion work in aged care. *Journal of Advanced Nursing, 31,* 892–899.

Gaydos, H.L. (2005). Understanding personal narratives: An approach to practice. *Journal of Advanced Nursing, 49,* 254–259.

Gewirtz, A., & Gossart-Walker, S. (2000). Home-based treatment for children and families affected by HIV and AIDS. Dealing with stigma, secrecy, disclosure, and loss. *Child & Adolescent Psychiatric Clinics of North America, 9,* 313–330.

Gray, R.E., Fergus, K.D., & Fitch, M.I. (2005). Two Black men with prostate cancer: A narrative approach. *British Journal of Health Psychology, 10,* 71–84.

Gullickson, T., & Ramser, P. (1996). Living with grief and mourning. *Contemporary Psychology: APA Review of Books, 41,* 847.

Hallberg, I.R. (2001). A narrative approach to nursing care of people in difficult life situations. In G.M. Kenyon, & P.G. Clark (eds), *Narrative Gerontology: Theory, Research, and Practice.* New York: Springer, pp. 237–272.

Harden, J. (2000). Language, discourse and the chronotope: Applying literary theory to the narratives in health care. *Journal of Advanced Nursing, 31,* 506–512.

Harter, L.M., Japp, P.M., & Beck, C.S. (2005). Vital problematics of narrative theorizing about health and healing. In L.M. Harter, P.M. Japp, & C.S. Beck (eds), *Narratives, Health, and Healing: Communication Theory, Research, and Practice.* Mahwah, NJ: Erlbaum, pp. 7–30.

Harter, L.M., Kirby, E.L., Edwards, A., & McClanahan, A. (2005). Time, technology, and meritocracy: The disciplining of women's bodies in narrative constructions of age-related infertility. In L.M. Harter, P.M. Japp, & C.S. Beck (eds), *Narratives, Health, and Healing: Communication Theory, Research, and Practice.* Mahwah, NJ: Erlbaum, pp. 83–106.

Hawkins, S.C. (2004). Emergency medicine narratives: A systematic discussion of definition and utility. *Academic Emergency Medicine, 11,* 761–765.

Hellstrom, O., Bullington, J., Karlsson, G., Lindqvist, P., & Mattsson, B. (1999). A henomenological study of fibromyalgia: Patient perspectives. *Scandinavian Journal of Primary Health Care, 17,* 11–16.

Hemphill, L., Uccelli, P., Winner, K., Chang, C., & Bellinger, D. (2002). Narrative discourse in young children with histories of early corrective heart surgery. *Journal of Speech, Language, & Hearing Research, 45,* 318–331.

Hendin, H., Lipschitz, A., Maltsberger, J.T., Haas, A.P., & Wynecoop, S. (2000). Therapists' reactions to patients' suicides. *The American Journal of Psychiatry, 157,* 2022–2027.

Hess, J.D. (2003). Gadow's relational narrative: An elaboration. *Nursing Philosophy, 4,* 137–148.

Hildingsson, I., & Haggstrom, T. (1999). Midwives' lived experiences of being supportive to prospective mothers/parents during pregnancy. *Midwifery, 15,* 82–91.

Horn, A., & Mehl, M.R. (2004). Expressive writing as a coping tool: A state-of-the-art review. *Verhaltenstherapie, 14,* 274–283.

Hoyt, M.F. (2000). *Some Stories are Better than Others: Doing What Works in Brief Therapy and Managed Care.* Philadelphia, PA: Brunner/Mazel.

Japp, P.M. (2005) Personal narratives and public dialogues: Introduction. In L.M. Harter, P.M. Japp, & C.S. Beck (eds), *Narratives, Health, and Healing: Communication Theory, Research, and Practice.* Mahwah, NJ: Erlbaum, pp. 53–59.

Japp, P.M., Harter, L.M., & Beck, C.S. (2005). Overview of narrative and health communication theorizing: Introduction. In L.M. Harter, P.M. Japp, & C.S. Beck (eds), *Narratives, Health, and Healing: Communication Theory, Research, and Practice.* Mahwah, NJ: Erlbaum, pp. 1–6.

Jaye, C., & Wilson, H. (2003). When general practitioners become patients. *Health: An Interdisciplinary Journal for the Social Study of Health, Illness & Medicine, 7,* 201–225.

Johnson, J.L., Lovato, C.Y., Maggi, S., Ratner, P.A., Shoeveller, J., Baillie, L., & Kalaw, C. (2003). Smoking and adolescence: Narratives of identity. *Research in Nursing and Health, 26,* 387–397.

Jones, D.W. (2004). Families and serious mental illness: Working with loss and ambivalence. *British Journal of Social Work, 34,* 961–979.

Jordens, C.L., Little, M., Paul, K., & Sayers, E.J. (2001). Life disruption and generic complexity: A social linguistic analysis of narratives of cancer illness. *Social Science & Medicine, 53,* 1227–1236.

Kalischuk, R.G., & Hayes, V.E. (2003–2004). Grieving, mourning, and healing following youth suicide: A focus on health and well being in families. *Omega: Journal of Death & Dying, 48,* 45–67.

Kameny, R.R. & Bearison, D.J. (1999). Illness narratives: Discursive constructions of self in pediatric oncology. *Journal of Pediatric Nursing, 14*(2), 73–79.

Kaptain, D.C. (2004). Narrative group therapy with outpatient adolescents. *Dissertation Abstracts, 65*(6-A), 2379.

Kaufert, J., & Koch, T. (2003). Disability or end-of-life? Competing narratives in bioethics. *Theoretical Medicine and Bioethics, 24*, 459–469.

Keeley, M.P., & Koenig Kellas, J. (2005). Constructing life and death through final conversation narratives. In L.M. Harter, P.M. Japp, & C.S. Beck (eds), *Narratives, Health, and Healing: Communication Theory, Research, and Practice*. Mahwah, NJ: Erlbaum, pp. 365–390.

Kirkman, M. (2001). Thinking of something to say: Public and private narratives of infertility. *Health Care for Women International, 22*, 523–535.

Kirkman, M. (2003). Parents' contributions to the narrative identity of offspring of donor-assisted conception. *Social Science & Medicine, 57*, 2229–2242.

Kirsi, T., Hervonen, A., & Jylha, M. (2004). Always one step behind: Husbands' narratives about taking care of their demented wives. *Health: An Interdisciplinary Journal for the Social Study of Health, Illness, & Medicine, 8*, 159–181.

Klein, K. (2002). Stress, expressive writing, and working memory. In S.J. Lepore & J.M. Smyth (eds), *The Writing Cure: How Expressive Writing Promotes Health and Emotional Well-being*. Washington, DC: APA, pp. 135–155.

Krieshok, T.S., Hastings, S., Wettersten, K., & Owen, A. (1999). Telling a good story: Using narratives in vocational rehabilitation with veterans. *Career Development Quarterly, 47*, 204–214.

Lichtenthal, W.G., Cruess, D.G., & Prigerson, H.G. (2004). A case for establishing complicated grief as a distinct mental disorder in DSM-V. *Clinical Psychology Review, 24*, 637–662.

Little, M., Jordens, C.F.C., & Sayers, E. (2003). Discourse communities and the discourse of experience. *Health: An Interdisciplinary Journal for the Social Study of Health, Illness, & Medicine, 7*, 73–86.

Loftus, L.A., & McDowell, J. (2000). The lived experience of the oncology clinical nurse specialist. *International Journal of Nursing Studies, 37*, 513–521.

Lule, J. (1990). Telling the story of story: Journalism history and narrative theory. *American Journalism, 7*, 259–274.

Lurier, A.C. (2004). Pathways and barriers to mourning: The lived experiences of grieving caregivers and their children in a group of inner-city African American families. *Dissertation Abstracts, 64*(7–B), 3531.

Lysaker, P.H., Clements, C.A., Plascak-Hallberg, C.D., Knipscheer, S.J., & Wright, D.E. (2002). Insight and personal narratives of illness in schizophrenia. *Psychiatry, 65*, 197–206.

Lysaker, P.H., Lancaster, R.S., & Lysaker, J.T. (2003). Narrative transformation as an outcome in the psychotherapy of schizophrenia. *Psychology and Psychotherapy, 76*, 285–299.

Lysaker, P.H., Wickett, A., & Davis, L.W. (2005). Narrative qualities in schizophrenia: Associations with impairments in neurocognition and negative symptoms. *The Journal of Nervous and Mental Disease, 193*, 244–249.

Mahera, J.M., & Souter, K.T. (2002). Midwifery work and the making of narrative. *Nursing Inquiry, 9*, 37–42.

Marchand, L., & Kushner, K. (2004). Death pronouncements: Using the teachable moment in end-of-life care residency training. *Journal of Palliative Medicine, 7*, 80–84.

Martins, A.J., Cardoso, M.H.C.A., & Llerena, J.C. (2004). In contact with genetic diseases: Norms and reason as cultural traditions in medical staff discourse. *Escola Nacional De Saude Publica, 20,* 968–975.

McAdams, D.P. (1990). Unity and purpose in human lives: The emergence of identity as a life story. In A.I. Rabin, R.A. Zucker, R.E. Emmons & S. Frank (eds), *Studying Persons and Lives.* New York: Springer, pp. 148–200.

McCreight, B.S. (2004). A grief ignored: Narratives of pregnancy loss from a male perspective. *Sociology of Health & Illness, 26,* 326–350.

Meeker, M.A. (2004). Family surrogate decision making at the end of life: Seeing them through with care and respect. *Qualitative Health Research, 14,* 204–205.

Meyer, B., & Carver, C.S. (2000). Negative childhood accounts, sensitivity, and pessimism: A study of avoidance personality disorder features in college students. *Journal of Personality Disorders, 14,* 233–248.

Milton, C.L. (2004). Stories: Implications for nursing ethics and respect for another. *Nursing Science Quarterly, 17,* 208–211.

Monk, G., Winslade, J., Crocket, K. & Epton, D. (1997). *Narrative Therapy in Practice: The Archaeology of Hope.* San Francisco, CA: Jossey-Bass.

Montello, M. (1997). Narrative competence. In H.L. Nelson (ed.), *Stories and their Limits.* New York: Routledge, pp. 185–197.

Morgan-Witte, J. (2005). Narrative knowledge development among caregivers: Stories from the nurses' station. In L.M. Harter, P.M. Japp, & C.S. Beck (eds), *Narratives, Health, and Healing: Communication Theory, Research, and Practice.* Mahwah, NJ: Erlbaum, pp. 217–236.

Murdoch, R.O. (1999). Working and "drugging" in the city: Economics and substance use in a sample of working addicts. *Substance Use & Misuse, 34,* 2115–2133.

Murphy, S.A., & Johnson, L.C. (2003). Finding meaning in a child's violent death: A five-year prospective analysis of parents' personal narratives and empirical data. *Death Studies, 27,* 381–404.

Murray, M. (2000). Levels of narrative analysis in health psychology. *Journal of Health Psychology, 5,* 337–347.

Myers, G.E. (2002). Can illness narratives contribute to the delay of hospice admission? *The American Journal of Hospice & Palliative Care, 19,* 32–330.

Nairn, S. (2004). Emergency care and narrative knowledge. *Journal of Advanced Nursing, 48,* 59–67.

Neimeyer, R.A. (2001). Reauthoring life narratives: Grief therapy as meaning reconstruction. *The Israel Journal of Psychiatry and Related Sciences, 38,* 171–183.

Nelson, S., & McGillion, M. (2004). Expertise or performance? Questioning the rhetoric of contemporary narrative use in nursing. *Journal of Advanced Nursing, 47,* 631–638.

Nilsson, M., Sarvimaki, A. & Ekman, S. (2000). Feeling old: Being in a phase of transition in later life. *Nursing Inquiry, 7,* 41–49.

Nochi, M. (2000) Reconstructing self-narratives in coping with traumatic brain injury. *Social Science & Medicine, 51,* 1785–1804.

Norbury, C.F., & Bishop, D.V.M. (2003). Narrative skills of children with communication impairments. *International Journal of Language & Communication Disorders, 38,* 287–313.

Ogle, K., Greene, D.D., Winn, B., Mishkin, D., Bricker, L.G., & Lambing, A.K. (2003). Completing a life. *Journal of Palliative Medicine, 6,* 841–850.

Olesen, F. (2003). A framework for clinical general practice and for research and teaching in the discipline. *Family Practice, 20*, 318–323.

Olofsson, B., & Norberg, A. (2001). Experiences of coercion in psychiatric care as narrated by patients, nurses, and physicians. *Journal of Advanced Nursing, 33*, 89–97.

Pals, J.L. (2001). Self-narratives of difficult life experiences in adulthood. *Dissertation Abstracts, 61*(7-B), 3891.

Park, C.L., & Blumberg, C.J. (2002). Disclosing trauma through writing: Treating the meaning-making hypothesis. *Cognitive Therapy & Research, 26*, 597–616.

Pennebaker, J.W. (2003). The social, linguistic, and health consequences of emotional disclosure. In J. Suls, & K.A. Wallston (eds), *Social Psychological Foundations of Health and Illness*. Malden, MA: Blackwell Publishers, pp. 288–313.

Penson, R.T., Partridge, R.A., Shah, M.A., Giansiracusa, D., Chabner, B.A., & Lynch, T.J. (2005). Fear of death. *The Oncologist, 10*, 160–169.

Porter, L.G. (2004). Personal narratives as reflections of identity and meaning: A study of betrayal, forgiveness, and health. *Dissertation Abstracts, 64*(9-B), 4666.

Rabin, S., Maoz, B., & Elata-Alster, G. (1999). Doctors' narratives in Balint groups. *The British Journal of Medical Psychology, 72*, 121–125.

Ragan, S.L., Mindt, T., & Wittenberg-Lyles, E. (2005). Narrative medicine and education in palliative care. In L.M. Harter, P.M. Japp, & C.S. Beck (eds), *Narratives, Health, and Healing: Communication Theory, Research, and Practice*. Mahwah, NJ: Erlbaum, pp. 259–276.

Ramos-Marcuse, F., & Arsenio, W.F. (2001). Young children's emotionally-charged moral narratives: Relations with attachment and behavior problems. *Early Education & Development, 12*, 165–184.

Rawlins, W.K. (2005). Our family's physician. In L.M. Harter, P.M. Japp, & C.S. Beck (eds), *Narratives, Health, and Healing: Communication Theory, Research, and Practice*. Mahwah, NJ: Erlbaum, pp. 197–216.

Rich, M., Lamola, S., Gordon, J., & Chalfen, R. (2000). Video intervention/ prevention assessment: A patient-centered methodology for understanding the adolescent illness experience. *Journal of Adolescent Health: Official Publication of the Society for Adolescent Medicine, 27*, 155–65.

Riessman, C. (2003). Performing identities in illness narrative: Masculinity and multiple sclerosis. *Qualitative Research, 3*, 5–33.

Robinson, J.A., & Hawpe, L. (1986). Narrative thinking as a heuristic process. In T.R. Sarbin (ed.), *Narrative Psychology*. New York: Praeger, pp. 111–125.

Romyn, D.M. (2003). The relational narrative: Implications for nurse practice and education. *Nursing Philosophy, 4*, 149–154.

Roth, N.L., & Nelson, M.S. (1997). HIV diagnosis and identity narratives. *AIDS Care, 9*, 161–179.

Rybarczyk, B., & Bellg, A. (1997). *Listening to Life Stories: A New Approach to Stress Intervention in Health Care*. New York: Springer.

Sakalys, J.A. (2000). The political role of illness narratives. *Journal of Advanced Nursing, 31*, 1469–1475.

Scherman, M.H., Dahlgren, L.O., & Lowhagen, O. (2002). Refusing to be ill: A longitudinal study of patients' experiences of asthma/allergy. *Disability & Rehabilitation: An International Multidisciplinary Journal, 24*, 297–307.

Schrank, R.C. (1990). *Tell Me a Story: A New Look at Real and Artificial Memory*. New York: Schribner's Sons.

Schwartz, L., & Drotar, D. (2004). Linguistic analysis of written narratives of caregivers of children and adolescents with chronic illness: Cognitive and emotional processes and physical and psychological health outcomes. *Journal of Clinical Psychology in Medical Setting, 11*, 291–301.

Sedney, M.A., Baker, J.E., & Gross, E. (1994). "The story" of a death: Therapeutic considerations with bereaved families. *Journal of Marital and Family Therapy, 20*, 287–296.

Sharf, B.F. (2005). How I fired my surgeon and embraced an alternate narrative. In L.M. Harter, P.M. Japp, & C.S. Beck (eds), *Narratives, Health, and Healing: Communication Theory, Research, and Practice*. Mahwah, NJ: Erlbaum, pp. 325–342.

Sharf, B.F., & Vanderford, M.L. (2003). Illness narratives and the social construction of health. In T.L. Thompson, A.M. Dorsey, K.I. Miller, & R. Parrott (eds), *Handbook of Health Communication*. Mahwah, NJ: Erlbaum, pp. 9–34.

Shiro, M. (2003). Genre and evaluation in narrative development. *Journal of Child Language, 30*, 165–195.

Siegel, K., & Meyer, I.H. (1999). Hope and resilience in suicide ideation and behavior of gay and bisexual men following notification of HIV infection. *AIDS Education & Prevention, 11*, 53–64.

Singhal, A., Chitnis, K., & Sengupta, A. (2005). Cross-border mass-mediated health narratives: Narrative transparency, "safe sex," and Indian viewers. In L.M. Harter, P.M. Japp, & C.S. Beck (eds), *Narratives, Health, and Healing: Communication Theory, Research, and Practice*. Mahwah, NJ: Erlbaum, pp. 169–188.

Skhorshammer, M. (2002). Understanding conflicts between health professionals: A narrative approach. *Qualitative Health Research, 12*, 915–931.

Skovdahl, K., Kihlgren, A.L., & Kihlgren, M. (2003). Different attitudes when handling aggressive behaviour in dementia—Narratives from two caregiver groups. *Aging & Mental Health, 7*, 277–286.

Skultans, V. (2003). From damaged nerves to masked depression: Inevitability and hope in Latvian psychiatric narratives. *Social Science & Medicine, 56*, 2421–2431.

Smyth, J., & True, N. (2001). Effects of writing about traumatic experiences: The necessity for narrative structuring. *Journal of Social & Clinical Psychology, 20*, 161–172.

Sorlie, V., Jansson, L., & Norberg, A. (2003). The meaning of being in ethically difficult care situations in paediatric care as narrated by female Registered Nurses. *Scandinavian Journal of Caring Sciences, 17*, 285–292.

Sorlie, V., Forde, R., Lindseth, A., & Norberg, A. (2001). Male physicians' narratives about being in ethically difficult care situations in paediatrics. *Social Science & Medicine, 53*, 657–667.

Sorlie, V., Kihlgren, A., & Kihlgren, M. (2005). Meeting ethical challenges in acute nursing care as narrated by registered nurses. *Nursing Ethics, 12*, 133–142.

Sorlie, V., Kihlgren, A.L., & Kihlgren, M. (2004). Meeting ethical challenges in acute care work as narrated by enrolled nurses. *Nursing Ethics, 11*, 179–188.

Sorlie, V., Lindseth, A., Uden, G., & Norberg, A. (2000). Women physicians' narratives about being in ethically difficult care situations in paediatrics. *Nursing Ethics, 7*, 47–62.

Squier, S.M. (1999). Narrating genetic disabilities: Social constructs, medical treatment, and public policy. *Issues in Law & Medicine, 15*, 141–158.

Stein, N.L., & Policastro, M. (1984). Concept of a story: A comparison between children's and teachers' viewpoints. In H. Mandl, N.L. Stein, & T. Trabasso (eds), *Learning and Comprehension of Text*. Hillsdale, NJ: Erlbaum, pp. 113–152.

Stern, S., Doolan, M., Staples, E., Szmukler, G.L., & Eisler, I. (1999). Disruption and reconstruction: Narrative insights into the experience of family members caring for a relative diagnosed with serious mental illness. *Family Process, 38,* 353–369.

Stiles, W.B., Honos-Webb, L., & Lani, J.A. (1999). Some functions of narrative in the assimilation of problematic experiences. *Journal of Clinical Psychology, 55,* 1213–1226.

Sunwolf, Frey, L.R., & Keranen, L. (2005). Rx story prescription: Healing effects of storytelling and storylistening in the practice of medicine. In L.M. Harter, P.M. Japp, & C.S. Beck (eds), *Narratives, Health, and Healing: Communication Theory, Research, and Practice*. Mahwah, NJ: Erlbaum, pp. 237–258.

Svedlund, M., Danielson, E., & Norbrg, A. (1999). Nurses' narrations about caring for inpatients with acute myocardial infarction. *Intensive & Critical Care Nursing, 15,* 34–43.

Tannen, D. (1988). Hearing voices in conversation, fiction, and mixed genres. In D. Tannen (ed.), *Linguistics in Context: Connecting Observation and Understanding*. Norwood, NJ: Ablex, pp. 89–113.

Tardy, R.W., & Hale, C.L. (1998). Bonding and cracking: The role of informal, interpersonal networks in health care decision making. *Health Communication, 10,* 151–173.

Thomas-MacLean, R. (2004). Understanding breast cancer stories via Frank's narrative types. *Social Science & Medicine, 58,* 1647–1657.

Ungar, M. (2000). Drifting toward mental health: High-risk adolescents and the process of empowerment. *Youth & Society, 32,* 228–252.

Ungar, M.T. (2001). Constructing narratives of resilience with high-risk youth. *Journal of Systemic Therapies, 20*(2), 58–73.

Valente, S.M., & Saunders, J.M. (2000). Understanding oncology nurses' difficulties caring for suicidal people. *Medicine & Law, 19,* 793–813.

Vegni, E., Zannini, L., Visioli, S., & Moja, E.A. (2001). Giving bad news: A GP's narrative perspective. *Supportive Care in Cancer, 9,* 390–396.

Warren, S.L, Emde, R.N., & Sroufe, L.A. (2000). Internal representations: Predicting anxiety from children's play narratives. *Journal of the American Academy of Child and Adolescent Psychiatry, 39,* 100–107.

Wear, D. (2002). "Face-to-face with it": Medical students' narratives about their end-of-life education. *Academic Medicine, 77,* 271–277.

Weick, K.E. (1995). *Sensemaking in organizations*. Thousand Oaks, CA: Sage.

Williams, L., Labonte, R. & O'Brien, M. (2003). Empowering social action through narratives of identity and culture. *Health Promotion International, 18,* 33–40.

Woolf, S.H., Kuzel, A.J., Dovey, S.M., & Phillips, R.L. (2004). A string of mistakes: The importance of cascade analysis in describing, counting, and preventing medical errors. *Annals of Family Medicine, 2,* 317–326.

Workman, T. (2005). Death as the representative anecdote in the construction of the collegiate "binge-drinking" problem. In L.M. Harter, P.M. Japp, & C.S. Beck (eds), *Narratives, Health, and Healing: Communication Theory, Research, and Practice*. Mahwah, NJ: Erlbaum, pp. 131–148.

Yamada, S., Maskarinec, G.G., Greene, G.A., & Bauman, K.A. (2003). Family narratives, culture, and patient-centered medicine. *Family Medicine, 35*, 279–283.

Young, A., & Flower, L. (2002). Patients as partners, patients as problem-solvers. *Health Communication, 14*, 69–97.

Zerwekh, J.V. (2000). Caring on the ragged edge: Nursing persons who are disenfranchised. *ANS: Advances in Nursing Science, 22*, 47–71.

Chapter 3

Supporting breastfeeding(?)

Nursing mothers' resistance to and accommodation of medical and social discourses

Emily T. Cripe

Kris is an educated woman in her mid-thirties with two sons—a nine-year-old Xander, and seven-month-old Aidan:[1]

> I think most doctors are *not* supportive of breast-feeding. It depends on what kind of obstetrician you have, whether or not you're going to have a positive experience with breast-feeding . . . It really made a difference for me with Xander, a big difference. And when I had Aidan, my doctor was very supportive, and I had the same kind of delivery with Xander that I had with Aidan, I had an emergency Cesarean . . . The doctor afterwards put me to sleep for 24 hours and then told the nurses to bottle feed him. So Xander got bottle-fed right away. The difference was, I-I had, um, local anesthetic, and I was *not* put to sleep after I had Aidan, and the doctor was *very* encouraging that I start breast-feeding right away. They sent in a lactation consultant as soon as possible to help me learn how to breast-feed around my Cesarean. The doctor really set the tone for how the staff treated me, and how the staff handled whether or not I was going to breast-feed or bottle-feed. Even though I was *very* clear both times, I wanted to breast-feed. So I think some doctors just aren't—either they're not convinced that it's so important or, you know they just aren't interested in finding out the importance for the relationship that breast-feeding can engender between the mother and child.
>
> Interview

Breastfeeding is viewed as an important public health concern in the United States, so much so that encouraging higher rates of breastfeeding has been included as one of the goals of the government's *Healthy People 2010* report (US Department of Health and Human Services [USDHHS], 2000). Experts such as the American Academy of Pediatrics (AAP) recommend that infants be fed exclusively on breastmilk for the first six months and that breastfeeding "should be continued for at least the first year of life and beyond for as long as mutually desired by mother and child" (2005, p. 499). However, currently only 60 percent of infants in the United States are breastfed exclusively after birth, and only 8 percent are exclusively breastfed by six months of age (Li et al., 2003).

Our failure to achieve breastfeeding goals is not as simple as needing newer, better health promotion campaigns. Breastfeeding is a health practice that is historically situated and is not universally supported for a number of complex social, political, and health reasons. There are several factors influencing breastfeeding rates. Breastfeeding is not always easy or uncomplicated for women. A variety of social constructions surround breastfeeding as a practice, rendering it as a seemingly off-limits practice for some women, and as almost compulsory for others if they are to be seen as "good mothers." Additionally, as Kris' quotation illustrates, breastfeeding can be problematic even for women who desire to practice it, sometimes (however unwittingly) because of the medical professionals they are involved with. Women can have dramatically different experiences with breastfeeding depending on the support and knowledge of medical practitioners who have appropriated breastfeeding as a health practice, often making it more difficult for women who wish to experience it as an embodied practice.

Viewing breastfeeding discourse in practice facilitates an understanding of breastfeeding as an embodied experience. In this chapter, I draw on data collected during participant observation and interviews with women participating in a breastfeeding support group in order to explore how the current medicalization of breastfeeding and the dialectical tensions embedded in breastfeeding discourses at both macro and micro levels have shaped it as a practice. In order to better understand the tensions and contradictions inherent in breastfeeding discourse, particularly in relationship to medicalized discourses, I discuss issues in breastfeeding literature. This is followed by analysis of the daily experiences of breastfeeding women.

Dialectical constructions of breastfeeding

The history of breastfeeding and its social and cultural construction has been documented by a number of scholars (e.g., Baumslag and Michels, 1995; Blum, 1999; Carter, 1995). While much public literature provides a monolithic view of breastfeeding as positive (see Wall, 2001), the decision of whether or not to breastfeed is problematic for many women. A myriad of factors constrain choice making, including the economic, social, and political ramifications of breastfeeding. These constraints lead to a disparity among different women's perceptions of breastfeeding and its feasibility in their lives.

Breastfeeding is generally lauded by health professionals and advocates (as seen in the power of La Leche League, a grass-roots movement that works to promote breastfeeding (Ward, 2000) as a "natural" and "fulfilling" choice for mothers). Women are frequently confronted with the many positive effects that breastfeeding has on the baby (which are documented and supported by science even as they are questioned by other scientific evidence[2]), but are often conflicted by a variety of issues involved with the breastfeeding experience itself, including the desire for independence, issues with the sexualization of the breast and breastfeeding, and uncertainty about the acceptability of breast-feeding in public, among others.

Riordan and Auerbach (1993) represent the dominant medical discourse surrounding breastfeeding, and call it "health promotion in its purest form," noting:

> Only a decade ago, the primary health benefit of breastfeeding was immunologic protection from gastrointestinal infection and disease. Indeed, some alternatives to breastfeeding have proven disastrous for babies. We now know that breastmilk reduces many other infections in the baby, as well as certain chronic diseases later in life and recognize that lactation also benefits mothers in both short- and long-term ways.
>
> (p. xv)

However, breastfeeding is far from the universally wonderful experience it is often depicted as. Schmied and Lupton (2001) examined mothers' qualitative experiences of breastfeeding and found that, while the mothers studied all agreed with the dominant "breast is best" discourse, individual experiences of breastfeeding differed. While some mothers experienced breastfeeding as a pleasurable, intimate connection with their babies, others had more conflicted experiences because they felt that they lost their independence and that breastfeeding confined them to the private world of domesticity. Some mothers even experienced breastfeeding as a distorting process that alienated them from their bodies and even their infants; these women "used metaphors of intrusion and devourment, talking of being 'suck[ed] dry' and the baby as 'the rotten sucking little leech' and 'the child from hell'" (p. 243). Thus, once the decision to breastfeed has been made, it still remains far from a universally positive experience and instead creates tensions and contradictions for mothers whose own experiences do not mesh with the dominant discourse of breastfeeding as "good mothering."

Nature/science

Breastfeeding is a messy practice, highlighting stigmatized issues such as bodily fluids and sexuality. In addition, breastfeeding also faces many of its problems from advocates of formula feeding and the general medicalization of pregnancy and breastfeeding. As Foucault (1978) notes, the medicalization of women was part of the discipline and regulation of sexuality. He notes that the hysterization of women "involved a thorough medicalization of their bodies and their sex, [which] was carried out in the name of the responsibility they owed to the health of their children, the solidity of the family institution, and the safeguarding of society" (pp. 146–147). The discourse surrounding breastfeeding as either a natural choice or a matter of science is documented by a number of scholars (e.g., Galtry, 1997; Nadesan and Sotorin, 1998; Palmer, 1988). As Palmer discusses, this battle began with the introduction of infant formula as a substitute for breastmilk, which was supported by the U.S. government and led many women to adopt the more "scientific" choice and feed their infants formula. However, the tides of public discourse concerning breastfeeding have again shifted, and now breastfeeding is being promoted as scientifically superior to formula (despite its messy and uncontrollable nature).

Nadesan and Sotorin (1998) argue that women's choice regarding breast-feeding is complicated by two competing discourses: the romanticization of breastfeeding as "natural" and the scientific or medical discourse of formula as "normal." Campaigns such as the Department of Agriculture's "breast is best" discourse are "deeply enmeshed in the cultural-political dynamics of maternalism" (p. 230). Thus, promoting breastfeeding as the "best" choice for women furthers dominant conceptions of a "good" mother as one who is devoted to her child and involved closely in its development, furthering its well-being above all else. Wall (2001) studied Canadian health promotion advertisements and educational literature aimed at increasing breastfeeding for underlying assumptions about motherhood and found that the literature primarily constructed breastfeeding as nature/natural. Recent public debates about breastfeeding in public places, or even images of breastfeeding, highlights this, with many arguments centering over whether a natural process such as breastfeeding should be conducted in public places, or whether it is "unnatural" for women to be engaging in an activity which could expose their breasts in public (e.g., "Eyeful" 2006). Regardless of the rhetorical framing of the choice, women are still faced with conflicting discourses surrounding breastfeeding versus bottle feeding. The sources of this discourse play an important role in framing how women view their role as breastfeeding mothers.

Medicalization/embodiment (who's the expert?)

Breastfeeding, though historically constructed in a variety of different ways, has more recently been positioned and appropriated as a medicalized form of infant nutrition. In contemporary Western culture, breastfeeding is also practiced by (and perceived to be available to) women who are privileged socially and economically—those more likely to feel comfortable with medical discourses. There are distinct and problematic racial and ethnic disparities among women who breastfeed, with the majority of breastfeeding women being white, educated, and affluent (Li et al., 2003; U.S. Department of Health and Human Services [USDHHS], 2000). According to the U.S. Department of Health and Human Service's (2000) *Healthy People 2010 Report*, women who were college graduates demonstrated the highest rates of breastfeeding, with 78 percent breastfeeding after birth and 40 percent still breastfeeding at six months (USDHHS). In contrast, "The lowest rates of breastfeeding are found among those whose infants are at the highest risk of poor health and development: those 21 years and under and those with low educational levels" (USDHHS, p. 47). A study of urban low-income mothers and found that many believed the prominent "breast is best" discourse, but still bottle-fed their infants for a number of reasons, including perceptions of the convenience of bottle feeding and seeing breastfeeding as correlated with socioeconomic privilege. They characterized a breastfeeding mother as "someone who 'has a lot of time on her hands,'" and "'one of those perfect, stay-at-home moms who doesn't have to work'" (Guttman and Zimmerman, 2000, p. 1467). Indeed, among the almost seventy women I met while observing these support groups, only three were African American, and one identified herself as Hispanic (although it should be noted that Hispanic women have the highest rates of breastfeeding of any minority[3]).

Yet even among mothers for whom breastfeeding is seen to be available societally, there is resistance to the medicalization of women's bodies and embodied practices. Physicians recommend breastfeeding in general, although the extent to which it is supported varies greatly. Thus medical practitioners, who often have little training or experience in the realm of breastfeeding and may not understand the individual struggles faced by nursing mothers, are positioned as experts and often give advice that fails to recognize the personal importance of breastfeeding to some mothers and the struggles they face to continue the practice.

While several scholars have attributed much of the decrease in breastfeeding rates to the medicalization of breastfeeding (Apple, 1987; Hausman, 2003; Ryan and Grace, 2001), arguing that placing the expertise about breastfeeding in the hands of medical practitioners (who often have little training or personal experience about the issue) disempowers women, little research has been done to explore how women themselves experience this medicalization and respond to it. Ryan and Grace (2001) document the historical medicalization (and briefly turn to the authority of women's experiences) in New Zealand through the narratives of women who had breastfed over a fifty-year period, but as Hauck and Irurita (2003) note, "information regarding infant feeding practices from different countries must be recognized as being relevant to their specific context and therefore cannot be transferred readily or accurately beyond cultural or social boundaries" (p. 63). However, Hausman (2003) and Bartlett (2002) argue that breastfeeding has been medicalized in the United States as well. Bartlett (2002) argues that the "plethora of changing ideas and cultural conditions in a relatively short time span (between generations and within a generation of mothers) have meant that knowledge of breastfeeding practices has been increasingly distanced from mothers, who are now largely positioned as novitiates in need of tuition on how to breastfeed" (p. 376). Both Hausman and Bartlett discuss the embodied position of women with regards to breastfeeding, but neither of these scholars supports their arguments with evidence from the actual lived experiences of breastfeeding women. Instead, both focus on criticism of published materials. Bartlett argues that the medicalization of breastfeeding has resulted in an exacerbation of the mind–body conflict that Babrow and Mattson (2003) argue health communication needs to address:

> This transfer of breastfeeding knowledge from its practitioners to the domain of the medical professional, from being embodied to requiring learning, involves a privileging of headwork that not only reinstalls the mind–body dichotomy of the Cartesian subject, but disempowers women as mothers at a time when their corporeality is most active and symbolically significant.
>
> (Bartlett, 2002, p. 376)

Thus, while breastfeeding mothers are facing changes in their bodies and their relationship to them, they are also often being told (implicitly or explicitly) that they do not have expertise about the process their bodies are involved in.

Embodiment/erasure

Much breastfeeding literature focuses almost exclusively on the benefits it provides to the child; little about the mother's role in the process is mentioned, and concerns that the mother might have about her own well-being and role in breastfeeding are rarely directly addressed. This is similar to Stormer's (2000) finding that discourse surrounding abortion tends to result in the erasure of the woman—the focus is instead on the fetal individual, which is seen as an autonomous being capable of self-creation. Breastfeeding discourse often exhibits these traits, as Wall (2001) found. She notes the child-centered nature of breastfeeding discourse in the Canadian public health materials studied and mentions that "the one benefit to women that was commonly mentioned, the fact the breastfeeding can help women lose weight and regain their pre-pregnancy shape more quickly, is one that plays to insecurities about the shape of the maternal body and reinforces current cultural conceptions of proper female body image" (p. 601).

Medical discourse about breastfeeding constructs women's bodies as "the ecosystem within which the child's optimum food source is produced" (Wall, 2001, p. 603). The construction of women's bodies as spaces or ecosystems functions to alienate women from their role in the process of breastfeeding, possibly exacerbating the need for independence experienced by many breastfeeding women (Schmied and Lupton, 2001) and also furthers the construction of breastfeeding as natural/nature (Nadesan and Sotorin, 1998). Schmied and Lupton's (2001) descriptions of women's experiences that breastfeeding distorted and alienated them from their bodies is also relevant here. In addition, the women interviewed by Stearns (1999) framed breast-feeding as either an embodied or disembodied process depending on the context. One woman framed breastfeeding *not* as "an embodied experience but simply a food service" (p. 318), while others argued for breastfeeding as a natural, embodied experience.

Breastfeeding as maternal/breasts as sexual

While breasts are sexualized in Western cultures, and this is a concern expressed by many breastfeeding women (Stearns, 1999), it often goes un-addressed in breastfeeding literature. Blum (1993) argues that feminists should embrace breastfeeding as a context in which the social construction of motherhood can be transformed. However, Blum admits that her analysis fails to reflect on the relationship between breastfeeding and women's sexual objectification. In her later work, Blum (1999) addresses more thoroughly the many dimensions of women's involvement in breastfeeding, including discourse surrounding breasts and sexuality. Breasts have been sexualized in Western culture to the extent that Stearns' interviewees expressed the fear that "the exposure of their breasts will be misread as a sexual invitation to male strangers and they fear potential consequences of that misreading" (1999, p. 316).

Women's bodies are inscribed with various power relations, most particularly the breast, which I argue contributes to many women's reluctance to breastfeed, particularly in public. In the United States, discussing sex from a male perspective (for instance, the proliferation of ads about various drugs to combat erectile dysfunction) is commonplace, but the exposure of a breast leads to a great deal of the discomfort many women have with the very idea of breastfeeding, much less breastfeeding in public where there is always a risk that one's breast will be exposed and there will be an ensuing furor. The ways in which breasts have been differently sexualized and singled out as a site of power relations influences strongly existing discourse surrounding breastfeeding. The prominence of the sexualization of breasts when discussing breastfeeding can be seen in the wording of laws that protect breastfeeding in public. For instance, eight states have enacted legislation that exempts breastfeeding women from public indecency laws even if there is exposure of the breast "during or incidental to breastfeeding" (United States Breastfeeding Committee [USBC], 2003, p. 1), because women breastfeeding needed to be protected from charges of obscenity in case their infant should happen to look away from the breast while feeding and inadvertently expose it.

When faced with the medicalization and contradictions in breastfeeding information, Hauck and Irurita (2003) indicate that women often find their own ways of determining how to act and approach breastfeeding. Trethewey (1997) documents the micropractices of resistance often engaged in by women. For example, Trethewey found that clients in a human service organization resisted authority through acts such as "bitching," breaking rules, and revisioning relationships. I was curious whether women placed in a position where their embodied identities were in flux would respond similarly.

Qualitative research and breastfeeding

Recently, there has been a call for more qualitative approaches to the study of health communication. Vanderford et al.'s (1997) call for a new focus in health communication research focusing on patients and their experiences as central. In addition to the need for a more patient-centered approach to health in communication and other disciplines, patients' voices need to be heard. Geist and Gates (1996) argue that there is a "crisis of representation" in health care where patients' voices are lost, and "the 'science-ing' (of our research, our medicine, our lives) is a silencing in the sense that it marginalizes aspects of our identities that we attempt to incorporate in our interactions with others" (pp. 219–220). Thus the strict biomedical focus of most health-care interactions serves to hide and potentially damage patients' identities as they are made absent in medical encounters. Vanderford et al. also argue that a patient-centered approach to health communication research can help health-care practitioners to better understand patients' experiences, which can contribute to better treatment through clarifying differences in understanding between patient and provider. A patient-centered approach also helps the provider facilitate the patient's negotiation of new identities and roles that come as a result of their medical diagnosis or care. Considering that breastfeeding is dealt with at the same time as becoming a new mother, a time of significant role adjustment and stress, it is particularly important that we have an understanding of what this experience is like for women in order to best help them.

Methods and analytic procedures

The main site of study is a breastfeeding support group held at a suburban hospital in a large Southwestern city. The Breastfeeding Mothers' Support Group meets weekly in a conference room of the hospital, holding one daytime meeting and one evening meeting a week, each of which lasts for an hour and a half. Membership is fluid, and "newbies" in the group (many of whom have recently delivered their babies) are present at virtually every meeting in addition to a core group of women who regularly attend ("returners"). The meetings are generally rather chaotic, with mothers arriving throughout, toting strollers, car-seats, and other baby paraphernalia, and various disruptions occur throughout the meetings as babies need to be changed, fed, or attempt to play with one another. The rattle of toys and the babble of infants is a constant backdrop to the discussions of the group. During the duration of my observation, some mothers attend one meeting a week regularly and others attend both. Approximately six to ten mothers are present at every meeting, but in the course of my observation I came into contact with about seventy women total. In addition to the women and their babies, at least one lactation consultant/group facilitator is present, and occasionally, women brought along guests such as their own mothers or another female relative (men and older children were not welcome except for meetings on special occasions such as the annual reunion). Members were primarily Caucasian and ranged in age from twenty-one to forty-three. Babies ranged in age from six days to thirteen months. Most participants were first-time mothers, but at least two had one older child, and two women who were pregnant and currently breastfeeding a toddler also attended the group.

The meetings are coordinated by the hospital's lactation consultants, Charlotte and Deborah, both nurses who have undergone a special certification process to assist women in breastfeeding. The hospital has two full-time lactation consultants on staff, and one or the other is always present at each meeting. In addition, another nurse who is a board-certified lactation consultant on staff at the hospital (and a veteran of the group) sometimes fills in and occasionally attends meetings. Topics for each meeting (e.g. "Breastfeeding after a Cesarean birth" or "Weaning—when and how") are designated by the lactation consultants ahead of time and are listed on a published schedule of meetings, but at all meetings the concerns and problems of the women present are also addressed. The women tend to feed off of each other's comments and provide advice to one another, as opposed to relying solely on the authority of the lactation consultants. Indeed, the lactation consultants often solicit the experiences of the women present when a question is posed instead of or in addition to answering it themselves.

Data sources and methods of collection

Data was collected using several methods. First, participant observation was conducted at meetings of the group. My level of participation in these meetings was somewhat limited by the fact that I myself do not have any children, but due to the fair amount of knowledge I have gained about the subject of breastfeeding through my research on the topic, I did participate in the meetings to some extent and provide support for mothers, meeting the description of "participant as observer" (Lindlof and Taylor, 2002, p. 147). I generally would announce my purpose as a researcher in the group during introductions at the meetings (unless everyone present was a returner and already was familiar with me), and when mothers came in late, I would explain my role to them one-on-one. As observation progressed, I became an accepted member of the group, with members occasionally directing comments at me and asking that I hold their babies (something of a sign of trust, as members have discussed being uncomfortable with strangers holding their babies). At times, it seems my status as a younger woman who is not yet a mother created an instructional relationship with the mothers in the group, where they felt they could provide help for me when I myself have children. As Weick (1985) notes, "for the participant-as-observer, normal rules do not apply. In this situation, researchers are free to act like naïve visitors or inexperienced 'boob[s]'" (p. 585)—a description particularly relevant considering the topic of my research. For instance, it might have seemed more bizarre for me to ask some of the questions I needed to for my research if the mothers thought that breastfeeding was something I had already experienced myself.

Although each meeting lasted approximately one and a half hours, observation for each meeting totaled two hours due to time spent before and after meetings. I attended twenty-seven group meetings over a period of nine months. In addition, I attended eleven meetings of another breastfeeding support group, Baby & Me, which meets in the evenings at another site, resulting in a total of approximately one hundred hours of participant observation research. These data may serve as a form of triangulation of sites, which serves to enrich the data I have collected.

In addition to participant observation, informant interviews (Lindlof and Taylor, 2003; Kvale, 1996) were conducted with twenty-three participants in the groups. Interview questions were designed based on information gained during participant observation, and served to obtain individual members' insights on the meetings that did not arise naturally through group conversations. The mothers interviewed reflected a variety of ages (of both mother and baby), as well as backgrounds, including two mothers for whom this is the second child and breastfeeding experience. During interviews, member-checking (as discussed by Stake and Trumbull, 1982) took place to provide data about member's perceptions of my emergent theories and categories. Interviews were audiotaped and transcribed, and lasted from 30 minutes to three and a half hours, with an average length of one and a half hours.

Data analysis methods

Data was organized using NVivo qualitative data analysis software and analyzed using a rigorous, iterative approach similar to grounded theory (Charmaz, 2001). As Lindlof and Taylor (2003) note, CAQDAS (Computer Aided Qualitative Data Analysis Software) neither independently codes nor theorizes data. All codes were created by the researcher, and there were several close readings of field notes and other data before formal coding began. Some relevant codes include medicalization, compliance with physician, and resistance—

direct or indirect. While codes primarily emerges from the scene, as Shaffir (1991) points out, I recognize that I was not a "blank slate" when beginning my research, and so by remaining cognizant of my research interests without imposing them on the scene, my previous knowledge served to sensitize me to potential issues in the data. At the same time, I do not wish to impose pre-defined categories and research questions on the scene that do not fit the data I collect, and so this approach, going back and forth between extant research and the scene to continue to clarify and hone my theories as they emerge, but remaining cognizant of pressing issues in the literature, provided me with a set of coherent codes and themes in the data (Miles and Huberman, 1994).

Findings and analysis

Women in the breastfeeding support groups studied emphasized that breast-feeding is an inherently tension-filled practice. Primary themes emerged around the topics of medicalization, receiving ambiguous or contradictory advice, and resistance strategies women used to cope with the tensions they faced.

Medicalization

The medicalization of breastfeeding brings to the forefront the tensions of nature/science and embodiment/erasure for many women. There were several ways in which breastfeeding is experienced as medicalized by the women in the group that appeared in my analysis of the data. Several manifestations of this medicalization include the distancing of physical implements from the embodied experience of breastfeeding and the variety of contradicting and ambiguous advice about breastfeeding, which was often rooted in medicalized discourses.

The role of machines

Perhaps the most common manifestation of the distancing of the self from the body with physical/medical devices is through pumping breastmilk, during which a machine is hooked up to the breasts to mechanically extract milk, either so the baby can be fed by a bottle or simply for the mother's comfort when her breasts become over-full, or engorged, with milk. One mother, Karen, described her first experience pumping as follows:

> We made it kind of a humorous situation. We're in an apartment, so there's not really a private area to go, so, my Dad's sitting there, my Mom's sitting there, and my husband, and I'm (laughs) sitting there with this machine going "argh, argh, argh" and I just, and we just kind of laughed. I went "moo," you know? And . . . I can't look at it when I'm pumping,

because psycholo[gically]—it doesn't hurt, but also, it's such a sensitive area, and your mind can play tricks on you. You look down, and you see your nipples like, being suctioned, and pulled really long, and it—when you look at it, you think "ow!" and so it makes it hurt. So, I just have to kind of cover it with my shirt, and not look, and not . . . it's not the most pleasant experience, but it's not really terribly painful. It's just kind of a weird sensation.

The distancing that Karen describes from her body, where her mind is playing tricks on her if she looks at the machine distorting her body, is indicative of the ways that this medically created machine serves to alienate her from the process of infant feeding as it naturally occurs. Pumping allows the milk to be separated from the body before going into the baby, providing a means for measuring how much the baby ingests—a practice that became common once formula became a common method of infant feeding. An alternative to pumping is a technique of hand-expressing breast milk, but this method requires more skill and is less reliable, sanitary, and scientific. Pumping is a somewhat conflicted practice in that it does allow women to be separated from their babies (for either convenience or out of necessity), but it also separates women from breastfeeding as an embodied practice allowing connection with their infants, which is often cited as one of the most rewarding aspects of breastfeeding as an experience.

In addition, overwhelmingly, participants described the experience of pumping as "feeling like a cow." Karen alluded to this metaphor when dealing with her discomfort through humor, mooing as she used the breast pump. However, this metaphor does more than provide humor—it indicates the depersonalized nature of pumping breast milk, where one is made to feel like a nameless, faceless animal that is being used for its production of food. Perhaps because of the often disembodied experience of breastfeeding, women seemed to seek back control of their bodies and the experience of breastfeeding through looking to other breastfeeding mothers for "expert" advice.

Expertise

Women felt the tension of expertise rather acutely, with many stating that they would rather receive advice from other women who had experience with breastfeeding. Kris demonstrated this in her response to the question "When it comes to people giving advice on breastfeeding when you're having difficulty, what sorts of things do you find most helpful?"

Well, I really hate it when people who haven't breastfed try to help. You know? Or people who don't have kids or, either don't have experience . . . it really just irks the sh- Irks me. (laughs) It really . . . (sigh) I mean, those are the same kind of who give you advice about how to raise kids, you know? And it's just out of ignorance comments happen that way. But if you've breastfed and you have experience, then I think there's—they also have a different approach in giving advice, I think. That somebody who's breastfed will say to me, well I don't want to tell you how to do it, because it's always different, *but* here's something you can try. Or here's something that worked for me. Instead of, "you should be doing this!" You know, there's always that different approach that breastfeeding—other breastfeeding women give, and that—it makes a difference.

Thus, advice regarding breastfeeding may be more useful to women if it is offered in less of a prescriptive manner than is typical of medical encounters, and mothers may be more receptive to advice that recognizes the diversity of breastfeeding experiences that women have.[4]

Breastfeeding and sexuality

The issue of the sexuality of breasts came up several times, but it was always touched on lightly and somewhat indirectly. For instance, when I asked "What are the most difficult or distressing aspects of breastfeeding?", Karen responded:

I guess just having . . . feeling like part of your body's not really your own. You know, it's hard to put into words. Um, it's just being used for a completely different function than it ever has before, and it's . . . I don't know, I think that a lot of people don't breastfeed because, in today's society, it- the function is so removed from how they're viewed now. I think the breasts are so sexualized, that people think of it as weird or icky, and it's hard to get over that, even though that really truly is what they're for. So it's kind of—that wasn't really something that I was expecting, that it's kind of . . .

Emily: That it felt weird for you?

Karen: It doesn't feel weird, but it just . . . (laughs). Like I said, just feeling like . . . something that's so private, and . . . like, it's just not really your own any more. It's being used for a different function.

Some women mentioned that there was a strange transition that they and their husbands experienced as the function or purpose of their breasts changed.

In addition, breastfeeding mothers themselves expressed contradictory feelings about breastfeeding in public, indicating an internalized understanding of the tension between desiring the rights to feed their infants in public settings while also keeping breastfeeding from being seen as sexual (despite breasts themselves being sexualized). While several mothers mentioned handling this tension by simply not breastfeeding in public at all, due to their own comfort levels, among women who did breastfeed in public this tension was still apparent. One mother told the following story about the "right way" to breastfeed in public:

> I was in the mall not too long ago, and there was this Mom with an older child, he was maybe one or so, but I had to do a double-take, because her— she had no blanket, and she had a tank-top on, and the side was just lifted up, she had no bra, so her whole breast was exposed . . . and the baby was older and he was kind of hanging down like this, so . . . her whole nipple almost was exposed too, except for this kid hanging off the end of it, and she was just sitting in the middle of the mall, like this (leans back, arms to side). And it was . . . gross! Like, I'm a breastfeeding mother, and it was gross. Like, you could see everything, and you don't want to see that. Also it was weird, like, there's her whole breast, and, a kid's hanging off the end! You know? So I think a lot of people maybe see stuff like that and that's what makes them have reservations about breastfeeding in public. But then, you can do it discreetly and it's not a problem.

This sort of "self censorship" that occurs among breastfeeding mothers may serve to increase the discomfort many women already feel about breastfeeding in public, and when such accounts become part of common discourse, they may discourage women from breastfeeding altogether.

However, some women felt that breastfeeding was a basic right, and the groups had several discussions centered around indignation at being relegated to restrooms to breastfeed when in public settings. Not only was the general feeling that this practice felt unsanitary, but a common comparison made was to eating one's lunch in the bathroom—a concept that seems foreign and wrong to most.

Women responded to the contradictions they faced regarding breastfeeding in a variety of ways, in part depending on the source of the contradictory advice. Contradictions that came from a concrete source, such as a physician, were often met with resistance, whereas contradictions from more general sources, such as societal norms about breastfeeding in public, were sometimes even reinforced by breastfeeding mothers, which in turn could reinforce their own subjugated status.

Ambiguity and contradicting advice

Due to the wide variety of information and advice available about breastfeeding, women often expressed confusion about topics surrounding breastfeeding and childcare, and went to the group to negotiate the ambiguity they perceived and decide what advice to follow. The knowledge of medical professionals was frequently undermined during group interactions when women asked for clarification about confusing advice or problems they were experiencing. For instance, when one working mother, Samantha, was experiencing problems getting her infant to sleep on nights when she was home, Charlotte asked if she'd tried giving him solids, and Samantha said that her pediatrician had said to give solids because he was feeding so frequently. "I did it and he spit up, and then I looked online and found the recommendation that you shouldn't give them solids until six months. The problems with the sleep cycle started then." Charlotte said, "The recommendation used to be four months and a lot of pediatricians haven't been updated. Most of the information they get is from formula reps and they have the wrong information." The notion that, when it comes to breastfeeding, physicians are *not* always the most knowledgeable was consistently repeated among group members.

Wary of receiving incorrect advice, sometimes mothers came to the group *before* seeing their physicians in order to "inoculate" themselves for the resistance they expected to face from their doctors regarding their breastfeeding experience. For example, one mother, Michelle, returned to the group when her child was a little over a year old after a slight pause in attending the group because she was pregnant again. She asked for advice from the group because she was still breastfeeding her toddler while pregnant, and had heard that her milk could change because of the pregnancy. She said she had not been to the doctor yet, and Charlotte asked, "Do you think the doctor will say you should stop breastfeeding?" Michelle said that her obstetrician was really supportive, but "I haven't been to a doctor since he turned one." Charlotte asked what she would do if the doctor told her to stop. Michelle said she figured she would arm herself with information. Charlotte seemed supportive of this approach, essentially advocating Michelle's plans to "educate" her doctor about breastfeeding.

Resistance

Mothers displayed resistance to medical expertise and dealt with contradictory and ambiguous advice through a number of tactics. The main manifestations of this resistance were through noncompliance, verbal criticism of physicians or questioning medical advice, embracing the ambiguity of breastfeeding knowledge and experience, and valuing advice that came through women's own embodied experiences.

Resisting through noncompliance

Sometimes when women felt criticized by their physicians for breastfeeding or disagreed with their advice, they responded by simply ignoring that advice. During a meeting of the Baby & Me group, one mother, Angela, shared the following story with the group:

> Angela stated, "I almost changed doctors." She told a story about how when she went for the one-week checkup, the baby had lost weight, which

is normal, and the nurse said, "Aren't you feeding her? She should be 9 lbs." Angela told her that all of the women in her family had been small babies, even premature, so it should be fine. The nurse said they should come in next week to weigh the baby again, but Angela said to us, "That's ridiculous. I'm not coming in. I know I'm feeding my baby." Maggie, the group leader, commented that they (medical practitioners) don't take family history into account.

The weight of a baby is frequently referred to as a measurement of their progress, but is a more medicalized and somewhat problematic one, because as leaders of both support groups noted, infant growth charts are based on formula-fed babies, which tend to gain more weight, whereas breastfed babies tend to be more lean. Additionally, by quantifying health and focusing on the numbers (a very scientific, medicalized approach), mothers are removed from the process of evaluating their own infants' health and growth. Thus, women in the groups were often told to simply watch their babies for cues and if the baby seemed healthy and was growing out of its clothes, not to worry. One mother, who had recently moved to the area and previously attended a different support group where weighing infants was a ritual, stated that she thought the practice was not a very good idea because "It tends to make you kind of neurotic." In addition to monitoring the infant's growth in this manner, sometimes women were encouraged to weigh the baby before and after feeding on an infant scale to determine how much milk they had taken in. This was generally resorted to as a method of comforting women who were concerned their infants were not eating enough, but occasionally served as another method of quantification requested by health professionals to ensure that the baby was eating "enough" by objective standards—something easily determined when babies are fed from bottles, which come equipped with measurements of the ounces of formula in them.

Women also discussed problems dealing with advice from their doctors or others about deciding when to wean their babies and whether to sleep with their infants in bed with them (referred to as "co-sleeping"), and when they disagreed with their doctor's advice, they typically discounted it and did what the group members suggested. Weaning was seen as problematic because, despite national recommendations to breastfeed for a minimum of one year, women were often pressured by family members, coworkers, or their physicians to stop breastfeeding much earlier. Additionally, breastfeeding mothers often found it more convenient to co-sleep because feeding their infants at night disturbed their own sleep less. This is a somewhat controversial issue, with some professionals strongly against it based on concerns about parents rolling over on their infants during the night. However, the group members generally seemed in favor of the practice, and cited evidence of lower rates of SIDS (Sudden Infant Death Syndrome) amongst co-sleeping babies.

"Ripping" doctors

Another direct form of resistance occurred through verbal criticism of physician advice. During one meeting, a new mother had experienced problems with nipple confusion (where the baby has difficulty latching onto the breast after bottle feeding because a different kind of skill is involved) after a doctor had advised that she use a bottle. Charlotte, the lactation consultant running the group that day, said, "Some time, if you're comfortable, you should tell the pediatrician what the baby did after you bottle fed her. Some people, I know I probably do this too, if you don't get feedback, you don't know that the advice you're giving isn't working, and think the advice worked." She said a lot of people never say anything so she could not know otherwise. Lacey said, "Not me! I've been ripping doctors lately." Kris said she had too. Her first son had asthma, "and they said, 'No, he couldn't be born with it!' I started saying, 'You're wrong!' Sometimes you have to be a pain in the butt parent, but you know when something's wrong with your kid!" This seems to be a form of "bitching" as resistance (Pringle, 1988; Trethewey, 1997). However, it is also significant to note that most of this resistance was more indirect, as it occurred outside of the doctor's offices—not many women actually confronted their physicians about problems they perceived, but chose "noncompliance" instead. Donovan and Blake (1992) note that noncompliance can be viewed more positively as a form of "reasoned decision making" instead of deviance.

Slightly more overt resistant stories also occurred. During one meeting, a new mother to the group was requesting advice because her baby was tongue-tied, and she had gotten conflicting advice on whether to get the baby's tongue clipped. Tongue-tied is a condition when the frenulum, or thin flap of skin under the tongue connecting it to the base of the mouth, attaches too near the end of the tongue, making it difficult for the baby to latch onto the breast properly. Deborah, the lactation consultant running the meeting, said this:

> I was talking one day with one pediatrician, who's really nice, and he was talking about how he didn't know why it was such a big deal (when babies were tongue-tied) and why people complained about it so much and so on. He didn't understand why people made such a big fuss about it. He said he didn't clip [tongues], but he mentioned that he did about 2000 circumcisions a year. And said he didn't know why tongue tied was a problem. I thought to myself, can I say this? And then I just went ahead. I said "the problem is that we don't have enough male doctors with sore nipples." He was quiet for second and I thought to myself "uhoh," but then he starts laughing and said that was probably right.

This story, offered by one medical professional (with personal of experience breastfeeding who is intimately experienced with the problems encountered by nursing mothers) about another, "higher ranking" medical professional provides an interesting critique of the knowledge provided by the medical community. It also illustrates how easily a layperson could become confused about breastfeeding-related advice when the "experts" themselves fail to agree.

Possibilities for change

As Kris' story in the introduction illustrates, though, there exists the potential for physicians and other medical practitioners to provide a great deal of significant support for breastfeeding mothers as well. She continued by saying

> I know our pediatrician was just—again, the difference between our pediatricians, with Xander's first pediatrician and Aidan and Xander's pediatrician now—just wildly different. When I said to the pediatrician, when I was having trouble breastfeeding and he was losing weight—I was crying, I was really upset and said I didn't want to go on the bottle because Xander was allergic, and I didn't, I was afraid that that would happen again . . . and she said, "Well, you don't have to go on the bottle." Whereas, you know, and he had lost a lot of weight, whereas I know many doctors would say "He's lost weight? Put him on a bottle. Stop breastfeeding, put him on the bottle." She said, "You know, you will work it out. You will get enough milk, if you just keep at it." And she was very encouraging for me to keep going. So, it made a difference.
>
> Emily: So you've had doctors give you bad advice in terms of breast-feeding?
>
> Kris: Well, Xander's first pediatrician—my obstetrician and Xander's first pediatrician, were—I mean, he was *allergic* to formula, throwing it up *all* the time, and we were having to go to these crazy, you know, extremes on formula, and I was trying all the different kinds, and very expensive kinds . . . and the doctor just seemed to think that that was OK. And I kept saying, there's gotta be something else. And never *once* did he say, "You know, you could always go back to breastfeeding. Let me help you."
>
> (Interview)

Thus, while some physicians are seen as impeding the breastfeeding process, at the same time, a doctor who is supportive can make a world of difference for a breastfeeding mother who is struggling.

Conclusions

Breastfeeding (as both practice and construct) is messy and complicated. While the medicalization of breastfeeding is problematic in that it can alienate women from their own embodied experiences, there is also a need for physicians and other health-care professionals to be educated about and involved in breastfeeding support practices if goals of increasing breastfeeding and thus improving health of both mother and baby are to be met.

Medical practitioners can perhaps improve both satisfaction in mothers and breastfeeding rates by recognizing that women experience confusion with much of the information and advice about breastfeeding and value solutions that are based on embodied knowledge and are compatible with their desires as mothers to be connected and bonded to their infants through breastfeeding. Also, if medical practitioners are willing to empower mothers to trust their own bodies and instincts (and admit where uncertainty lies), it will likely lead to a healthier, happier provider–patient relationship.

Further, monolithic advice that "breast is best" seems to be problematic for women who are not the "typical" breastfeeding mother as well as for those who breastfeed and find themselves facing tensions that they were not expecting surrounding their own bodies. By recognizing and acknowledging tensions and contradictions in women's own experiences, we can learn to help women breastfeed in ways that are more sensitive to the issues they are facing. Of course, there are limitations to the current study, which only examines breastfeeding mothers in one metropolitan area, and further, only looks at those who are able to (and/or feel the need to) attend support groups. More research should be done to find out what kinds of advice would be most helpful to "nontraditional" breastfeeding mothers, as well as what specifically medical practitioners can do to help increase breastfeeding rates and duration. Hopefully, this research offers a starting point.

Breastfeeding attitudes among women (and consequently breastfeeding rates) will be very difficult to change without first understanding and validating women's own experiences with their bodies. By recognizing that breastfeeding is a complex experience and is influenced by a myriad of often conflicting discourses, we can begin to make necessary changes to facilitate healthier, happier experiences with breastfeeding among a wider range of the population.

Notes

1 All organization and participant names are pseudonyms
2 For example, numerous studies have been conducted regarding the linkage between breastfeeding and obesity, with contradictory findings (e.g. Agras et al., 1990; Grummer-Strawn and Mei, 2004).
3 As there is a large Hispanic population in the area where this study was conducted, cultural differences such as social support from family members who have breastfed may account for the absence of Hispanic women participating in the support groups.
4 There were few discussions of race or class in the support groups I observed, probably because they were primarily attended by women who were educated, middle class, and white. The only times these issues were really touched on was when women reflected on the cultural influences they perceived about breast-feeding, and some women noted that in more collectivist cultures (Mexican Americans, in particular) there is more support in families for breastfeeding

women. Additionally, the cost of formula feeding was frequently cited as an incentive for women to breastfeed, even though most participants could have afforded formula for their infants. Indeed, many women found it paradoxical that lower-class women are less likely to breastfeed given the cost of formula (though the cultural influences surrounding breastfeeding differ by class, not to mention constraints that differ—for instance, employment being mandatory rather than optional, shorter maternity leave, and employers being less accommodating of the needs of lower-level, "replaceable" employees).

References

Agras, W.S., Kramer, H.C., Berkowitz, R.I., and Hammer, L.D. (1990). Influence of early feeding style on adiposity at 6 years of age. *Journal of Pediatrics, 116,* 805–809.

American Academy of Pediatrics. (2005). Breastfeeding and the use of human milk. *Pediatrics, 115,* 496–506.

Apple, R.D. (1987). *Mothers and Medicine.* Madison, WI: University of Wisconsin Press.

Babrow, A.S., & Mattson, M. (2003). Theorizing about health communication. In T.L. Thompson, A.M. Dorsey, K.I. Miller, & R. Parrott (eds), *Handbook of Health Communication.* Mahwah, NJ: Erlbaum, pp. 9–34.

Bartlett, A. (2002). Breastfeeding as headwork: Corporeal feminism and meanings for breastfeeding. *Women's Studies International Forum, 25,* 373–382.

Baumslag, N.M. & Michels, D.L. (1995). *Milk, Money, and Madness: The Culture and Politics of Breastfeeding.* Westport, CT: Bergin & Garvey.

Blum, L.M. (1993). Mothers, babies, and breastfeeding in late capitalist America: The shifting contexts of feminist theory. *Feminist Studies, 19,* 291–311.

Blum, L.M. (1999). *At the Breast: Ideologies of Breastfeeding and Motherhood in the Contemporary United States.* Boston: Beacon Press.

Carter, P. (1995). *Feminism, Breasts, and Breastfeeding.* New York: St. Martin's.

Charmaz, K. (2001). Grounded Theory. In R.M. Emerson (ed.). *Contemporary Field Research.* Prospect Heights, IL: Waveland Press, pp. 335–352.

Donovan, J.L., & Blake, D.R. (1992). Patient non-compliance: Deviance or reasoned decision-making? *Social Science & Medicine, 34,* 507–513.

Eyeful of breast-feeding mom sparks outrage. (2006, July 27). Retrieved on August 15, 2006, from www.msnbc.msn.com/id/14065706/.

Foucault, M. (1978). *The History of Sexuality: An Introduction.* New York: Vintage.

Galtry, J. (1997). Lactation and the labor market: Breastfeeding, labor market changes, and public policy in the United States. *Health Care for Women International, 18,* 467–481.

Geist, P. and Gates, L. (1996). The poetics and politics of re-covering identities in health communication. *Communication Studies, 47,* 218–228.

Grummer-Strawn, L.M., & Mei, Z. (2004). Does breastfeeding protect against pediatric overweight? Analysis of longitudinal data from the Centers for Disease Control and Prevention Pediatric Nutrition Surveillance System. *Pediatrics, 113,* e81–e86.

Guttman, N. & Zimmerman, D.R. (2000). Low-income mothers' views on breast-feeding. *Social Science & Medicine, 50,* 1457–1474.

Hauck, Y.L., and Irurita, V.F. (2003). Incompatible expectations: The dilemma of breastfeeding mothers. *Health Care for Women International, 24,* 62–78.

Hausman, B. (2003). *Mother's Milk: Breastfeeding Controversies in American Culture*. New York: Routledge.

Kvale, S. (1996). Thematizing and designing an interview study (Chapter 5). In *InterViews: An introduction to qualitative research interviewing*. Thousand Oaks, CA: Sage, pp. 83–108.

Li, R., Zhao, Z., Mokdad, A., Barker, L., & Grummer-Strawn, L. (2003). Prevalence of breastfeeding in the United States: The 2001 National Immunization Survey. *Pediatrics*, *111*, 1198–1201.

Lindlof, T.R., & Taylor, B.C. (2002). *Qualitative Communication Research Methods*, 2nd edn. Thousand Oaks, CA: Sage.

Miles, M.B., & Huberman, A.M. (1994). *Qualitative Data Analysis*. Thousand Oaks, CA: Sage.

Nadesan, M.H., & Sotorin, P. (1998). The romance and science of "breast is best": Discursive contradictions and contexts of breastfeeding choices. *Text and Performance Quarterly*, *18*, 217–232.

Pringle, R. (1988). *Secretaries Talk*. London: Verso.

Palmer, G. (1988). *The Politics of Breastfeeding*. London: Pandora.

Riordan, J., & Auerbach, K.G. (1993). *Breastfeeding and Human Lactation*. Boston: Jones and Bartlett Publishers.

Ryan, K.M., & Grace, V.M. (2001). Medicalization and women's knowledge: The construction of understandings of infant feeding experiences in post-WW II New Zealand. *Health Care for Women International*, *22*, 483–500.

Schmied, V., & Lupton, D. (2001). Blurring the boundaries: Breastfeeding and maternal subjectivity. *Sociology of Health & Illness*, *23*, 234–250.

Shaffir, W.B. (1991). Managing a convincing self-presentation. Some personal reflections on entering the field. In W.B. Shaffir, & R.A. Stebbins (eds), *Experiencing Fieldwork: An Inside View of Qualitative Research*. Newbury Park, CA: Sage, pp. 72–81.

Stake, R.E., & Trumbull, D.J. (1982). Naturalistic generalizations. *Review Journal of Philosophy and Social Science*, *7*, 1–12.

Stearns, C.A. (1999). Breastfeeding and the good maternal body. *Gender & Society*, *13*, 308–325.

Stormer, N. (2000). Prenatal space. *Signs: Journal of Women in Culture and Society*, *26*, 109–144.

Trethewey, A. (1997). Resistance, identity, and empowerment: A postmodern feminist analysis of clients in a human service organization. *Communication Monographs*, *64*, 281–301.

United States Breastfeeding Committee (2003). State breastfeeding legislation. Retrieved on May 5, 2003 from www.usbreastfeeding.org/Issue-Papers/Legislation.pdf.

U.S. Department of Health and Human Services. (2000). *Healthy People 2010: Conference Edition*. Vols I and II. Washington, DC: US Governmental Printing Office, pp. 47–48.

Vanderford, M.L., Jenks, E.B., & Sharf, B.F. (1997). Exploring patients' experiences as a primary source of meaning. *Health Communication*, *9*, 13–26.

Wall, G. (2001). Moral constructions of motherhood in breastfeeding discourse. *Gender & Society*, *15*, 592–610.

Ward, J.D. (2000). *La Leche League: At the Crossroads of Medicine, Feminism, and Religion*. Chapel Hill: University of North Carolina.

Weick, K. (1985). Systematic observation methods. In G. Lindsey & E. Aronson (eds), *Handbook of Social Psychology: Vol. 1. Theory and Method*, 3rd edn. New York: Random House, pp. 567–634.

Chapter 4

Communicating healing holistically

Patricia Geist-Martin, Barbara Sharf, and Natalie Jeha

We are nothing but angels
who gave up their wings
to touch divinity
through human skin

Wingless
we dance
in the same blue dream
under the same limitless sky
we caress
flying
              (Cangemi, 2002)

We begin with a poem by a practitioner that reflects epistemological dimensions of holistic healing. For many users of complementary/alternative medicine
(CAM), healing modalities based on beliefs about spirituality, balance and
energy flow within the body, and interactions among nature, individuals, and
social systems have served as a parallel, preferred and/or more affordable
approach to treating illness and promoting health. Others seek answers to
problems for which the powerful institutions of allopathic and osteopathic
medical care cannot provide adequate, satisfying responses. In this chapter, we
begin with the premise that health communication research has barely
skimmed the surface in understanding the role of communication in healing
processes undertaken by holistic practitioners and those who seek their help.

  We start with an exploration of the various, sometimes confusing, terminologies (Caspi et al., 2003; Gaudet, 1998; Turner, 1998) used to describe the care
provided by "other healers" (Gevitz, 1988). These include such terms as
complementary, *alternative*, *integrative*, *holistic*, and *healing*. Our discussion will
touch upon the implications of these vocabularies for public perception,
professionalization, and communication scholarship.

  Using two case studies based on in-depth interviews with three holistic
healers working in Hawaii and Texas, our objectives are to identify

commonalities and distinctions in terms of epistemologies, definitions of healing, ethnocultural influences, and therapeutic practices. We conclude with an expanded agenda for health communication scholarship that can contribute to understanding what healing means, and how and why healing practices work.

Holistic medicine: a review of literature

We embark on this research by reviewing literature that defines and explains holistic medicine. By briefly tracing its history, we seek to explore the various and confusing terminologies (Caspi et al., 2003; Gaudet, 1998; Turner, 1998) used to describe the care provided by "other healers" (Gevitz,1988), that is, healers who draw from knowledge, beliefs, and modalities beyond the biomedical model. As holistic medicine is constantly changing, we also seek to describe its current, evolving status of acceptance in today's health care. These explorations provide the foundation for our investigation of the epistemologies, therapeutic and communication practices of three providers who utilize complementary and alternative medicine. We end this section with a statement of our research questions.

Defining holistic medicine

Discussing and researching biomedicine and holistic medicine is complicated by the fact that there are a wide variety of terms used to refer to each category. For example, the former is sometimes called conventional or allopathic medicine, while the latter is often referred to as *alternative, complementary, unconventional, nontraditional,* and *unorthodox* (Bascom et al., 2003). These different terminologies are used interchangeably in popular media and medical literature, yet often seem to reflect varying attitudes and levels of acceptance. For instance, Turner (1998) claims that as therapies outside of the biomedical approach have increased in popularity, *complementary* has replaced *unconventional* as a descriptive term. In this essay, we prefer the term *holistic*, since it refers to what healing encompasses (that is, wholeness or a sum of the wellness of mind, body, and spirit), whereas *unconventional* is a judgment of how common or accepted a treatment is. Therefore, we refer to health therapies in two main categories: *biomedical* or *holistic medicine*. Our choice acknowledges that the distinction is not absolute, insofar as some practitioners combine aspects of both worlds, hence the terms *complementary* and *integrative*.

The first of these categories, *biomedicine*, is the predominant model taught to and used by physicians, focusing primarily on physiology, biochemistry, genetics, and other basic or so-called "hard sciences." For centuries, biomedicine has been extremely useful in diagnosing and treating disease. However, this model is limited by the fact that social, psychological, or cultural factors are often not considered (Filc, 2004; Verhoef & Sutherland, 1995).

Holistic medicine, the other category of healing therapies, refers to "health practices, approaches, knowledge and beliefs incorporating plant, animal and mineral-based medicines, spiritual therapies, manual techniques, applied singularly or in a combination to treat, diagnose, and prevent illness or maintain well-being" (World Health Organization, 2003). What diverse holistic therapies share is an emphasis on prevention and maintaining health. Biomedicine, in contrast, is perceived as more focused on disease and cure (Verhoef & Sutherland, 1995).

Tracing the history of holistic therapies

Holistic therapies date back centuries; however, widespread use within modern industrialized society has only recently been recognized (Barrett et al., 2003). The word "holism" was first used in relation to medicine in 1952 (Weil, 1952). "Alternative medicine" has been more frequently used to describe the set of diagnostic and therapeutic modalities considered in contrast to conventional medicine (Caspi et al., 2003; Whorton, 1999). The terms "complementary" and "integrative" medicine emerged in the 1990s as holistic and allopathic medical systems were employed together or alongside of each other (Caspi et al., 2003; Coates et al., 1998; Gaudet, 1998; Zollman & Vickers, 1999).

The rising popularity of CAM, an acronym for complementary/alternative medicine(s), has been documented in the United States (Dossey, 2004). Caspi et al. (2003) offer a description of the evolution of terms for holistic medicine as representing changes in societal and cultural attitudes:

> In 1992, as a response to the increasing interest . . . the U.S. Congress instructed the National Institutes of Health (NIH) to create the Office of Unconventional Medical Practices. . . . As societal attitudes have continued to change, the funding for this center [now called the National Center for Complementary and Alternative Medicine (NCCAM)] has grown from an initial $3 million in 1993 to more than $100 million today. Indeed CAM is no longer a term used by the medical fringe but has entered the mainstream.
>
> (p. 59)

In 1997, there were 629 million visits to holistic practitioners, compared to less than 390 million visits to biomedical physicians in 1996 (Eisenberg et al., 1998). Nearly 75 percent of American adults have used some form of holistic medicine (Huggins, 2005) and Americans spend $12 billion annually out-of-pocket on alternative therapies (Donnelly, 2003). Holistic medicine's popularity is rising in other countries as well. In Canada, Europe, and Australia, between 20 and 49 percent of people have reported using holistic medicine (Astin, 1998; Verhoef & Sutherland, 1995).

There is growing integration of CAM in U.S. hospitals. In 1998 only 6 percent of hospitals reported that they offered CAM, yet by 2001 that percentage had increased to 15 percent (Institute of Medicine, 2005). One study found that two-thirds of heath maintenance organizations offer at least one form of alternative care, with chiropractic and acupuncture being the most common (Landmark Healthcare, Inc., 2006). Prominent cancer centers utilize CAM, such as music therapy, massage therapies, reflexology, acupuncture, meditation, guided imagery, and yoga (Cassileth, 2002; Dana-Farber Cancer Institute, 2006; M.D. Anderson Cancer Center, 2006).

As holistic therapies have become more prevalent, a growing body of related literature has emerged. Research has examined correlates of patients' use (Conroy et al., 2000; Furnham & Forey, 1994) and disuse of (Jain & Astin, 2001), as well as physician–patient communication about, holistic medicine (Sibinga et al., 2004; Sleath et al., 2001; Wynia et al., 1999).

Findings indicate that people who turn to CAM are dissatisfied with physicians' reliance on prescription medications and lack of a holistic approach (Kroesen et al., 2002; Mercer & Reilly, 2004), feel that CAM modalities are less invasive than those of allopathic medicine (Swartzman et al., 2002), and perceive CAM as more consistent with personal values and general life orientation (Astin, 1998; Biesanz et al., 1999; du Pré, 2000; Furnham & Kirkcaldy, 1996; O'Callaghan & Jordan, 2003; Siahpush, 1999) There appears to be a pattern of more women using CAM than men (Buchbinder et al., 2002; Cherkin et al., 2002; Jain & Astin, 2001). It is not yet clear to what degree cost is a determining factor in people's decision to opt for CAM therapies. Insurance coverage for acupuncture varies (Medicare does not reimburse for acupuncture); while data on the influence of cost is scanty, there is some support for finances not being a primary factor in decisions to use CAM (Goldbeck-Wood et al., 1996; Buchbinder et al., 2002).

Relationships between patients/clients and their practitioners have been highlighted as a key reason for people choosing to use CAM. Listening seems to be key to what people want and gain from their relationships with their health providers. When people talk about the differences between holistic and biomedical practitioners, they indicate that they feel more listened to by the holistic practitioners (Barrett et al., 2003). A study of acupuncture health outcomes found that people experienced positive changes in their mental and emotional health even if they were being treated for physical ailments (Gould & MacPherson, 2001). People who were interviewed for the study used the words "*listening, respect, acknowledgement, trust,* and *working together*" (p. 266) to describe their relationships with providers.

For most patients, the perception of being carefully listened to by the doctor can make them feel better, resulting in a reduction in the secretion of stress hormones (Adler, 2002). Essentially, medical communication is a relational activity constituting the therapeutic process wherein the doctor and patient "create the illness, its meaning, and the solutions" *together* (Massad, 2003,

p. 13). Although the importance of the "human side" of medicine is now widely acknowledged, patient–provider relationships generally remain less a focus in biomedical clinics than in holistic practices. It is not surprising that patients of holistic medicine have been reported to feel that the environment is more patient-centered, caring, empathic, and warmer as compared to biomedical medicine (Lowenberg, 1989).

Holistic healing emphasizes health practices such as spirituality or manual techniques that accentuate communication in patient–provider interaction (WHO, 2003). It is not surprising then that research reveals that the healer–patient relationship is a greater predictor of healing than the particular therapy or the scope of the healer's training (Herman, 1993; Horvath & Symonds, 1991; Luborsky et al., 1986; Orlinsky & Howard, 1985; Strupp & Hadley, 1979).

A few health communication researchers have indicated the significance of spirituality in provider–patient interaction (Gonzalez, 1994; Parrott, 2004a). However, more research is needed that explicitly examines the role of patient–practitioner communication in the context of holistic medical settings. "Research to date on spiritual and energetic healing has treated the medicine and the practitioner as 'black boxes,' and has not explored the implications of the practitioner as an integral part of the medicine" (Sutherland & Ritenbaugh, 2004, p. 14). Despite the variety in healing modes now available and the therapeutic value of holistic healer–patient relationships, these therapies remain highly under-researched (du Pré, 2000), in part due to the hegemony of the biomedical model.

Tracing the history of holistic therapies, then, necessitates a brief consideration of how and in what ways holistic medicine has been marginalized in mainstream medicine. The evolution of societal beliefs regarding holistic medicine is represented in the personal account of C. Norman Shealy, M.D., regarding the prejudice that surrounded his work.

> When I began the first holistic clinic for management of chronic pain and stress illnesses in 1971, I was told that I was ruining my career. That clinic became the most successful pain clinic in the country and allowed me to explore the comprehensive approaches that are the foundation of holism.
>
> (2003, p. 334)

Larry Dossey, M.D. (2004) reflects on why CAM has been so threatening. In his view, it is human nature to withdraw from what is foreign. He provides a brief historical account of acupuncture:

> When news of this therapy reached the West from China during the early 1970s, American physicians enjoyed a good belly laugh at the idea of relieving pain by sticking needles in someone. The ridicule was premature. Following decades of research, in 1998 acupuncture was vetted by a panel

of experts at the National Institutes of Health as an effective intervention in a variety of conditions (Villaire, 1998). There was "clear evidence," the panel concluded, for the efficacy of acupuncture in treating postoperative and chemotherapy-related nausea and vomiting, the nausea of pregnancy, and postoperative dental pain.

(p. 10)

Dossey goes on to mention examples of other holistic therapies such as homeopathy, therapeutic touch, meditation, yoga, and nutrition that were disparaged by critics initially, but have now become mainstream because of the realization that the positive effects of these therapies are stronger and more pervasive than previously imagined.

Darwin (1999) argues that what holistic therapies emphasize—meaning, perception, and discourse being the core of health and healing—challenges the foundations of biomedicine, namely that focus on disease in the bodily organs takes precedence over the subjective, lived experience of illness. The politics of holistic medicine challenges biomedicine's hierarchal power to allow specialized knowledge of diseases to take precedence over, often to the exclusion of, patients' voices. Advocating a more equal and active role for patients, holistic therapies are premised on people having "agency in deliberation over their own health and healing" (p. 1052). While medical research and education has become more accepting of the importance of provider–patient communication, certain related topics remain sources of tension.

One such tension is the topic of spirituality in conversations between health providers and patients. Spirituality is defined "as a search for what is sacred or holy in life, coupled with a transcendent (greater than self) relationship with God or a higher power or universal energy" (Kliewer, 2004, p. 616). There is a long history of spirituality in medicine; some of the earliest "healers" were spiritual leaders. Today, such talk between health-care professionals and patients in practice situations is not widely accepted. Physicians trained to treat biological diseases have ethical concerns with discussing spiritual issues with patients for fear of crossing boundaries and touching on matters in which they have no expertise (Ellis et al., 1999; Graigie & Hobbs, 1999; Sloan et al., 1999). For many physicians, "spirit remains almost as isolated from medicine and psychology as it has been since Descartes led the scientific community to discard spirit and separate body and mind" (Shealy, 2003, p. 333).

Nonetheless, many people want physicians to address issues of spirituality in their medical care (Kliewer, 2004; Ehman et al., 1999; Daaleman & Nease, 1994; Weaver et al., 2003). For many, spirituality "profoundly impacts and is impacted by, illness" (Kliewer, 2004, p. 616). When they are ill, people want the kind of relationship with their health-care providers that allows them to be treated as a whole persons, "addressing not only physical, but also social, emotional, and spiritual issues" (ibid., p. 621). The emphasis here is on a caring rather than curing model of communication in which the provider is open to what the patient has to say and is willing to dialogue with them to discover what they need, no matter what the topic (Widdershoven, 1999). Dossey (2004) indicates that when Americans have been surveyed about why they chose holistic therapies, many said they did so for spiritual reasons:

> They had experienced events in their own lives that shifted them toward a holistic worldview in which the disparate pieces of reality seemed to fit together. They sensed that CAM provides a stronger affirmation of this vision than does modern medicine, in which the emphasis is on separate things and parts—organs, molecules, atoms, specific drugs etc. In increasing numbers, they seem to be arriving at an understanding expressed by the Dalai Lama: "If I am to eliminate my own sufferings, I must act in the knowledge that I exist in dependent relationship with human beings and the whole of nature."
>
> (p. 86)

As it turns out, research has indicated that a patient's spirituality and the opportunity to discuss it has a positive influence on coping with illness, preventing illness, and aiding treatment (Kliewer, 2004; Larson et al., 1997; Miller, 1999).

Among the array of questions raised when considering the work of holistic providers, in particular we asked, "What are the purposes and forms of communication?" Our investigation is designed to deepen understanding of the role of communication in holistic healing encounters. Through interviews with practitioners who utilize CAM therapies, the research investigates the following related study questions: What epistemology guides the work of each practitioner? How is epistemology communicated in healing practices?

The narratives of providers offer insight into what they seek to expand or redefine in their conversations with patients. The research questions are designed to explore, in part, their epistemological and ontological assumptions and communication used in therapeutic practice.

Methodology

The two case studies that are the basis for this analysis were chosen because they represent a range of unconventional health-related practitioners. All our participants[1] began with a background in medical education and a concern for helping others through periods of suffering, but one decided to forgo medicine altogether in order to pursue a different approach to healing, while the other two continued as physicians, albeit with an enlarged repertoire of methods. All are well-traveled people and are practicing in a place far from their ethnic and national origins. In this sense, the interviewees bring a blend of contrasting cultural influences to their respective work: urban Italian Sophia mellowed and gained self-knowledge and an array of healing practices through her experiences in Mexico, Guatemala, Costa Rica, California, and now, Hawaii. Aparna and Suresh Shah, whose values were formed in the multicultural national character of India and the religious precepts of Hinduism, adapted to relatively small town life in Texas. The Hawaii case study illuminates a place where people of many traditions are drawn to explore issues of spirituality; in contrast, the Texas case study demonstrates that complementary healers, perhaps unexpectedly, practice in more conventional settings as well.

The Hawaii interview is part of a larger data collection focused on alternative healers conducted by Patricia, the first author (Becker et al., 2005). The Texas interview, separately conducted by Barbara, the second author, used the same interview guide, including items on cultural and educational background, definition of health, description of current practice, recollections of enjoyable and difficult practice situations, and views on the process of communication taking place between practitioner and patient/client.

For the three authors, research interests together with personal use of holistic health therapies prompted involvement in this study. Both Patricia and Barbara have developed research in CAM as an extension of past work in patient–provider communication and cultural aspects of health; Patricia has collected comparative data in California, Hawaii, Mexico, Cuba, and Costa Rica. Furthermore, both have personally experienced a broad range of CAM therapies. In conjunction with this study, each author participated in healing experiences with one of the informants: Patricia engaged in Watsu and Dolphin Dance with Sophia, and Barbara has received acupuncture treatment from Aparna. Natalie's interest in holistic health communication research stems from her personal experience as a reiki practitioner and yoga instructor, but had no personal encounters with the research participants, thereby providing a welcomed element of triangulation. Thus, this study is not autoethnographic, but our interpretation of the data is certainly informed by our respective personal experiences. Transcripts were read by all three authors, who each did her own version of open coding, which were exchanged via email, followed by several discussions to negotiate agreement about interpretation of data.

Results

The results of this investigation are presented in six sections. First, we offer a brief narrative biography of the participants. Second, we present the providers' healing epistemologies. Third, the providers' definitions of healing are discussed. Fourth, we describe the ethnocultural influences that are integral to their epistemologies. Fifth, we offer providers' perspectives of patient characteristics and the pathways to healing. Sixth and finally, we offer the pragmatics of holistic healing described by the practitioners who participated in this study.

Practitioners' biographies

The presentation of the results begins with a short narrative biography of our participants. Their backgrounds framed our understanding of their epistemologies and practices. Their names and identifying information have been changed to preserve confidentiality, but the descriptive information offered comes directly from our interviews with them.

Aparna and Suresh Shah

> After I moved here, I was very depressed. I first went to a doctor who prescribed anti-depressants. They didn't help and there were a lot of side effects. A friend recommended that I see Dr. Aparna because she does acupuncture. I think the acupuncture did gradually help, but, really, getting a hug from her is the best medicine.
>
> (Sue Ellen, a patient)

In a small, unpretentious waiting room, the TV is tuned to CNN as the space fills up with a broad spectrum of people, reflecting varied races, ethnicities, socioeconomic levels, religions, and occupations. This is the office of Aparna and Suresh Shah, respectively, a family practitioner and a geriatric psychiatrist, who have shared a medical practice for nearly twenty-five years. The bright yellow walls are decorated with photos of flowers grown in Aparna's garden, framed handwritten notes of gratitude from patients, and small individual gifts of thanks, such as a luminous portrait of Jesus with Arabic writing. Behind the waiting area is a corridor leading to three exam rooms, a multi-function open area, and a nicely furnished private office at the rear.

Born in west India, each came from a conservative, Hindu, closely knit, supportive family. In Suresh's words, "The significant challenges were reduced to only moderate challenges because of such parental support . . . that way we learned the value of family and how it could be a rock for the future generations." After completing their medical educations, they married and came to the United States for residency and fellowship training at major medical centers. They then decided to establish their practice in a small north Texas city within an hour of the Dallas-Ft. Worth Metroplex, and where they knew a few other Indian physicians. The city is a location for a private university, two hospitals, several small businesses, and a multitude of churches, while cattle ranching dominates the surrounding rural areas. From social, political, and religious perspectives, the region is predominantly white, conservative, Republican, and Protestant.

About fifteen years ago, Suresh and Aparna came to a realization that allopathic medicine was not sufficient for treating the range of ailments and pain they were seeing among their patients. Making a decision that involved economic sacrifice, the couple went to UCLA to study acupuncture with a master teacher, and have continued to partake in advanced instruction in acupuncture and other techniques. After returning to Texas, they gradually began incorporating into their practice other modalities, such as moxabustion, therapeutic oils and herbs, from traditional Oriental medicine and the Ayurvedic healing system that they had experienced growing up in India. They refer to both the allopathic and the less-visible alternative practitioner networks in their community. While acupuncture has recently become available though other health professionals, notably chiropractors, the Shahs remain the only medical doctors in the area who practice acupuncture and are among the very few to be open to complementary therapies.

Sophia

The steady rain falls punctuated by the bird-like calls of the frogs. In this remote part of one of the Hawaiian Islands, Sophia, a holistic healer, originally from Italy, works at a healing center, practicing both land and aquatic therapies. Her specialty is Watsu (an abbreviation for water-shiatsu), which is aquatic bodywork that combines passive movement with gentle shiatsu massage. In warm hot spring pools people are cradled, swirled, and relaxed as the practitioner gently supports them through a series of movements and stretches (Bodywork, 2006). She pioneered her own form of Watsu called Dolphin Dance (2006), a variation of Watsu that includes music, dance, and Water-shiatsu.

At the beginning of the interview, Sophia states that she was interested in healing works since she was a child and that it was a calling:

> I call it a calling because I knew it from the beginning in some way. I was a pioneer of the Red Cross when I was twelve. I was the youngest pioneer in Europe, with my sister. And then I started reading the medical encyclopedias since I was like sixteen. . . . And then I continued to be interested in, in healing in general throughout my life. During medical school anyway, I realized that this really wasn't only the physical aspect of this that I was interested in and that there were some problems in what the Western approach was about. And that really, hospitals weren't the places where people would heal. . . . I also had problems with some of the conceptions of the Western medical interpretation, like the brain cannot reproduce itself or it cannot heal. . . . Every year I found that some of my doubts were confirmed in the sense that science of medicine really didn't exist as they were trying to communicate to us.

Sophia stayed in medical school until her final year, when she shifted into a masters program in journalism because she believed it was "a better vehicle" to study what she was most interested in, though medical school had served as a good foundation for the research and writing she did on health issues.

She walked away from journalism as well and found herself in Oaxaca, Mexico, where she explored shamanic healing. This third-world country offered her an opportunity to escape the consumerism of first-world countries. She learned about healing traditions and worked closely with Zapotec Indians as an interpreter for a master weaver. In her words, she was "learning about being more than having." Since then, she has explored the culture and traditions of the Navajos in New Mexico, the Mayans in Guatemala, the BriBris in Costa Rica, and the Bon shamans in Nepal. In each place, she learned that the secrets of happiness are about valuing simplicity and community life, living in a rhythm that is slower and more natural. When asked if she plans to stay in Hawaii, she said "I never know. I really go with the flow. (laughs) I always go with the flow and I'm never really planted you know. It's kind of my condition, it's where I feel best."

These brief biographies set the stage for what we learned about our participants' epistemologies, as the next section reveals.

Epistemologies

The epistemologies guiding the practices of the holistic healers view humans as the physical world representation of divinity. By relating human experience to divinity, day-to-day life incorporates people's spiritual aspirations toward a specified state, ultimately one not defined by physicality. For example, Suresh explains that the Hindu aspects of Dharma, Artha, Karma, and Moksha are the foundation for Aparna's and his spiritual beliefs and everyday life:

> Dharma is about the virtuous ways of life. The Artha is the means to arrive at those virtues. . . . Karma means the human fulfillment of the desires and the Moksha means reaching ultimately a state where the individual from within is free of those desires, which is a state of peacefulness that he would attain. In Hinduism, they call it nirvana state. But it is kind of practiced in a day-to-day life within the family.

As Suresh details, a person strives to attain a state of peace or liberation from physical or worldly desires. However, this aspiration occurs over many lifetimes, because of the Hindu belief in reincarnation. In a way, it is not accurate to state that a "person" strives to attain peace, because it is not the physical person that makes the spiritual endeavor, it is the soul's quest. Aparna adds that all Hindus are "God-fearing," meaning that they "believe in God" and "follow the rules laid down in the holy books." In this sense then, the Shahs base their own lives on the four Hindu aspects and this world view extends out into their medical/healing practice.

Another guiding principle of the Hindu epistemology is Ahimsa, the practice of nonviolence. As Suresh describes, "There is no violence extended to any living being. And basically it means that you are nonviolent toward nature. Anything that comes naturally to you, you don't violate that and particularly the living beings." An important aspect of the Hindu perspective, because nonviolence toward all living things includes the body, the physical self in its entirety. Although the soul strives for liberation from physical desires over the course of lifetimes, deep respect is shown toward the physical body, because it represents the divinity of nature.

As Sophia views the human experience, divinity is omnipresent but may only be realized by a person who strives to integrate the immortal reality of the soul with the experience of the physical world. She describes the human experience as a "divine paradox," where "we can be intermediaries and we can live in both worlds. The timeless one of the spirit and the space–time reality of duality. And that being aware of both we can also reconcile ourselves without continuing to struggle." The "struggle" refers to the conflict of trying to comprehend mentally an awareness of "oneness" that may only be experienced. Once she relinquished the quest to gain more tactical knowledge of the relationship between divinity and physicality, she was able to accept the "mystery" of the experience.

While in the Shahs' perspective, the soul strives to find peace or liberation from the physical world over lifetimes, in Sophia's view, the peaceful state comes from reconnecting with the divine realm, then reconciling the two realities within the person's lifetime. She describes being "whole" as the "natural state" of a person, in which the person accepts and connects with both the physical human experience and the immortality of the soul. Sophia's view indicates the possibility of finding a state of peace *in* the physical existence, not *outside* of it.

Definitions of healing

Holistic health practitioners use therapeutic modalities on the physical body in order to restore the "whole" person—all aspects including both the body and the soul. The desire to approach healing from this perspective stems from a perception of the scientific view of health and healing as somewhat limited. Sophia describes her frustration with the training she received in medical school when she says that "medical studies were more about statistics" while "healing . . . happens in the human spirit." Whereas Sophia decided to pursue other modalities in order to access a different perspective on healing, Suresh describes his and Aparna's holistic health education as a means to "broaden [their] experience of medicine and bring it to the benefit of [their] patients" because "medicine is all about help, in helping the patient come to wellness." Aparna describes their integrated approach to wellness as "providing more avenues for patients to get better." She explains that "every form of healing is complementary if you just do it the right way." Aparna and Suresh incorporate other healing modalities into their biomedical experience as physicians, while Sophia's approach to healing very much diverts from the biomedical perspective.

Nonetheless, Sophia also underscores the importance of having a variety of modalities for treating a person. She explains that a fundamental component of treating a person is the use of the most appropriate approach, which she refers to as "vehicles," capable of creating a "trance state" for the person seeking treatment. As a holistic healer, Sophia has many potential techniques for reaching a person on a level of consciousness that will foster a profound shift in awareness, because her view of healing focuses on such significant life transformations. As Sophia explains, she specializes in "emergencies of the soul" to effect healing that is vital to the rest of the person's life. To this end, Sophia's approach emphasizes the "psychology of healing" in which she focuses on issues, emotional traumas, or disturbances people have experienced throughout the course of their lives that influence the body's state of health. Personal crises such as conflict in close relationships, the death of a loved one, or severe fear, in Sophia's perspective, often manifest as illness in the body. Within this view is the notion of such crises rising up as a means of challenging a person to grow or evolve. Indeed, Sophia describes a person seeking treatment as being "stuck," that is, the person's "soul [is] screaming, crying for an expression at the highest level." For example, Sophia explains that a person must be "willing . . . to do the journey and to find themselves at the other part, at the other point." According to Sophia, the healing process is a journey and the emergencies of the soul surface as a way of challenging a person to evolve, to "get to another level in your soul's development." Sophia perceives healing as movement along a path that challenges a person to gain new awareness of the self on both the physical and the spiritual levels.

Aparna and Suresh explain the healing process as one of restoring equilibrium between the body, mind, and spirit, in addition to the body being free from disease. Aparna describes health as a "dynamic state" due to fluctuations incorporated in the state of equilibrium. Suresh explains that "ultimate health should have both a perfection of the mind, body, and spirit and the freedom from the disease process." He proposes the visualization of three sticks that represent the body, mind, and spirit, each of which supports the others. This notion illustrates the perspective that "our spirit is living within our body, our body is living within our mind, and our mind is living within our spirit. It is all one connected, functioning system." Suresh explains that one cannot be separated or distinguished from the other. He emphasizes that he must view a person seeking treatment as a "whole" person, therefore incapable of being divided out into the body aspect or the mind aspect. Suresh describes this perspective as viewing the person as "a representation of the whole universe, that the patient or myself are just a replica of the whole universe that we live in." This perspective highlights the inherent perfection of the person as a system in that everything that is needed for a state of wellness is already present within the person. The person is not seeking to arrive anywhere; rather the person is in need of healing because of an imbalance that is representative of the world.

Ethnocultural influences

The cultural beliefs, traditions, and practices of the Shahs' native India significantly impact their perceptions of holistic health. In his description of Indian culture, Suresh explains that it "is made up of many different philosophies and religions" that naturally have different beliefs and practices, all of which are honored within India's health-care system. Suresh describes the integration of India's population as stemming from the connection between people and their native environment. He states that "minorities and majorities lived together because they were bound by "years of culture that grew up within that land." Respecting the traditions of the different beliefs systems necessitates the integration of various potential health treatments. Additionally, India's ancient healing system of Ayurvedic medicine broadly defines the Shahs' perception of health, because Ayurveda is based on maintaining balance between the three doshas of vata, pitta, and kapha. Each of the doshas has qualities that represent the body, mind, and spiritual health of a person. Illness, then, is due to an imbalance of one or two of the doshas. Furthermore, the remedies that Ayurvedic medicine uses to treat the imbalance or illness are, as Suresh states, "naturally occurring substances." Undoubtedly, the reverence for nature, tradition, and equilibrium representative of Indian cultural traditions is fundamental to the Shahs' negotiation of biomedical and holistic health practices.

While influenced by the traditions of their native country and trained in Western medicine, the Shahs integrate aspects of both systems into their perceptions of health. They were trained as physicians under the British curriculum of medicine, yet combined their formal education with the holistic healing principles of their culture. Whereas Indian or Eastern representation of health stresses balance, Suresh explains that Western medicine has distinguished body from mind and spirit in order to address illness. He explains that holistic medicine addresses the interconnectivity of mind, body, and spirit because "the spiritual part of the medicine and the mental or mind part of the medicine [make] you stronger, your patient can do well here on the health side." However, Suresh continues:

> Western medicine . . . [has] taken that body side and divided it into different parts and whenever we go to the medical practicing physician, we take of only that part without strengthening those other two parts. If we simultaneously strengthen those other two parts, a lot of people with chronic illnesses may not have to suffer as much as they do now.

The Shahs' native Indian culture greatly influences their perception of health, but aspects of U.S. culture and medical practice also affect how they construct an integrated approach to health care.

Because holistic and biomedical medicine are not used interchangeably by health practitioners in the United States, difficulties emerge for those who attempt to combine the two systems. Suresh describes the widespread practice of acupuncture, noting that "it is practiced a lot less in the United States. In many other countries, in Europe, in Latin America, Australia, India, China, people use that for the advantage of their patients along with . . . Western medicine training." He cites "lack of exposure and lack of willingness to change" as possible causes for attitudinal differences in the United States. Another issue restricting physicians from fully integrating health treatments is the medical licensing board. As Suresh explains, "License means living. That one small piece of paper means a lot. So you have to work within the guidelines prescribed by the board." Whereas in other countries such as "China and India and Sri Lanka, they use acupuncture for treatment of depression, anxiety, and even manic depression," Suresh states that he "would be very careful in using it here simply because that treatment may not have been approved." As a result, U.S. health regulations limit the comprehensive use of holistic health practices.

The restrictions that the Shahs describe stem from the American perspective on medical practice. Suresh explains that "holistic medicine is not a very profitable medicine" and cites the "economic incentives" intrinsic to the biomedical model. As Suresh notes, "the amount of surgical interventions done in the United States are tremendously much more than other places." His assertion is that the biomedical approach is taken elsewhere in the world, but that "people use holistic medicine as a part of their total medical practice just like [we] are doing in [our] practice." Suresh suggests that an integrative medical approach is complicated because "economic motives do direct to some level the medical practice in the United States, more than maybe other countries." The relationship between health care and profit or capital seems to be a shared perception among holistic health practitioners because Sophia cites her aversion to the consumer mentality of Western culture as influential to her practice of holistic health.

For Sophia, the cultures of first-world countries stress values that are not consistent with her perspective of health. She explains that she prefers the culture of third-world countries to the "whole consumer aspect and . . . arrogance aspect" of the first-world cultures. She describes her experience in third-world countries as being more enriching to her life because they "teach the secrets of happiness" by emphasizing the importance of "simplicity and community life . . . and love" over money. The pace of locations such as Mexico were much more appealing to Sophia because they are "slow and much more natural," differing dramatically from the fast-paced atmosphere of her native city of Milan. The lifestyle typical in cultures of first-world countries appears to diverge from Sophia's perspective of health.

For Sophia, the environment that a person lives in is critical to a person's ability to heal. Indeed, she remarks that her decision to pursue holistic health modalities stems from the experience of living in "an establishment where the values are somewhat dysfunctional" because "it's difficult to be functional in a dysfunctional environment." Because the focus of her holistic health practice emphasizes a view of health as a person's natural state, she is attracted to cultures that value simplicity and emphasize the importance of family, community, and love. For example, Sophia comments that the big island of Hawaii, the current location of her practice, "invites the soul to rest," a quality suggestive of an environment that would facilitate the healing that Sophia practices. The values that characterize the surrounding environment impact her practice as healer, and accordingly, the experience of the person seeking treatment. Similarly, the Shahs' location considerably shapes the degree to which they, as physicians, are able to use holistic medicine. As such, culture appears to be a significantly influential aspect of holistic health practices.

Knowledge gained about epistemologies, definitions of healing, and ethno-cultural influences provide insight into the foundation for communication between provider and patient. The next section offers more specific insights into what providers believe that their patients bring to the healing encounter. Finally, the results section will offer providers' perspectives on communication within the therapeutic practices of holistic healing.

Participant attitudes and the path to healing

The three providers offered insight into what they believe individuals bring to the healing encounter and what they believe the patient needs to face, control, or change. Implicit within each statement of the characteristics of people who seek holistic healing is the recommended path to healing. The three characteristics most emphasized include fear, skepticism, and resistance.

Fear

Both Suresh and Sophia indicate that fear is a characteristic of patients that holistic healing must address. Describing one patient in particular, Suresh indicates that fear—of losses, of death, of everything—comes into the picture, leading patients to seek answers for their illnesses. The path to healing must address these human fears and the accompanying pain in the context of what is happening to that person. In this patient's case, he had everything going for him in terms of finances, family, and children, but he was unhappy, obsessed with looking into the future. Suresh tells us that for this patient "the root cause was fear of loss of what he had" and that the path to healing was for him "to look at what was really going on . . . and attack those human fears." In Suresh's view, fear must be examined and controlled or eliminated in order for the patient to move forward on the path to healing.

Similarly, Sophia describes fear and pain as "an important part of our make-up." Mirroring Suresh's statements, Sophia says that "fear of the unknown" can block the way. In her view, fear is not a negative entity, but instead something positive, to be respected, and integrated into the healing path. In her view, "without pain we wouldn't be able to know when to withdraw our hand from the fire. Same with fear." While fear can be "an obstacle to the full expression of yourself and your spirit and your potential," healing requires taking in the fear and using it for understanding and healing. While fear is not an uncommon characteristic of patients, skepticism and doubt are even more frequently part of what patients bring to their encounters with these providers.

Skepticism

Suresh, Aparna, and Sophia talk a great deal about patients' doubts, suspicion, skepticism, hesitance, and angst. Suresh declares, "There are always going to be doubts;" Aparna states that "they may be hesitant in the beginning;" and Sophia asserts, "There is a place within us that loves the angst and that's why we create it."

Suresh points out that skepticism can be in both patients and providers: "There is a tremendous amount of skepticism . . . that is changing slowly, but it will take a critical mass of physicians to embrace that and accept that." For him, every patient can be difficult because of the doubts they harbor, but, "to me, they are the best patients because they have a lot of questions and a lot of skepticism." He uses this opportunity to tell patients about holistic healing: "Look, this is just another way of helping you." He provides the example of one skeptical patient who was suffering from "heaviness in the chest with sharp pain" and "excruciating headaches." While doctors had been able to alleviate her depression after the death of her husband, the cardiologist and two neurologists had not been able to alleviate the chest pain and headaches. Suresh described the situation in this way:

> She was saying that this was not going away and she was already on three medicines by the neurologist and one by the cardiologist for treating chest pain and headache. So I just asked her, "Would you let me try acupuncture to see if . . .?" And she said, "That's not going to work. All these people have done these things and it's not going to work." I said, "Why don't you talk to your neurologist and see if he would be in agreement with it." But by this time, the neurologist just laughed it off. And so she didn't receive the treatment. Almost three or four months later she had the similar complaints, so I asked her again, "Why don't you talk to him again." . . . By this time, I had an idea why she could be hurting, but I didn't say anything to her. And he had already gotten her Neurontin to almost thirty-six hundred milligrams and there was nothing happening. So he said, "Well give the guy a try. What's wrong with it? You can put a bunch of needles." She was extremely skeptical, "I'm not going to get well." So what I did was, I placed a needle in her head, five in the center and four needles around and I put the two needles here for the heart points. Immediately, as I put the needles in the heart point, what she said was, "Doctor, something burst inside my chest." And she said her headache was

gone that day. And almost a year now, there has been no headache and no chest pain. And what you have is an extremely resistant patient. Now the neurologist thinks it's just a coincidence. He just said that I'm lucky that it happened. I have a retrospective theory which I kind of started developing is that as she went through this grief period; now this is where you can't have a double blind study but I believe it got stuck in her chest and her loss got stuck in her mind, in her head. And this is a soul point that communicates to the universe and the heart point, it communicates with the grief part. We allowed the grief and the loss through those needles to be relieved.

Suresh recognizes that the path to healing is complicated by a wide range of interrelated emotions that may block the path. It is clear from this example that he chooses to meet the patient's resistance with encouragement and patience.

Interestingly, Suresh indicates that as a provider trained in biomedicine he experienced a similar skepticism about holistic therapies. First, referring to treating patients, he states that "as you break through the skepticism, they experience a new world." Then shifting to his own perspective as a provider, he notes, "And it is basically the same way how we learn these branches of medicine. You know you started out with the skepticism and until you see the other side and say 'Oh my goodness, what a vast difference;' we have in front of our very eyes through these treatments."

As a way to explore patients' skepticism, Sophia talks about the reasons why people tend to "love the angst." She posits that "sometimes we feel empty without the angst . . . and so we create it." Sophia suggests that sometimes we find ourselves stuck in a particular stage. In her view, "sometimes we are stuck in a stage because it's comforting. Even if it's painful, it's comforting." Yet people often struggle with the question "is my life going to get boring if I don't have the angst," and Sophia suggests that "if we realize that we can have life without that angst, we can find out that it's really amazing."

These providers recognize that the angst of doubt, skepticism, or hesitance is a natural, maybe even comforting state. Yet in their view, leading the patient to embrace and or move through these characteristics to the healing path means that perhaps they find "a new world," "a vast difference," that is "really amazing." However, beyond skepticism, the patient may bring to the healing encounter a resistance that is difficult for the provider to address.

Resistance

Resistance is a patient characteristic the providers discuss, often in the same breath as skepticism. While they are very interrelated, resistance is frequently talked about in terms of "stuck up energy," difficulty in "giving up control," and "emergencies of the soul."

"Being stuck" is a phrase used to describe patients by both Sophia and Suresh. The problem with most attempts to heal is a problem of resisting it. Part of this stuckness, according to Sophia, is a combination of things—our rational mind not able to let go, the dysfunctional environments we live in, the double binds that bombard us, and generally not feeling safe. Sophia suggests that the holistic intuitive body work "is so immediate" that it becomes "a shortcut to the spiritual realm." In her view, people have "difficulty resisting it" insofar as body work is a modality where spiritual, physical, and psychological come together in a "good synthesis." The environment of holistic healing, then, is one where the rational mind has difficulty resisting it and "lots happens without the person realizing it."

Suresh used the phrase "stuck up energy" to describe the patient with the chest pain referred to earlier. In his view, this was "an extremely resistant patient" who became opposed to treatment because "her loss got stuck in her mind, in her head." He elaborates:

Now there are no technical, medically certified dictionary words for this but you can only see from the experience. This woman is off all those medicines and everything and hasn't had that experience again. So here we were communicating with her body and her soul and her mind through the use of those needles.

Similar to Sophia's description, Suresh describes acupuncture as what allowed for the release of the patient's resistance. Sophia adds to that by saying in the environment of holistic healing a provider can help a patient to "give up their control," and thus release their resistance. In many cases, Sophia suggests that resistance is tied to fears about which people may or may not be conscious. When resistance is released through holistic healing, it is unbelievable to patients that "a lifetime of fear is gone in an hour and 15 minutes."

"Emergencies of the soul" (Grof & Grof, 1989) is a phrase that Sophia utilizes to describe the surfacing of an emergency, where "the soul is screaming, crying for an expression at the highest level" and the person "is stuck in a place" where he or she does not want to be anymore. Resistance signals the beginning of the crisis as issues are brought to the surface. Often this is the point at which the pragmatics of holistic healing can be revealed.

Pragmatics of holistic healing: theory into practice

Clearly, Sophia and the Shahs have distinctive purposes as practitioners, specialize in separate modalities, and thus do different things with people who come to use their services. In this section, we will highlight our interviewees' self-identification as healers and detail how they view communication intrinsic to their healing practices. Though the CAM research literature has combined "complementary" and "alternative" medicine, our two case studies demonstrate that there is some separation between the two. At the same time, there is also notable overlap in the discussions of the practical applications of their work.

Self-identity

The Shahs consider themselves regular physicians. States Aparna, "I think medicine is medicine. There are ways of practicing. . . . In general I don't think I'm doing anything different. I'm still a medical doctor, just providing more avenues for patients to get better. Adds Suresh, "To me, these are all tools. You can use one tool at a time, you can use two or three simultaneously at a time. . . . I think the ultimate goal is to serve the best interest of your patient and help them reach a higher level of health than what they are at." More specifically, whatever "tools" are used, they are all components of a physician's repertoire, integrated with the biomedical model. Explains Aparna:

> No, I don't think there is any conflict between any forms of healing. I think every form of healing is complementary if you just do it the right way. You do the medical diagnosis first and if you think this just a plain muscular skeletal problem you can offer them physical therapy, you can offer them medication, you can offer them massage, you can offer them acupuncture, you can offer them herbal medicines to help their pain and it would all be complementary and . . . they would be at a different level.

Still, there is strong remnant of conventional allopathic medicine insofar as the Shahs do not express beliefs about patient responsibility, empowerment, or joint decision making. Their discourse still emphasizes doctors performing procedures or offering options to patients.

Sophia is alternative, that is, separate from the biomedical system of healing. Still, like the Shahs, she also sees herself as helping people to move to another level, though from a psychological, rather than a physical, perspective: "They're stuck in a place where they don't want to be anymore. . . . So it's looking for initiation." Similarly, she describes that "what I was interested in in my life was to have many tools so they would be able to connect to . . . people at different stages." She calls herself a "facilitator" though "the water is the teacher." She refers to those who seek her services not as patients or clients, thus avoiding medicalizing, psychologizing, and even commodifying her work, even though she charges fees. Furthermore, she perceives the people who come to her as co-equals, partners engaged in enacting positive change: "I feel that everybody is a healer, OK? We all have a natural ability to heal. It's our trust in that ability that can change . . . because we are really partners and really who dances the healing is the person." She explains that people may not know, at first, that they are entering a partnership: "You might not feel that you are partners in the beginning, but you are. Just the decision to step into that pool makes you a partner. It's your decision to try and to dare."

She has pushed the art of Watsu past "passive receiving, while dolphin dance [her original creation] is based also on unwinding and interactivity." The starting point for Sophia is her own experience. What she encourages others to do is a product of her own self-learning: "First, you know, I experiment on myself and I explore myself and I feel, you know, how it feels like and then if I feel OK with sharing it and if people can benefit from it, then they will."

Communication as an essential tool

For the Shahs and Sophia, communication is practiced as interpersonal connection in a multi-sensory approach, including talk, sight, sound, touch, and mutual contact though media such as acupuncture needles, and water. For Aparna, interpersonal exchange is a basic clinical skill, essential to any decisions about medical care. She declares:

> Well, I think communication is the first step to medicine. If you don't talk to your patient, how would you know what's going on? Talking is very, very important. It is time consuming, I would say that, but I think it is the first step. If you can't communicate with your patient, you really cannot take care of them. . . . Every patient who comes to the doctor wishes they are able to communicate good.

Both Shahs emphasize observation as an essential clinical skill. For Suresh,

> Listening is to me, more powerful than talking to the patient. If you just keep your ears open the patient is going to tell you how to treat him, in most of the cases. . . . I think that is the first thing a physician must always do is use his skill of observation through listening, seeing, feeling, touching, whatever.

Aparna elaborates:

> Listening to the patient, eye to eye contact with the patient, not looking at the computer screen. . . . But sitting down, making the patient feel at home, asking, not being in a rush and let the patient vent out. I tell Suresh that a patient can walk and I can diagnose the person's problem. It's come to that level that you can just walk in and know how sick the patient is, what's going on, how much time this patient is going to take.

Beyond the typical forms of communicating through speaking and listening, Suresh notes that communication occurs in more subtle ways:

> For example, the acupuncture needles; people just think of them as going into the body but really these needles as you use the points, you're actually

talking to the body's organ system. As physicians we forgot the touch. The healthy touch with the patient. . . . So here we're communicating with her body and her soul and her mind through the use of those needles.

He explains that even the cheerful yellow walls and even the parking lot communicate positive messages to the patients.

By definition, Sophia's modality of collective dance in the water is a powerful nonverbal communicative format. She elaborates: "They're three different change-inducing factors in dolphin dance. One is the water. One is the music. And one is me." Beyond her interpersonal connection, she describes the aquatic environment as essential. Using a spiritual metaphor, she states, "I'm a minister of the large universal church . . . the warm pond has been my office for three years." As for the music:

> Most of the techniques that I use actually are designed to induce the trance state. And, the variety of this is that, you know, you can reach many people. So, a person that is not very auditory, for example, would not be induced to play music. But, they will be induced by the water . . . And then the loss of orientation that comes with the water. And then the music is a vehicle and is used in shamanist states.

The three healers affirm elements of relational process that have been long established in both the communication and health-care literatures: the importance of identifying psychosocial and spiritual needs, and in so doing, taking time to listen. Yet, they also underscore issues that have not received ample attention in previous research, namely, the power of acute sensory observation and the importance of environmental, tactile, and other forms of nonverbal communication.

Discussion

The results of this investigation raise questions and provide some answers about communication in holistic health interactions. We identified commonalities and distinctions in terms of epistemologies, definitions of healing, ethnocultural influences, participants' attitudes, and therapeutic practices. In this final section we discuss a few conclusions and an agenda for health communication scholarship that contributes to understanding what healing means, and how and why healing practices work.

Conclusions

From the two case studies presented, several dialectical tensions materialize that indicate contradictory aspects of providing holistic health treatment. First, the dialectic of specialization versus integration illustrates the tension between expertise in one particular health perspective and sphere of treatment and the merging together of holistic and biomedical perspectives to provide various treatment options. Sophia, having withdrawn from the biomedical health perspective, immersed herself in the holistic health perspective, and specifically aquatic healing because of the profound effects that water has for spiritual healing. Her specialization requires close proximity to natural bodies of water as a practice environment, and she finds that the focus on healing that exists on the big island of Hawaii fosters a greater capacity to develop her expertise. The Shahs are physicians who effectively blend acupuncture and other holistic health principles with their biomedical training to provide medical care. While their work thrives even in a socially conservative environment, they find difficulty in maintaining an integrative practice within the United States due to licensing regulations. The experiences of these three practitioners provide insight into the issues that holistic health providers may face in developing a practice that suits the ethnocultural advantages and limitations of their respective environments.

A second notable dialectic tension is the opposition between the holistic and biomedical health perspectives and the therapeutic approaches they entail. All three participants describe the biomedical model as focused on treatment of the physical body, a reality that encouraged their interest in holistic health modalities which are designed to provide healing to the "whole" person. Features of holistic healing may include the communicative faculties of listening and talking with the person, and possibly their family members, about personal experiences and concerns in an effort to understand the spiritual, psychological, and physical features of the person's health. Holistic and biomedical perspectives may not absolutely contradict one other, but the differences suggest the presence of a distinctly oppositional framework for conceptualizing the treatment of illness and the enhancement of health.

A third dialectic represented in this research is the degree to which healing is scripted versus improvisational. While we see in these case studies epistemological patterns that might be considered scripts for communicating in holistic encounters, it is clear that for the most part providers and patients negotiate and improvise their communication partnership with one another based on patients' needs and characteristics. During the encounter, the providers strive to make the patient comfortable in order to facilitate the healing experience. For example, when presented with a patient who is not inclined to be at ease in the water, Sophia abandons her primary modality of treatment and offers a modality that is more suited to the patient. Similarly, when the presence of family members alleviates the stress of treating a chronic condition, Aparna arranges to meet with the patient in the company of the patient's extended family. Essentially, this research suggests that holistic health providers recognize the utility of modifying the script of a treatment session in order to calm the patient. Once anxieties have been placated, the patient becomes more susceptible to benefiting from the treatment session.

One final conclusion, then, that can be drawn from this research related to these dialectic tensions is the notion of *dynamic equilibrium* in the healing process. Both the Shahs and Sophia talk about healing as a breakthrough or release. While the path to healing is one of creating equilibrium in the "three sticks" or mind, body, and spirit, there always exists a dynamic fluctuation within this equilibrium. Change is expected, welcomed, and even a natural part of this equilibrium we call health. We turn now to questions that have been raised by our research and a brief agenda for future research.

Holistic healing and future research

We agree with Parrott's (2004b) assessment that there is a "collective amnesia" concerning the role of spirituality and religious beliefs in health communication scholarship. However, while Parrott's work focuses on how these beliefs are embedded in lay discourse, in this chapter we have explored how three holistic practitioners attempt to connect with human spirit and pain to relieve suffering and bring people to a different level—of health, self-awareness, and wholeness. A review of social science research on the relationship of spirituality and religiosity to health care (Egbert et al., 2004) reveals that the preponderance of scholarship has been devoted to finding ways to measure attitudes and correlations. We have used qualitative inquiry in an effort to better understand what healing means, and how and why healing practices work.

Of course, our analysis of these two case studies is just a beginning, limited by the particular practitioners and circumstances we have chosen to study. As a result of this work, certain questions have come to the forefront of our thinking. We share them as a way of concluding and, in part, as a way of encouraging health communication scholars to expand their research agendas to include CAM as a focus of study.

As communication scholars and specialists, our tendency is to gravitate toward and privilege the verbal in terms of what kinds of data we identify, collect, and study. What we have learned in the current work is that silent observation, movement, touch, sound, environment, even materials such as needles, are an important part of the currency of holistic healing. How can we best adapt our expectations, perceptions, methods, and analyses to better comprehend these forms of data and the phenomenological patterns that they generate?

In examining the stories of these three healers, we note that one of their primary distinctions from other practitioners reported in the research literature (and in our own experiences) is a persistent willingness to delve into areas of physical and psychic pain that are frequently downplayed or ignored in biomedicine, and generally not addressed in health communication research, except perhaps in illness narrative work. What are the language and symbol systems, as well as behavioral skills, that enable holistic practitioners to communicate about pain, and to break through the interpersonal barriers of fear, skepticism, and resistance? How can health communication as a discipline better prepare to turn its gaze in the direction of the expression of suffering as a conduit to understanding healing?

Finally, this study has helped to clarify the extent to which cultural beliefs and values affect the ways in which practitioners conceptualize their work and shape their practices. In what ways can health communication research be designed to demonstrate how modes of healing are both embedded in and reflective of cultural influences?

Note

1 While all quotations are verbatim, names and identifying information of participants resemble actualities, but have been fictionalized to assure confidentiality.

References

Adler, H.M. (2002). The sociophysiology of caring in the doctor–patient relationship. *Journal of General Internal Medicine*, *17*, 883–890.

Astin, J.A. (1998). Why patients use alternative medicine. *Journal of the American Medical Association*, *27*, 1548–1553.

Barrett, B., Marchand, L., Scheder, J., Plane, M.B., Maberry, R., Appelbaum, D., et al. (2003). Themes of holism, empowerment, access, and legitimacy define complementary, alternative, and integrative medicine in relation to conventional biomedicine. *Journal of Alternative and Complementary Medicine*, *9*, 937–947.

Bascom, A., Kowalek, J.P., Chohan, N.D. & Follin, S.A. (2003). *Nurse's Handbook of Alternative and Complementary Therapies*, 2nd edn. Philadelphia: Lippincott, Williams, & Wilkins.

Becker, C., Geist-Martin, P., Carnett, S., & Slauta, K. (2005). Exploring the rhythms of healing on the Big Island of Hawai'i. Paper presented at the annual meeting of the Western States Communication Association, San Francisco.

Biesanz, M.H., Biesanz, R., & Biesanz, K.Z. (1999). *The Ticos: Culture and Social Change in Costa Rica*. Boulder, CO: Lynne Rienner.

Bodywork (2006). Available www.kalani.com/learn/bodywork.htm (accessed March 26, 2006).

Buchbinder, R., Gingold, M., Hall, S., & Cohen, M. (2002). Non-prescription complementary treats used by rheumatoid arthritis patients attending a community-based rheumatology practice. *Internal Medicine Journal*, *32*, 208–214.

Cangemi, L. (2002). *Magic*. Unpublished poems.

Caspi, O., Sechrest, L., Pitluk, H.C., Marshall, C.L., Bell, I.R., & Nichter, M. (2003). On the definition of complementary, alternative, and integrative medicine: Societal mega-stereotypes vs. the patients' perspectives. *Alternative Therapies*, *9*, 58–62.

Cassileth, B.R. (2002). The integrative medicine service at Memorial Sloan-Kettering Cancer Center. *Seminars in Oncology*, *29*, 585–588.

Coates, J.R., Jobst, K.A., Fielding, S., Fisher, F., Holgate, S., Mills, S., et al. (1998). Integrated healthcare: A way forward for the next five years? *Journal of Alternative and Complementary Medicine*, *4*, 209–247.

Conroy, R.M., Siriwardena, R., Smyth, O., & Fernandes, P. (2000). The relation of health anxiety and attitudes to doctors and medicine to use of alternative and complementary treatments in general practice patients. *Psychology, Health & Medicine, 5*, 203–213.

Dana-Farber Cancer Institute. (2006). *Zakim Center for Integrated Therapies*. Available: www.dana-farber.org/pat/support/zakim_default.asp (accessed March 14, 2006).

Darwin, T.J. (1999). Intelligent cells and the body as conversation: The democratic rhetoric of mindbody medicine. *Argumentation & Advocacy, 36*, 105–143.

Dolphin Dance (2006). Available: www.aquaticdance.com/ (accessed March 26, 2006).

Donnelly, G.F. (2003). From the editor: The White House embraces holism. *Holistic Nursing Practice, 17*, 19.

Dossey, L. (2004). Snow on the equator: Reflections on the CAM wars. *Alternative Therapies in Health and Medicine, 10*, 10–13, 86–87.

du Pré, A. (2000). *Communicating about Health: Current Issues and Perspectives*. Mountain View, CA: Mayfield.

Egbert, N., Mickley, J., & Coeling, H. (2004). A review and application of social scientific measures of religiosity and spirituality: Assessing a missing component in health communication research. *Health Communication 16*, 7–27.

Ehman, J.W., Ott, B.B., & Short, T.H. (1999). Do patients want physicians to inquire about their spiritual or religious beliefs if they become gravely ill? *Archives in Internal Medicine, 159*, 1803–1806.

Eisenberg, D.M., Davis, R.B., Ettner, S.L., Appel, S., Wilkey, S., Van Rompay, M., et al. (1998). Trends in alternative medicine use in the United States, 1990–1997. *Journal of the American Medical Association, 280*, 1569–1575.

Ellis, M., Vinson, D., & Ewigman, B. (1999). Addressing spiritual concerns with patients: Family physicians attitudes and practices. *Journal of Family Practice, 48*, 105–109.

Filc, D. (2004). The medical text: Between biomedicine and hegemony. *Social Science & Medicine, 59*, 1275–1285.

Furnham, A., & Forey, J. (1994). The attitudes, behaviors and beliefs of patients of conventional vs. complementary (alternative) medicine. *Journal of Clinical Psychology, 50*, 458–469.

Furnham, A. & Kirkcaldy, B. (1996). The health beliefs and behaviours of orthodox and complementary medical clients. *British Journal of Clinical Psychology 35*, 49–61.

Gaudet, T.W. (1998). Integrative medicine: A new approach to medicine and medical education. *Integrative Medicine, 1*, 67–73.

Gevitz, N. (1988). *Other Healers: Unorthodox Medicine in America*. Baltimore: Johns Hopkins University Press.

Goldbeck-Wood, S., Dorozynski, A., Lie, G.L. (1996). Complementary medicine is booming worldwide. *British Medical Journal, 313*, 131–133.

Gonzalez, M.C. (1994). An invitation to leap from a trinitarian ontology in health communication research to a spiritually inclusive quatrain. In S.A. Deetz (ed.), *Communication Yearbook 17*. Thousand Oaks, CA: Sage, pp. 378–387.

Gould, A., & MacPherson, H. (2001). Patient perspectives on outcomes after treatment with acupuncture. *Journal of Alternative and Complementary Medicine, 7*, 261–268.

Graigie, F., & Hobbs, R., III. (1999). Spiritual perspectives and practices of family physicians with an expressed interest in spirituality. *Family Medicine, 31*, 578–585.

Grof, S., & Grof, C. (eds). (1989). *Spiritual Emergency: When Personal Transformation Becomes a Crisis.* New York: Tarcher/Putnam.

Herman, K. (1993). Reassessing predictors of therapist competence. *Journal of Counseling and Development, 72*, 29–32.

Horvath, A.O., & Symonds, B.D. (1991). Relation between working alliance and outcome in psychotherapy: A meta analysis. *Journal of Counseling and Psychology, 38*, 139–149.

Huggins, C.E. (2005). Mainstream medicine diversifies; But what does CAM have to do with it? *The Network Journal, 12*, 14.

Institute of Medicine of the National Academies. (2005). *Complementary and Alternative Medicine in the United States.* Washington, DC: The National Academies Press.

Jain, N., & Astin, J.A. (2001). Barriers to acceptance: An exploratory study of complementary/ alternative medicine disuse. *Journal of Alternative and Complementary Medicine, 7*, 689–696.

Kliewer, S. (2004). Allowing spirituality into the healing process. *The Journal of Family Practice, 53*, 616–624.

Kroesen, K., Baldwin, C.M., Brooks, A.J., & Bell, I.R. (2002). US military veterans' perceptions of the allopathic medical care system and their use of complementary and alternative medicine. *Family Practice 19*: 57–64.

Landmark Healthcare, Inc. (2006). Established 1985, Sacramento, CA. Available www.landmarkhealthcare.com (accessed March 24, 2006).

Larson, D.B., Swyers, J.P., & McCullough, M.E. (1997). *Scientific Research on Spirituality and Health: A Consensus Report.* Rockville, MD: National Institute for Healthcare Research.

Lowenberg, J.S. (1989). *Caring and Responsibility: The Crossroads Between Holistic Practice and Traditional Medicine.* Philadelphia: University of Pennsylvania Press.

Luborsky, L., Cris-Chrisoph, P., McLellan, A.T., Woody, G., Piper, W. Liberman, B., Imber, S., & Pilkonis, P. (1986). Do therapists vary much in their success? Findings from four outcome studies. *American Journal of Orthopsychiatry, 56*, 501–512.

Massad, S. (2003). Performance of doctoring: A philosophical and methodological approach to medical conversation. *Advances, 19*, 6–13.

Mercer, S.W. & Reilly, D. (2004). A qualitative study of patients' views on the consultation at the Glasgow Homeopathic Hospital, and NHS integrative complementary and orthodox medical care unit. *Patient. Education & Counseling; 53*, 13–18.

M.D. Anderson Cancer Center. (2006). *Place . . . of wellness.* Available: www. Mdanderson.org/departments/wellness (accessed March 14, 2006).

Miller, W.R. (ed.) (1999). *Integrating Spirituality into Treatment.* Washington, DC: American Psychological Association.

O'Callaghan, F.V., & Jordan, N. (2003). Postmodern values, attitudes, and the use of complementary medicine. *Complementary Therapeutic Medicine, 11*: 28–32.

Orlinsky, D.F., & Howard, K.I. (1985). Therapy process and outcome. In S. Garfield, & A. Bergin (eds), *Handbook of Psychotherapy and Behavior Change.* New York: John Wiley & Sons.

Parrott, R. (ed.) (2004a). Spirituality in Health Communication. A special issue of *Health Communication* 16 (1).

Parrott, R. (2004b). "Collective amnesia:" The absence of religious faith and spirituality in health communication research and practice. *Health Communication* 16, 1–5.

Shealy, N.C. (2003). Holism in evolution. *The Journal of Alternative and Complementary Medicine*, 9, 333–334.

Siahpush, M. (1999) Why do people favour alternative medicine? *Australia–New Zealand Journal of Public Health*, 23, 266–271.

Sibinga, E.M.S., Ottolini, M.C., Duggan, A.K., & Wilson, M.H. (2004). Parent–pediatrician communication about complementary and alternative medicine use for children. *Clinical Pediatrics*, 43, 367–373.

Sleath, B., Rubin, R.H., Campbell, W., Gwyther, L., & Clark, T. (2001). Ethnicity and physician–older patient communication about alternative therapies. *Journal of Alternative and Complementary Medicine*, 7, 329–335.

Sloan, R.P., Bagiella, E., & Powell, T. (1999). Religion, spirituality, and medicine. *Lancet*, 343, 664–667.

Strupp, H.H., & Hadley, S.W. (1979). Specific vs. nonspecific factors in psychotherapy: A controlled study of outcome. *Archives of General Psychiatry*, 36, 1125–1136.

Sutherland, E.G., & Ritenbaugh, C.K. (2004). The practitioner as medicine. *Journal of Alternative and Complementary Medicine*, 10, 13–15.

Swartzman, L.C., Harshman, R.A., Burkell, J., & Lundy, M.E. (2002). What accounts for the appeal of complementary/alternative medicine, and what makes complementary/alternative medicine "alternative"? *Medical Decision Making*, 22, 431–450.

Turner, R.N. (1998). A proposal for classifying complementary therapies. *Complementary Therapies in Medicine*, 6, 141–143.

Verhoef, M.J., & Sutherland, L.R. (1995). Alternative medicine and general practitioners. *Canadian Family Physician*, 41, 1005–1011.

Weaver, A.J., Flannelly, K.J., Stone, H.W., & Dossey, L. (2003). Spirituality, health and CAM: Current controversies. *Alternative Therapies in Health and Medicine*, 9, 42–46.

Weil, J. (1952). The holistic attitude in medical consultation. *American Practitioner Diagnostic Treatment*, 3, 1.

Whorton, K. (1999). The history of complementary and alternative medicine. In W.B. Jonas, & J.S. Levin (eds), *Essentials of Complementary and Alternative Medicine*. Baltimore: Lippincott, Williams, & Wilkins.

Widdershoven, G.A.M. (1999). Care, cure and interpersonal understanding. *Journal of Advanced Nursing*, 29. Downloaded 9/4/04 from EBSCOhost.

Wynia, M.K., Eisenberg, D.M., & Wilson, I.B. (1999). Physician–patient communication about complementary and alternative medical therapies: A survey of physicians caring for patients with human immunodeficiency virus infection. *Journal of Alternative and Complementary Medicine*, 5, 447–456.

World Health Organization (2003). *Traditional medicine: Fact sheet*. Retrieved September 24, 2004 from www.who.int/mediacentre/factsheets/fs134/en/print.html.

Zollman, C., & Vickers, A. (1999). ABC of complementary medicine: What is complementary medicine? *British Medical Journal*, 319, 693–696.

Chapter 5

'You feel so responsible'

Australian mothers' concepts and experiences related to promoting the health and development of their young children

Deborah Lupton

Introduction

Promoting the health of infants and young children is a central plank of contemporary public health. It is regularly argued in public health forums that if health-promoting habits and good health can be established in early childhood, then the groundwork is laid for optimal health in later life. Government-sponsored health communication mass media campaigns and other mass-distributed media such as pamphlets, as well as privately published materials such as pregnancy and parenting manuals, are frequently employed to convey to parents the importance of promoting their children's health and development.

In Australia at both the national and state levels of government there are numerous documents setting out policy frameworks for promoting children's health. In order to implement such policies, the Australian government has funded many programs and initiatives, including the National Breastfeeding Strategy, the National Child Nutrition Program and the National Immunisation Strategy, that specifically address the health and development of young children. These programs draw on a mixture of traditional individualistic approaches to public health and health promotion and what has been termed the "new" public health, which takes a broader ecological approach and addresses the role played by communities in promoting the health of individuals (Lupton, 1995; Petersen & Lupton, 1997).

Immunization provides an example of the action of public health and government policy in relation to parents' choices about their young children's health. Since the early 1990s in Australia initiatives increasingly have been put in place to persuade (or from the perspective of some, coerce) parents to have their children immunized. For instance, since 1994 in New South Wales, Australia's most populous state, under that state's Public Health Act parents have been required to provide evidence of age-appropriate immunization to childcare facilities and to present an immunization certificate at the time of school entry. In the event of outbreaks of the infectious diseases covered by the immunization schedule, children who are not immunized may be excluded from school or childcare. At a national level, all new parents are provided after the birth of their children with booklets that, among other actions related to health promotion, outline the immunization schedule with sections to be completed by medical professionals when they have completed the immunizations and present immunization as the automatic decision of parents. Further, the Australian government provides financial incentives both to families to encourage immunization and to general practitioners, who are seen as the key players in promoting immunization among individual families. All of these discourses and practices assume that parents will make the "right" and "rational" choice to immunize their children.

Interestingly, however, in the health promotion literature there has been limited in-depth examination or understanding of the reasons behind the decisions that parents make in relation to immunization. It is often assumed, for example, that parents fail to immunize because of ignorance, irrationality, neglect or apathy rather than acknowledged that their reasons to avoid immunization may be founded on fully considered reasons that make good sense to the parents (see below for further discussion of this).

Directing attention at the health of infants and young children presupposes that their parents will take particular actions, including seeking out relevant information, to ensure that their children maintain good health and achieve optimal development. Because women tend to undertake the vast proportion of childcare, much expert advice and health communication materials are directed at them in their role as caring mothers. Recent years have witnessed an intensification of emphasis upon women's behaviors in pregnancy and as the mothers of infants and young children. Medical research on the relationship between the intrauterine environment, foetal development and later outcomes in life has ensured a continuing focus on a mother's health status and behaviors during pregnancy. For example, women are exhorted to carefully control their diet, avoid drug intake, engage in regular exercise, ensure appropriate medical supervision and treatment, undergo screening tests such as ultrasound and engage in antenatal education to ensure the optimal health and development of their foetuses (Lupton, 1999a). After the birth of their children, women are expected to take on the major responsibility for protecting and maintaining the health of their offspring, including having them immunized and ensuring a nutritious diet, commencing in infancy with breastfeeding. Opportunities for children to exercise are emphasized, together with maintaining a child-safe environment, educating children about basic hygiene practices, seeking medical care when illness strikes and so on.

In this chapter, I critically examine the discourses that surround maternal practices relating to the health and development of young children, exploring the notions of maternal responsibility and child vulnerability that underpin these discourses and give them meaning. My interest in this topic stems not only from years of research and writing in the sociology of health, medicine, and risk (see, for example, Lupton, 1995, 1999a, 1999b, 2003; Petersen & Lupton, 1997; Tulloch & Lupton, 2003) but also from my own recent experience as the mother of two young children (the first born in 1998, the second in 2005). After entering the world of motherhood, it became increasingly apparent to me how pervasive and persuasive was the network of information and health-promoting messages that surrounded pregnancy and the mothering of young children. It made me wonder how other mothers of young children were dealing with this network and to what extent they were adopting, or indeed challenging, the messages and exhortations of health communication media in their everyday practices as the carers of their children, and I designed a research study to investigate these issues.[1] As is common in sociological research, therefore, I held both an academic and a personal interest in the research topic I was investigating.

My intention in undertaking this research was to go beyond standard health promotion research that is merely interested in identifying "gaps" in people's knowledge as a precursor to filling these "gaps" with methods of health communication such as mass media campaigns or pamphlets. Rather, I was interested in critically exploring mothers' concepts, experiences, and practices relating to the health and development of their children, seeking to place these concepts, experiences, and practices in their broader sociocultural milieux. The research took a discourse analysis approach, with a central focus upon identifying the broader sets of meanings (discourses) that underpin women's explanations of their health-promoting beliefs and practices. In doing so, the study drew upon sociological research and theorizing related to the discourses circulating concerning "good health," "good motherhood," risk, child development, the maternal body, and the infant and child's body.

Previous research

Despite the plethora of information directed at mothers discussed above, few studies exist that are able to examine the ways in which they respond to public health and health communication imperatives relating to their children's health and development. While some sociological studies have been conducted that explore parents' views on and experiences of illness in their young children, little is known, for example, about what aspects of their children's health mothers give priority to over others, how they make decisions about health-related behaviors, what risks they perceive as threatening their children's health, or upon what sources of information they draw when forming their beliefs and acting upon them. Nor have many in-depth empirical research studies using qualitative methods been conducted which have sought to examine the ways in which parents of infants and young children conceptualize their children's bodies or the notions of health parents ascribe to their children.

One Scottish study by Cunningham-Burley (1990), involving interviews with mothers with preschool-aged children, found that the mothers closely observed their children for signs of illness, particularly in relation to their sleeping and eating habits. The women's negotiation of their children's behavior and illness was embedded in common-sense assumptions and individual experiences about what they considered normal and acceptable in a child. Thus, understandings and practices were grounded in social and cultural context.

The importance of social and cultural context in shaping ideas about the care of children is further underlined by a cross-cultural study comparing views and practices of mothers from Swedish, Italian, and Anglo-American cultural backgrounds (Welles-Nystrom et al., 1994). This study identified the differences that may exist between different cultures in relation to the bodily management of infants. It found, for example, that the Italian mothers were concerned about their babies not eating enough and their cleanliness and protection from the elements, while the American women worried about such aspects as sleeping and their babies' achievement of independence, and the Swedish mothers focused on ensuring their babies had plenty of fresh air and a child-safe space to explore, both indoors and out.

A study of English mothers' decisions about immunizing their infants (Poltorak et al., 2005) found that the mothers' decisions were influenced by such diverse aspects as the women's personal histories of immunization, their birth experiences and related feelings of control over the health of their children, their own family health histories, their interpretations of their infants' health and particular strengths and vulnerabilities, the mothers' experiences of using health services and by friendships and conversations with others. For example, some mothers recalled catching childhood diseases with few serious effects, others held philosophical or political attitudes which made them suspicious of government intervention and drug companies, some had had negative experiences with medical professionals that rendered them less likely to seek a medical intervention for their child, while others believed in the concept of "natural immunity."

Social class differences also may be found in the same cultural setting. Middle-class parents, for example, often are highly concerned that their infants are breastfed and that their young children consume "natural" and "healthy" foods and avoid sugary confections or foods that contain additives or preservatives (Miller, 1997). Backett-Milburn (2000) researched ideas of health in middle-class families living in Edinburgh in the late 1980s. She noted a general ethos of personal responsibility for health, including related to diet and exercise among both children and their parents. The parents she interviewed saw their children's health as more important than their own, and the majority said that they carefully monitored and observed their children's states of health and well-being.

These studies suggest that while the bodily needs of the child are inescapably biological, the ways in which these needs are met (or not met), and the meanings that surround them, are the products of acculturation into social and cultural norms. Health beliefs, including those related to the health of one's child, are constructed through a complex interaction with personal experience, discussions with others and positioning within a broader sociocultural context. Notions of motherhood are also central to ideas about how infants and young children are cared for.

Research methods

As noted above, my own research study was directed at identifying mothers' concepts, beliefs, and practices related to maintaining good health and encouraging optimal development in their infants and young children. To do so, a qualitative approach was adopted, using in-depth, semi-structured interviews with a total of ninety mothers who were caring for at least one young child aged between 0 and 5 years old. Sixty of the mothers lived in Sydney, Australia's largest city, while the remaining thirty were resident in Bathurst, a small rural town in the far west of the state of New South Wales, about three hours' drive west from Sydney.

The intention of including both Sydney and Bathurst residents was to compare and contrast the concepts, experiences, and practices of urban with rural women. Because of space limitations, however, the discussion in this chapter will focus solely upon the interview data derived from the Sydney interviewees. These sixty women were a heterogeneous group. They lived in various parts of Sydney, including both socioeconomically advantaged and disadvantaged suburbs. They ranged in age from 19 to 48 and had between one and eleven children.

The interviews with these women produced much rich data on aspects relating to their concepts and experiences concerning the health and development of their young children. In this chapter, I will focus on a number of major topics emerging from the data, including the mothers' sense of responsibility for their children's health, their belief in the importance of good health and the concept of the vulnerable child. Throughout the women's discussion of these topics, a number of major discourses intertwined relating to notions of health, the "good mother" and "bad mother," and the child's body. These discourses are discussed in greater detail in the discussion section that concludes the chapter.

Findings

One of the central findings of the study was the extent to which the participants had internalized the notion that they, and they alone, held responsibility for the health of their children. The mothers frequently used the term "my responsibility" when referring to the maintenance and promotion of their children's health. The notion was expressed that children's health required constant monitoring and vigilance from their mothers: such aspects as the child's eating, bowel and sleeping habits, their energy levels, their progress in growth and development, and their general demeanor were observed and considered in relation to whether mothers thought their children were feeling well or ill. Even such aspects of brain development and the level of intelligence of the child were considered to be a direct outcome of how well the mother had provided enough "stimulation" for her or him. As a mother of a 10-month-old baby said:

> She's our responsibility, and you want to make sure that she gets the best out of everything, you want to make sure that she learns as much as she possibly can, you want to make sure that she's getting enough stimulation, trying to provide an environment for her where she can develop to her best potential. So everything you do revolves around it, I guess.
>
> (administrator on maternity leave, aged 28)

Similarly, a stay-at-home mother, aged 39, with seven-year-old and three-year-old children commented that:

> I think that is definitely a mother's job, or part of a mother's job, to manage their [children's] health. I think it's wrong to not manage it, to not give them the right guidance in life.

Good health was positioned by the mothers as of extremely high importance for the child's well-being and future prospects in life:

> Well obviously you want your children to be healthy, you want them to have a healthy diet, you want them to be active, and obviously it's always a concern if they do get sick, you hope that it's something minimal. So absolutely, health is very important.
>
> (part-time recruitment consultant, aged 27,
> four-year-old and two-year-old children)

> It's probably the most important thing, they have to be healthy. There are so many overweight children out there and children that have disabilities and stuff like that. You're really lucky to have three healthy children—no, I don't think a lot of it is luck. We're lucky that they don't have a disability and stuff like that, they are healthy children, but you've got to keep them healthy and maintain a healthy lifestyle for them to stay healthy.
>
> (stay-at-home mother, aged 25, eight-year-old,
> five-year-old and three-year-old children)

Notions of the child's body as expressed in the interviews with the mothers positioned the child as vulnerable, constantly open to the threat of ill health, particularly in the case of infants. This sense of their child's vulnerability contributed to women's feelings of responsibility and need for constant vigilance in preserving and protecting their child's health:

> They're so little for sure, from day one they've been vulnerable. And if you don't do the right things to stop stuff, like immunization for example, if you don't give them that and they catch something, you pay for it for life.
>
> (sole-parent-pensioner, aged 22,
> four-year-old and two-year-old children)

> I felt very unprepared for that aspect, [my first child] was so vulnerable, I responded to her completely different to the way I would myself. I ignore illness and things in myself, but with her I was very concerned often that I was doing it all the right way and she was learning the right things and being cared for well enough. I think I was a bit neurotic in the beginning.
>
> (marketing executive on maternity leave, aged 33,
> 15-month-old and one-month-old babies)

Due to their concept of their children's bodies as vulnerable and open, the mothers tended to worry if they heard that a virus was "going around," and there was quite a lot of talk in the interviews about the germs that are "out there" waiting to attack children. Several women, especially those with babies and very young children, talked about not letting their children be near or play with other children who may have colds or other illnesses that could be infectious. Media coverage of outbreaks of viral illnesses such as meningococcal or pneumococcal disease particularly aroused concern in the mothers because they felt that there was little they could do to protect their children from such illnesses:

> I suppose there's always anything that could threaten their health. All these viruses that are always around, that's always a worry, you always worry in winter time with all these deadly flus and stuff like that. Just things like that I tend to worry about a little bit, not excessively, but if you hear on the news that there is a new deadly virus going around you sort of panic a little bit.
>
> (stay-at-home mother, aged 31, six-year-old,
> four-year-old, two-year-old and eight-month-old children)

> These days there's so many new diseases, you've got meningitis and pneumococcal and all of those kinds of things. And they worry me because I can't prevent those things from happening, besides having immunization

or whatever. I don't know, those kinds of diseases worry me, the things that you can't prevent.

(part-time recruitment consultant, aged 29, 13-month-old baby)

In addition to the threat of external invaders such as viruses and bacteria, the mothers were extremely concerned about their children's diet and exercise. There has been much publicity over the past five years or so in Australia concerning childhood obesity and growing rates of overweight in young children (Lupton, 2003). The women in this study were highly aware of this publicity, and all of them made some reference to the importance of a healthy diet to protect their child from overweight problems and to maintain good health.

Part of the concern about overweight was the idea, expressed by many of the women, that children today spend too much time in sedentary pursuits such as watching television, and not enough time exercising. The mothers saw it as their responsibility to ensure that their children ate a healthy diet and engaged in exercise:

I don't want my kids to be obese, because that brings problems in their life. Also with my daughter it's a confidence issue, but the most important thing is it's just health, you want your kids to be healthy. These days our heart disease rates and our cholesterol rates are skyrocketing, they're not as they used to be before and it's all because of this junk food that we have available.

(stay-at-home mother, aged 28, seven-year-old, four-year-old and two-year-old children)

As far as I'm concerned, high quality diet also goes without saying. It's important to have a diet that's free of processed foods as much as possible, at least for the first year, then it gets out of your control. Diet affects their behavior, growth—physical growth, immune system, skin, their intelligence, I definitely think that their brain is growing and developing and you want to give them the right foods to help that.

(receptionist and student on maternity leave, aged 28, nine-month-old baby)

Media reports of childhood obesity have tended to lay the blame for overweight in children at the door of their mothers (Lupton, 2003), and this acceptance that it was up to mothers to control their children's diet was widespread in the interview data. However, monitoring their children's diet and level of exercise involved much vigilance from the mothers. They found themselves contending with "fussy eaters"—children who were reluctant to eat such foods as meat, fruit or vegetables—and the seductive pull exerted by television and other sedentary pursuits. The women were largely determined to attempt to overcome these barriers to ensuring their children's good health, but found it a continuing struggle.

Breastfeeding was a practice around which there was much discussion, particularly for those mothers still with young babies and who had recently grappled with difficulties concerning breastfeeding. It was universally acknowledged that breastfeeding was best for the baby in terms of promoting their health and development. Those women, therefore, who struggled with breastfeeding their babies, and especially those who were not successful at establishing and maintaining breastfeeding, felt guilty and positioned as "bad mothers."

For example, one woman (a 28-year-old administrator on maternity leave), despite her best efforts, had only managed to breastfeed her baby for her first month of life. She spoke of the crushing disappointment and guilt she felt about not being able to successfully breastfeed for longer:

> I felt very guilty, because, well to be honest my husband wasn't much of a support, he really wanted her to be breastfed for as long as possible, so did I, but he didn't understand that it just wasn't working. I didn't have any breast milk there, I didn't have a choice, but I felt that he wasn't really supportive. I do think that there's still very much, it's like if you take your baby out somewhere and see another mother, for example in shopping centres where they have those mothers' rooms to change and feed, and people would say "Are you still breastfeeding?" and I'd feel really guilty about saying no. And I found I'd start telling the whole story about why I had to stop, almost like I felt I had to justify myself. So you do feel really guilty because people expect you to be breastfeeding, I mean that's the best thing for the baby.

This mother's words denote the pressure that women feel to breastfeed, the lack of support they may feel even from their partners if they have difficulties in establishing breastfeeding and the need women may feel to justify themselves to others, whom they see as judging them negatively because they have not done what is "best" for the baby. It is clear that in this case, the baby's needs are positioned as more important than those of the mother, even if the mother is suffering from lack of supply, mastitis, or painfully cracked nipples.

The idea that children needed to be provided with the resources for optimal development was prevalent in the interviewees' accounts. Rather than infants and children being left to reach developmental milestones at their own pace and without requiring intervention, it was assumed by many of the women that it was their responsibility to provide their children with stimulation, maternal attention, appropriate toys, and so on to ensure that they would develop appropriately.

Sometimes this interest in their child's development would result in feelings of inadequacy if the child did not seem to be "measuring up" to others of the same age. Women with infants, in particular, frequently talked about a competitiveness between each other as to how well their child was progressing in terms of reaching developmental milestones. As one mother with a two-year-old child living in a middle-class suburb (aged 33, working part time as a cashier) said about her mothers' group: "I found that there was a lot of competition, a lot of 'My child does this and why isn't yours doing that?' And very, very, very child and baby focused." Another woman with a young baby commented that:

> You're looking at other parents and other babies, just to try to collect the evidence to say "OK, where is she on this?", "Is there something I'm missing?" I guess it's what you don't know that you don't know that's the really terrifying thing, you could just miss something. You could be missing something that you're supposed to be doing, if you didn't read up on it you could be missing something critical . . . I guess you go through the whole development thing and [wondering] whether I'm talking to her enough, or talking to her clearly enough, just things like that, so you know that she's developing appropriately.
>
> (part-time accountant, aged 36)

Mothers can be made to feel as they are not measuring up to the ideal of "good motherhood" if their baby or young child is not developing or reaching "milestones" according to others' expectations of appropriate behaviors at certain ages. Mothers themselves may experience a sense of failure, as if they have not done enough to stimulate their child to ensure optimal development. As the women quoted above suggest, pressure to conform to these expectations often comes from other mothers.

The women also talked about how they felt pressure from others, including family members and friends, but also strangers, concerning the ways they parented and how these had an impact on their children's well-being:

> I think other people can judge you and judge your parenting abilities and that's the pressure. For example I was in a shop yesterday and my baby is tiny and she can wiggle herself out of her pram, she actually wiggled herself out of her strap and was standing up in her pram. Now I was standing with her and I knew she was safe and she was fine. And the sales assistant turned around to me and said "She's going to fall out, you'd better strap her in." She made a judgment on me. And I said "No, she's fine—I'm with her." And she gave me the filthiest look I've ever seen and gave it to the other sales assistant. I've never had that experience before and it was the first

time I actually thought she thinks I'm a bad mum, and I didn't like that feeling at all.

(part-time recruitment consultant, aged 29,
13-month-old baby)

Yeah, the thing that worries me the most is my son's diet. And I've felt a lot of pressure, just 'cause I feel like he's not eating as well as other children. And because my husband's away I don't have a lot of time to self-prepare things for him and I have relied too much on the commercial foods, and I feel like I'm a bad mother because I've done that. Because there's so much bad press about the baby foods, even though when I read on the labels, I always try to choose the healthy ones . . . I think it mainly comes from me, but also does come from other mums.

(part-time teacher, aged 35, 11-month-old baby)

Being represented as a "bad mother" by other people does much to affect women's own views of their mothering qualities. External disapproval may be internalized, so that again women feel guilt for not conforming to general expectations about being a "good mother."

As noted above, it was evident from the interviews that nearly all the mothers felt that they had a major role to play in promoting the health and development of their children. This was the case whether women were older or younger, had high or low educational qualifications or lived in socio-economically advantaged or disadvantaged parts of Sydney. A significant social class difference was not noticeable in the extent to which mothers valued the health and development of their children, although it was evident that mothers from middle-class backgrounds tended to be somewhat more concerned about their children's intellectual development and exposure to "stimulation" than mothers from working-class backgrounds.

Nearly all the mothers, therefore, felt more or less empowered to take responsibility for their children's health and development. The case of a very young single mother (aged 21) from a working-class area with two children, one aged five, the other three years, is a notable exception. This young woman had had her first child at 16, and thus had not completed her secondary education. Her eldest child had a mild developmental and speech delay, which she worried might be autism, and she felt powerless to do anything to help him: "Nothing I try works. I've done everything the paediatrician told me to do and I've tried things and nothing works."

This mother's experiences of encounters with medical staff had left her feeling that she was doing the wrong thing, albeit often through lack of knowledge, which reduced her confidence further. For example, after having her first child "I was only 16 when I had him, it made things worse. In the hospital I felt like they had no respect or nothing for me." Unlike other mothers, this woman had no plans for how she might promote her children's health and development as they grew older. Her life experiences and lack of cultural and economic capital had positioned her as a mother who was concerned about her children's health, but felt disempowered to be able to do anything to help them. This young woman was extremely aware of how others, especially health professionals, looked upon her as an inadequate mother because of her youth, lack of education and general feelings of powerlessness when it came to her children's health and development.

Discussion

In sociology, much has been written over the past two decades or so about the body and social theory. Drawing in particular upon Foucauldian writings, theorists have argued that the body is subject to a network of discourses and related practices that shape that ways in which we deport, present, and care for it. Medical and public health discourses and practices have been particularly influential in dictating the ways in which bodies are experienced and cared for (see, for example, Turner, 1992, 1996; Lupton, 1995, 2003; Petersen & Lupton, 1997; Petersen & Bunton, 1999).

For scholars drawing on Foucault's work on govermentality (see, for example, Foucault, 1984, 1991), the centrality of risk discourse in relation to childhood can be related to apparatuses of "biopolitics" in neoliberal societies, efforts on the part of the state, and other agencies to discipline and normalize citizens. Foucault argued that governmentality is a system of social regulation that began to emerge in the sixteenth century in Europe and which now dominates the attempts of modern Western societies to manage their populations. By the eighteenth century, the early modern states of Europe had begun to think of citizens as part of a social body requiring a central system of management to ensure social order and maximum productivity. Integral to governmentality is the notion of political rule which attempts to avoid direct state intervention and coercion for more subtle systems of power relations.

Normalization, or the method by which norms of behavior and physical health of members of populations are measured and reproduced, is a central technique of governmentality. Mass surveillance is a major means by which normalization takes place, including the regular recording of statistics about human behavior and health status. Expert knowledges are also vital to normalization, used to collect, interpret, and apply data about populations and give advice to citizens about how best to deport themselves, including how to compare themselves against the established "norm." Foucault uses the term "biopower" to describe the ways in which strategies such as normalization work to reproduce and exert power relations at the site of the human body.

Another central aspect of governmentality and biopower is the idealized figure of the autonomous, self-regulated citizen. Such individuals voluntarily seek to maximize their life opportunities and minimize the risks to which they are exposed. They police their own behavior and need only guidance from "expert" knowledges to engage in activities that serve their best interests (Gordon, 1991).

This emphasis on self-regulation is strongly evident in discourses on health and risk emerging from public health institutions (Lupton, 1995; Petersen & Lupton, 1997). In the case of infants and young children, who to varying degrees (depending on their age) are unable to care for and take responsibility for the health of their bodies, it is the mother as responsible citizen who is charged with conforming to guidelines concerning their health.

Mothers' responsibility for the health status and development of their children has been a central focus of medicine and public health for over a century. The problem of "the child" was constructed from the middle of the eighteenth century through discourses on the regulation of the family, with parents—and in particular, mothers—charged with the responsibility of monitoring and facilitating their children's development, growth, and health. Since then, women have been constructed as active citizens not through participation in the public sphere, as is the case with men, but rather predominantly through their responsibilities in caring for the health and well-being of others, in their roles as wives and mothers (Petersen & Lupton, 1997; Lupton, 1999a, 2003; Christensen, 2004; Craig & Scambler, 2006).

It was clear from the interview data presented above that the notion of mothers' responsibility for their children's health and development had very much been internalized by women themselves. Foucault argues that self-regulating citizens do not need externalized systems of power to "force" them into actions deemed desirable by state and other institutions. Rather, through the process of internalization, citizens come to take responsibility for protecting their health—and in the case of mothers', their children's health—because they give value to doing so and it becomes part of their identity and way of life. Governmental power relations are not just about deportment of the body, but also about how people constitute ideas of selfhood. Thus, the mothers interviewed in the study strongly believed both in the importance of good health and optimal development for their children and in their own role in promoting their children's health and development. The mothers' beliefs were based not simply on a desire to ensure that their children were as healthy as possible, but also to constitute themselves as "good mothers," a central part of which notion was the idea that a "good mother" takes responsibility for protecting her children's health.

It was evident from the interview data that it is no longer considered a product of fate or "good luck" whether one's children are healthy or advanced in their development. Rather, good health and optimal development in children are viewed as a direct result of mothers' endeavors to ensure that their children are breastfed as babies, eat a good diet when older children, are protected from "germs" as much as possible, engage in regular exercise, receive immunization, are exposed to adequate mental stimulation, and so on. Even while babies are developing *in utero*, their good health and optimal development are considered primarily the responsibility of their mothers. To give birth to a baby with health problems or to have a young child who is sickly or does not reach developmental milestones at the age considered normal, therefore, may be seen not as the unfortunate outcome of a fickle fate, but rather as a failure of the mother to protect or stimulate her child adequately.

As these data demonstrate, in concert with an increasing focus on the health of children there has emerged in Western societies a preoccupation with children and their development and accomplishments. Recent sociological writings on the family in late modern Western societies have noted that the child has been given greater prominence than ever before. Due to smaller families and the acceptance that life is malleable to individual agency, children are now often seen as planning objects, requiring the investment of much care and attention as well as economic resources on the part of their parents (Beck & Beck-Gernsheim, 1995). There is an emphasis in contemporary societies on how parents can actively improve their children's abilities and life-chances, and they are expected to become experts on child development and management by consulting books and other sources of information. Even playing with one's child is now seen as a means to an end, a way of stimulating cognitive development to promote high intelligence. Many parents actively seek to produce a perfect child, for the child has come to stand as the tangible outcome of parental labour and care (Urwin, 1985; Beck & Beck-Gernsheim, 1995; Beck-Gernsheim, 1996; Miller, 1997). Part of this view of the child is the notion that all children should be in excellent health and achieve developmental "milestones" at the appropriate ages.

Finally, the data suggest that not only do women themselves internalize the messages of responsibility conveyed to them by such institutions as medicine and public health, as well as in the mass media, but they also place pressure, however well meant, on other women to conform to expectations of maternal responsibility. Women as the mothers of young children, are positioned, and, importantly, position themselves and other mothers as responsible for the health of their children through a complex and intersecting network of discourse, practice, and power relations. The nature of the power relations contributing to this network is rendered largely invisible because of the ideal of the "good mother"—the selfless woman who lavishes unstinting care and attention upon her children—that underpins dominant discourses that give meaning to mothering beliefs and practices. Under this system of beliefs and network of power relations, disadvantaged mothers who have low levels of access to education and material resources may find themselves cast in the role of "bad mother" despite their best efforts to conform to expectations concerning promoting their children's health and development.

Note

1 This research was funded by an Australian Research Council Discovery Grant awarded to the author.

References

Backett-Milburn, K. (2000) Children, parents and the construction of the "healthy body" in middle-class families. In Prout, A. (ed.), *The Body, Childhood and Society.* Houndsmills: Macmillan, pp. 79–100.

Beck, U., & Beck-Gernsheim, E. (1995). *The Normal Chaos of Love.* Cambridge: Polity.

Beck-Gernsheim, E. (1996) Life as a planning project. In Lash, S., Szerszynski, B., & Wynne, B. (eds), *Risk, Environment and Modernity: Towards a New Ecology.* London: Sage.

Christensen, P. (2004) The health-promoting family: A conceptual framework for future research. *Social Science & Medicine*, 59, 377–387.

Craig, G., & Scambler, G. (2006) Negotiating motherhood against the odds: Gastronomy tube feeding, stigma, governmentality and disabled children. *Social Science & Medicine*, 62, 1115–1125.

Cunningham-Burley, S. (1990) Mothers' beliefs about and perception of their children's illnesses. In Cunningham-Burley, S., and McKeganey, N. (eds), *Readings in Medical Sociology.* London: Tavistock/Routledge.

Foucault, M. (1984) The politics of health in the eighteenth century. In Rabinow, P. (ed.), *The Foucault Reader.* New York: Pantheon Books.

Foucault, M. (1991) Governmentality. In Burchell, G., Gordon, C., & Miller, P. (eds), *The Foucault Effect: Studies in Governmentality.* Hemel Hempstead: Harvester Wheatsheaf.

Gordon, C. (1991) Governmental rationality: An introduction. In Burchell, G., Gordon, C., & Miller, P. (eds), *The Foucault Effect: Studies in Governmentality.* Hemel Hempstead: Harvester Wheatsheaf.

Lupton, D. (1995) *The Imperative of Health: Public Health and the Regulated Body.* London: Sage.

Lupton, D. (1999a) Risk and the ontology of pregnant embodiment. In Lupton, D. (ed.), *Risk and Sociocultural Theory: New Directions and Perspectives.* Cambridge: Cambridge University Press, pp. 59–85.

Lupton, D. (1999b) *Risk.* London: Routledge.

Lupton, D. (2003) *Medicine as Culture: Illness, Disease and the Body in Western Societies*, 2nd edn. London: Sage.

Miller, D. (1997) How infants grow mothers in North London. *Theory, Culture & Society*, 14(4), 67–88.

Petersen, A., & Bunton, R. (1999) (eds) *Foucault, Health and Medicine.* London: Routledge.

Petersen, A., & Lupton, D. (1997) *The New Public Health: Health and Self in the Age of Risk.* London: Sage.

Poltorak, M., Leach, M., Fairhead, J., & Cassell, J. (2005) "MMR talk" and vaccination choices: An ethnographic study in Brighton. *Social Science & Medicine*, 61, 709–719.

Tulloch, J., & Lupton, D. (2003) *Risk and Everyday Life.* London: Sage.

Turner, B. (1992) *Regulating Bodies: Essays in Medical Sociology.* London: Sage.

Turner, B. (1996) *The Body & Society*, 2nd edn. London: Sage.

Urwin, C. (1985) Constructing motherhood: The persuasion of normal development. In Steedman, C., Urwin, C., & Walkerdine, V. (eds), *Language, Gender and Childhood*. London: Routledge & Kegan Paul.

Welles-Nystrom, B., New, R., & Richman, A. (1994) The "good mother": a comparative study of Swedish, Italian and American maternal behaviour and goals. *Scandinavian Journal of Caring Sciences*, 2, 81–86.

Chapter 6

Destigmatizing leprosy

Implications for communication theory and practice

Srinivas R. Melkote, Pradeep Krishnatray, and Sangeeta Krishnatray

Public health challenges such as leprosy, AIDS, tuberculosis, and plague have implicitly assumed stigmatization of patients. A frequent response has been the isolation of patients (Krishnatray & Melkote, 1998). Thus, for persons infected with these diseases it is both a medical and a social problem. The publicity given to HIV/AIDS patients in the last fifteen years has had the positive effect of systematically examining stigmatization of the disease and persons affected by it. Public communication campaigns have addressed issues of stigmatization and discrimination and ways to destigmatize affected individuals (Pryor & Reeder, 1993).

This chapter is about leprosy in Madhya Pradesh state in India. This state is one of the areas in the country with high endemicity (www.who.int/lep/en). Leprosy is one of the oldest diseases known to humankind. It involves physical disfigurement and negative social consequences. It is manifestly visible, progressively deforming, chronic, and of unusually long duration. Persons suffering from it often have been neglected, avoided, segregated, and ostracized (Skinsnes, 1964). Today, leprosy is curable if detected early. However, the social problem of stigma still persists.

> In its most recent report, the World Health Organization reported that the global registered prevalence of leprosy at the beginning of 2006 stood at 219,826 cases, while the number of new cases detected during 2005 was 296,499 (excluding the small number of cases in Europe). The number of new cases detected globally has fallen by more than 111,000 cases (a 27% decrease) during 2005 compared with 2004. During the past four years, the global number of new cases detected has continued to decrease dramatically, by about 20% per year. Most previously highly endemic countries have now reached elimination and those few that remain are very close to eliminating the disease. However, pockets of high endemicity still remain in some areas of Angola, Brazil, Central African Republic, Democratic Republic of Congo, India, Madagascar, Mozambique, Nepal, and the United Republic of Tanzania.
>
> (www.who.int/lep/en/)

What are the implications for communication theory and practice in dealing with negative ramifications of health challenges such as leprosy, where the infected person faces both a medical and a social/cultural problem? What should be the role of the health system and the health workers in such situations? How do we involve the local community as an important stakeholder in this process? In this chapter, we wish to touch upon several core themes that explore these questions in greater depth within the Indian national context with special reference to Madhya Pradesh state. We will discuss the dominant framework as used in neoliberal/modernization perspectives in health as well as general development areas and the inherent biases associated with it. An alternative framework anchored on the principle of empowerment is provided as a contrast to the dominant framework. We will attempt to find agency in the local communities and explore the value of participation in health-related activities and the positive impact of *creating experiences of cure* within local contexts. We will also discuss the implications of these on the role of health worker and health-care system in the treatment/eradication of leprosy and its stigma.

Leprosy and its stigma

Skinsnes (1964), a leprologist, constructed a hypothetical scenario expressing the ultimate in physical disfigurement and negative social consequences. Such a disease would be manifestly visible, progressively deforming, chronic, and of unusually long duration. It would have an insidious onset, long incubation period, high endemicity, and appear to be incurable. Persons suffering from it would be neglected, avoided, segregated, and ostracized. Leprosy's characteristics fit Skinsnes' description above. It is described as a chronic disease caused by a bacterium, Mycobacterium leprae, which is normally contracted through the respiratory tract. The Mycobacterium leprae have a long generation time. The clinical revolution of the disease is slow, often extending many years (Browne, 1985). One of the two types, the multibacillary (MB), is considered contagious. Leprosy had no effective therapeutic treatment until recently. The disease develops insidiously for years, infiltrating skin and nerve cells before causing permanent damage to limbs and eyes. The disfigurement often associated with the disease leads to stigmatization of the patient (Hirmani, 1992).

Until recently, leprosy patients in India suffered from several penalties that were inflicted by the dominant social structure. In India, the Indian Christian Marriage Act (1872), the Muslim Marriage Act (1939), and the Hindu Marriage Act (1956) granted divorce on grounds of leprosy. The electoral laws disqualified patients from contesting elections, and the various local accommodation acts authorized owners to evict them. The Motor Vehicles Act (1939) prohibited them from obtaining a driver's license, although only about 25 percent suffer from sensory loss of the limbs. Provisions in the legal manuals of public transport companies imposed travel restrictions. Insurance companies charged them a higher premium. Leprosy patients continue to be quarantined at home and sometimes evicted from a village. Incidents of patients' dead bodies being buried rather than cremated, as in the Hindu custom, have also been recorded (Patankar, 1992).

The concept of stigma

Today, leprosy is curable if detected early. However, the social problem of stigma still persists for leprosy patients. The disfigurement often associated with it only serves to increase stigmatization of the infected person. Stigma may be defined as negative attitudes and prejudice toward a person that results in avoidance of social interaction. According to Goffman (1963) stigma does not reside in the attribute but is ascribed by "normal" others to those whose characteristics are seen as not fulfilling normative expectations. The perception of "undesired differentness" typically relates to attributes of physical disfigurement, blemishes of individual character or personality or both, and social categorization such as race, national origin, and religious affiliation (Goffman, 1963). The first, that is, physical disfigurement, is the focus of stigma in this chapter and it includes physical handicaps and somatic conditions.

The crux of the communication problem is whether public campaigns promote behavioral involvement between the so-called normals and others. Freidson (1970) and Scambler (1989) argue that even when an individual apparently no longer possesses a particular characteristic, he or she may have to bear the cross of "spoiled identity." Research into twenty-seven stigmatizing conditions, mostly health related, led to similar conclusion, that "stigma itself is chronic. Regardless of the person's present behavior, individuals are not likely to accord him or her the status of a normal" (Albrecht, Walker, & Levy, 1982, p. 1326).

Leprosy communication

In the case of leprosy, a deliberate focus on the processes of destigmatization and change began in earnest with the onset of AIDS, and it mainly took the form of public health education/communication programs. In India, the government-based health-care agencies have developed educational/communication programs to destigmatize and eradicate leprosy. In the Indian state of Madhya Pradesh, which has the highest incidence of leprosy, the health-care agency has employed the Survey-Education-Treatment (SET) model. SET is a health system innovation over the earlier hospital-based treatment of leprosy patients. It emphasizes case detection by surveying every family, disseminating information about early signs and symptoms, and performing treatment on an out-patient (home-based) basis. At the heart of the model is the diffusion of an idea, a social behavioral innovation: acceptance of the person with leprosy. The model aims to achieve this by (Directorate General of Health Services [DGHS], 1992, 1993):

1 developing *knowledge* on the nature of leprosy, its amenability to cure, recognition of early signs of the disease, and prevention of deformities;
2 creating a reasoned and rational *attitude* toward patients, so that they are not ostracized from society, displaced from their homes, jobs, marriages, etc.;
3 promoting *social integration* of the leprosy patients [emphasis added].

SET was introduced in the 1960s around the time the classical diffusion of innovations (DOI) model was beginning to impact adoption of agricultural innovations in India. The model, therefore, shares many of DOI's structural and theoretical underpinnings. Its three interrelated innovation diffusion sub-systems are patterned on the diffusion model: the Gandhi Memorial Leprosy Foundation is the innovation-development system; the district level leprosy education society, the chain of primary health centers and subcenters, and the patients' families constitute the diffusion network; and the armies of leprosy health workers constitute the change agents. This structure ensures that the health system is represented at all levels. In terms of theoretical orientation, both SET and DOI are unilinear message-based persuasion processes. Both believe knowledge is the first step in bringing about attitudinal and behavioral change. The foci of the communication campaign are to tackle low awareness knowledge, low exposure to expert knowledge, low recognition of problem conditions, and a low priority to the "problem" by the local actors. The health worker is the disseminator of expert knowledge and is beholden to the state health system and its priorities and messages. The voices heard are that of specialists, experts, and celebrities (see Table 6.2). The bias in these systems and models is that they are slanted in favor of the state health apparatus and toward the project goals. The assumption is that local people lack a logical understanding of the concepts, cause, and cure of leprosy, and that the diffusion of "expert" knowledge will overcome low awareness and effectively destigmatize leprosy.

Krishnatray and Melkote (1998) showed through a field-based experiment in Madhya Pradesh, India that the diffusion approach utilized by the state health system generated lower behavioral involvement (of the subjects) when compared with a participatory communication campaign. The limited efficacy of the diffusion model in generating greater behavioral involvement can be better appreciated by situating it in the information-education perspective. This perspective is predominantly informed by clinical construction of disease. It derives its persuasive thrust from the message-based theories that postulate that dissemination of medical information will bring about desirable change

(Devine & Hirt, 1992). Anchored in the presumption that people do not know, do not know enough, or know incorrectly, the diffusion model strategizes information with the explicit purpose of "exposing," "creating awareness," and "imparting knowledge." The monologic nature of the dissemination of communication in which the health workers delivered what they believed to be the correct knowledge about leprosy has precluded the recognition and incorporation of the voices and contexts of the local people and their communities.

Local voices and context

What is missing in the diffusion of innovations approach employed by the state health care agencies is the absence of the voices and ideas of the local people. Essentially, these top-down approaches deny agency to the subaltern Indian people in Madhya Pradesh. The participatory approaches to communication and cure discussed later in this book invoke the arguments of the culture-centered approach (Airhihenbuwa, 1995; Dutta-Bergman, 2004, 2006). Dutta-Bergman (2006) posits:

> With an emphasis on speaking from the margins, on building episte-mologies from the margins, on creating alternative discursive spaces for the conceptualization of health, the culture-centered approach provides a theoretical framework for participatory communication projects, reversing the traditional one-way flow of communication from the core to the periphery.

Leprosy is a classic example of the tensions and contradictions between the expert's and the layperson's cultural–symbolic systems. The experts such as the medical doctors and leprologists posit that anesthetic skin patches are an early sign of the disease while the local people identify it with ulcers and deformity. The expert public health system pronounces that leprosy is curable. But, people believe leprosy is not curable. In any case, their concept of cure is very different from cessation of bacterial activity. The public health system believes that with the new multidrug therapy (MDT), segregation of persons with leprosy is a thing of the past. Despite the availability of the drug, sections of the local population consider it safer to isolate the person with leprosy. Whereas the diffusion of innovations model advocates the dissemination of medical knowledge of the disease and its symptoms, the local community is more interested in addressing social concerns such as fear and stigma. Rather than diffuse clinical information, the community is interested in creating experi-ences of cure with the active participation of the local people and the leprosy affected persons. Table 6.1 highlights the tension between the expert's and the layperson's cultural–symbolic system.

Table 6.1   Differences in perception of leprosy between the state health agencies and the local community

Variable	Expert system	Local cultural–symbolic system
Concept of leprosy	Disease	Curse or act of God; past sins
Cause	Bacteria	Mysterious
Contagiousness	Paucibacillary: no Multibacillary: yes	Highly contagious
Early signs	Anaesthetic skin patches; swollen nerves	Disease associated with physical pain; early signs of anaesthetic skin patches ignored due to lack of pain
Ulcers and deformity	Are a consequence of neglect; avoidable by early detection	Are causes of transmission of disease; no healing observed
Concept of cure	Both types of leprosy are curable	Not curable
Method of cure	Medication, hospitalization, rehabilitation	Segregation from community
Definition of cure	Cessation of bacterial activity ("bacteria kill")	Regain lost parts of body
Communication objectives of the program/ campaign	Disseminate correct information about cure and early signs; dispel myths and create reasoned and rational attitude toward patients; promote social integration of patients	Address social concerns such as fear and stigma; create experiences of cure; facilitate social interaction through three-way interaction between local community, patients, and the expert health workers on nature of disease, cure, and destigmatization

Participatory approaches to communication and cure

A discussion of the divergent frameworks adopted by the experts and the local communities brings into sharp focus the communication models used by change agencies including health-care agencies. Communication models have traditionally looked at communication as a process of moving a message through some channel with the hope that it will reach the receiver and that there will be an effect. The process is usually linear, top-down (from a health expert down to a receiver), and the message itself is prescriptive, preachy, and quite often very technical in nature. The intention in most communication situations related to health matters is to provide an effective mechanism of providing medical cure. However, this transmission communication model that is so widespread is not true to the real intention of communication. The root of the word "communication" is "communicare" or to build commonness and closeness between participants. Especially, in health-care situations such as eradication/treatment of leprosy, communication should involve the objectives of building understanding, empathy, and partnerships between the members of a community and between the health-care system and the community. Foregrounding the voices of the local community members and locating this agency within the local community praxis is paramount. After all, it is the local community that stigmatizes persons with leprosy and, therefore, it should be the community that must lead in destigmatization. This idea calls for a different model of communication. We advocate an organizing function for communication (besides the transmission function) that brings together the local community, the persons suffering from leprosy, and the state health-care system in a "trialogue" to collectively interact on the nature of leprosy, its cure, and destigmatization of persons with leprosy.

In a participatory approach to communication and cure, the individuals in the community are active in all the programs and processes; they contribute ideas, take initiatives, articulate their needs and problems, and assert their autonomy (Ascroft & Masilela, 1989). There is great diversity in participatory research methodologies. The following description brings together many of its tenets (Servaes, 1989; Kronenburg, 1986):

- It rests on the assumption that human beings have an innate ability to create knowledge and that this is not the prerogative of experts or professionals.
- It is an educational process for the participants as well as the health workers. It involves the identification of community needs, awareness regarding constraints, an analysis of the causes of glitches and the designing and execution of solutions.
- There is a conscious commitment of the health worker to work for the cause of the community.
- It is based on a dialectical process of dialogue between the worker and the community.
- It is a problem-solving approach. The objective is to discover the causes of problems by involving all the stake holders and to mobilize the creative human potential to solve social problems by clarifying the underlying conditions to those problems.

The model's major asset is its heuristic value. The close cooperation between the health worker and the community fosters an atmosphere in which all participants analyze the social environment and formulate plans of action. Most importantly, it recaptures the voices and context of the local actors and communities. Table 6.2 summarizes the participatory communication approach

Table 6.2 Comparison of the Diffusion of Innovations and Participatory Communication Models in leprosy communication, cure, and its destigmatization

	Diffusion of Innovations Model	Participatory Communication Model
Paradigm	Dominant (Ex. Diffusion)	Alternative: communicative social action (participatory)
Value/model	Transmission	Organizing
Belief	Lack of correct knowledge, attitude and behavior on the part of receiver of communication	Lack of sustained access to and availability of resources
Bias	Toward project goals	Toward community empowerment
Main issues addressed	Low awareness Low exposure Low recognition Low priority	Critical inquiry, collective action-reflection, *trialogue* (3-way interaction), emphasis on interpersonal contact, and cultural interpretations of disease
Objective	Create awareness— dissemination/education	Encourage empowerment and integration
Audience	Stakeholders, general public	Local community, families, caretakers, doctors, paramedics, social support network, traditional healers
Message	Intent: Disseminate "expert" information Content: Scientific information about disease, types of disease, treatment/curability, whom to consult and when	Intent: Skill acquisition and enhancement, capacity building, integration of stakeholders, redefine medical illness. Action: Create experiences of cure, build self-esteem, identify and train change agents, mobilize community groups, NGOs, media, etc., train for case detection and advocacy
Media	Mass media	Groups, volunteers, persons who have conquered disease, and other champions
Health worker	Expert; health system-faced	Co-learner and community-faced
Spokesperson	Specialists, experts, celebrities, leading writers, artists and journalists	Community members, cured persons, caretakers, researchers, NGOs

and compares it with the diffusion of health innovations model actively used by the state health-care system.

Krishnatray and Melkote (1998) directly compared the participatory approach to cure and destigmatization with the diffusion model through a field-based experiment in Madhya Pradesh, India. The participatory approach showed lower perception of risk, a higher knowledge of cause (of leprosy), and higher behavioral involvement of the subjects as compared with the target group in the diffusion approach. This evaluative study found several strengths with the participatory approach. Unlike the medical/scientific orientation of the diffusion strategy, the participatory model directly addressed people's fear of contracting leprosy by its dialogic and action components. These two components take as their premise the position that because the community stigmatizes the patient, it is the community that first needs to be released from fear of ulcers and deformity before the patient can be influenced to seek treatment (Patankar, 1992). The participatory strategy's dialogic component draws sharp distinctions between experts' scientific understanding and people's cultural interpretation of the disease. Thus, it recognizes different constructions of leprosy and creates space for contest and convergence between them. The immediate positive outcome of the participatory approach was dialogue between the health worker and the members of the community. A dialogue involves the group in a serious engagement on issues of concept, cause, and cure of leprosy. The health workers abet the participatory process by refraining from directing attention to themselves, that is, questions are deflected to the group, answers are avoided, clarifications are withheld, and conclusions are discouraged; instead, questions are raised to keep the dialogue going. The main arguments tend to be based on analogy. The purpose of the dialogue is threefold: to remove the health worker from occupying a position of centrality, to energize the group to collectively analyze multiple conceptualizations of leprosy by a process of cognitive agitation (Patankar, 1992), and to create redundancies in the communication situation so that an open and free environment built by this process reinforces the action component.

The action component of the participatory strategy rests on hydro-oleo-physio-therapy (HOPE), an inexpensive water-oil massage of ulcers and wounds patients undertake three times daily. The purpose of HOPE is also to let the group see for itself that ulcers, perceived to be sources of infection, gradually heal. However, the latent function of the therapy is more powerful. The act of seeing the health worker scrubbing and applying medication on ulcers raises doubts and questions on infectivity and patient-avoidance behavior. These doubts and questions are explained by an additional component of the action strategy: live case demonstrations. Unlike the diffusion approach that uses video film and slides, the participatory method strategizes its main arguments and attention around patients. Patients display their wounds and skin patches and narrate their trial and tribulation in dealing not only with the disease but also its social consequences. The sharing of life stories and personal experiences often creates strong emotional bonds between the community and the patients.

The effectiveness of the participatory strategy is additionally explained within the framework of the contact hypothesis (Allport, 1954). This suggests that health behavioral changes occur due to experiential learning. In contrast to modeling, which is essentially learning by imitation, contact can be hypothesized as learning by direct personal interaction with stigmatized categories of people (Miller & Brewer, 1984). Contact is not merely a structural property of communication as having the health worker, community members, and the patients together in the camp. Rather, it is the open, equal, and transactional quality of interaction between the three actors that is the defining characteristic of contact. In the case of the diffusion approach, the monologic nature of communication in which the health workers delivered what they believed to be the correct knowledge of leprosy precluded the real possibility of a dynamic three-way learning interaction. An obvious implication for health communication campaigns is de-emphasizing technical content and contextualizing information in the personal and social experiences of the group.

Discussion

The foregoing case study about leprosy, its cure and destigmatization, and the role of participatory and culture-based approach has to be subsumed within the larger discussion of the dominant and alternative frameworks used by change agencies in development-related initiatives in the third world. We will present the dominant approaches influenced by neoliberal/modernization policies and contrast them with alternative approaches that will need to be seriously examined and incorporated in eradication and/or treatment of persons with leprosy, a disease that involves both medical as well as social dimensions.

We have summarized in Table 6.3 some of the core ideas and practices in the dominant framework and contrasted it with the empowerment and resistance approaches. The *goal* in the dominant framework has been to promote community improvement or people development through the eradication of debilitating diseases or by provision of specific health development programs. This is good but not sufficient. In the alternative framework, the goal is building social justice, capacity, and equity in the community. The underlying *belief* in the dominant framework has been that the present conditions are mostly due to cultural and individual inadequacies and that there is a universal standard available for health development. This standard is usually articulated by the experts and is nonnegotiable. On the other hand, in the alternative framework, the belief is that the present conditions are usually due to a general lack of power and control of the people, especially their lack of power and control to access resources that are important for their survival or betterment. Additionally, there is a diversity of standards that may be set up by the community as opposed to the single standard of the experts.

The combined above-mentioned goals and beliefs have led to a distinct *bias* in the dominant framework. In general, there is insensitivity to the local cultures and their practice, the change directed is always by the sources external to the community, the process is deterministic and is usually toward a pre-determined end dictated by an external agency. The individual or the local community is the locus of change and blame and any anomalies are attributed to the inadequacies of individuals or local contexts. In other words, we see evidence of the victim-blaming hypothesis. On the other hand, in the alternative framework, the process and the solutions are culturally proximate to the community, the change directed is influenced by local ideas and sources, the process itself is open-ended and ongoing, and the locus of control is the local community.

The *context* is also important. In the dominant framework, there is little interest in the power relationships and structural constraints in the host community but in the alternative framework these factors become very important. The *role of the health worker* or the change agent in the dominant framework has been to consider him or her as an expert, a benefactor, and a nonparticipant. In the alternative framework, the change agent plays the role of a collaborator, facilitator, participant, and advocate for the people or the community, risk-taker or even an activist.

The *best examples* of work in the dominant framework have included the prevention of debilitating diseases or illnesses, remedy through/by experts, and use of mass media to diffuse standard messages that are usually prescriptive. In the alternative framework, the best examples include the activation of social support systems, social networks, mutual help and self-help activities; facilitate critical awareness; facilitate community and organizational power; and importantly, use communication to build and strengthen interpersonal relationships between members of the community. Finally, in the dominant framework the outcomes desired have been modernization, infrastructure development, and change in people's attitudes and behavior toward modernizing objectives. In the alternative framework, the outcomes have included an increased access of all community members to material, psychological, cultural, and informational resources; the honing of individual and group competence, leadership skills, and critical awareness skills; and, the building of empowered organizations and communities (Jacobson & Kolluri, 1999; Servaes, 1999; Tehranian, 1994).

Empowering the community

What then are the implications for practice in health communications? Empowerment requires more than just information delivery and diffusion of technical innovations. The objective of health professionals and other change agents is to work with individuals and communities at the grassroots so that they may eventually enter and participate meaningfully in the political, cultural, and economic processes in their societies. This calls for grassroots

Table 6.3 Comparison of development communication theories and approaches in the modernization and empowerment frameworks

	Development communication in the neoliberal/modernization frameworks (Diffusion of Innovations, social marketing)	Development communication in the empowerment/resistance frameworks (Participatory action research, empowerment strategies)
Goals	National and regional development, people development, community improvement	Empowerment of people, social justice, building capacity and equity
Belief	Underdevelopment due to economic, political, cultural, geographic, and individual inadequacies; existence of a single standard (as articulated by experts)	Underdevelopment due to lack of access to economic, political and cultural resources; underdevelopment due to lack of power and control on the part of the people; diversity of standards
Bias	Cultural insensitivity, environmentally unsustainable; standardization; change directed by external sources and ideas; deterministic process toward a predetermined end dictated by an external agency; pro-innovation bias; individual as locus of change and blame; victim-blame hypotheses	Cultural proximity, ecological; diversity; change directed and controlled by endogenous sources and ideas; open-ended and ongoing process of change; system-blame hypotheses; community or group is paramount
Context	Macro and micro settings; very little interest in local cultures or power relationships and structural impediments in host society	Local and community settings; cognizant of formidable power inequities and systemic constraints
Level of analysis	Nation, region, individual	Individual, group or organization, community
Role of change agent	Expert, benefactor, nonparticipant	Collaborator, facilitator, participant, advocate for individuals and communities, risk-taker, activist.

Communication model	Linear, top-down, transmission of information using big mass media; media treated as independent variables with direct and powerful effects; pro-source bias; asymmetrical relationship (subject–object)	Nonlinear, participatory, used to convey information as well as build organizations; increased use of small media, indigenous media, group as well as interpersonal communication; media treated as dependent variables; communication used for transaction, negotiation, understanding and not for powerful effects of a source; symmetrical relationship (subject–subject); horizontal flows of communication influence
Type of research	Usually quantitative (surveys), some use of focus groups, contextual or evaluation research	Quantitative and qualitative, longitudinal studies, labor-intensive participatory action research
Best practices	Prevention of underdevelopment; remedy through/by experts; blame the victim; individual adjustment to a dominant norm; use of mass media to spread standardized messages and entertainment; messages that are preachy, prescriptive, and/or persuasive	Activate social support systems, social networks, mutual help and self-help activities; participation of all actors; empower community narratives; facilitate critical awareness; facilitate community and organizational power; communication used to strengthen interpersonal relationships
Outcomes desired	Modernization; economic growth; political development; infrastructural development; change in people's attitudes and behavior toward modernization objectives	Increased access of all citizens to material, psychological, cultural, and informational resources; honing of individual and group competence, leadership skills, useful life and communication skills at the local level; honing of critical awareness skills; empowered local organizations and communities

organizing (Kaye, 1990) and communicative social action on the part of the individuals suffering from debilitating diseases, the poor, women, and others who have been marginalized in the process of social change. The implication then is a reconceptualization of the role of health communication. Greater importance will need to be directed to the organizing value of communication and the role of communicative efforts in empowering people.

So, what are the best practices the community can follow to deal with leprosy and its social ramifications? We have already pointed to practices such as the activation of social support systems, social networks, mutual help and self-help activities; facilitating critical awareness; facilitating community and organizational power; and, importantly, using communication to build and strengthen interpersonal relationships between members in the community. Thus, it is important that with the active use of practices such as the ones listed above, the community members need to be empowered to deal with the social stigma issue on their own even as the health-care system aggressively attacks the issue as a medical problem and provides methods of cure. Additionally, there are other ways in which communities may achieve empowerment in general. First, empowerment is achieved through organizational effectiveness (Speer & Hughey, 1995). Communities need effective organizations of their own that work for their self-interest, network with similar organizations, and compete effectively for resources. This provides a niche for community workers. They may be used to help local leaders in forming or strengthening local organizations, develop communication and problem-solving skills, and help in information gathering and networking. Second, effective organizations are sustained by strong interpersonal relationships (Speer & Hughey, 1995). Participatory approaches described earlier help in creating viable and self-sustaining organizations that are built through interactions with people based on shared values. The third tenet relates to individual empowerment and involves the concept of action–reflection. Individuals must activate their critical consciousness (Freire, 1970); however, they need to go beyond reflection to social action as part of an organized group. Organized groups provide a context and process for cognitive and emotional insights, for challenging new ideas and for testing and evaluating actions and behaviors. Over time, increased participation and reflection on the part of individuals are associated with their empowerment (Speer and Hughey, 1995).

Role of the health/community workers in eradicating leprosy and its stigma

In terms of general recommendations from the empowerment model in communication research, there are several factors that contribute to an effective intervention on the part of the workers. The role of the health worker would be as a facilitator. It requires the practical commitment of the external facilitator to the goal of social transformation. This may be achieved by the immersion of the worker in the praxis adopted by the community and by the rejection of an asymmetrical relationship between the health worker and the community members, that is, the subject–object relationship and its replacement by a subject–subject relationship. These steps are hard to achieve. Hence, some have argued that individual personality and motives are crucial in this type of work, and that only a selected few may be capable of sufficient sensitivity, humility, and self-reflexivity to do this work (Patai, 1999; Fals-Borda, 1991). However, in the end, the health worker's role will become redundant. Successful campaigns will mean that social change process moves forward with the momentum created by community dynamism and without the presence of the worker. Thus, the locus of control in this process rests with the community leaders, groups or individuals involved and not with the health worker, doctors, experts, or the sponsoring external organizations. While the professionals may have an important role to play in designing intervention strategies, they are not the key players. The key players are the people of the community, handling their problems in local settings and honing their competencies in the concrete experiences of their existential realities.

The community worker plays a very important role in the empowerment process. This person may be employed to work with the community as equal partners and help its members to:

- Perceive and articulate their social, cultural, historical, economic, and political realities
- Operationalize their needs
- Identify resources they need
- Identify, articulate, and operationalize possible solution alternatives
- Identify and gain access to individuals, agencies or organizations that are crucial to meeting their needs or solving their problems
- Build communication skills such as presenting issues cogently, resolving conflicts, negotiate and arbitrate
- To help the community members to organize and lead.

The model shown in Figure 6.1 may be used to illustrate the role of the important actors in the cure and destigmatization process. It suggests a *trialogue* with the health-care system, the community, and persons with leprosy constituting the three vectors. The health-care system through a cadre of health workers and health clinics forms the first vector. The health worker is in contact with the community through a dedicated community worker (or workers). Meanwhile, the health worker is in direct contact with persons with leprosy to provide the medical advice and cure. However, destigmatization takes place within the community. The second vector represents the local community with the community worker, community organizations, and leaders

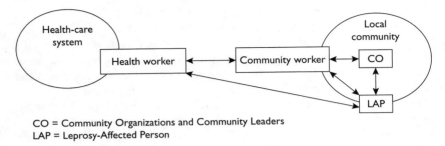

CO = Community Organizations and Community Leaders
LAP = Leprosy-Affected Person

Figure 6.1 Relevant actors in leprosy cure and its destigmatization

constituting the important actors. This highlights the community-orientedness. Destigmatization and rehabilitation of the cured persons will occur within the community and individual families. The health workers and the community workers are the most important catalysts in the process. Sometimes, the health worker and the community worker could be the same person or persons. The health/community workers can assist local groups and organizations and persons with leprosy in identifying and articulating possible solution alternatives, identifying resources that may solve their security problems, and identifying and gaining access to relevant authorities external to the system that are crucial to meeting their needs or solving their problems.

Conclusion

While the medical cure of leprosy may be a relatively straightforward process (www.who.int/lep/en), destigmatization of the disease is not. This chapter points to the possibility of reducing stigma using participatory communication and culture-based approaches. It suggests that strategies that address local cultural ideologies, engage patients, community and health workers in triadic dialogue, and incorporate action components have greater potential of reducing stigma.

We recommend public policy measures that would focus on resource reallocation, which would entail gradually scaling down assistance to voluntary efforts that permanently segregate patients and increase support for initiatives such as community-based preventive, promotive, and rehabilitative efforts to educate members about early signs, early detection, and early treatment of cases; community participation in delivery and referral systems; training of members of the newly formed village health committees and the village health worker; and, public efforts that offer hitherto neglected services such as reconstructive surgery, and rehabilitation of patients by training them in income generating professions. After all, an economically independent and self-reliant person can be the best spokesperson for desegregation.

References

Airhihenbuwa, C.O. (1995). *Health and Culture: Beyond the Western Paradigm.* Thousand Oaks, CA: Sage.

Albrecht, G.A., Walker, V.G., & Levy, J.A. (1982). "Social distance from the stigmatized: A test of two theories." *Social Science & Medicine,* 16: 1319–1327.

Allport, G.W. (1954). *The Nature of Prejudice.* Cambridge, MA: Addison-Wesley.

Ascroft, J., & Masilela, S. (1989). From top-down to co-equal communication: Popular participation in development decision-making. Paper presented at the seminar on Participation, University of Poona, Pune, India.

Browne, S.G. (1985). The history of leprosy. In R.C. Hastings, (ed.), *Leprosy.* London: Churchill Livingstone, pp. 1–13.

Devine, P.G., & Hirt, E.R. (1992). Message strategies for information campaigns: A social psychological analysis. In C.T. Salmon, (ed.), *Information Campaigns: Balancing Social Values and Social Change.* Newbury Park, CA: Sage.

Directorate General of Health Services (1992). *National Leprosy Eradication Programme: Status Report.* New Delhi: Ministry of Health and Family Welfare.

Directorate General of Health Services (1993). *National Leprosy Eradication Programme in India; Guidelines for Multidrug Treatment in Endemic Districts.* New Delhi: Ministry of Health and Family Welfare.

Dutta-Bergman, M. (2004). "The unheard voices of Santalis: Communicating about health from the margins of India," *Communication Theory,* 14(3): 237–263.

Dutta-Bergman, M. (2006). "The radio communication project in Nepal: A culture-centered approach to participation," *Health Education & Behavior,* 20(10): 1–13.

Fals-Borda, O. (1991). Some basic ingredients. In O. Fals-Borda, & M.A. Rahman (eds), *Action and Knowledge.* New York: Apex Press.

Freire, P. (1970). *Pedagogy of the Oppressed.* New York: Seabury Press.

Friedson, E. (1970). *Profession of Medicine: A Study of the Sociology of Applied Knowledge.* New York: Russel Sage.

Goffman, E. (1963). *Stigma: Notes on the Management of Spoiled Identity.* Englewood Cliffs, NJ: Prentice Hall.

Hirmani, A.B. (1992). Health education for early detection of "leprosy." In *Leprosy: A Reference Guide.* New Delhi.

Jacobson, T.L., & Kolluri, S. (1999). Participatory communication as communicative action. In T. Jacobson, & J. Servaes (eds), *Theoretical Approaches to Participatory Communication.* Creskill, NJ: Hampton Press, pp. 265–280.

Kaye, G. (1990). A community organizer's perspective on citizen participation research and the researcher-practitioner partnership. *American Journal of Community Psychology,* 18(1).

Krishnatray, P., & Melkote, S. (1998). Public communication campaigns in the destigmatization of leprosy: A comparative analysis of diffusion and participatory approaches. A case study of Gwalior, India. *Journal of Health Communication,* 3(4), pp. 327–344.

Kronenburg, J. (1986). Empowerment of the poor: A comparative analysis of two development endeavours in Kenya. As cited in Jan Servaes (1989), Participatory communication research within social movements. Paper presented at the seminar on Participation, University of Poona, Pune, India.

Miller, N., & Brewer, M.B. (1984). *Groups in Contact: The Psychology of Desegregation.* New York: Academic Press.

Patai, D. (1991). US academics and third world women: Is ethical research possible? In S.B. Gluck, & and D. Patai (eds), *Women's Words: The Feminist Practice of Oral History*. New York: Routledge.

Patankar, P. (1992). *Innovative Approaches to NLEP in Madhya Pradesh: Case Studies of Rajnandgaon and Durg, January 1987 to July 1992.* Report submitted to the Department of Health, Government of Madhya Pradesh, India.

Pryor, J.B., & Reeder, G.D. (1993). Collective and individual representations of HIV/AIDS sigma. In J.B. Pryor and G.D. Reeder (eds), *The Social Psychology of HIV Infection*. Hillsdale, NJ: Lawrence Erlbaum.

Scambler, G. (1989). *Epilepsy*. London: Tavistock.

Servaes, J. (1989). Participatory communication research within social movements. Paper presented at the seminar on Participation, University of Poona, Pune, India.

Servaes, J. (1999). *Communication for Development: One World, Multiple Cultures.* Creskill, NJ: Hampton Press.

Skinsnes, O.K. (1964). Leprosy rationale. *Military Medicine*, 130: 927–929.

Speer, P.W., & Hughey, J. (1995). Community organizing: An ecological route to empowerment and power. *American Journal of Community Psychology*, 23(5), pp. 729–748.

Tehranian, M. (1994). Communication and development. In D. Crowley, & D. Mitchell (eds). *Communication Theory Today*. Stanford, CA: Stanford University Press, pp. 274–306.

Part II

Culture in health communication

Introduction

Mohan J. Dutta and Heather M. Zoller

The growing racial and ethnic diversity within the United States as well as shifts in cultural processes in the realm of globalization have led to increasing attention to the concept of culture in health care. Attending to this broader call for incorporating culture in health care, health communication scholars have articulated the importance of addressing culture in the study and application of communication processes and messages in health settings (Airhihenbuwa, 1995; Dutta-Bergman, 2004a, 2004b). The relevance of addressing cultural issues through health communication programming has become particularly important within the United States as empirical evidence on racial distribution of health resources and outcomes has documented widening gaps between the haves and have-nots, with the health disparities often falling along racial lines such that African Americans and Hispanics experience poorer health outcomes compared to Caucasians (Dutta et al., in press). In the face of these widening disparities, health communication scholars have pointed out that perhaps understanding and addressing the cultures of underserved communities would provide an entry point for improving the health outcomes of these communities.

It is worth noting that much of the earliest discussions of culture in health communication started with a critical lens, directed as a critique of the lack of cultural responsiveness in existing health communication processes and interventions. As early as the 1990s, Lupton (1995) criticized the eurocentric assumptions driving health communication efforts and articulated the importance of addressing culture in health communication. Along similar lines, Airhihenbuwa (1995) pointed out that health communication interventions often suffer from eurocentric biases of individualism and Cartesian dualism, and therefore, fail to address the characteristics of cultural communities that often serve as the target audiences of these interventions. Responding to this call for addressing culture, two streams of health communication scholarship evolved that sought to theorize and develop health communication applications around the concept of culture: (a) the cultural sensitivity approach, and (b) the culture-centered approach.

The widely circulated cultural sensitivity approach is one of the predominant responses to the question of culture in health communication. In the cultural sensitivity approach, the emphasis is on developing culturally appropriate health communication programs. In the realm of physician–patient interactions, the cultural sensitivity approach focuses on developing culturally appropriate communication strategies for delivering health-care services. In the area of health campaigns, culturally sensitive health communication programs seek to develop culturally appropriate health messages that would be persuasive in the target community in promoting a specific health behavior. In both of these cases, the objective is to develop and fine tune health communication programs that are responsive to the characteristics of the culture. Culture becomes a point of entry for understanding, interpreting, and developing health communication interventions.

In contrast to the goal of the cultural sensitivity approach to develop culturally meaningful health messages and processes, the culture-centered approach engages dialogically with cultural communities to situate the meanings of health at the intersections of culture and structure (Dutta-Bergman, 2004a, 2004b). In other words, cultural contexts are explored in the realm of the social structures that constrain access to usage of health-care services and resources. These structures also simultaneously create openings for enacting agency; these avenues for enacting agency range from everyday practices of health that operate within the limited social structures to collective mobilization processes that seek to transform the unhealthy structures of health. Aligned with its goals of exploring the intersections of culture, structure, and agency, the culture-centered approach to health communication articulates the violence in dominant structures that create conditions of poor health, and simultaneously seeks to alter these structures with the goal of creating greater health capacities in local communities.

As opposed to the emphasis on tweaking health messages to cultural characteristics, the culture-centered approach emphasizes a dialogical journey with cultural community members that foregrounds the voices of cultural members in articulation of health issues and relevant health solutions. Culture-centered approaches seek to understand the co-constructions of health meanings through participatory engagement with cultural members. Participatory communication processes take the centerstage in order to create avenues for voicing the meanings of health through dialogues with cultural community members.

Although the two different strands of culture-based health communication theorizing, research, and practice followed different trajectories based on their epistemological commitments, they also share certain commonalities, and often interpenetrate each other. For instance, a health communication application that is designed to be culturally sensitive might evolve into a culture-centered framework after noting the necessity to address structural features of the environment through participation of local community members. Similarly, a

starts as a culture-centered program and articulates certain
nmitments might emerge into a culturally sensitive intervention
elements of the social structure have been recognized, and
n strategies need to be developed to promote a set of health
e community. In other instances, health communication efforts
might embody both elements of culture-centered and culturally sensitive
frameworks in addressing a specific health problem in a community.
Furthermore, across the spectrum of culture-based health communication
projects, there are some key issues that have continued to receive increasing
attention in recent years. These issues include questions of voices of local
communities, the emphasis on local contexts, the role of structures in health
communication processes, and the commitment to participatory health
communication strategies as entry points for engaging with cultures.

Health communicators have increasingly realized that local communities
need to play a vital role in the ways in which health decisions are made,
resources are allocated, messages are developed and delivered, and programs are
evaluated. This increasing emphasis on the voices of cultural community
members has led to research into communicative strategies that engage with
local community participants. This attention to voices of local communities
has influenced the ways in which health communication theories are
articulated, the development of methods for studying health communication
phenomena, as well as the applications that are developed to meet community
needs. This emphasis on community voices is seen in wide-ranging health
communication scholarship addressing the concept of culture. Post-positivistic
scholars working on culture-based health interventions address the voices of
local communities through formative research; interpretive scholars emphasize
local meanings articulated through the voices of cultural members; and critical
scholars attend to the question of voice by investigating the dominant erasures
of marginalized communities and by seeking to resist these dominant structures
by suggesting alternative epistemological entry points articulated through the
voices of hitherto marginalized communities (Dutta, 2008, 2007).

Culture-based health communication scholarship also suggests the relevance
of understanding health communication processes in the realm of the local
contexts within which they are situated. The emphasis here is on locating the
local context as an axis for interpreting and critiquing health-care systems. In
contrast to the universal assumptions of dominant health communication
theorizing, interpretive and critical scholars studying culture argue that health
meanings need to be understood within the local contexts within which they
are situated. Therefore, instead of searching for grand narratives of health, these
scholars emphasize the locally narrated stories of health through which health
meanings come to be constituted and understood (Dutta & Basu, 2007).
Interpretive scholars focus on meanings articulated within the local contexts,
and critical scholars study the local contexts in the realm of the structural
processes within which health is situated.

Structure is yet another point of emphasis in current scholarship on culture in health communication. Culture-centered health communication also draws our attention to the interpenetrations of structure and culture, noting the structural inequities that often play out in the constructions of culture in traditional health communication approaches, and suggesting entry points for introducing cultural voices that have hitherto been ignored by traditional health communication approaches (Dutta, 2006; Dutta-Bergman, 2004a, 2004b). The role of health-care structures in the realm of health is documented in a growing body of literature on health-care disparities that points out that racial and ethnic minorities systematically experience limited access to health-care solutions. The cultural sensitivity approach also seeks to address these disparities by focusing on developing effective health communication messages and processes that would appeal to the culture and hence be able to address the disparities by changing individual-level behaviors that put underserved communities more at risk. For instance, digital divide research in health communication targeted at underserved communities seeks to promote internet use in the context of specific disease states as a way of addressing disease-specific disparities.

Finally, with the focus on voice and context, much culture-based health communication work addresses participatory platforms for listening to the voices of local communities, articulated within the local contexts of health. Therefore, one of the common features of much of the culture-based work in current scholarship is the examination of participatory systems (Dutta & Basnyat, 2006). It is through these participatory platforms and spaces that alternative discourses are introduced and circulated, and points of change are articulated in the realm of the broader social structures within which health gets situated. Each of the chapters presented here in this Part II explore some combination of the culture, context, structure, and participation ingredients outlined here. They nicely demonstrate the theoretical, methodological and pragmatic contributions of this emerging body of work on culture and health.

In their chapter titled "Teach-with-stories method for prenatal education: using photonovels and a participatory approach with Latinos," Susan Auger, Mary E. DeCoster and Melida D. Colindres explore the role of stories in cultures, and the ways in which stories can be used to create culturally sensitive health education efforts. As an alternative to the more top-down "medical model" of health education efforts, the authors propose empowerment-based models of prenatal education with Latinos that emphasized cultural appropriateness and participatory learning. Drawing on the oral tradition of *teaching with stories* (TWS) and using *photonovels*, the authors suggest that culturally meaningful stories can offer entry points for addressing health disparities and improving health literacy.

Chapter 8 on "Ethical paradoxes in community-based participatory research" authored by Virginia M. McDermott, John G. Oetzel, and Kalvin White also addresses the issue of empowerment in the realm of a community-based effort to develop a peer-led multimedia prevention campaign directed at American Indian early adolescents. Through the example of the community-based effort, the authors explore the ethical paradoxes in the development of community-based participatory research (CBPR). McDermott et al. discuss the paradox of power, paradox of participation, and paradox of practice. The paradox of power plays out in community-driven but researcher-initiated participatory research, the sharing of financial responsibility but researcher-initiated funding access, and developing equal partnership but protecting the community and individuals. The paradox of participation is evident in the competing needs to value the community but also change the community, the decision about who participates, and the need to balance collaboration and participation with leadership and direction. Finally, the paradox of practice is manifest in long-term versus short-term goals of the project, research-oriented versus community-oriented directions of the project, and the supportive versus critical natures of the project. The paradoxes identified in this chapter provide valuable insight into the complexities of theory and practice in participatory health communication efforts that engage with the concept of culture, and align with the tensions between the culture-centered and cultural sensitivity approaches identified earlier.

Chapter 9 titled "*Voces de Las Colonias*: dialectical tensions about control and cultural identification in Latinas' communication about cancer", Melinda Villagran, Dorothy Collins, and Sara Garcia utilize the principles of the culture-centered approach to health communication to explore the ways in which economically disadvantaged Latinas living along the Texas–Mexico border interpret, co-construct and negotiate meanings of cancer through their communication with others. Building on the interactions among culture, structure, and agency outlined in the culture-centered approach, the authors suggest two dialectical tensions that emerge from the interviews around the concepts of control and cultural identification. The dialectical tension around the issue of control emphasized the views of the participants regarding the role of nature as opposed to the role of God. The tension around the theme of cultural identification was constituted around identification with Mexican culture and the Mexican medical system as opposed to concerns with the U.S. medical systems. The findings of this chapter suggest the relevance of exploring the interactions among culture, structure, and agency in the realm of understanding health disparities and finding ways of addressing such disparities.

In Chapter 10 titled "*El Poder y La Fuerza de la Pasión*": toward a model of HIV/AIDS education and service delivery from the "Bottom-Up," Ariana Ochoa Camacho, Gust A. Yep, Prado Y. Gomez, and Elissa Velez utilize the concepts of critical health communication praxis, "third-order" research, and collaborative community dialogue to describe the communicative strategies utilized by Proyecto ContraSIDA Por Vida (PCPV) that was created, implemented, and evaluated in Latino communities in San Francisco, CA. The authors outline a "living theory" of wellness, health behavior, and HIV/AIDS education constituted by Proyecto, and driven by a commitment to listening and organizing that would create a culturally affirming, holistic, grassroots, and alternative HIV/AIDS organization. The RICCA (Receptacle, Individual, Community, Crossings, Atmosphere) model was developed on the basis of extended engagement with the staff at Proyecto and was directed toward developing a model-in-practice that informs their work with the community. Through its articulation of bottom-up grassroots strategies, the chapter demonstrates the ways in which cultural engagement may facilitate transformative participatory action, aligned with the goals of the culture-centered approach to create discursive openings for social change.

The last chapter in this section, "Interrogating the Radio Communication Project in Nepal: the participatory framing of colonization," draws on the key concepts of the culture-centered approach to health communication to examine the participatory nature of an entertainment–education project that is often cited in the communication literature as an exemplar of the participatory genre of entertainment education projects. Through their critical analysis of the discursive constructions in the tactical materials of the Radio Communication Project (RCP) in Nepal, Mohan Dutta and Iccha Basnyat examine the communicative processes through which the concepts of agency and context play out in the project that is typically presented as an alternative to the more top-down models of health communication based on the diffusion of innovations framework. The authors argue that the project uses participatory language and participatory strategies to co-opt the participatory capacities of local communities into a dominant agenda, and instead pushes the agenda of population control as defined by mainstream actors such as the United States Agency for International Development (USAID) in ways that are much more aligned with the traditional diffusion of innovations framework. The chapter concludes by pointing out the importance of examining the nature of participation in health communication efforts that claim to be participatory.

In summary, each of the chapters in Part II focuses on understanding and engaging with the concept of culture in health communication. Part II highlights some of the tensions and paradoxes inherent in culture-based health communication work. It suggests that culture is constituted through the processes of meaning making that cultural members engage in, and is rendered meaningful in the realm of the social structures that constrain and enable the possibilities of health. Agency is enacted at these intersections of structure and culture, and is realized in the discursive processes of cultures. The chapters suggest the importance of creating, sustaining and supporting participatory structures and processes in communities that create openings for listening to the voices of cultural communities, and engaging with these voices in health communication practice. Part II provides insight into the nuanced nature of participation and ultimately suggests the need for additional health communication scholarship that theorizes about and conceptualizes the ways in which participatory processes might be mobilized in communities.

References

Airhihenbuwa, C. (1995). *Health and Culture: Beyond the Western Paradigm*. Thousand Oaks, CA: Sage Publications.

Dutta, M. J. (2008). *Communicating Health: A Culture-centered Perspective*. London: Polity.

Dutta, M. J. (2007). Communicating about culture and health: Theorizing culture-centered and cultural sensitivity approaches. *Communication Theory, 17*(3), 304–328.

Dutta, M., & Basnyat, I. (2006). The Radio Communication Project in Nepal: A critical analysis. *Health Education and Behavior*, 8 2006; vol. 0: pp. 1090198106287450v1 (http://heb.sagepub.com/cgi/rapidpdf/1090198106287450v1). Retrieved on July 5, 2007.

Dutta, M. J., & Basu, A. (2007). Health among men in rural Bengal: Exploring meanings through a culture-centered approach. *Qualitative Health Research, 17*(1), 38–48.

Dutta-Bergman, M. (2004a). Poverty, structural barriers, and health: A Santali narrative of health communication. *Qualitative Health Research, 14*(8), 1107–1123.

Dutta-Bergman, M. (2004b). The unheard voices of Santalis: Communicating about health from the margins of India. *Communication Theory, 14*, 237–263.

Dutta, M. J., Bodie, G. D., & Basu, A. (in press). Health disparity and the racial divide among the nation's youth: Internet as an equalizer? In A. Everett (ed.), *The MacArthur Foundation Series on Digital Media and Learning: Race and Ethnicity*. Cambridge, MA: MIT Press. http://heb.sagepub.com/cgi/rapidpdf/1090198106287450v1. Retrieved on July 5, 2007.

Lupton, D. (1995). *The Imperative of Health: Public Health and the Regulated Body*. London: Sage Publications.

Chapter 7

Teach-with-stories method for prenatal education

Using photonovels and a participatory approach with Latinos

Susan J. Auger, Mary E. DeCoster, and Melida D. Colindres

Prevailing studies in health care and health communication show that patient-centered or culture-centered approaches and empowerment-based strategies can significantly improve patient satisfaction, compliance, and health outcomes (Trummer et al., 2006; Massey et al., 2006; Institute of Medicine [IOM], 2003; DeCoster, 2002). These approaches, now being incorporated in the definition of "quality health care," have been shown to improve health literacy and reduce health disparities (Johnston Lloyd et al., 2006; IOM, 2004). At present there is a lack of empowerment-based health education and prevention programs that are culturally sensitive and linguistically appropriate. Most are based on traditional "medical model" pedagogy and clinician-centered models of care. They can be ineffective, or worse, can disempower and further marginalize women and ethnic minority groups, especially those who are poor and have low literacy skills (IOM, 2003, 2004).

DeCoster, a co-author and international board certified childbirth educator, shares a teaching experience that led her to seek alternative health communication approaches in order to be more responsive to the needs and interests of the Latino families she serves:

> I was at a community health center teaching a prenatal education class in Spanish. The group included Latinas with a wide range of education and experience. I used a traditional curriculum, with classic childbirth education materials and pamphlets. I was feeling particularly frustrated because many of the members couldn't relate to the materials ... even to my usually popular Spanish videos. Some couldn't even relate to the pictures in my most basic posters. Several women sat quietly, seeming to listen, but I didn't feel like I was reaching them. Others sat lifeless, looking quite bored. The few men in attendance had completely disengaged, and sat in the back of the room, talking in low voices among themselves. I remember a young mother-to-be from Guatemala struggling to understand since

> Spanish was her second language . . . that was the day I knew what I was
> doing wasn't working . . . I needed a different approach.

Patient-centered care is now recognized as a core health professional competency, central to meeting patients' evolving needs, improving the quality of care, and transforming the healthcare system (IOM, 2003). The IOM (2003) stresses that this approach is especially important given the ethnic and cultural diversity in the United States. Skills related to patient-centeredness identified through research to date include: sharing power and responsibilities with patients and caregivers; taking into account patients' individuality, emotional needs, values, and life issues; implementing strategies for reaching those who do not present for care on their own, including care strategies that support the broader community; and enhancing prevention and health promotion (ibid.). Community-based research is needed to translate science and recommendations like those in the IOM reports into interventions and programs that work in communities, where cultural and social factors are addressed, as well as practice needs (Baker et al., 2001).

In 1998, we began a community-based, interpretative inquiry into implementing the health promotion recommendations central to quality prenatal care, in a culturally and linguistically appropriate way for Latinas and their families in public health clinics (United States Public Health Service, 1989). Effective prenatal education can positively affect a woman's health and her infant's health through behavior change and self-care, self-monitoring, and initiation of timely intervention; foster the active participation of her and her family in prenatal assessment and decision making, and shape her expectations of pregnancy and prenatal care and increase her understanding of the scope and limitations of care (ibid.). The goal was to experiment with using the oral tradition of storytelling, a culturally appropriate strategy for Latin American cultures, in an innovative way (Airhihenbuwa, 1995). The proposed concept was to use photonovels (or photo-stories), a popular media format in Latin American countries, in combination with a facilitation process that incorporated theories on empowerment, culture, gender, and change.

The study examined two research questions. First, we explored ways to develop a simple, flexible, participatory educational process that can be used effectively in clinics with Latinos with diverse backgrounds and educational levels. Second, we tested approaches to helping clinic staff members with different backgrounds and training make the shift to a power-sharing way of relating and educating.

We used an existing series of easy-to-read, bilingual, culturally appropriate photonovels on prenatal care, created through a community-based approach by co-authors, Auger and Colindres. The spirit of inclusion, mutual respect and valuing of differences that fueled the development of the photonovels extended into our exploration of methods for teaching with them. Interpretative inquiry, having evolved in the attempt to give voice to the needs, interests and perspectives of the poor and marginalized segments of society, is a particularly fitting way to study and share what we have learned (Hubbard & Power, 1999). In addition, it supports the exploratory process and nature of learning through dialogue, practice, and the mutual negotiation and balancing of ideas, needs, and constraints (Dutta-Bergman, 2004; Hubbard & Power, 1999). Consistent with the theory and aims of the study, interpretive inquiry values a sense of connection to the participants and their unique experiences and embraces participants' stories as significant sources of meaning (Dutta-Bergman, 2004). These aspects are typically devalued in a quantitative evaluation process and lost in that type of reporting (Hubbard & Power, 1999).

To successfully develop an alternative educational approach that can improve the quality of prenatal care for Latinos could make an important contribution to on-going efforts to reduce health disparities (March of Dimes, 2002). Despite progress in recent years, health disparities among Hispanics exist related to access and quality of prenatal care (Centers for Disease Control, 2004). Hispanics also experience disparities in critical health conditions, such as high blood pressure, obesity, and diabetes, which can negatively impact pregnancy and delivery and adversely affect a woman's health across her lifespan (Regenstein et al., 2005). An additional contribution would be an educational model that could be tested and adapted for use with other topics and with other marginalized groups or those from other oral tradition-based cultures.

In this chapter, we present 1) a theoretical framework for the approach (henceforth called the "Teach-With-Stories (TWS) Method") based on a review of the literature, 2) the methodology, 3) the results, including a description of the TWS Method, findings from the groups, and highlights of lessons learned during implementation, 4) a discussion regarding tensions related to culture and change, benefits of this approach, and limitations of the study, and 5) the conclusion.

Literature

In this section, we first identify critical elements of participatory and culture-centered approaches, along with essential components related to empowerment and gender in order to establish a theoretical framework for the TWS Method. Second, we examine the characteristics of effective empowerment-based, culture-centered approaches and change to help assess the successfulness of the TWS Method in achieving the intended objectives.

Participatory and culture-centered approaches

The continuum of teaching approaches, that is, teacher-centered versus learner-centered, provides a helpful model for understanding the clinician-centered versus patient-centered continuum of care in health, and the types of changes that could be useful in making the shift to a patient-centered approach (Knowles, 1990). A didactic, teacher-centered approach, referred to as "pedagogy" in adult learning theory, is the most dominant form of education in the United States and Europe (Knowles, 1990; Hiemstra, 1990). It is commonplace in health professional education and training, with principles similar to clinician-centered care. The teacher is the "expert" who determines and organizes information to be disseminated in a logical sequence and presented through transmittal techniques, such as lectures. Participants are placed in a submissive role requiring obedience to the teacher's instructions (Knowles, 1990).

A participatory, learner-centered approach, also referred to as "andragogy," encompasses the principles and practices of adult learning theory and patient-centered care (Knowles, 1990). A participatory approach typically draws on participants' own experiences; actively engages them in the learning process to build knowledge and take action to solve and/or prevent problems (ibid.). It encourages teamwork and group problem solving around issues that are important to the participants, and emphasizes experiential "learning through doing" (ibid.). These aspects correspond closely to the key elements of a culture-centered approach to health communication (Airhihenbuwa, 1995; IOM, 2003). Also, participatory and culture-centered approaches emphasize that the participants' views, needs, and cultural values should be central in the design, implementation, and evaluation of the learning process (Dutta-Bergman, 2004; Knowles, 1990).

Empowerment

The use of power in relationships is a critical dynamic to understand, as the IOM's recommendation that health professionals enhance their skills in "sharing power" suggests. Cultural–relational theorists examine closely the use of power in relationships. Miller (2003) describes *power-to* as "the capacity to make change in a situation, large or small, without restricting or forcing others" (p. 5). The term *power-over* applies "to situations or structures in which one group or person has more resources and privileges and more capacity to force or control" (p. 5). *Mutual empowerment*, an alternative to power-over practices, is defined as "a two-way, dynamic process in which all people in a relationship move toward more effectiveness and power, rather than one moving up while the other moves down" (p. 8).

In relational–cultural theory, self-efficacy is viewed within the context of relationships and the multidimensions of culture (Hartling et al., 2003). This dovetails with the concept of *cultural empowerment* (versus self-empowerment) in culture-centered approaches. *Cultural empowerment* recognizes that health behaviors and outcomes are not just within the domain of individuals but occur and are influenced by political, social, historical, economic, and cultural factors (Airhihenbuwa, 1995). In a culture-centered approach, this broader context of decision making of individuals and families must be incorporated in health promotion and prevention strategies (ibid.).

Miller (2003) contends that mutual empowerment is possible in all relationships, even those that may be unequal due to differences in age, experience, knowledge, access to resources, etc. In relationships with power imbalances, such as parent–child, teacher–student, or therapist–patient, the more powerful member supports the other person and facilitates change toward mutuality and, eventually, equality. This is not to say the other person is powerless or that the person with more power "gives" the other person power (Airhihenbuwa, 1995). Jordan (1986) explains that mutuality implies "joining together in a kind of relationality in which all participants are engaged, empathic, and growing" (as cited in Miller, 2003, p. 2). There is a fundamental respect for the inherent dignity and equality of each other as human beings.

Participatory approaches are based on these empowerment principles. The teacher is a facilitator who shares power with participants and joins them in the learning process. Arnold et al. (1991) suggests that participants build and use power-with others, while drawing out and/or tapping into their power-from-within; for example, their own creativity, strengths, confidence, and/or spiritual source. According to Freire (1970), active participation and critical thinking are essential parts of empowerment-based education. The spiral model of action and reflection illustrates the key elements in any empowerment-based, participatory approach (Arnold, 1991, p. 38–39). Figure 7.1 shows how the learning process begins with participants sharing an experience. Participants move through a cycle involving reflection, adding new information, thinking critically, practicing new skills, developing plans of action, and taking action. Taking action leads to new experiences, and eventually to new knowledge, skills, and behaviors, in an iterative process of action and reflection.

Gender appropriate

Fishback (n.d.) and Collard and Stalker (1991) call for the use of techniques to help women identify their own concerns and develop their own strategies, using their personal experience. Collaborative, non-confrontational learning, such as sharing stories, is important for women in general, as well as being culturally appropriate for Latinos (Fishback, n.d.). Women also benefit from the chance to explore their identities in relationship with others and their societal roles (ibid.). Linking information to emotional content by acknowledging feelings in the classroom, through self-disclosure, storytelling, role playing, and literature, may be beneficial to the learning process too (ibid., p. 2). These more nurturing, "feminine" ways of knowing and learning, typically devalued or absent in traditional pedagogy, help validate and empower women learners (Collard & Stalker, 1991).

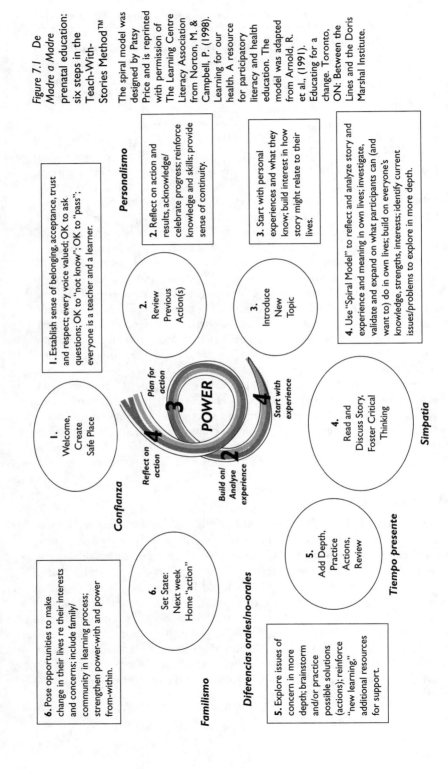

Figure 7.1 De Madre a Madre prenatal education: six steps in the Teach-With-Stories Method™

The spiral model was designed by Patsy Price and is reprinted with permission of The Learning Centre Literacy Association from Norton, M. & Campbell, P. (1998). Learning for our health. A resource for participatory literacy and health education. The model was adapted from Arnold, R. et al., (1991). Educating for a change. Toronto, ON: Between the Lines and the Doris Marshal Institute.

Personalismo

1. Establish sense of belonging, acceptance, trust and respect; every voice valued; OK to ask questions; OK to "not know"; OK to "pass"; everyone is a teacher and a learner.

2. Reflect on action and results, acknowledge/ celebrate progress; reinforce knowledge and skills; provide sense of continuity.

3. Start with personal experiences and what they know; build interest in how story might relate to their lives.

4. Use "Spiral Model" to reflect and analyze story and experience and meaning in own lives; investigate, validate and expand on what participants can (and want to) do in own lives; build on everyone's knowledge, strengths, interests; identify current issues/problems to explore in more depth.

1. Welcome, Create Safe Place

2. Review Previous Action(s)

3. Introduce New Topic

4. Read and Discuss Story, Foster Critical Thinking

5. Add Depth, Practice Actions, Review

6. Set State: Next week Home "action"

Plan for action 3

POWER

4 Start with experience

Reflect on action 4

2 Build on/ Analyse experience

Confianza

Simpatia

Tiempo presente

Diferencias orales/no-orales

Familismo

6. Pose opportunities to make change in their lives re their interests and concerns; include family/ community in learning process; strengthen power-with and power from-within.

5. Explore issues of concern in more depth; brainstorm and/or practice possible solutions (actions); reinforce "new learning," additional resources for support.

Characteristics of effective empowerment-based, culture-centered approaches and change

Empowerment-based approaches are cooperative, dynamic, and potential-releasing, in contrast to competitive, control-oriented, disempowering pedagogy (Knowles, 1990). They aim to cultivate what Miller (Hartling et al., 2003) describes as "five good things" characteristic of growth-fostering relationships. These outcomes include: *zest*—a sense of vibrant energy; *action*—enhanced sense of power to act; *clarity*—knowing oneself and others; *sense of worth*—when others important to us recognize and acknowledge our experience; and *desire for more connection*.

The Transtheoretical Model of Change (or stages-of-change theory) provides insight into how to facilitate and evaluate culture-centered behavior change interventions. People can be at different stages of readiness to make behavioral changes (Prochaska et al., 2002). The goal of the facilitator is to meet and support participants at whatever stage they may be, and provide an environment where they mutually support each other in making progress through the stages of change, that is, precontemplation, contemplation, preparation, action, and maintenance (Prochaska et al., 2002).

Culture-centered approaches have two main aims with participants: 1) to deepen understanding of environmental forces (personal, institutional, and societal), influencing an individual and/or group, and 2) to foster a willingness and ability to act on those forces to transform one's reality (Airhihenbuwa, 1995). Airhihenbuwa (1995) stresses that the resulting changes are as varied as the contexts—for example, individuals, groups, organizations, communities—where empowerment occurs.

Method

Participants

A convenience sample of 122 pregnant Latinas volunteered to participate in this four-phase study. The women were from diverse Hispanic backgrounds (Mexico, Central and South America), had a low socioeconomic status, and typically had low literacy skills in English and/or Spanish.

Phases I–III group members

Eighty Latina participants at various stages of pregnancy participated in the first three study phases. They were recruited from two community health centers and a rural health department in North Carolina. These women were typically in their twenties; however, there were a few teen mothers and some women in their early thirties. Some women were first-time mothers and others were mothers with children. A few husbands attended, as well as female relatives.

Some participants brought young children; childcare was provided. In Groups 2–5, families attended a weekend community session, with hospital and birthing center tours and a meal.

Phase IV group members

Latinas with high-risk pregnancies were recruited from the Neighborhood Health Plan of Rhode Island (NHPRI), a Medicaid health plan that partners with local community health centers. Of the forty-seven women contacted, forty-two participated at least once; twenty-two attended at least four of seven sessions. Some brought family and friends. Those who brought young children received childcare on-site.

Facilitators/participant observers

A total of ten facilitators with different backgrounds and skills participated in the study. Health education consultants facilitated the groups in Phase I and II. Although the consultants did not have prior formal training in participatory approaches, they did have experience in group facilitation and prenatal education with Latinas.

In Phase III and IV, staff members designated by the hosting agencies facilitated the groups and the consultants served as mentors. The educational backgrounds of the facilitators ranged from high school through graduate level social work and nursing degrees; most had no or limited prior group facilitation experience; a few had experience with traditional didactic health education classes.

Project coordinators/observer participants

In Phases I–III, the NC project coordinator and the two consultant facilitators formed the research team. The project coordinator brought experience in health professional training and curriculum development. She had a master's degree in social work, specializing in family and child health. Although her ability to speak Spanish was limited, she could understand, read, and follow the group dialogue in Spanish. In Phase IV, the RI project coordinator was a monolingual (English) nurse and manager for NHPRI. During the sessions, she observed the facilitators and group dynamics, and provided medical information as needed. She had no previous experience with participatory approaches.

Training of Trainers (TOT) participants

Twenty-seven participants attended the two Train-the-Trainer (TOT) workshops. The invitational TOT workshops, conducted in English, included the new facilitators, other educators, and selected staff and community members who could help support the TWS groups and assist with recruitment.

Materials

In all phases, groups used the *De Madre A Madre Prenatal Care Photonovel Series™*. There are seven photonovels, each with a unique story focus. The key topics include: conception, visit to clinic, nutrition, risks during pregnancy, labor, immediate postpartum care, and breastfeeding. The TWS Method and training materials evolved over the four phases of testing. In Phase I, formal facilitator materials were not developed in advance. The photonovels provided the content focus, while the Spiral Model provided a conceptual framework. In Phase II, the facilitators had an informal set of questions for each photonovel based on the actual questions and dialogue from Group 1. In Phase III, we developed a traditional, stand-alone training manual for facilitators in English. However, during the TOT practice sessions, participants found the manual design to be impractical and too cumbersome to use in the dynamic process. So for Groups 4–5, the team improvised and created a simple guide in Spanish, with informal questions for each photonovel. In Phase IV, we revised the TOT materials based on the experiences and feedback from Phase III, including creating a more concrete description of the approach, now called the six-step 'Teach-with-Stories Method,' and a facilitator guide prototype in English with a new user-friendly, highly functional, customizable design.

Procedure

We adopted the Plan, Do, Study, Act (PDSA) Cycle methodology since our focus was practice oriented. The PDSA Cycle is a quality improvement model with four iterative steps for continuous improvement and learning (Speroff et al., 2004, p. 34). Using the PDSA process throughout the four phases, the team tried out small changes under a variety of conditions. As shown in Table 7.1, the PDSA cycles are summarized for each phase. The planning step includes the changes to be tested which helped determine the core questions guiding the inquiry process. The study drew from the collective experiences, observations, reflections and dialogue with Latino participants, facilitators, observers, clinic staff members, as well as research team members. This resulted in a rich, participatory learning process.

Results

In this section, first we present the six-step TWS Method, followed by a discussion of cultural appropriateness and dealing with differences. Second, we outline and discuss seven themes that emerged across groups related to group characteristics and member participation. Third, we highlight findings related to the facilitators' experiences and staff observations. Fourth, we summarize lessons learned related to implementation. We conclude the results section with findings related to sustainability.

Table 7.1 Summary of PDSA cycles

Phase I (1998)

Plan:	• Shift from pedagogical to participatory process; test facilitation process with 2 facilitators.
Do:	• **Conduct Group 1**—8 weekly sessions with 17 pregnant Latinas.
Study:	• Data included: attendance log, field notes of session observations, and participant feedback (oral). Research team reviewed results and process through reflection and dialogue after each session and at end of Phase I.
Action:	• Document concerns, interests, questions asked; refine logistics and facilitation techniques. Conducted informal interviews with clinic staff including nurse, MCC supervisor, van driver, and receptionist. Conducted focus group with 7 participants three months later.

Phase II (1999)

Plan:	• Test applicability of questions/ideas from Phase I; 2 new groups; new site; effectiveness with 1 facilitator and a community session.
Do:	• **Conduct Groups 2 and 3**—9 weekly sessions each. A total of 35 pregnant Latinas participated.
Study	• Data included: attendance logs, field notes of session observations, and participant feedback (oral). Research team reviewed results and process through reflection and dialogue after each session and at end of Phase II.
Action:	• Refined group process, logistics further. Conducted TWS in-service for new staff at one site to enhance recruitment efforts. Conducted periodic informal interviews with MCC supervisor and nurse midwife.

Phase III (2000)

Plan:	• Test applicability of questions/ideas from Phases II; 2 new groups; new site; how to train and mentor new facilitators; effectiveness of 3 new facilitators; community sessions with different facilitators and at a new site; effectiveness with different incentives.

Do:
- **Conduct Training Of Trainers (TOT) Workshop I. Conduct Group 4**—7 weekly sessions; **Group 5**—9 weekly sessions; **Group 6**—never started due to staff shortage. A total of 28 pregnant Latinas participated.

Study:
TOT data: written evaluations and field notes of participant feedback (oral); 5-month follow-up telephone interviews of 4 TOT participants; research team review of results. **Groups 4–5** data: attendance logs and field notes re coaching/observations of mentors; session observations; participant feedback (oral). Research team review of process and results throughout series and at end of Phase III.

Action:
Refined facilitator skills; developed simpler facilitator guide; conducted informal interviews with clinic staff and observers. Conducted informal interviews of Group 4 MCC Supervisor & Group 5 facilitator 3 years later (2003).

Phase IV (2005)

Plan:
- Test revised TOT program and materials based on Phase III results; how to mentor new project coordinator and facilitators in a different type of organization and state; 4 new groups; 1 new site; new facilitators; biweekly sessions; new data collection strategies.

Do:
- **Conduct TOT Workshop II. Conduct Groups 7-11**—7 biweekly sessions each. 42 pregnant Latinas (high-risk only) participated.

Study:
TOT data: feedback from participants (oral) and written evaluations. **Groups' 7-11** data: attendance logs; meetings with facilitators; session observations; focus group with 8 participants (from Groups 7-11) and written "staff reflections" survey 3 months after project completed. Field notes of technical assistance provided re facilitator training, logistics, and evaluation.

Action:
Added 3 practice sessions before implementation since no on-site mentoring; ongoing refinements re facilitator skills; trained 2 new facilitators internally due to staff turnover. Currently completing additional evaluation activities.

Teach-With-Stories (TWS) Method

Overview

Everyone is a teacher and a learner in the TWS Method. In a typical session, group members volunteer to be the characters in the photonovel, or "photo-story," and together, read their parts like in a play. Teaching points and health issues are embedded in the stories. These give the facilitator natural openings and "*chispas*," or sparks, to stop and discuss. The characters' *and* the participants' life experiences, feelings, and beliefs are a vital part of the group dialogue. Those who cannot read can listen and participate in the discussion.

Six-step facilitation process

A facilitator, using six basic steps, actively engages participants in the mutual planning, implementation, and ongoing evaluation of the learning process. The six steps of the TWS Method are listed in Figure 7.1. Participants come together in a safe place. During the check-in process when the sessions are conducted in a series, they share how their week(s) went as they "practiced" doing something new or differently, celebrate successes and problem-solve issues encountered. Participants can work on the behavior change process with the support and resources of the group. This is a critically important component for those who may be isolated emotionally, mentally, and physically.

When introducing a new topic, the key is to start with the perspectives, personal experiences and knowledge of participants to build interest in how the story might relate to their lives. While discussing a story, a facilitator can explore and validate feelings, cultural norms, and beliefs; identify current issues and concerns of group members; tailor health messages and even terminology so it is culturally and linguistically appropriate for participants; and facilitate critical thinking. The dialogue can be adapted easily to the needs and interests unique to that group. After reading a story, there is an opportunity to review and reinforce health messages, add additional information and explore areas of interest in more depth; for example, through videos, role plays, and guests from community programs. In the final step, participants are invited to think of ways to practice making change and to create new meaning in their lives. In the next session, participants spiral through the six steps again, as the learning and relationships deepen.

Cultural appropriateness

The six steps occur in a way that honors and builds on primary Latino cultural values and norms. See Table 7.2 for list of definitions. As illustrated in Figure 7.1, the TWS Method incorporates these values and norms as members move through a session. The group is founded on respect or *respeto*. The TWS Method emphasizes and facilitates personal connections, *personalismo*, in the

Table 7.2   Definitions of common Latino cultural values and norms

Latino cultural values and norms	Definition
Respeto	Involves deference based on age, sex, social position, position of authority. Respeto in social hierarchy is not about politeness. It is a keen sense of mutual obligation between individuals. That "obligation" is founded on caring—caring for family, for elders, for children
Personalismo	Value of personal relationships and connections over impersonal, institutional ones
Simpatía	Kindness and caring
Tiempo presente	Present rather than future time orientation
Familismo	Reflects the high value placed on family, including the extended network of blood relatives, in-laws, close friends
Confianza	Trust based on relationships and established over time

Source: adapted from Randall-David (1989).

spirit of *simpatía*. These steps make the learning process feel "personal" easily and naturally. Kindness is the cornerstone of how the group listens, shares, challenges, and learns from each other as they read the photonovels and tell their stories.

The participatory process helps keep the focus on group members' present realities, immediate needs and priorities or *tiempo presente*. Learning that is relevant and can be applied immediately to one's life, is important not just from a Latino cultural perspective but also for women as adult learners and those who live in a culture of poverty.

The facilitator training, room set-up, and TWS Method are designed to help ensure that different verbal and nonverbal communication styles and norms, *diferencias orales/no-orales*, are accommodated. Latino norms for verbal communication include being emotionally expressive; nonconfrontational; not expressing negative feelings; and hesitant to disclose personal/family information to a stranger. So, for example, even if participants do not feel comfortable disclosing personal information, learning and a productive dialogue can still occur by discussing sensitive issues and key health messages through the characters in the story.

Nonverbal communication norms among Latinos include touching people with whom they are talking; sitting and standing closer than Anglos; shaking hands; engaging in an introductory embrace, kissing on cheek, back slapping (Randall-David, 1989). The circle format of chairs, for instance, allows for expressive movement and closer physical contact between group members than a traditional classroom setup.

The TWS Method invites inclusion of family members in the learning process whenever possible. This includes bringing to the sessions friends and relatives who may be a support for the pregnant mother; asking about the impact/feelings of family members during the dialogue process; involving family in "home action" activities; sharing information with others in their community, thus incorporating *familismo*. By following the six steps in the TWS Method each session, *confianza* builds among the facilitators and participants over time and is supported by respect, caring, and kindness. The bonds that develop often extend outside of the groups and last after the sessions are over.

Dealing with differences

We used the photonovel, a universal story, as the starting point for group dialogue about similarities and differences in knowledge, perceptions, and the past and present experiences of participants. Individuals became actors, literally and figuratively, in the learning process. Space was created for cultural dynamics, such as communication codes, meanings and context, to be explored and affirmed for each group of participants, a critical element of cultured-centered approaches (Airhihenbuwa, 1995). The TWS Method, emphasizing oral communication, invites all members to be storytellers and story listeners as they produce meaning and new connections rooted their cross-cultural exchange. A dialectical dance unfolded in the groups between themes of universality and locality/difference, between Western "science" and traditional views, and multisensory modes of communication. Adopting a salad bowl (versus melting pot) mentality, facilitators were able to harness heterogeneity in a constructive way and avoided disempowering, "culturally universal solutions" (Airhihenbuwa, 1995).

Group characteristics and member participation

In Phase I, we studied the process of making the shift to a participatory approach and observed the results, with attention to the following questions. 1) Did the group reflect the empowerment-based characteristics, such as vitality, mutuality, an enhanced sense of connection and motivation to learn? 2) How did group members participate; for example, were they actively engaged, did they ask questions? 3) Did the dynamics foster critical thinking, relevant content, a deeper understanding of the health messages, and changes in thoughts, attitudes and behavior? We continued to study the group characteristics and participation in the subsequent phases.

The results observed were consistent across groups and time, even with different facilitators, sites, and frequency of sessions. Participant experiences, team and staff member observations included many examples of these empowerment-based characteristics and participatory group dynamics. The major themes we found across groups are as follows.

1 Group members participated actively in the sessions, with a sense of "vitality" in the group

> At first, I felt "tentativeness" in the air, a shyness or timidity. Once the women got the hang of the photonovel process, members were quick to volunteer to read the parts. The groups had a dynamic energy, with a lot of enthusiasm in the group interaction.
>
> (Phase I: Observer field notes)

The "zestful" energy of the groups is characteristic of motivated participants and the empowerment process at work. Most significantly, these participants were from the same target population as those who were described as typically difficult to recruit, engage, and/or retain in traditional prenatal education classes by health-care providers in the study sites.

2 Participants built strong connections with each other

> The mothers in the class bonded quickly and formed a very supportive and cohesive group. They were soon calling each other outside of class time, and even giving each other rides, and so on.
>
> (Phase II: Group 3 facilitator field notes)

> Here we developed a "comadrearía" (friendship among mothers) that helped us through the pregnancy.
>
> (Phase IV: Translation—focus group participant)

> At the Beaufort classes, one mother was paying a taxi $30 per week so she could attend classes. Everyone seemed very eager to learn, and participated actively in the discussion. They also seemed hungry for contact with their peers. Some planned to visit the next series with their babies to help other pregnant women learn from their experiences.
>
> (Phase III: Group 5 mentor field notes)

These responses reflect an experience of social support and "desire for more connection" that was a common occurrence in all phases. In some instances, members did return to the sessions after they had their babies. In Group 5, they wanted to continue meeting after the series was over so they started a breastfeeding support group. According to studies (Beck et al., 1997; Goldenberg & Rouse, 1998; Rice & Slater, 1997; Sadur et al., 1999; Taylor et al., 1997) cited by Massey et al. (2006), "women with more social support and less stress were less likely to experience pregnancy complications, postpartum depression and adverse neonatal outcomes" (p. 288). Studies by Feldman et al. (2000) and Rickheim et al. (2002) (as cited by Massey et al., 2006) indicate that improved fetal growth and greater infant birth weight is also associated with prenatal social support.

3 Participants expressed a change in their experience and feelings of self-worth

Here (in the US), women are worthy. In our country we barely have some rights. Now I know that I am valuable as a woman, mother, and friend.

(Phase IV: Translation—focus group participant)

The women indicated that this renewed sense of worthiness and that they found "support in one another and no longer felt alone" were the biggest benefits of the program.

(Phase IV: draft focus group report, March, 3, 2006)

I am no longer scared to ask questions to my doctor.

(Phase IV: Translation—focus group participant)

As a maternity care coordinator, I spend a great deal of time discussing childbirth and related topics with prenatal patients. I have noticed a remarkable difference in the women who have attended the classes taught using this model. When discussing birth plans with these women, I have noted a great sense of confidence regarding the information that they have learned. One first-time mom explained the labor process to me as if she were teaching me how it is.

(Phase I: MCC supervisor, February 19, 1999, correspondence)

As these self-reports and observations suggest, participants were developing and strengthening their voice as women and mothers. In addition, their increased confidence and evolving sense of self translated into action and changes in behavior, such as a greater willingness to ask questions and share their thoughts and feelings during the group dialogue and with others outside of the group.

4 Participants learned new information and changed some beliefs and practices

In our countries we place our babies on their bellies when asleep and now I know that is not good. Now I know that babies should sleep on their backs.

(Phase IV: Translation—focus group participant)

During a discussion of the photonovel "Going to the Clinic," one woman reported that she was not going to prenatal visits every month because she didn't think it was necessary. Her previous baby had been healthy without prenatal care. The other women in the group advised her that she should go every month, and that it is very important to go. The facilitator explored with the group about some of the reasons why it is important to go to prenatal visits. The next week the woman was late to class because she had followed-through and went to her scheduled prenatal appointment. The other women gave her a round of applause and a lot of verbal approval and affirmation for keeping her appointment.

(Phase III: Group 4 mentor field notes)

In the "nutrition" class, one woman talked about really loving the taste of beer and wanting to continue to drink beer while pregnant. The other participants talked about how this was not safe for her baby and strongly encouraged and advised her not to drink beer while pregnant. This offered the opportunity for the facilitator to talk more about the effects of alcohol on fetuses and also the availability of support for her if she wanted to stop drinking beer but couldn't by herself. The next week the photonovel topic was *Risks During Pregnancy*, which specifically raised the issue of the dangers of drinking while pregnant and the availability of treatment programs for addiction problems. This reinforced the women's advice and the facilitator's information shared the week before. During one of the following sessions, the woman reported that now she was not drinking because she wanted to have a healthy child.

(Phase II: Group 4 facilitator field notes)

These anecdotes help illustrate four important dynamics: 1) the role of flexibility of the facilitator and participants and the value of putting into practice the principle that "everyone is a teacher and a learner"; 2) the critical thinking process fostered by the spiral model; 3) the resulting connected learning context, that is, matching of health information to the participants' logic, language, and experience; and 4) the group members' movement through the stages of change.

5 Participants found the sessions relevant to their lives and concerns

When discussing the *Risks During Pregnancy* photonovel, the women initiated and carried out a very honest discussion about the pain of growing up being abused as children and they do not want to repeat this and inflict this suffering on their own children. The discussion also included the connection of domestic violence between parents. They offered one another a lot of validation, support, and empathy. I added pertinent information about parenting, the dynamics of domestic violence and encouragement to seek help if the women are in this type of situation now. The group discussed places and people who could provide help.

(Phase II: Group 3 facilitator field notes)

Unlike a control-oriented, didactic format, the "*chispas*" or sparks create a way for participants to speak spontaneously about issues and concerns pertinent in their lives, as illustrated in this example. The group dialogue format creates a safe space for women to voice underlying feelings and perceptions about their relationships, dreams, and difficulties. Just being heard and accepted can be therapeutic. When resources and ideas for possible action are discussed in this type of context, a move toward action is more likely. For example, in one group after a similar discussion, a participant encouraged a neighbor in a domestic violence situation to seek help. With the assistance of community resources, the mother and her two children relocated to another state to safety.

> We feel much less anxiety about having our baby. Many of our questions were answered about practical things—like parking, where to go and how to get around in the hospital, and who can attend the birth.
> (Phase III: Translation—couple who attended the community/family
> session Group 4 facilitator field notes)

Practical, hands-on learning experiences, such as the family session with a hospital and birthing center tour, enhanced the sense of relevance and value of the sessions among the whole family. These sessions in particular helped bridge cultural and language differences, making the local health-care resources more accessible and user-friendly.

6 Participants shared what they were learning with others

> Another great benefit I have noticed is the communication that continues beyond the classroom. As many of the women ride on the prenatal van, they have to wait for a while after the class is over for other women to be seen by the provider. On several occasions, I have heard the women discussing the topics with each other and with other pregnant women who did not attend the classes. Not only have the women formed a bond amongst themselves, they are also reaching out to other women indicating their level of confidence with the information.
> (Phase I: MCC supervisor, February 19, 1999, correspondence)

Observations and self-reports of "teach-back" examples were common among group members across all four phases. When people "teach back" new information in their own words to someone else, it indicates comprehension and that they have assumed "ownership." Their interaction with the information enhances and reinforces long-term retention (Doak et al., 1996).

7 Participants' often brought or referred other women to the groups

Unanimously, these women indicated that they wanted more classes and some of them have already "referred" some friends.

(Phase IV: project coordinator field notes, telephone debriefing-focus group facilitator)

The participants' willingness to bring and refer their family and friends in their community is a strong indicator of acceptance and satisfaction with the TWS Method and use of photonovels for prenatal education. Their feedback during the series debriefings and observations of facilitators and observers were consistent with these actions.

Facilitator experiences and staff perceptions

Facilitators across the groups expressed feeling a closeness and bond with group members and a greater sense of empathy and understanding of their life circumstances and needs.

I was attending the groups as an observer and at the end all the moms came by, hugged me, and thanked me for my help. And I don't even speak Spanish!

(Phase IV: facilitator reflections survey)

Regardless of your Spanish speaking abilities, you must be open and try to understand the participant's needs. Some women have left children in their native countries trying to make it here! If you are not sympathetic to their plights, then you fail as a facilitator.

(Phase IV: facilitator reflections survey)

The TOT workshops and group experiences have also helped the facilitators and clinic staff members deepen their understanding of the dimensions of effective education, especially for marginalized groups and people with low literacy skills. They reported a greater appreciation of the power of the participatory-based TWS Method to meet these needs in a culturally appropriate way.

Working with the photonovels has given me a broader picture of what effective communication is. Latinas not only need information but also need to have a sense of community and to feel empowered and respected . . . to feel that people are truly interested in their well-being . . . Pamphlets may have accurate information and say to do this or that but these (information dissemination only) approaches leave all the other pieces out of the picture.

> (Phase IV: NC project coordinator field notes,
> facilitator "reflections" interview)

I have been very impressed with the results I have seen in the patients attending these classes. Having taught childbirth classes myself using a traditional childbirth class curriculum, I would like to highly recommend this model . . . the participants are able to learn the material and feel more confident rather than fearful. I feel this is a vital part of promoting healthy pregnancies.

> (Phase I: MCC supervisor, correspondence, February 19, 1999)

The team observed that for some facilitators, especially those with more health professional training, making a shift to the participatory process was quite anxiety provoking. However, the facilitation guides and mentoring in Phase III and the concrete steps of the method developed in Phase IV, along with the practice sessions, helped provide enough structure to make the change easier.

> I'm afraid of letting go and losing control . . . what if no one talks or what if the members do talk and just go off on tangents?
> (Phase III: Group 4 mentor field notes—dialogue with facilitator)

Facilitators expressed a greater sense of personal and professional sense of satisfaction with the heightened sense of mutuality and shift to a power-sharing, growth-fostering way of relating. Facilitators experienced and others observed that they could transfer this way of relating and the associated skills to relationships outside of the prenatal groups.

> The TWS method has provided valuable lessons for us at NHPRI relating to the benefits of a high-touch approach in member education. We plan to apply these lessons to additional targeted member groups in 2006. Our goal is to partner with provider practices to implement high-touch participatory member education. Areas of opportunity for NHPRI include adolescent well-care, teen pregnancy prevention, weight management, and women's health issues.
> (Phase IV: RI-project coordinator, correspondence,
> December 22, 2005)

Implementation issues and feasibility of replication

We tested the feasibility of replicating the TWS Method at four sites: three in NC and one in Rhode Island. In several sites, groups were launched successfully despite some difficult circumstances, such as budget constraints, lack of trained Spanish-speaking staff, lack of transportation, and historically poor attendance to other types of classes by Latinos.

We experienced how critical building alliances and collaborating with community partners can be for starting up and sustaining a program. For example, an interview with facilitator "E" (Group 5) three months after the project ended revealed:

> The co-facilitation of a health department staff member and volunteer from the Episcopal Hispanic Ministry worked out very well. They were excited about the success of the first series and are looking forward to doing another series together. The Episcopal Hispanic Ministry provided some funds for the community session and is planning to help financially support another series in the fall . . . (In addition to the strong agency partnerships that evolved) Facilitator "E" reports that the network among the mothers and their families in the communities has also deepened.
>
> (Phase III: Group 5 project coordinator field notes)

However, a successful start-up is not always guaranteed, even with resources and training. For instance, despite having a willing, interested, and trained facilitator, an existing infrastructure, including transportation for prenatal clients, and having already held two successful TWS groups, Group 6 was not launched due to staff shortages. The other educators who attended the TOT I workshop (who were not involved in Groups 4 or 5) did not start up a series either. Some of the reasons they gave in a five month follow-up telephone interview included no time, other priorities, no organizational support or interest.

We learned that orienting clinic staff members about the groups can help recruitment. Touching base with key staff members, such as maternity care coordinators, medical providers, and receptionists, throughout the series can help with evaluation and attendance. For example, we encouraged them to ask participants about their experiences and reinforce attendance. Incentives were used in all phases, although they varied. For example, in Phase I participants received small baby gifts. In Phases II–III, participants received a new car seat at the end of the series if they attended a designated number of sessions. In Phase IV, participants received grocery store gift cards, along with other smaller gifts. While participants expressed enthusiasm about receiving incentives, their impact on enrollment and attendance is not clear.

Factors related to sustainability

We identified three factors that suggest that the TWS groups are sustainable. First, the TWS groups were still being offered at both Phase III sites three years after the grant funds ended. For example, at the Beaufort site, they continued to offer TWS groups in the spring and fall in partnership with the Episcopal Hispanic Ministries, a breastfeeding support group, along with a cookout and family gathering. The program had a strong reputation in the community, and the facilitator reported that it was considered to be a "real privilege" to attend (2003 Phase III follow-up: project coordinator field notes).

Second, when there was staff turnover, the project team/facilitators were able to train other facilitators themselves. In Phase IV, the positive participant feedback indicated that this was done successfully. However, at the Carrboro site, we were not able to assess or substantiate the level of training effectiveness.

Third, the organizations offering the TWS groups received feedback from participants that their experience with the TWS approach improved the public perception of their organizations.

> All participants were thrilled with the experience provided by NHPRI. They raved about the facilitators, especially their sincere concern for the participant's well-being. According to these women, the staff's courtesy, and attention to individual needs as well as education provided makes NHPRI "lo mejor que existe" (the best there is).
> (Phase IV: draft focus group report, March 3, 2006)

Discussion

Our findings suggest that the use of photonovels and the TWS Method does offer an effective empowerment-based, educational alternative that respects and reinforces important Latino cultural values and builds on women's strengths. Its simplicity and flexibility make it possible to implement in public health settings with the support and leadership of clinic staff and management. Despite changes in facilitators, sites, and group members, reports from participants, facilitators, and observers were consistent across the four phases. They described experiences and observations reflective of the five "good things" characteristic of growth-fostering relationships.

Tensions related to culture and change

One question raised at the outset of this study concerned the cultural appropriateness and effectiveness of this approach given Latino cultural norms regarding respect and deference to authority figures, such as doctors. Some Latinos can be reluctant to ask questions or engage in dialogue that may appear critical for fear of appearing disrespectful. Also, some may fear retaliation or negative consequences for themselves or their families due to one's legal status or the perception that they are challenging existing power-over dynamics. A related, but opposite, power-over dilemma is that some clients desire and expect the doctor or other health professional to be the "expert." In this instance, being directive and telling clients what to do is perceived as competence since, for example, the doctors are the ones with a medical education.

Perhaps this desire and expectation are truly cultural norms, or simply personal preferences, and/or maybe they reflect underlying issues of internalized oppression at individual and/or sociopolitical levels. Regardless, a culture-centered approach requires respect and consideration of the participants' needs, feelings, and perceptions. Health care is seen as more than medical care, health and health-related decisions are recognized as a multidimensional phenomenon (Airhihenbuwa, 1995). Therefore, health-care providers and educators must find innovative ways to include the views of individuals, the community, and traditional health beliefs and practices, as well as scientific views and Western, biomedical beliefs and practices.

The shift from a disease-focused, clinician-centered approach to a wellness-focused, culture-centered model of care and communication is an evolving process. It requires a change in paradigms and action for everyone involved. The TWS Method is not designed to force empowerment on others but rather to create the space for individuals to come together in a spirit of mutual respect and caring, to foster reflection and critical thinking about choices they have made and are presented with in their daily life experiences and the multiple cultures in which they dwell. The team took these concerns seriously, recognizing that participants may also need support to make the shift to a power-sharing process. The TOT workshop, training materials, and facilitator guides help raise awareness of these issues, along with strategies to address them.

Benefits

Health literacy is more than the ability to read and write; it involves a person's ability to obtain, understand, effectively use basic medical instructions and health information, and make informed choices (IOM, 2004). True appreciation for the complex dynamics that influence health literacy requires understanding the interconnections of culture at individual and societal levels (ibid.). The TWS six-step participatory approach helps address these types of health literacy needs in a safe and responsive environment. Participants can explore and think critically about feelings, perceptions, and needs related to issues, problems, and desired changes relevant to their daily lives. They can also give and receive practical support, such as sharing rides and childcare, as well as informational and emotional support.

The emphasis on participation and critical thinking may have also enhanced the way participants learned and retained information. When information is verbally transmitted (traditional lecture), only 20 percent of the material is retained, but the amount retained can increase up to 90 percent when people "hear, see, talk, and do" (Arnold et al., 1991, p. 40). Health information embedded in the stories and participatory process also put into practice effective health literacy strategies, especially for poor readers and nonreaders. Research shows that information learned in context and connected to what the participants already know is more likely to be understood, remembered, and used by learners than facts disseminated in a pamphlet or a didactic lecture (Doak et al., 1996).

In addition, our findings suggest that, through the use of TWS groups, health professionals can enhance their skills and competencies, increase their satisfaction, and accomplish the objectives related to patient-centered care. The training and TWS Method provided support and a practical way to shift to a power-sharing paradigm to actively engage clients in their own care. Finally, health professional feedback points to many other potential applications of the TWS Method.

Limitations and implications for future research

The major limitation to this study is its sampling method. The convenience sample of participants recruited through local clinics or a health plan membership may not represent Latinas who do not have access to health care, who do not seek prenatal care and/or do not self-select for prenatal education. Although once group members experienced the process, they often referred other women to the sessions. This suggests that the TWS Method may be an effective outreach strategy. However, resource constraints did not permit us to follow up members who attended only once. This kind of follow-up in future groups could provide valuable information for refining the method, materials, and implementation strategies to further improve quality and outreach capabilities.

Other limitations include the relatively small sample sizes which may have limited the external validity, and possible observational biases which may have compromised the study's internal validity. The collaborative study process between Latina participants, facilitators, and project coordinators helped minimize the risk of over-interpreting the results.

Further study is needed on how to improve implementation efficiency and capacity building. Additional information regarding cost effectiveness and the program's impact on individuals, staff members, and the community could help advocate for funding and system changes to support using the photonovels and TWS Method. Further research regarding the effectiveness of the TWS Method with other groups, in other languages and other topics could prove to be beneficial given the pervasive problems related to health literacy needs and health disparities.

Conclusion

Our findings support the use of the *De Madre a Madre* photonovels and the Teach-With-Stories Method for prenatal education as a practical and effective approach to improve the quality of prenatal education for Latinos. It proved to be an effective way to connect with and provide meaningful support to pregnant Latino women and their families with a wide range of literacy levels. Group members were able to build relationships with each other, while they explored their feelings, needs, and interests as mothers, Latinas, and women. Participants shared and learned about information and resources that could be used and applied immediately in their lives and to real-life problems. These dynamics appeared to be instrumental in supporting and fostering behavior change. Working *with* the women and their families, health professionals were able to identify problems and potential barriers to care early, make appropriate referrals, and assist women in navigating the health-care system, while improving their skills and job satisfaction. The TWS Method, with potential applications for other health issues and populations, does appear to provide a feasible, innovative option for improving health literacy, reducing health disparities, and supporting the health-care system transformation currently underway.

References

Airhihenbuwa, C.O. (1995). *Health and Culture: Beyond the Western Paradigm.* Thousand Oaks, CA: Sage.

Arnold, R., Burke, B., James, C., Martin, D., & Thomas, B. (1991). *Educating for a Change.* Toronto, Canada: Doris Marshall Institute for Education and Action.

Auger, S., & Colindres, M. (1997). *De Madre a Madre/From Mother to Mother Prenatal Care Photonovel Series.* Durham, NC: Aprendo Press.

Baker, E.L., White, L.E., & Lichtveld, M.Y. (2001). Reducing health disparities through community-based research: A commentary. *Public Health Reports, 116,* 517–519.

Beck, A., Scott, J.,Williams, P., Robertson, B., Jackson, D., Gade, G., et al. (1997). A randomized trial of group outpatient visits for chronically ill older HMO members: The Cooperative Health Care Clinic. *Journal of the American Geriatrics Society, 45,* 543–549.

Centers for Disease Control. (2004, October). Health Disparities Experienced by Hispanics—United States. (Electronic version). *MMWR Weekly, 53*(40): 935–937.

Collard S., & Stalker, J. (1991). Women's trouble: Women, gender, and the learning environment. In R. Hiemstra (ed.), *New Directions for Adult and Continuing Education.* San Francisco: Jossey-Bass, pp. 71–80.

DeCoster, M.E. (2002). Empowerment education for promoting breastfeeding among Latinas: A pilot evaluation. Master's thesis, University of North Carolina, Chapel Hill, School of Public Health, Department of Health Behavior and Health Education.

Doak, C., Doak, L., & Root, J. (1996). *Teaching Patients with Low Literacy Skills,* 2nd edn. Philadelphia, PA: J.B. Lippincott Company.

Dutta-Bergman, M.J. (2004). The unheard voice of Santalis: Communicating about health from the margins of India. *Communication Theory, 14,* 237–263.

Feldman, P.J., Dunkel-Schetter, C., Sandman, C.A., & Wadhwa, P.D. (2000). Maternal social support predicts birth weight and fetal growth in human pregnancy. *Psychosomatic Medicine, 62*, 715–725.

Fishback, S.J. (n.d.). Professional tips for adult and continuing educators: Tips on teaching women. Retrieved on December 20, 2005 from http://home.twcny.rr.com/hiemstra/tips.html

Freire, P. (1970). *Pedagogy of the Oppressed.* New York, NY: The Seabury Press.

Goldenberg, R.L., & Rouse, D.J. (1998). Medical progress: Prevention of premature birth. *New England Journal of Medicine, 339*, 313–320.

Hartling, J.M., Miller, J.B., Jordan, J.V., & Walker, M. (2003). Introducing relational-cultural theory: A new model of psychological development. Retrieved December 20, 2005, from www.tribal-institute.org/2004/handouts/C10%20-%20Pamela%20Burgess-Responding%20to%20Violence%20Against%20Native%20LGBT-All%20Handouts.pdf

Hiemstra, R. (1990). Moving from pedagogy to andragogy. *Instructional Developments, 1*(3).

Hubbard, R.S., & Power, B.M. (1999). *Living the Questions: A Guide for Teacher-researchers.* Portland, ME: Stenhouse Publishers.

Institute of Medicine. (2003). *Health Professions Education: A Bridge to Quality.* Washington, DC: National Academies Press.

Institute of Medicine. (2004). *Health Literacy: A Prescription to end Confusion.* Washington, DC: National Academies Press.

Johnston Lloyd, L.L., Ammary, N.J., Epstein, L.G., Johnson, R., & Rhee, K. (2006). A transdisciplinary approach to improve health literacy and reduce disparities. *Health Promotion Practice, 7*(3), 1–5.

Jordan, J. (1986). The meaning of mutuality, *Work in Progress*, No. 23, Wellesley, MA: Stone Center Working Paper Series.

Knowles, M. (1990). *The Adult Learner: A Neglected Species.* Houston, TX: Gulf Publishing Company.

March of Dimes. (2002). Obstetrics and diversity in the US: Se habla español? (Electronic version). *Contemporary Ob/Gyn, 9*, 102–111.

Massey, Z., Rising, S.S., & Ickovics, J. (2006). Centering pregnancy group prenatal care: Promoting relationship-centered care. *Journal of Obstetric, Gynecologic, and Neonatal Nursing, 35*, 286–294.

Miller, J.B. (2003). Telling the truth about power. (Electronic version). *Work in Progress*, No. 100. Wellesley, MA: Stone Center Working Paper Series.

Prochaska, J.O., Redding, C.A., & Evers, K.E. (2002). The transtheoretical model and stages of change. In K. Glanz, B.K. Rimer, & F.M. Lewis (eds), *Health Behavior and Health Education: Theory, Research, and Practice*, 3rd edn. San Francisco: Jossey-Bass, pp. 99–120.

Randall-David, E. (1989). *Strategies for Working with Culturally Diverse Communities and Clients.* Washington, DC: Association for the Care of Children's Health.

Regenstein, M., Cummings, L., & Huang, J. (2005). *Barriers to Prenatal Care: Findings from a Survey of Low-income and Uninsured Women who Deliver in Safety Net Hospitals.* Washington, DC: National Public Health and Hospital Institute.

Rice, R.L., & Slater, C.J. (1997). An analysis of group versus individual child health supervision. *Clinical Pediatrics, 36*, 685–689.

Rickheim, P.L., Weaver, T.W., Flader, J.L., & Kendall, D.M. (2002). Assessment of group versus individual diabetes education: A randomized study. *Diabetes Care, 25,* 269–274.

Sadur, C.N., Moline, N., Costa, M., Michalik, D., Mendlowitz, D., Roller, S., et al. (1999). Diabetes management in a health maintenance organization: Efficacy of care management using cluster visits. *Diabetes Care, 22,* 2011–2017.

Speroff, T., James, B.C., Nelson, E.C., Headrick, L.A., & Brommels, M. (2004). Guidelines for appraisal and publication of PDAS quality improvement. *Quality Management in Health Care, 13*(1), 33–39.

Taylor, J.A., Davis, R.L., & Kemper, K.J. (1997). A randomized controlled trial of group versus individual well child care for high-risk children: Maternal-child interaction and developmental outcomes. *Pediatrics, 99,* E9.

Trummer, U.F., Mueller, U.O., Nowak, P., Stidl, T., & Pelikan, J.M. (2006). Does physician–patient communication that aims at empowering patients improve clinical outcome? A case study. *Patient Education and Counseling, 61,* 299–306.

United States Public Health Service. (1989) *Caring for Our Future: The Content of Prenatal Care.* Washington, DC: DHHS.

Chapter 8

Ethical paradoxes in community-based participatory research

Virginia M. McDermott, John G. Oetzel,
and Kalvin White

> Powerlessness is a significant health risk factor and conversely, oppor-
> tunities to experience power and control in one's life contribute to health
> and wellness.
>
> (Bergsma, 2004, p. 152)

Powerlessness, for both disadvantaged and advantaged populations, is a key
element in health-risk behavior, especially substance use and abuse (Petoskey
et al., 1998; Rissel et al., 1996; Wallerstein & Sanchez-Merki, 1994).
Recognizing that a sense of personal efficacy is an important step in addressing
health risks (Witte, 1994), researchers have begun to transition from traditional
health promotion research paradigms, in which researchers develop and deliver
prevention and intervention programs, to paradigms in which the culture and
learning styles of the recipients are reflected, and the community included, in
the development and dissemination of the health-risk programs (Wallerstein
et al., 2004; Wallerstein & Sanchez-Merki, 1994).

The development of researcher–community collaborations has become a
much more common practice in the last twenty-five years (Butterfoss & Kegler,
2002). Community-based participatory research (CBPR) practices are
considered increasingly important in health research because of a "gap between
the concepts and models professionals use to understand and interpret reality
and the concepts and perspectives of different groups in the community" (de
Koning & Martin, 1996, p. 1). Additionally, researchers recognize that cultural,
historical, economic, geographic, political, and social factors influence the
outcomes and need consideration before, during, and after implementing a
health program (Airhihenbuwa, 1995; de Koning & Martin, 1996; Dutta-
Bergman, 2004; Wallerstein & Duran, 2003).

Unfortunately, though CBPR initiatives are usually driven by the best of
intentions, the actual processes of the researcher–community collaboration
are difficult and often ethically challenging (Goldstein, 2000; Nama & Swartz,
2002). Stohl and Cheney (2001), in exploring democratic participation in
organizations, identified participation in the workplace as growing into a
"fundamental social right" filled with "provocative ironies, contradictions, and

paradoxes" (p. 351). However, though there is growing attention to the paradoxes of organizational life (Stohl & Cheney, 2001; Wendt, 1998) and interpersonal relationships (Baxter, 1990), outside of ethical dilemma case studies (Brugge & Kole, 2003) and practitioners' recommendations for working ethically in underprivileged countries (Hyder et al., 2004), little attention has been focused on how ethical paradoxes affect the initiation of CBPR endeavors.

The purpose of this chapter is to identify key ethical paradoxes in the initiation and development of CBPR. To provide a context for understanding the ethical paradoxes, and possible ways to address these issues, we use our experiences in developing a community-based effort involving a peer-led multimedia drug-prevention campaign aimed at American Indian (AI) early adolescents. Understanding these paradoxes will help practitioners and community members approach this relationship with more sensitivity and provide scholars a lens through which to explore future collaborations.

Community-based participatory research

Healthy People 2000 and 2010 set as goals the elimination of racial/ethnic health disparities in the United States (Abuse, 2001). To successfully address these disparities, researchers are realizing that they must not only understand the nature of the community, but also involve community members in the research process (Minkler & Wallerstein, 2003). Though several different terms for this research paradigm have been used, including participatory research (de Koning & Martin, 1996), participatory action research (Whyte, 1991), empowerment research (Rappaport, 1994), and community coalition building (Wolff, 2001b), we use the term community-based participatory research (CBPR). Minkler and Wallerstein (2003) proposed this overarching term to capture the collaborative, democratic processes of the three inter-connected goals: research, action, and education.

Community-based participatory research is an approach that "equitably involves ... community members, organizational representatives, and researchers in all aspects of the research process ... to enhance understanding of a given phenomenon and the social and cultural dynamics of a community and integrate the knowledge gained with action to improve health and well-being of community members" (Israel et al., 1998, p. 177). CBPR is rooted in research traditions of the action research school (Lewin 1948/1997) and participatory research (Fals-Borda, 1991; Freire, 1970). Wallerstein and Duran (2003) described these as the Northern and Southern traditions respectively. Lewin emphasized that researchers did not study a world objective from themselves, but rather the intersubjective meanings of participants with their world was critical. Through his approach, he challenged scholars to bridge the gap between theory and practice "to solve practical problems through an action research cycle involving planning, action, and investigating the results of action" (Wallerstein & Duran, 2003, p. 29). The Southern tradition arose in

Latin American, Asia, and Africa, receiving impetus to address structural crises of underdevelopment and to search for ways to work with communities vulnerable to globalization by the dominant society. These researchers adopted goals of critical consciousness, emancipation, and social justice to help the poor and oppressed progressively transform their communities by their own actions.

CBPR is an orientation to research rather than a method per se and refers to a set of principles and approaches to research rather than encompasses a variety of quantitative and qualitative methods (Israel et al., 1998). The core principles of CBPR are as follows:

> it is participatory; it is cooperative, engaging community member and researchers in a long-term joint process to which each contributes equally; it is a co-learning process; it involves systems development and local capacity building; it is an empowering process through which participants can increase control of their lives; and it achieves a balance between research and action.
>
> (Minkler, 2004, p. 685)

Effective community-based participatory research requires attention to a variety of issues, which Foster-Fishman et al. (2001), in a qualitative analysis of eighty articles and guides, summarized as member capacity, relational capacity, organizational capacity, and programmatic capacity. Member capacity refers to the capacity of participants to perform the tasks and work together. Thus, collaborative efforts are enhanced when participants have the skill, knowledge, and attitudes to support the program. Relational capacity recognizes that collaboration is about developing social networks and refers to the capacity to build both internal and external relationships. Beyond relationship development, successful collaborations require organizational capacity, which is the capacity to engage members to achieve goals, including the capacity for decision making, leadership, and communication (Wolff, 2001a). Finally, effective collaborations require programmatic capacity or the capacity to develop and implement changes according to the program's mission.

Unfortunately, not all community-researcher collaborations have been successful in all capacities (Hancock et al., 1997; Wolff, 2001b). Kreuter et al. (2000) analyzed approximately one hundred articles describing collaborative research approaches and reported that although some programs had strong, positive outcomes, many failed to achieve the target goals. They concluded that, in addition to unrealistic expectations and a lack of clear mechanisms for detecting effects, participants underestimate the complexity and commitment required in effective collaborations. It seems reasonable to assume that collaborative research partnerships are fraught with the contradictions and paradoxes inherent in any relationship or organizational endeavor (Baxter, 1990; Stohl & Cheney, 2001). Given the differences between researchers and community members in power and the personal salience of the issue, this process may be especially prone to ethical paradoxes.

We use our experiences in developing community-based effort to develop a peer-led multimedia drug-prevention campaign aimed at American Indian (AI) early adolescents as one context for identifying and addressing the ethical paradoxes. The larger goal of this current project is to develop and test a Manual of Procedures for a school-based intervention for preventing, reducing, or delaying substance use by American Indian adolescents. This program will train high school juniors as health advocates to deliver culturally appropriate messages using communication campaigns (audiovisual, brochures, and speaking) to younger peers (i.e., middle-school students). This process will be used to help prevent adolescent drug-use by developing their personal (e.g., normative beliefs and self-efficacy), interpersonal (e.g., refusal skills and social support skills), and advocacy skills (e.g., advocating for change in the school or community).

Ethical paradoxes in CBPR

CBPR has been utilized most frequently by researchers in community and public health, epidemiology, sociology, and anthropology (Minkler & Wallerstein, 2003), and less frequently by communication scholars. However, CBPR is largely a communicative and relationship practice and our understanding of the dilemmas inherent in the process can be informed by interpersonal and organizational communication research that investigates dialectics (Baxter, 1990; Martin & Nakayama, 1999) and paradoxes (Stohl & Cheney, 2001; Wendt, 1998). We first describe what paradoxes are and then focus specifically on ethical paradoxes in CBPR.

Paradoxes in organizations and relationships

The study of simultaneous, yet contradictory desires, messages, and/or forces can be broadly categorized as the study of paradoxes (Wendt, 1998) or dialectics (Baxter, 1990). Though conceptually similar, there is a subtle difference between a paradox and dialectic. A paradox exists when your need to fulfill a goal requires you to act in a way contrary to that goal (e.g., workers most interested in achieving a workplace participatory goal are the ones who ignore the participation process to be more efficient) (Stohl & Cheney, 2001). A dialectic tension exists when a person wants both conflicting ideas at the same time (e.g., I want to be open with you so you will really know me, but I want to protect my privacy and guard myself against hurt) (Baxter, 1990). Though both these contradictions can manifest in action, dialectical tensions are internal to a person and paradoxes are structural and organizational. Though we recognize that individuals can and do experience ethical dialectics in CBPR, we use the term paradox to capture the structural ethical dilemmas faced in CBPR.

Participative structures and management are a contributing factor to organizational paradoxes (Wendt, 1998), and even with the best of intentions, collaborative research involves myriad ethical issues (Goldstein, 2000). Understanding organizational and interactional paradoxes can lead to more successful leadership and relationships (Baxter, 1990; Farson, 1996).

Ethical paradoxes

Scientific endeavors and ethical considerations are intertwined. As modern scientists, we are guided by the fundamental principle of "do no harm" and adhere to the standards of informed consent and voluntary participation. Institutional Review Boards (IRBs) developed to ensure that research is conducted in an ethical fashion. IRBs, however, are focused on protecting the rights of individual subjects and not of communities, and often do not take the culture of the participants into consideration (Brugge & Kole, 2003) or the risk of harm to entire communities (Wing, 2002). One reason why attention to ethical dilemmas is an important first step is that in CBPR, cooperative relationships are dependent on trust and trusting (the behavioral consequences of trust) (Das & Teng, 2001).

CBPR should be a genuinely empowering process, not simply an outcome where community members work within the agenda of university researchers. However, when university researchers and community members collaborate, the structure of the endeavor will entail a number of tensions. Three ethical paradoxes, especially with marginalized populations, need to be assessed and clarified for all involved: the paradox of power, the paradox of participation, and the paradox of practice.

To highlight the complexity of these issues, we provide examples from the initiation of our current project. This project, developed in conjunction with members of an AI community, proposed to develop and test a school-based, peer-developed and led, intervention for preventing, reducing, or delaying substance use by AI adolescents. Specifically, this intervention focuses on universal prevention of substance use by training high school students as health advocates to deliver culturally appropriate messages using communication campaigns (audiovisual, brochures, and speaking) to middle-school students.

The paradox of power

The basis for much of the concern about ethics in community-based research stems from the frequent, and often unavoidable, power imbalance between researchers and community members (Nama & Swartz, 2002; Trickett, 1998). Researchers and community members struggle to balance the power differences with equality and equity in the process. These issues are compounded when working in resource-poor locations and when dealing with cultures very different from one's own. In CBPR, the community is not the "subject" but an equal partner. However, while the term "partners" implies equity and equality in all stages of the process, CBPR members also need to be aware of oppression and racism that are often a factor for the communities. Issues of racism (Jones, 2000) can impact the CBPR process in many ways including (but not limited to) the following: a) being the group studied, rather than those doing the studying; b) "White" researchers dominating the process and direction of the research; c) misunderstanding between researchers and communities' members because of different lived experiences; and d) team members not participating fully because they feel that the university researchers know what is best for them.

Negotiating these power dynamics and differences in CBPR underlie the entire process and require that there is clarification and equality of roles, mutual openness to dialogue, mutual compensation, and evaluation of the process. The first step to consider in the research process is for researchers and community members to address issues of roles and responsibility. When university- and government-funded researchers enter a community, there is often a perceived imbalance in authority, and a real imbalance in education and socioeconomic status. However, community members and stakeholders have key roles in the research—they are the cultural informants and keys to understanding what works and what does not. The roles are necessarily different (e.g., you would not expect most community members to be able to do statistical analyses), but equally important. One way to ensure the equality of collaboration is to discuss roles and responsibilities directly. Additionally, members of the community should be key personnel on the project.

In developing our collaboration, three specific paradoxes of power were identified and addressed: a) CBPR needs to be community driven but is researcher initiated; b) we need to share fiscal responsibility but our expertise allows us to access the funding; and c) we need to be equal partners but protect the community.

COMMUNITY DRIVEN BUT RESEARCHER INITIATED

Sharing control is an essential aspect of participatory research and it starts with the decision to initiate research. The typical research process that most of us follow is an orderly sequence of phases in which we first think about the problem, we then find whom the problem influences, and we then develop our plan to address the issue. This linear model is problematic in CBPR, because the community needs to be part of identifying a need and designing how the need will be addressed (Israel et al., 2003; Minkler, 2004). Thus, to employ CBPR, community representatives need to be part of the process from the very beginning. The entire process is evolving and synergistic with "both partners offer[ing] unique contributions and complementary expertise to the joint enterprise (Jensen et al., 1999).

The first paradox between power and equality is that to begin a collaborative and organized process, a person needs to take the lead and continue to provide vision and leadership (Zoller, 2000). The initial step of the CBPR process is deciding on the research topic—something that is of importance for the community. Reason (1994), however, noted that many CBPR projects would not be undertaken "without the initiative of someone with time, skill, and commitment, someone who will almost inevitably be a member of a privileged and educated group" (p. 334).

Even if the research question initially comes from a noncommunity researcher, the community stakeholders should be part of identifying and clarifying the problem and deciding what should be done to address the problem (Minkler, 2004). This collaboration requires that all participants clarify their needs and goals, and then negotiate what gets done. In some cases, the community advances the idea and in others it is the university research team. Both cases can result in a true collaboration so long as the research question truly addresses a community problem and the community wants to use the approach proposed by the researchers.

In our particular case, we had a member from the tribe who was interested in partnering with university researchers to address adolescent school and social problems. The university team was interested in creating a peer-led substance use intervention and we discussed the procedures and processes for making such a collaboration work. However, the key was to make sure that the project would not simply involve research about a problem, but that it would result in some type of intervention that would benefit the community. It was also critical that whatever was created would be sustainable. To ensure that peer-developed, peer-presented drug prevention curriculum will reflect the experiences of current students, we built in training of teachers in how to implement the curriculum after the research project was over. To that end, each school will be provided computers and software, our manual of procedures will include all information for teachers to instruct new students to develop a health campaign (including use of all audio-visual equipment), select teachers from each school will participate in the hands-on training, and our department will continue to offer classes in broadcast and editing.

Thus, the purpose of the research has to be community-based and not simply community-placed (Israel et al., 2003; Chavez et al., 2003). The initial idea can come from researchers, but the focus has to be on community benefit and be community driven, not on researcher careers. In our case, the idea came from both the community and the researchers and the collaboration resulted in something that all parties agreed upon and support.

SHARE FISCAL RESPONSIBILITY BUT PROVIDE THE FUNDING

Money is power. Though oft heard, this statement is a major dilemma in CBPR: community-based research, especially with underserved and under-represented, populations, requires funding, typically provided through mechanisms external researchers can access. In addition to providing the start-up financing, this group is usually responsible for monitoring expenses and compensating participants. At minimum, this inequity can lead to dilemmas of shared control and joint governance. More importantly, if the financial management is one-sided, community members may fear that questioning the researchers and objecting to processes could have financial consequences. To address this, researchers and communities must understand, and respect, the importance of social capital (Krueter & Lezin, 2002), as well financial capital.

Compensation is another way that power differences may become clear. Though identifying effective health promotion and prevention strategies may be indirect benefits from research, both researchers and communities need to share direct benefits as well. Researchers benefit from the process by presenting and publishing their research, thus enhancing their careers. Funded researchers may also receive monetary benefits through extra salary and associated compensation. In CBPR, it is imperative that community participants also directly benefit. Starting our partnership with the tribe required that we not only share publication credit with community partners but also that we share resources with the schools and individuals involved, including computers, printers, software, and media equipment, in addition to monetary compensation for participating in the survey stage and implementation of the program. Most importantly, tribal compensation and resources will not be handled through the university; instead, the tribe will be subcontracted as a partner and tribal representatives responsible for monitoring their own compensation and expenses. All in all, about 45 percent of the funds will go to the community with 55 percent going to the university.

Sharing financial responsibility during the research process helps equalize the power, but the act of paying communities, and individuals, poses another dilemma: in treating the community as partner, and individuals as resources, we may also treat them as commodities. We need to first consider the needs of the community and protect against inducements that may cause people to take disproportionate risks (Dickens & Cook, 2003). Second, we need to attend to the cultural norms of the community and not insult them by treating people as objects "available for purchase and sale in the marketplace" (p. 82). Though many communities are based on the market principle of reciprocity, we need to remember that the importance of equality and reciprocity are not only about financial considerations but also about respect and appreciation. In our partnership with the tribe, we recognize that while we provide monetary compensation to participants, our partners coordinate and provide space for our meetings, which, in an open marketplace, is a personal and financial burden.

BE EQUAL PARTNERS BUT PROTECT THE PARTICIPANTS

Though CBPR is crucial to developing targeted and effective health risk prevention campaigns, researchers and community members need to balance inclusion of the community with protection of the community, individuals, and research processes. The first issue we encountered is: Is it possible to protect the anonymity of community participants when community participants are co-researchers (Lax & Galvin, 2002)? Additional issues involve data sharing and the dissemination of the results.

A part of consent is protecting participant confidentiality and, if possible, anonymity. Community partners should be equal participants in the process, with equal access to the results, but to protect individual participants, researchers may need to limit access to any identifying information. In health research, information provided by participants is often sensitive and potentially stigmatizing, so protection requires that community partners, who may know the subjects, not access all information. In straightforward situations, this process may simply require stripping all identifying information from data files; however, in situations where participants are asked to disclose very sensitive, stigmatizing, or even illegal, information, researchers may need to take additional steps to assure participants that their information will remain confidential and anonymous. In our case, the tribe owns the data, while the university team maintains the individual consent forms. In this manner, individual confidentiality is protected, while the tribe controls the data and ensures that the community benefits.

How researchers and communities benefit is not only an issue of power, but also of protection. An important outcome of research is public dissemination of the findings through publication; however, this need may conflict with community members' desire for privacy and rights to confidentiality. University and community partners are both obligated to protect the integrity of publication outcomes: to ensure that the publication is an accurate representation of the research while at the same time not causing undue harm to the community.

The relationship between researchers and communities is often threatened by issues surrounding the ownership and control of programs, and these issues subsequently affect the sustainability of the program (Altman, 1995). In CBPR, it is crucial that data protection questions are clearly addressed: Who owns the data at the end of the project? What happens to the data? Lack of agreement about control of the data can jeopardize the process and outcomes and may result in researchers publishing reports without the knowledge or inclusion of the community or communities vetoing the rights of researchers to publish. Both of these scenarios are problematic because they violate the collaborative and equality basis of CBPR. For our collaboration, we follow a code similar to that used in the Kahnawake Schools Diabetes Prevention project (Macaulay et al., 1998), which is:

> No partner can veto a communication. In the case of disagreements, the partner who disagrees must be invited to communicate their own interpretation of the same data as an addition to the main communication, be

it oral or written. All partners agree to withhold any information if the alternative interpretation cannot be added and distributed at the same time, providing the disagreeing partner(s) do not unduly delay the distribution process.

(p. 107)

Additionally, we agree that all publications will be multiauthored and both the tribe and university team need to approve its contents. Finally, we have a responsibility to take the results back to community members and schools to ensure that those who need the data get it. Thus, we will hold community forums to share results and train teachers to ensure a sustainable project.

In sum, in the initial stages of CBPR two primary objectives are a) to work toward reducing the power typically held by researchers and b) to empower the community. However, these objectives are often in contrast to research goals and requirements; thus, we need to understand and address these issues. This sets up an ethical paradox because in order to start the collaborative project, one person needs to take charge, one group usually provides the resources, and one group may need to protect the community and individuals. We must also be cognizant that our attempts to equalize resources and participation may have the unintended consequence of strengthening existing power bases, and increasing existing power differentials, in the community (Hancock et al., 1997). Once the project has been initiated, the next objective of CBPR is to manage researcher and community participation.

Paradox of participation

Using community-based frameworks for any research project is a complex and time-consuming process that requires coordination and flexibility from researchers and community members. As the importance of employing CBPR increases (as it does when addressing health risk behavior with marginalized populations), so does the complexity of the process. In CBPR, researchers respect the rights of individuals but require the participation of a community. In requiring participation, issues around self-determination develop and we may overlook the demand that we place on community partners and fail to appreciate that sometimes collaboration and partnership become burdensome and exhausting (Stohl & Cheney, 2001). Although participation is intended to empower people, the structure of the participation may prevent people from feeling free to express their thoughts by formalizing a process that needs to be informal (i.e., advisory board meetings). In developing our collaboration, three specific paradoxes of participation were identified and addressed: a) the competing needs to value the community and attempt to change the community; b) the decisions about who participates; and c) the need to balance leadership and direction with collaboration and participation (Zoller, 2000).

VALUE THE COMMUNITY BUT CHANGE THE COMMUNITY

A primary ethical paradox of participating in CBPR is managing the respect and appreciation for the community and community partners against the goal of changing the community in some way. As researchers, we have to recognize that the CBPR activities involve cost to the individuals and communities involved (Hancock et al., 1997), and that activities aimed to improve conditions in communities also intrude on the lives of individuals and groups (Trickett, 1998). In our own proposal, we are aiming to reduce substance use and abuse in adolescents, which is a goal of the community as substance use is considered counter to traditional culture. However, building on recommendations for reaching adolescents about health issues (Payne & Schulte, 2003; Rich, 2004), we are proposing the use of a multimedia campaign which is more mainstream than many traditional AIs in the community might prefer.

At best, CBPR is not only designed to address, but hopefully improve, existing problems. One ethical dilemma in attempting to change something in a community may arise by simply identifying a group as "a population at risk" (Trickett, 1998). As researchers address "problems," individuals may alter their perceptions of the group, and even of themselves. Addressing substance use and abuse in tribal communities is difficult for some community members because it "paints a negative picture" of the community. While most community members know the issue needs to be addressed, and want to address it, they resent the negative publicity and changes to traditional culture. We address this paradox by designing a program that will empower adolescents and schools to *prevent* substance use as a way to strengthen the community, bring skills to adolescents and helping to avoid the problems in the first place.

WHO DECIDES WHO PARTICIPATES?

Communities need to be defined carefully, since "'localities' may not represent cohesive identities" (Hancock et al., 1997) and there are a variety of groups and individuals who need to be considered. As university- and government-funded researchers, in our research we face the prospect of partnering with AI adolescents and community members to develop peer-created and peer-led communication campaigns to reduce and prevent adolescent substance use. Our situation necessitates that we consider and address a variety of community groups and individual stakeholders, including the tribal nation, the Department of Education, the schools, the community, the family, and the individual.

When partnering with a sovereign nation, especially one that has been historically mistreated by researchers, researchers need to follow the appropriate channels for starting the research process. Once an idea has some support, the next step is to address a formal governing body, which might include a tribal research board, tribal council, and a department council. In our case, the tribe has a research board and education council and both are gateways to any research done on tribal land or with tribal members. The first step was to get

DUE DATE

_____

_____

_____

_____

IMPORTANT NOTICE ABOUT ITEMS BORROWED FROM I-SHARE LIBRARIES

This item belongs to a CARLI member library (Consortium of Academic and Research Libraries in Illinois).

You are subject to the owning institution's loan and fine policies.

The lending institution may charge lost book fees for failure to return or renew this material by the due date. Failure to return this material in good condition or to pay the lending institution's fees may result in suspension of *all* borrowing privileges.

To renew:
    click on My Account at
https://www.library.illinois.edu
Central Access Services
217-333-8400
circlib@library.illinois.edu

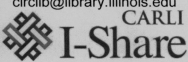
CARLI
I-Share

approval of the education council who will allow research to be done in schools. The second step will be to receive approval of the research process and procedures by the research board. Both entities are there to protect the tribe from unethical researchers and to ensure the rights of the tribe and tribal members are protected. They also want to ensure that the research is collaborative and that community members will be consulted and involved in the research (e.g., having members of the tribe as researchers—our proposal includes four tribal members as researchers).

This entire consenting process is only the first step in answering the "who participates" question. CBPR requires more than consent of the community; it requires participation. It would, however, be an unwieldy process if everyone participated, so a common alternative is the creation of a community advisory board (CAB) (Minkler, 2004), with members selected by their community, not by the researchers. The CAB should be composed of representatives from all stakeholder groups, which in our case is teachers, parents, students, health professionals, elders, and community leaders. The size will be approximately ten to fifteen members and the composition and membership will be determined by consultation with all members of the research team (but with the tribal members having a stronger say since they have more understanding and knowledge about who is need to make the project successful). Additionally, individual students, identified by teachers, will be invited to join the research team as partners in designing the campaigns. These students will be responsible for delivering and disseminating the campaigns.

The final members of the CBPR process are the researchers. The usual competencies should be considered here—that is, who has the requisite skills to complete the work proposed. However, another two other core considerations are necessary. First, do the researchers have skills in engaging in truly collaborative projects? Many researchers are used to "dictating" the process and if this is the only type of research with which they are comfortable, they are not good choices for CBPR. Second, given the context, the researchers need to be culturally sensitive (Airhihenbuwa, 1995; Chavez et al., 2003; Dutta-Bergman, 2004). Research team members need to have some knowledge about intercultural communication in general, but also about the specific community. Thus, some of the researchers should be members of the community and others should have experience working with the community previously. Researchers who are new to the community need to at least be self-reflexive and aware of power differentials and be willing to discuss such issues.

BE A PARTNER AND LEADER

Research demonstrates that the most creative, participative, and high-performing groups have strong leaders and that "a central challenge of participation revolves around the issue of how to facilitate, foster, and lead participation efforts without controlling them" (Stohl & Cheney, 2001,

p. 387). The fundamental elements of CBPR are collaboration, equality, and equity in which the community and the researcher work together to develop and implement a program. This process, however, requires a leader, and similar to the power issues surrounding the initiation of the project, the project leader is often a highly trained, professional researcher. In addition to keeping the group on task and facilitating decisions, the partner/leader also needs to "provide guidance and vision without controlling that vision" (p. 389).

In our project, the principal investigator (PI) and one of the co-PIs (a member of the tribe) have created a structure in which decision making, meeting management, and research duties are shared. Briefly, in the first step the co-PI, working from a list of requisites and collaborating with schools, determines the appropriate choices and suggest CAB members. Once the group is set, initial meetings focus on the project, but more importantly, the collaborative process and constructing a set of communication guidelines for the meetings (e.g., respect, sharing opinions, what to do if you do not feel if you have a voice, etc.). After the guidelines are determined, the group work begins. The PI (and university research team) set agendas and bring research information to the table. The co-PI organizes the CAB members and arranges meeting places and times. The meetings are cooperatively facilitated by these two individuals and a research assistant. Finally, rigorous process evaluation is conducted by a research team member, who is also from the tribal community. She is responsible for observing the meetings and interviewing participants to ensure that we are following stated communication guidelines. In this manner, we can use research to improve the CBPR process.

The final and potentially most complicated task of the leader is recognizing the need to relinquish the leadership position. The goal of CBPR is for communities to become self-sufficient in sustaining the program, so a true leader may need to make him/herself irrelevant (Stoecker, 2003). By partnering on all fiscal, design, and implementation tasks throughout our process, and then transferring all accumulated resources to the community, we hope to increase the sustainability of the project.

In sum, the participation considerations are complex and paradoxical. To facilitate collaboration, we need to maintain respect, equity, and equality in the process, but the process requires that the community change. Additionally, researchers struggle with competing ethical demands about the protection of participants and communities with the inclusion of community researchers and dissemination of result. The third participation paradox is that the process requires a leader to provide vision while at the same time allowing the community to make decisions. To balance participation dilemmas, we recognize that there will be people whose participations is much more consultative (e.g., review boards) and those whose participation is active (e.g., CAB members, research team members). The membership needs to consider the requisite skills, but also cultural competence and willingness to engage in a complex and lengthy collaboration. Understanding and addressing these participation paradoxes are crucial if the practice of CBPR is to be successful.

Paradox of Practice

In addition to the contradictions in power issues and participatory roles, CBPR requires that we manage the paradoxes of practicing collaborative research. Researchers and community participants are likely to have different agendas and goals that must be addressed and managed at the start of the process. To ensure that role differentiation and ongoing dialogue are not strongly affected by racism and prior history, we need to engage in some checks and balances through ongoing evaluation of the process. Specifically, we need to focus on how different needs and perspectives are negotiated. Since researchers and community members may have different end goals, and different timelines, process problems are likely to arise. Anticipation of these differences is crucial to the success of the partnership, and this requires that the process begin with a clarification of how different issues are negotiated. The guidelines of issue resolution should be agreed to by all involved prior to the start of the research. All partners should take an active role in crafting an issue resolution document. Advisory groups are crucial to this process, as is a trained facilitator. Clarification of the issue and dispute resolution process is an important as a mechanism to equalize power differences but is an equally important step in protecting the CBPR process. In our project, we will have a research assistant, who is a member of the community, conduct a process evaluation to make sure dialogue and collaboration is followed and disputes are resolved fairly.

BE LONG TERM AND SHORT TERM

In CBPR there is often a conflict in the need of the researchers to conduct scientifically sound research and the need of the community to see results (Altman, 1995; Hancock et al., 1997). Promoting participatory and "bottom-up" processes is often in opposition to the need to meet funding and publication deadlines (Lax & Galvin, 2002). In addition, tribal communities have a long-term focus and want to slowly establish trust and ensure the researchers are trustworthy. This focus is counter to some researchers' short-term focus to get the project done.

In our project, we have built in time for establishing the CBPR process. If both researchers and communities know that the CBPR process will take time, but it is part of the scope of work, short- and long-term goals can be combined. Further, three members of the university research team are highly experienced in CBPR processes having engaged in such processes with a number of tribal communities (including the one we are working with). The key is to ensure that there are realistic expectations and time allotted for the CBPR process.

When meeting the needs of the community, researchers need to make ensure that results be published and presented in all appropriate venues, which includes channels community members can access and language appropriate to the readers. For researchers, this will require more than sending a final paper; it will involve oral presentations, local radio and television broadcasts, and other culturally appropriate media outlets. This dissemination can be time-consuming and work-intensive, and resources must be allocated for this. In past projects, we approached this in several stages. First, we provided a summary of the results to the overseeing body (e.g., tribal council, education council, etc.). This summary includes descriptive statistics and identifies key patterns in the data, but is presented in lay language. Second, we provided community forums where we discuss the findings with community members (all data that was approved by the overseeing body). We included a short summary paper in lay language as well. Third, we then developed presentations for professional associations and articles for publications. These presentations and articles were collaboratively developed with a sharing of tasks based on experiences (e.g., statistical analysis by the university team, writing by all with formal writing backgrounds, etc.). Authorship is inclusive with both researchers and tribal community members and all have the opportunity for review. The final presentation and articles must be approved by the tribal council and/or IRB.

BE RESEARCH ORIENTED AND COMMUNITY ORIENTED

Science is predicated on the assumption of the transparency of the process. A tenet in science is that replication should not only be allowed but also encouraged. In CBPR, however, we need to balance the transparency of the process with the protection of the community. Wing (2002) recounted his experience of the conflict between the openness of research and his responsibility to his community-partners in a community-driven study of the environmental effects of industrialized hog production. When, after publication of initial findings, lawyers for the hog industry requested copies of all his research (under the public records statute), he had to balance his obligation to protect the individuals, and communities, from identification against a threat by the university attorney that "the university would call the State Bureau of Investigation and have me arrested for stealing state property" (p. 441) if he did not turn over all records. For our purposes, the approval process of the research by the IRB and educational council ensures that we are being community oriented. The members of these bodies appreciate the need for research, but balance the research orientation with community focus and protection.

BE SUPPORTIVE AND CRITICAL

Researchers need to provide an atmosphere that makes participants feel safe and encourages and respects their collaboration. Community members need to provide ideas and opinions. Researchers need to address the complexity of the community and learn to ask the right questions and not anticipate the "correct" answer. Community members need to ask the right questions and be willing to question the "correct" answer. The researchers need to be willing to learn from the community and the community needs to be willing to learn from the researchers. To establish and sustain this dialogue, we have protocols for discussions with the advisory board, opportunities for groups from the community, including elders, parents, teachers, and students, to evaluate the materials and process.

Further, the researchers and CAB members need to be critical and supportive of the research findings. The tribal community may wish to "hide" negative findings about the community just as researchers might like to "hide" negative findings about the effectiveness of an intervention. However, these negative findings, and subsequent community concerns, must be addressed honestly and critically if health problems are to be truly addressed.

In sum, practicing CBPR is time-consuming and sometimes difficult. Researchers and community members are faced with a variety of competing needs, including focusing on long-term outcomes while meeting the immediate needs of the community, understanding the need to adhere to the best research practices while adhering to the needs of the community, and being both supportive and critical. The key thing we need to know is that how these dilemmas are handled is a crucial aspect of the CBPR process.

Addressing paradoxes

Organizational paradoxes and relational dialectics are likely inevitable (Baxter, 1990; Stohl & Cheney, 2001). In dealing with relational dialectics, it is not the presence or absence of dialectical tensions that predict relational satisfaction, it is how the dialectics are handled (Baxter, 1990). Similarly, some responses to organizational paradoxes seem to be more effective than others (Tracy, 2004). Whether dealing with relational dialectics or structural paradoxes, ignoring or avoiding the contradictions, withdrawing from the partnership, or selecting one extreme of a contradiction to guide actions, is often maladaptive. Instead, partners need to recognize that "out of the crucible of paradox can emerge creativity, innovation, and excitement" (Stohl & Cheney, 2001, p. 391).

In our work, we attempt to address ethical paradoxes in CBPR through a three-step communication process: recognition, reflection, and reframing. Partners must first recognize that there are multiple perspectives both within the partnership and between the partners. This requires that all stakeholders know and communicate their goals and needs while at the same time understanding the goals and needs of other stakeholders. Once we can recognize the differences and contradictions, we need to individually and collectively reflect on these paradoxes and understand how they influence the process and partnership. This requires that together we create a communication environment that allows people to communicate freely and in ways that they are most comfortable. Through initial meeting and CAB interactions, we attempt to clarify the paradoxes. Finally, we attempt to reframe the seemingly incompatible goals and needs by using the paradox as a "fulcrum for constructive organizational change" (Stohl & Cheney, 2001, pp. 395–396). Reframing requires "movement to a different level of analysis or to a new attitude toward the paradox that is perceived to be a problem" (p. 396). We believe that it is through addressing and reconciling these tensions that the collaborative process begins, the partnership is strengthened, and the success of the program enhanced. Contrary to viewing these issues as problems or threats, we view them as opportunities to communicate and learn. For example, we recognize that though power differentials may exist at the onset, power is a "dynamic and fluid force . . . not possessed but is exercised; that it emerges from the grassroots rather than coming from the top down" (Martin, 1996, p. 89). We do not think any person or group needs to "give up" power; instead, it is our goal to facilitate community members' willingness and skill to exercise their voice and implement their ideas. When there is equality (and in the end, community sustainability) we have achieved our goals.

Conclusion

As researchers, we have long understood the need for ethical guidelines. Though community-based research can result in successful health prevention and intervention programs, it can also be harmful to those involved. Trickett and Espino (2004), in their selective review of collaborative research, reference the Tuskegee experiments (Thomas & Quinn, 1991) and research with the Inupait Indians of Barrow, Alaska (Foulks, 1989a, 1989b) as to why "vigilance around outside researchers, particularly when race and power issues are involved, represent an adaptive rather than paranoid response" (Trickett & Espino, 2004, p. 5).

We do not seek to prescribe specific ethical codes of conduct for community-based research. The range and scope of CBPR is too diverse and idiosyncratic to achieve such a goal, and as the collaborative process develops, and alters perceptions and expectations about roles and status, new issues emerge (Trickett & Espino, 2004). We seek, instead, to highlight the need for addressing ethical paradoxes at the start of projects. By considering and addressing foreseeable ethical dilemmas at the start of a project, we enhance our chances of a successful partnership and effective program. Additionally, though the recognition, reflection, and reframing process is crucial in the initiation of CBPR, it is also imperative that it is an ongoing dialogue as well.

CBPR involves a multitude of people on a variety of levels, which is necessary but also complicated. How does CBPR operate in an ethical manner? First, by developing a process that addresses issues of power by including all relevant community members in all stages of the process, identifying and targeting research agendas that are important to the community and including measures of protection for all involved. Second, researchers need to appreciate that collaboration requires respect for the community and understanding of their need to change, discussion about who participates and where accountability lies, and recognition that participative practices requires leadership. Finally, we need to understand that implementing CBPR requires a balance between the short-term and long-term needs of the partners, a respect for the research demands and the community needs, and the willingness of all partners to be both supportive and critical.

It is important, however, to understand that CBPR is not a panacea for all the problems in a community. Real material and political gains will happen over time and with changes in federal and state policies. However, the CBPR process may effect change by providing important data and by training community members and researchers to address key problems. Addressing ethical paradoxes at the initiation of a program, as well as dealing with them as they arise, is crucial to the sustainability of any intervention.

References

Abuse NIoD. (2001). *Strategic Plan on Reducing Health Disparities*. National Institute on Drug Abuse.

Airhihenbuwa, C.O. (1995). *Health and Culture: Beyond the Western Paradigm*. Sage.

Altman, D.G. (1995). Sustaining interventions in community systems: On the relationship between researchers and communities. *Health Psychology, 14*, 526–536.

Baxter, L.A. (1990). Dialectical contradictions in relationship development. *Journal of Social and Personal Relationships, 7*, 69–88.

Bergsma, L.J. (2004). Empowerment education: The link between media literacy and health promotion. *American Behavioral Scientist, 48*, 152–164.

Brugge, D., & Kole, A. (2003). A case study of community-based participatory research ethics: The healthy public house initiative. *Science and Engineering Ethics, 9*, 485–501.

Butterfoss, F.D., & Kegler, M.C. (2002). Toward a comprehensive understanding of community coalition: Moving from practice to theory. In R.J. Di Clemente, R.A. Crosby, & M.C. Kegler (eds), *Emerging Theories in Health Promotion Practice and Research: Strategies for Improving Public Health*. San Francisco: John Wiley, pp. 157–193.

Chavez, V., Duran, B., Baker, Q.E., Avila, M.M., & Wallerstein, N. (2003). The dance of race and privilege in community based participatory research. In M. Minkler & N. Wallerstein (eds), *Community Based Participatory Research*. San Francisco: Jossey-Bass, pp. 81–97.

Das, T.K., & Teng, B.S. (2001). Trust, control, and risk in strategic alliances: An integrated framework. *Organization Studies, 22*, 251–283.

de Koning, K., & Martin, M. (1996). Participatory research in health: Setting the context. In K. de Koning & M. Martin (eds), *Participatory Research in Health: Issues and Experiences*. London: Zed Books, pp. 1–18.

Dickens, B.M., & Cook, R.J. (2003). Challenges of ethical research in resource-poor settings. *International Journal of Gynecology and Obstetrics*, 80, 79–86.

Dutta-Bergman, M.J. (2004). Poverty, structural barriers, and health: A Santali narrative of health communication. *Qualitative Health Research*, 14, 1107–1122.

Fals-Borda, O. (1991). Some basic ingredients. In O. Fals-Borda, & M.A. Rahman (eds), *Action and Knowledge: Breaking the Monopoly with Participatory Action Research*. New York: Apex, pp. 3–13.

Farson, R. (1996). *Management of the Absurd: Paradoxes in Leadership*. New York: Simon and Schuster.

Foster-Fishman, P.G., Berkowitz, S.L., Lounsbury, D.W., Jacobson, S., & Allen, N.A. (2001). Building collaborative capacity in community coalitions: A review and integrative framework. *American Journal of Community Psychology*, 29, 241–261.

Foulks, E.F. (1989a). Misalliances in the Barrow Alcohol Study. *American Indian and Alaska Native Mental Health Research*, 2, 7–17.

Foulks, E.F. (1989b). Rejoiner to the comments on the misalliances of the Barrow Alcohol Study. *American Indian and Alaska Native Mental Health Research*, 2, 88–90.

Freire, P. (1970). *Pedagogy of the Oppressed*. New York: Seabury.

Goldstein, L.S. (2000). Ethical dilemmas in designing collaborative research: Lessons learned the hard way. *Qualitative Studies in Education*, 13, 517–530.

Hancock, L., Sanson-Fisher, R., Redman, S. and the CART Project team (1997). Community action for health promotion: A review of methods and outcomes. *American Journal of Preventive Medicine*, 13, 229–239.

Hyder, A.A., Wali, S.A., Khan, A.N., Kass, N.E., & Dawson, L. (2004). Ethical review of health research: A perspective from developing country researchers. *Journal of Medical Ethics*, 30, 68–72.

Israel, B.A., Schulz, A.J., Parker, E.A., & Becker, A.B. (1998). Review of community-based research: Assessing partnership approaches to improve public health. *Annual Review of Public Health*, 19, 173–202.

Israel, B.A., Schulz, A.J., Parker, E.A., Becker, A.B., Allen, A.J., & Guzman, J.R. (2003). Critical issues in developing and following community based participatory research principles. In M. Minkler, & N. Wallerstein (eds), *Community-based Participatory Research for Health*. San Francisco: Jossey-Bass, pp. 53–79.

Jensen, P.S., Hoadwood, K., & Trickett, E.J. (1999). Ivory towers or earthen trenches? Community collaboration to foster "real world" research. *Applied Developmental Science*, 3, 206–212.

Jones, C.P. (2000). Levels of racism: A theoretical framework and a gardener's tale. *American Journal of Public Health*, 8, 1212–1215.

Kreuter, M.W., & Lenzin, N.L. (2002). Social capital theory: Implications for community-based health promotion. In R.J. Di Clemente, R.A. Crosby, & M.C. Kegler (eds), *Emerging Theories in Health Promotion Practice and Research: Strategies for Improving Public Health*. San Francisco: Jossey-Bass, pp. 228–254.

Kreuter, M., Lenzin, N.L., & Young, L. (2000). Evaluating community-based mechanisms: Implications for practitioners. *Health Promotion Practice*, 1, 49–63.

Lax, W., & Galvin, K. (2002). Reflections on a community action research project: Interprofessional issues and methodological problems. *Journal of Clinical Nursing*, 11, 376–386.

Lewin, K. (1997). *Resolving Social Conflict and Field Theory in Social Science*. Washington, DC: American Psychological Association. (Original work published in 1948).

Macaulay, A.C., Delormier, T., McComber, A.M., Cross, E.J., Potvin, L.P., Pavadis, G., et al. (1998). Participatory research with Native Community of Kahnawake creates innovative code of research ethics. *Canadian Journal of Public Health, 89,* 105–108

Martin, M. (1996). Issues of power in the participatory research process. In K. de Koning, & M. Martin (eds), *Participatory Research in Health: Issues and Experiences.* London: Zed Books, pp. 82–93.

Martin, J.N., & Nakayama, T.K. (1999). Thinking dialectically about culture and communication. *Communication Theory, 9,* 1–25.

Minkler, M. (2004). Ethical challenges for the "Outside" researcher in community-based participatory research. *Health Education and Behavior, 31,* 684–697.

Minkler, M., & Wallerstein, N. (2003). Introduction to community based participatory research. In M. Minkler & N. Wallerstein (eds), *Community-based Participatory Research for Health.* San Francisco: Jossey-Bass, pp. 3–26.

Nama, N., & Swartz, L. (2002). Ethical and social dilemmas in community-based controlled trials in situations of poverty: A view from a South African project. *Journal of Community and Applied Social Psychology, 12,* 286–297.

Payne, J.G., & Schulte, S.K. (2003). Mass media, public health, and achieving health literacy. *Journal of Health Communication, 8,* 124–125.

Petoskey, E.L., Van Steele, K.R., & De Jong, J.A. (1998). Prevention through empowerment in a Native American community. *Drugs and Society, 12,* 147–162.

Rappaport, J. (1994). Empowerment as a guide to doing research: Diversity as a positive value. In E.J. Trackett, R.J. Watts, & D. Birman (eds), *Human Diversity: Perspectives on People in Context.* San Francisco: Jossey-Bass, pp. 359–382.

Reason, P. (1994). Three approaches to participative inquiry. In N.K. Denzin, & Y.S. Lincoln (eds), *Handbook of Qualitative Research.* Thousand Oaks, CA: Sage, pp. 324–339.

Rich, M. (2004). Health literacy via media literacy. Video intervention/prevention assessment. *American Behavioral Scientist, 48,* 165–188.

Rissel, C.E., Perry, C.L., Wagenaar, A.C., Wolfson, M., Finnegan, J.R., & Komro, K.A. (1996). Empowerment, alcohol, 8th grade students and health promotion. *Journal of Alcohol and Drug Education, 41,* 105–119.

Stoecker, R. (2003). Are academics irrelevant? Approaches and roles for scholars in community based participatory research. In M. Minkler, & N. Wallerstein (eds), *Community-based Participatory Research for Health.* San Francisco: Jossey-Bass, pp. 98–112.

Stohl, C., & Cheney, G. (2001). Participatory processes/Paradoxical practices: Communication and the dilemmas of organizational democracy. *Management Communication Quarterly, 14,* 349–407.

Thomas, S.B., & Quinn, S.C. (1991). The Tuskegee Syphillia Study, 1932 to 1972: Implications for HIV education and AIDS risk education in the Black community. *American Journal of Public Health, 81,* 1498–1505.

Tracy, S.J. (2004). Dialectic, contradiction, or double-bind? Analyzing and theorizing employee reactions to organizational tension. *Journal of Applied Communication Research, 32,* 119–146.

Trickett, E.J. (1998). Toward a framework for defining and resolving ethical issues in the protection of communities involved in primary prevention projects. *Ethics and Behavior, 8,* 321–337.

Trickett, E.J., & Espino, S.L.R. (2004). Collaboration and social inquiry: Multiple meanings of a construct and its role in creating useful and valid knowledge. *American Journal of Community Psychology, 34,* 1–69.

Wallerstein, N., & Duran, B. (2003). The conceptual, historical and practice roots of community-based participatory research and related participatory traditions. In M. Minkler, & N. Wallerstein (eds), *Community-based Participatory Research for Health.* San Francisco: Jossey-Bass, pp. 27–52.

Wallerstein, N., Sanchez, V., & Dow, L. (2004). Freirian praxis in health education and community organizing: A case study of an adolescent prevention program. In M. Minkler (ed.), *Community Organizing and Community Building for Health,* 2nd edn. Mahwah, NJ: Rutgers University Press.

Wallerstein, N., & Sanchez-Merki, V. (1994). Freirian praxis in health education: Qualitative research on adolescent alcohol prevention. *Health Education Research, 9,* 105–118.

Wendt, R.F. (1998). The sound of one hand clapping: Counterintuitive lessons extracted from paradoxes and double binds in participative organizations. *Management Communication Quarterly, 11,* 323–371.

Whyte, W.F. (1991). *Participatory Action Research.* Newbury Park, CA: Sage.

Wing, S. (2002). Social responsibility and research ethics in community-driven studies of industrialized hog production. *Environmental Health Perspectives, 110,* 437–444.

Witte, K. (1994). Generating effective risk messages: How scary should your risk communication be? *Communication Yearbook, 18,* 229–254

Wolff, T. (2001a). A practitioner's guide to successful coalitions. *American Journal of Community Psychology, 29,* 173–191.

Wolff, T. (2001b). Community-coalition building: Contemporary practice and research. *American Journal of Community Psychology, 29,* 165–172.

Zoller, H. M. (2000). "A place you haven't visited before": Creating the conditions for community dialogue. *Southern Communication Journal, 65,* 191–207.

Chapter 9

Voces de Las Colonias

Dialectical tensions about control and cultural identification in Latinas' communication about cancer

Melinda Villagran, Dorothy Collins, and Sara Garcia

The role of communication in producing health disparities is well-documented in research from a variety of disciplines (Ashton, et al., 2003; Kreps, 2006; Villagran et al., 2005). One potential source of these disparities is the lack of culturally and linguistically appropriate messages about the cancer-care process (Office of Minority Health [OMH], 2003). Many times Latino cancer patients who enter into the health-care system must overcome unique barriers that arise from cultural and linguistic differences between themselves and their providers (Villagran & Hoffman, 2006). Health-care interactions are then shaped by culturally recognized communicative and behavioral practices of Latino patients that do not necessarily coincide with a biomedical approach to treatment and prevention. In this manner, the dynamic nature of culture in health-care interactions influences communication between patients and providers.

As the fastest growing minority in the United States, Latinos are especially susceptible to illnesses stemming from ineffective communication about available treatment and prevention measures. This chapter uses the culture-centered approach to health communication (Dutta-Bergman, 2004, 2005) to explore how economically disadvantaged Latinas interpret, manage, and create meaning about cancer through their communication with others. Specifically, interview data from socioeconomically disadvantaged persons living along the Texas–Mexico border were examined to reveal the ways in which communication enmeshes with culture to foster health-care barriers related to cancer.

Literature review

Cultural approach to health communication

The cultural approach to health communication offers a framework for analyzing and interpreting data from marginalized populations (Dutta-Bergman, 2005). Dutta-Bergman's (2004, 2005) cultural perspective serves as a framework to begin developing shared meanings about cancer experiences and grounded theories about ideological and power differences. The cultural framework is appropriate because it helps examine structure and cultural as the core of health communication processes and behavior. Marginalized populations tend to be limited by structural issues such as lack of basic resources including information. These structural issues have the potential to explain the reflexive nature of health-related human behavior and communication. Culture is also the framework by which members of a community construct and explain health-related problems. Specific structural issues draw attention to surface-level disparities currently present for Latino/a patients in the health-care context. The concept of cultural issues will be a lens for discussing how unique tendencies of the Latino/a community affect how the members interpret and understand their experiences with cancer.

Even though structure and culture may help explain communication and behavior, this does not guarantee that people respond to these issues consistently. Dutta-Bergman (2005) suggests that polymorphism is also an important aspect of the cultural framework that allows researchers to explore how members of a community use communication to negotiate multiple meanings of events. Polymorphism opens the door to begin searching communication for dialectical tensions that the members of a cultural community must negotiate.

Agency and culture-centered communication

At the heart of the culture-centered framework for health communication is the goal to raise the level of agency for the members of the marginalized population (Dutta-Bergman, 2005). In this model, experiences are defined within the culture of the patient based on a constructed meaning for each health-care interaction (Dutta-Bergman, 2004). O'Hair et al. (2003) also propose a framework for understanding how communication in the cancer experience can lead patients to have enhanced empowerment and agency. In O'Hair et al.'s model, choice is a preeminent concern for cancer patients, and communication and agency are critical for helping patients negotiate difficult choices.

From a culture-centered perspective, choice would be tempered by perceptions of social and political constraints based on the cultural interpretation and construction of meaning. O'Hair et al. (2003) point out that the patient's level of agency is "often restricted and undermined by institutional and social forces" (p. 198). These "institutional and social forces" are the ideologies present in the health-care setting. Research about communication of cancer patients' experiences reveals important themes of control, power, and patient resources (Bowker, 1996; Ellingson & Buzzanell, 1999; Gibbs & Franks, 2002) that fit in with the O'Hair et al. (2003) model. Bowker (1996) defines her struggle as a cancer patient as a "struggle between having cancer and finding a way to respond to the condition" (p. 97). In their research to conceptualize patients' satisfaction with providers, Ellingson and Buzzanell (1999) link surface themes (physicians' amount of respect, care, and reassurance of expertise) and root themes of power, control, and the importance contextualizing the cancer experience to the rest of their lives. Cancer communication is an area of health communication that explores the role communication plays in the unique experiences of cancer patients and survivors.

Lupton (1994) challenges the health communication discipline to incorporate a critical perspective that considers how language acts to perpetuate the interests of some groups over others. She suggests that a critical perspective could begin to consider several questions including the meaning of the illness and treatment experience to the individual "by considering how personal experiences subscribe to or resist wider ideologies present in culture" (p. 58). The messages that come from the Latina women about their cancer experiences may reveal their ideologies and values. These ideologies and values can be discussed by using Dutta-Bergman's (2005) cultural framework. Social and political disparities can be examined as structural issues that impact health communication. Latino/a values and practices can be examined based on their transformative impact on health communication and behavior.

Ethnic and racial disparities in health care

The structure of health care is one factor that contributes to social and political disparities for racial and ethnic minorities (Kreps, 2006). The National Institutes of Health (n.d.) defines health disparities as "differences in the incidence, prevalence, mortality, and burden of diseases and other adverse health conditions that exist among specific population groups in the United States." Health-care disparities among Latinos have been linked to patients' knowledge levels, attitudes, organizational factors in the health-care system, and cultural and social values (Thomas et al., 2004). Research also suggests that health disparities are associated with higher mortality rates among lung cancer patients (Bach et al., 1999). Moreover, minorities including Latinos have poorer health status and receive lower quality of health care than non-minorities (Solis, 2003). Comparing Latinos to non-Latino Whites, Latinos are 152 percent more likely to die from cervical cancer, 107 percent more likely to die from stomach cancer (63 percent higher for males and 150 percent for females), and 20 percent less likely to receive ongoing health care (U.S. Cancer Statistics, 2003). Health organizations are less likely to provide clinically necessary and routine procedures for minorities, and are more likely to deliver low-quality health services to these patients (Smedley et al., 2003).

While some research links health disparities to sociodemographic characteristics of minority patients, other researchers demonstrate that racial and ethnic disparities exist even when patients' ages, income levels, insurance status, and severity of medical condition are consistent (OMH, 2003). Given that at least 35.5 million persons in the United States are Latino (U.S. Census,

2000), the need to eliminate racial and ethnic disparities in health is evident. Culturally competent communication that more fully incorporates patient needs could play a central role in helping to overcome health disparities among racially and ethnically diverse patients.

The relationships among communication, culture, and health disparities are especially salient for two major reasons. First, disparities may occur because of providers' inability to co-create culturally sensitive interactions with patients and their families. If patients receive and manage health information in culturally specific ways, it is important to understand this process clearly. For example, efforts to increase the number of mammograms performed on Latino women may be hindered by familial roles of women in Latino culture.

Second, communication between patients and providers is the fundamental means through which high-quality medical care occurs. Patients experiencing disparities may differ in their communication with providers based on culture (Ashton et al., 2003). If there are treatment barriers that originate from culturally specific issues, then providers interested in reducing health disparities for Latinos must identify those issues. Specific areas of concern are such issues as how to create culturally and linguistically appropriate care for Latinos, and the role of family in cancer care.

Finally, since information management plays such an important role in a cancer patient's health experience, Brashers et al. (2002) encourage researchers to examine how patients' cultural beliefs affect patient information seeking and avoiding behaviors. They also suggest researchers examine how patient behaviors vary in terms of directness and indirectness, and whether patients or family members should be the primary recipients of health information. An awareness of socioeconomic characteristics and Latino cultural values can be incorporated by providers to enhance cultural competencies about the manner in which health messages are constructed and disseminated.

Latino cultural values and characteristics affecting cancer care

Although many communication models offer culture as a barrier to effective communication, the culture-centered approach to health communication highlights the voices of marginalized people as a central force in health-care decision making. In this manner, culture "is conceptualized as both transformative and constitutive, providing an axis for theorizing the discursive processes through which meaning are socially constructed" (Dutta-Bergman, 2004, p. 241). The fluidity of Latino culture creates a lens through which cultural values influence, and are influenced by, health concerns. Issues such as language barriers and cultural values including *fatalismo, familiaism, machismo, marianismo, respeto,* and spiritualism all have a potential impact on the way patients experience cancer care.

Language

Perhaps the most obvious barrier to quality health care for many language. Language barriers impede access to health organizations, diminis. potential quality of health-care services, and increase the risk of unintended health outcomes due to miscommunication (Lu & Flores, 2005). Spanish-speaking patients face a multitude of obstacles in health organizations where English is the primary language for spoken and written communication. In addition to problems interacting with providers, language barriers for Spanish-speaking patients might include making appointments, locating appropriate health-care facilities, reading signage in provider offices, completing patient intake forms, interacting with providers, and reading prescription and drug interaction information.

Although Title VI of the Civil Rights Act requires U.S. medical facilities to provide translators for patients with limited English proficiency, translators are not typically involved in every aspect of patient care and decision making, and many are poorly trained or inexperienced with translating medical information (Lu & Flores, 2005). In some cases, family members who attend doctor visits with their parents act as translators (McGorry, 1999). Even though their language skills allow them to speak in both English and Spanish, patient family members are not typically experienced with using specific medical jargon, or detailing treatment options and drug protocols. Moreover, family members may be a barrier to openness between patients and providers if they need to translate sensitive or embarrassing information for the patient. For example, Latina women being screened for breast cancer are less likely to share personal information about their symptoms if their child is asked to act as the translator.

Latino cultural values and the health-care context

Members of the Latino population co-construct meaning about their health-care experiences in terms of structural and cultural issues. Language barriers help explain some health disparities for Latinos, yet cultural issues move beyond language differences. A third feature of Dutta-Bergman's cultural framework is polymorphism, which suggests that events have possible multiple meanings. Members of the Latino community struggle with dialectical tensions related to structural and cultural issues common in many Latino communities. Values such as fatalismo, personalismo, familiaism, and gender roles affect communication about cancer as patients negotiate meanings of their health-care experiences through a cultural lens.

Fatalismo is a cultural and religious belief that leads many Latinos to believe that illnesses such as cancer are predetermined by God, and should therefore be accepted or endured in accordance with God's will (Antshel, 2002). Latinos who have a strong sense of fatalismo are more likely to feel anxiety and psychological distress about illness (Ross et al., 1983). They are also less likely to comply with treatment recommendations by providers or seek treatment for themselves or their families (Baquet & Hunter, 1995).

An emphasis on personal relationships in Latino culture is referred to as *personalismo* (Antshel, 2002). Interactions with physicians may be influenced by respect, or *respeto*, and a high context communication style. Personalismo explains the value that the Latino culture places on warm, sincere, and relational communication (Cora-Bramble & Williams, 2000). Underscoring this need for personalization of care, Trevino et al., (1991) report that when discussing health care, Latinos are more likely to refer to their medical care provider than they are the institution where they receive care. If a provider moves out of the area, Latinos families sometimes stop receiving health-care services until they can receive an introduction to a new provider and build a relationship with him or her (Trevino et al., 1991).

A sense of respeto for persons in positions of power may lead to fewer questions asked in medical interviews because the patient is concerned about challenging the doctor's authority (Cora-Bramble & Williams, 2000; Kakai et al., 2003). Personalismo as a cultural belief is antithetical to the current trends of short physician–patient interactions and fewer long-term relationships between providers and patients.

Although Latino culture is comprised of persons from several races and nationalities, a central cultural value among many Latinos from various backgrounds is *familiaism*, a strong emphasis on both nuclear and extended family (Antshel, 2002). The collectivistic orientation of Latino culture leads to behaviors such as a sense of responsibility and sacrifice for the benefit of the family, generous assistance for family members, and expected obedience, loyalty, and respect toward senior members of the family.

Gender roles within Latino families often highlight the patriarchal nature of Latino culture. *Machismo* is often treated as a negative value referring to "male domination" (Antshel, 2002, p. 439), and "aggressiveness, sexual domination, risky behavior" (Neff, 2001, p. 173) among Latino men. However, machismo also can refer to such positive masculine ideas as courage, honor, fearlessness, pride, and charisma (Neff, 2001; Stevens, 1973). *Marianismo* refers to the corresponding female ideal of a nurturing, caretaker who takes the primary role in social support and care for immediate and extended family members (Antshel, 2002). Origins of Marianismo as a behavioral pattern come from deep-rooted Catholic beliefs of the traditional Latin female as related to the Mary, the mother of Christ (Wood & Price, 1997). Implications of marianismo create an ideal of women who are morally superior and spiritually stronger than the man. In terms of health care, this may mean that Latino women choose not to undergo treatments that would take them away from family responsibilities, or fail to disclose negative health information to family or providers.

This research explores stories of Latinos' cancer experiences as voices from the margin. Members of this population share their experiences to create meaning about cancer care through the negotiated tensions between the margin and the hegemonic center. In this tension we find inconsistencies and gaps that reveal power and ideological differences (Dutta-Bergman, 2004; Martin et al., 1997). Cultural values are present in varying degrees, and various interpretations of Latino values are present in each negotiated experience.

We want to understand and examine these experiences because they reveal ideological differences and power differences, especially for traditionally marginalized populations. We have met Latina women (and one male) who were willing to talk about their experiences with cancer. From their stories, we can begin to understand the tensions that they deal with when negotiating their cancer experiences from the margins. Dutta-Bergman's cultural framework of health communication is a starting point to begin legitimate theory building from the marginalized spaces. This study may have a small population, but the dialectical tensions in the stories serve as a starting point for beginning to understand constructs and their relationships for how Latinas negotiate their understandings of cancer and how it should be treated. As we begin to understand these processes, then health-care professionals can use this information to communicate with patients from this population in more culturally appropriate ways.

Given the unique forms and functions of communication about cancer among socioeconomically disadvantaged Latina residents along the Texas–Mexico border, we ask:

- RQ1: How do Latino residents of the colonias conceptualize and communicate about their experiences with cancer?
- RQ2: What are the inherent gaps and inconsistencies in the dialectical tensions in their stories?
- RQ3: What do these gaps reveal about access and agency for Latinos in their experiences with cancer?

Method

Background

As health communication scholars living in South Texas, we are consistently reminded by news reports and personal experiences of the growing need for health communication research on marginalized Latinos in this area of the country. Our initial introduction to the people of the colonias came as part of an interdisciplinary research team examining health disparities among Latinos in the South Texas region. Our co-researcher on a previous project was a radiation oncologist from Laredo, Texas, who had several contacts at community centers in the colonias near Laredo, including El Cenizo. The community center in El Cenizo was familiar and accessible, and therefore became the location of our interviews for this study. Two members of the research team have close family members who immigrated to the United States from Mexico, and who share many of the cultural values of the Latino people in the colonias. Although our families come from more privileged backgrounds than our participants, the desire to explore the cultural realm of cancer care comes in part from our own backgrounds.

Setting of colonias

For this study, we traveled to the Texas–Mexico border region to interview residents of a *colonia* about their experience with cancer. El Cenizo is a Texas colonia located 15 miles south of the city of Laredo on the banks of the Rio Grande River (Wilson & Guajardo, n.d.). According to the US Department of Housing and Urban Development, the definition of a colonia is a rural community or neighborhood located within 150 miles of the Texas–Mexico border that lacks basic infrastructure and services, that is, potable water and paved roads. There are more than 1,400 colonias along the Texas–Mexico border.

While each colonia is different, many share the same set of challenges, from a need to improve housing quality to a need for improved infrastructure. The great majority of the families have extremely low incomes. Most colonias suffer from unpaved and poorly paved streets, a sewer system which is in very poor condition, lack of garbage collection, police and fire services, and other basic city services. As an economically poor community, residents of the colonias struggle with very limited resources and a state government not entirely responsive to their needs.

Residents of the colonias face challenges including isolation from city services and transportation, extremely low wages, a steady increase in the number of people competing for jobs, and high unemployment rates. Almost one-third of the entire region lives below the poverty line, and at least 38 percent of children living in the Texas border counties live below the poverty level (Strayhorn, 1998). Meanwhile, the population is still increasing at rapid rate. According to the North American Free Trade Agreement (NAFTA), the region will see an accelerated migration to the area and by the year 2020 the region is expected to have 6.3 million residents (Strayhorn, 1998). The rapid population growth and prevailing low incomes contributes to the housing problems in the region. Low-income border families are not able to obtain affordable housing in border cities so many families buy lots in rural colonias and build homes for themselves from whatever supplies they can procure. The inadequate housing and infrastructure services create some of the worst health conditions in the country. Tuberculosis, hepatitis, salmonella, and water-related disease are found at elevated levels (Wilson & Guajardo, n.d.). The Texas state government has made some efforts to improve living conditions in the colonias, but modernization of the infrastructure has occurred much more slowly than in most other parts of the state (Wilson & Guajardo, n.d.).

Research participants

Residents of the El Cenizo colonia participated in the study. Seven women, ages 19–65, and one man, age 42, participated in the voluntary interviews, which lasted approximately 25 minutes each. Of the eight participants, two had cancer themselves and six experienced cancer of a close family member. A 19-year-old female participant successfully waged a battle with leukemia, and a 42-year-old female participant was undergoing chemotherapy for breast cancer at the time of the interview. Table 9.1 offers a description of each participant in the study.

Significant research highlights Latino males' reluctance to communicate about illness. For this reason, the original goal of this study was to explore women's narratives about their cancer experiences. In the end, however, one male participant was included because of his strong desire to talk with the research team about his family member's cancer diagnosis. His narratives helped illuminate how his female family member dealt with her cancer through dialogue with her male cousin. Because his narrative came from the perspective of a male receiver of communication from a female cancer patient, the male participant was especially helpful in illuminating how gender roles influence perceptions of the cancer experience.

Procedures

The research team contacted the Catholic Archdiocese of Laredo to help solicit volunteers for this study. A nun who was working in the colonias provided a list of potential participants who she knew had personally experienced cancer, or had a close family member who had experienced cancer.

Table 9.1 Research participant demographics

Participant	Gender	Age	Marital status	Characteristics or circumstances
A	Female	55	Single	Lump in breast possibly has breast cancer
B	Female	57	Married	Aunt died of cervical cancer & sister died of uterine cancer
C	Female	65	Married	Brother-in-law had stomach cancer
D	Female	42	Married	Diagnosed with breast cancer
E	Female	64	Married	Husband had lung cancer
F	Male	42	Married	Female cousin has breast cancer
G	Female	58	Widowed	Husband died of lung cancer
H	Female	19	Single	Had leukemia beginning at age 12

Members of the research team contacted potential participants by telephone to set up interviews. To be sensitive to the needs of a few participants who were undergoing treatment for cancer at the time of the study, the nun contacted them directly to inquire about their desire and ability to participate in the project. To show gratitude for their participation in the study, each participant was paid $25.

The general protocol for the interviews was conducted at the El Cenizo Community Center in a private office to ensure participant confidentiality. To increase participants' comfort levels and willingness to share their stories, the third author served as lead interviewer because she is a first-generation Mexican American from South Texas. The first author was also present and participated in the interview process. The use of open-ended questions was used to elicit participant narratives for the project. Since all eight interviews were conducted in Spanish, the interview guide was also translated into Spanish to avoid conversational lags due to translation issues.

The interviews were audio recorded for transcription, following participants' permission. Interviews lasted between 20 and 45 minutes, with an average of 25 minutes. In total, over 10 hours of audio tape were collected. Both narrative and thematic analytic techniques were used to transcribe the interviews. Researchers used interview data from participants to systematically examine personal narratives about experiences with cancer. Finally, the researchers examined each extracted phrase to formulate meanings of significant statements, issues, and concerns discussed by participants (Ellingson & Buzzanell, 1999). Finally, consistent with Ellingson and Buzzanell's (1999) methodological approach, words and phrases from each participant's narratives were grouped together based on common root issues, semantic issues, and examples of cultural barriers to cancer care.

Existing research on Latinas' communication about cancer was used in combination with the research questions for this investigation to create an interview protocol comprised of four primary categories with probes. Table 9.2 outlines the specific areas of inquiry and goal issues to be discussed during the interviews. Three categories dealt with personal experience with cancer, religiosity and fatalismo, and medical establishment barriers. An additional category examined cultural identification (marianismo) among the participants.

In the first category, participants were asked to describe cancer based on their own experiences. Participants were asked to define cancer and share a story about their own experience with the disease. These questions sought to address goal issues of knowledge of cancer, sources of information, and experience with interaction.

The second category asked participants if they felt they could play a role in preventing cancer, what they would do if they had cancer, and where would they go for guidance. To explore perceptions of fatalismo, participants were also asked to describe their view of God's role in a person getting and surviving

Table 9.2 Interview guide

Major theme	Narrative	Goal issues
Personal experience with cancer	1 How would you describe cancer to someone who has never had it? 2 Tell me the story about your experience with cancer?	• Knowledge of cancer • Sources of information • Experience of interaction
Religiosity and fatalismo	1 Do you feel you can play a role in preventing cancer? 2 Based on your experience, do you think God plays a role in getting cancer? What about surviving cancer?	• Perceived risk of cancer • Perceived physical risk of cancer • Perceived social support • Perceived efficacy • Perceived prevention
Cultural identification (marianismo)	1 Describe a typical day in your household. In your neighborhood. Who is there? What happens? What do you do? 2 Do you feel your family is a traditional sort of Mexican–American family? Why or why not?	• Role in household • Type of marital relationship • Self-image/Self-esteem • Sacrifice
Medical establishment barriers	1 Tell me about the experience you had with the cancer doctors. What was it like? How did you (and/or they) feel? 2 Did your doctors speak Spanish? Did they listen to you? 3 Was payment an issue?	• Language

cancer. The goal of these questions was to tap into their perception of risk, physical risk, social support, efficacy and prevention.

The third category requested a description of a typical day in the participants' household. They were asked to describe who is there, what happens and what they do. Also, we asked if their households are traditional Mexican-American family and why or why not. Finally, participants were asked to share what types of things they do for themselves. Again, these questions sought to address their role in the household, type of marital relationship, self-image/self-esteem and sacrifice.

The final category asked participants to share an experience they had with a doctor; more specifically, what the experience was like and how it made them feel. Here, the goal was to gain insight to their views of physicians, power differences, language and insurance.

Results and interpretation

The data from the interviews were analyzed to understand how the participants negotiate dialectical tensions while trying to decode and interpret messages about cancer. Such an analysis reveals the interdependent and complementary aspects of seeming opposites. The juxtaposition of these opposites reveals both the presence or absence of certain ideologies. Messages of power and resistance are located in the boundaries of the competing meanings of the messages (Martin et al., 1997).

The original areas of inquiry from the interview guide helped elicit participant accounts about their experiences with cancer. The purpose of reconfiguring themes based on data obtained was to organize accounts in such a way to privilege participants' experiences over our a priori categories. The resulting analysis revealed a set of dialectical tensions present in two major themes from participant narratives. The dialectical approach stresses the contradictory and sometimes oppositional nature of communication (Martin et al., 1997).

The two emergent themes of dialectical tensions present were control and cultural identification. The poles of the theme of control were based on "the balance of nature" versus "a good God theory." The poles of the theme of cultural identification were identification with the Mexican medical system and barriers to health care in the U.S. medical system.

Control: balance of nature versus the good God theory

Discourse about their cancer experiences revealed cultural influences on participants' views about the role of God and nature in illness. This theme illuminates perceptions about personal control in preventing, treating, and surviving cancer. A dialectical tension seems to exist between controlling cancer through harmony in the natural environment, and God's ability to supersede nature to act whenever necessary.

Balance of nature

The term *bienstar*, reflects the Latino belief about maintaining well-being by balancing emotional, physical, and social contexts (Cora-Bramble & Williams, 2000). At one end of the issue of control was the participants' ideas that cancer is a natural process that can sometimes be avoided by maintaining balance in the psychological, physical, and spiritual aspects of life. This perspective suggests the balance of nature allows for some level of control in preventing and treating cancer, but lack of moderation can cause cancer. Participant F described cancer by saying, "It's bad. They're bad things one asks for from a drunken night, a fight, if one doesn't take care of their body—that's how illness enters. A wisdom tooth that one doesn't take care of . . . that can cause cancer." In this case a lack of balance results in lack of control over body and mind. Participant A also noted, "Cancer is of natural things. It comes from nature, but we can prevent it by what we do."

Contrary to Anglo-American culture, Latino cultural norms dictate that mind and body are inseparable. There is also a belief that strong emotional states cause physical illness (Maduro, 1983). Many Latinos feel that the human body is healthy when it has balance and harmony of opposing qualities such as hot and cold, or wetness and dryness (ibid.). In other words, maintaining health is related to maintaining balance and moderation. In this view, cancer comes from an imbalance of dietary, social, or emotional inputs. These beliefs illustrate a view that cancer patients may have played a significant role in getting cancer based on their own "unnatural" behaviors; however, cancer itself is seen as being a very natural process.

The view of cancer as natural seems to be in opposition with a purely fatalistic view of cancer. Fatalismo, the belief that an individual can do little to change fate, may explain cancer in seemingly innocent patients such as children who appear to have no control over their own fate. Participant H described her battle with leukemia at a very young age as, "a test to go ahead— we're getting another chance if we pass. It's a test from God, not something natural. The only thing natural is that God always gives people tests. Mine was just cancer."

Good God theory

Among all participants, the issue of control of cancer was intertwined with beliefs about God. All participants reported a strong belief in God, but the role of God in cancer treatment and prevention varied slightly. This finding connects previous research that suggests that patients and their families tend to define their cancer experiences more by issues of control and social support rather than the biology of the disease (Bowker, 1996; Ellingson & Buzzanell, 1999; Gibbs & Franks, 2002; Keeley, 1996).

Except for Participant H, who viewed cancer as a test, the common theme among other participants' descriptions of God was that of a healer—the only one who can cure cancer. This "good God theory" is defined as a sense that cancer is not a punishment from God, but rather something that occurs in nature that can only be cured by God. This approach means that control of cancer outcomes lies with a benevolent God who has the power to alleviate pain and suffering, and ultimately heal cancer patients.

The control theme was also exemplified by participants' narratives about their information needs related to cancer. Consistent with existing literature, some participants reported avoidance of information about cancer as a means of control and as a demonstration in the power of God. Information avoidance may be a result of trust in God or health-care providers, fear of the information, and a belief that other patients have greater need of the doctor (Leydon, 2000; Rees & Bath, 2001). In this study, participants generally felt that while they did not have control of the cancer in themselves or their family member, they could control the information they chose to receive about diagnosis and treatment options. Moreover, Participant D who was undergoing chemotherapy at the time of our interview stated, "I haven't asked my doctor what comes next. And my husband doesn't ask me what is happening either. We are just praying that everything will be alright." Information avoidance as a means of control may be affected by the tendency of Hispanic patients to be more afraid of cancer (Grenier, 1995) or attributions of "fatalismo" to their desire to know little information about terminal illness (Sullivan, 2001).

Although research links religious coping strategies with improvements in the physical and mental health of patients (Pargament, 1997), few studies examine the role of religion in cancer patients' and their families sense of control over their disease. Participants in this study described a very strong sense that God was the source of all cures, not just a source of strength in the survivorship process. As Participant C noted, "God is like a very special doctor because he has healed people with cancer." Similarly, Participant E stated, "I think curing cancer is a miracle that only God can perform."

Finally, consistent with existing literature that indicates Latinos use prayer as an active form of seeking help (Guarnaccia et al., 1992), participants noted the importance of families (*familiaism*) in the prayer process. For example, Participant C explained, "Our whole family prayed to God every day for a cure. We all had to pray." Prayer was a way for family members to actively seek to control and *luchar* (fight) for their family members' health.

Cultural identification: Mexican identity versus the US approach to health care

Reflecting the collectivist orientation associated with Latino culture, group and social roles was a major theme discussed by participants. The poles of this theme were identification with Mexican culture and the Mexican medical system versus confusion from barriers to healthcare in the US medical system.

Identification with Mexican culture and the Mexican medical system

A major topic area posed to all participants was about their potential views about marianismo among Latina cancer patients. The first significant finding in this area came as all participants except one identified themselves as Mexican, not Mexican American, in terms of their citizenship and their view of life. For example, Participant B whose two close female relatives died of cancer described her family by saying, "We are a Mexican family, with Mexican customs that we already had with us ... that we brought. We all keep our customs now." Similarly, when Participant C was asked if her family is a traditional sort of Mexican-American family she answered "yes" as the interviewer was still speaking so as to cut off the word American. She then stated, "We are Mexican. Not American. It's a Mexican household because we're from Mexico." This explanation reveals a resistance to prevailing U.S. cultural norms.

The second major issue related to maintenance of cultural roles was the consistent discussion of traditional gender roles by cancer patients. Participant D offered perhaps the most poignant narrative by describing her struggle with cancer as a struggle to maintain her identity as a mother and wife. She felt that it was important to continue caring for others during her cancer treatment, and that loss of her role as nurturer for others was as painful as the cancer treatment itself. Discussing her struggle with breast cancer, she explained,

> I cannot sweep or mop. I try, like yesterday I was trying to fold clothes for my four children. It's not hard, I think I can do it, but I can't, I don't have the strength. If I push myself, the next day is really hard for me. I'll wake up the next day swollen and I felt a stinging pain. It's not strenuous, I think it's not hard, but my body cannot handle it. My husband helps me. I put the clothes to wash, but the laundry basket has to be up high and presorted. It has to be ready to be put in. I can't lift the bottle of bleach. How hard is it to fold clothes? It's not hard, I just can't do it.

Participant D also noted that although her husband presorted the laundry for her so she could wash it, she did not discuss her cancer treatment with him and he did not take over her responsibilities, even when she was undergoing chemotherapy. Her discourse reveals a need to maintain her identity and traditional gender role in her family.

Concern about U.S. medical system

A major finding in this area was the concern about cultural identity as it relates to dealing with what Beck (2001, p. 15) describes as "a widespread commitment to medical absolutism and institutional authority." Participants' decisions about how and whether to use alternative forms of health-care treatment seem to relate in part to their levels of acculturation.

Acculturation is defined in the medical literature as acquisition of cultural elements of a dominant society (Lara et al., 2005). Sabogal et al. (1987) found that although more acculturated Latino people continue to perceive high support from their family, they often demonstrate less behavior associated with familismo. Low acculturated persons, on the other hand, are more likely to share the medical experience with family members. Participant H noted that her entire family often went with her to doctor visits because, "We're a united family. We encourage each other."

Some participants discussed patients' reliance on Curanderos as an alternative to traditional American cancer treatments. Curanderos are Mexican folk healers who often attribute illness to the person's acculturation and will encourage them to resist this change (Maduro, 1983). Whereas American physicians typically treat only the body of a person, curanderos treat the soul of the person separate from the body. For example, prayers, penance, miracles and vows are part of curandismo because of the Latino beliefs of the inter-penetration of the natural and supernatural worlds. Moreover, Curanderos value the family as part of the treatment process (Maduro, 1983).

Participant B described how financial barriers led her family to go to Mexico for alternative treatment. She added, "I haven't needed to but I have seen a doctor before. No (I didn't have insurance) but I went to Mexico. We go to Mexico and pay cash and (get care from doctors and Curanderos) at a much lower rate." Financial barriers were also a major issue for Participant A, who was concerned about a potentially cancerous lump in her breast. Her sense of frustration was due to her inability to get medical attention despite consistent attempts to do so. She explained,

> I don't have the money for a biopsy. They ran all sorts of screenings that ranged from $5, $10, $15 and $40, but I just can't afford a biopsy. Even with the smaller fees for the other tests, I had to arrange payment plans. I have a pap every year and I've had over twenty mammograms, but I'm stuck right now. There's no help. Lots of programs come to the community center. They tell you to check yourself and they bring information, but no resources. We need monetary help. What is the program? Where is the program? Where do I/we go from here? It is not free help—it's no good.

The final significant finding from participant narratives related barriers to the U.S. medical care was the prevalence of Spanish physicians in the border region. Although many Spanish-speaking patients face obstacles due to language differences during the medical interview and treatment procedures, all participants reported that medical providers in and around the colonias spoke Spanish. Since Spanish is so predominant in the area, it makes sense that providers speak Spanish. However, this finding is still surprising in light of the small number of Latino physicians and Spanish-speaking physicians in the United States. It is not likely that all Latina cancer patients have access to Spanish-speaking providers. Participant C explained, "All of our health-care workers speak Spanish. How else would we be able to talk to them?"

Latino health-care providers may themselves face barriers to effective patient care. For example, Hargraves et al. (2001) found that almost 15 percent of

Latino physicians reported difficulty in getting specialty referrals for their patients, compared to less than 8 percent of white physicians. This finding highlights potential sources of health disparities for Latina patients.

Discussion and conclusion

This study focused on how low-income Mexican American's communicate their experiences with cancer treatment and prevention. Specifically it asked questions about how Latinas communicate about their cancer experiences, the gaps and inconsistencies present in these inconsistencies, and the power and ideological differences revealed by these gaps. The data collected during the interviews revealed dialectical tensions between two prominent themes that emerged: control of nature balance in environment versus a good God theory, and cultural identity versus socioeconomic barriers to health care. These tensions illustrate how discourse shapes ideologies to enhance or reduce individuals' status as agents in the cancer-care continuum. The roles of nature, God, family, socioeconomic status, and culture in participants cancer-care experiences reside within the larger structure of communication about cancer. Patients and their family members use narratives to make sense of the inherent tensions between these concepts in their cancer experiences. In this way, cancer became one manifestation of identity situated in the larger sociocultural context of their lives.

Conceptualization and communication of cancer

The first research question considers how Latino residents of the colonias conceptualize and communicate about their experiences with cancer. From Dutta-Bergman's (2004) framework, the cultural perspective highlights perceptions of incongruities the health-care setting related to issues such as familiaism, marianismo, and fatalismo. The structural perspective highlights how members of the Latino population negotiate the roles of health information and financial barriers with their cultural identities.

Aspects of the Latino culture, familialism, marianismo, and fatalismo shape how its members co-construct meaning about health issues, including their experiences with cancer (Dutta-Bergman, 2004). Family is the structure through which the cancer-care process occurred. As co-agents in the cancer-care process, the family members expressed true concern and interest in their loved ones' illnesses and recovery. The patients were not perceived as individuals with cancer, but rather as group members in need of additional social support and consideration. Within this context of family, the Latina women's roles as caretakers for their families were difficult to maintain in the face of a cancer diagnosis. Nevertheless, participants demonstrated that to take on the identity of "cancer patient" was to give up the identity associated with marianismo.

Finally, although there was evidence of fatalism among some participants, findings about God as a source of hope offered an interesting glimpse at religiosity in the cancer context. Specifically, participants did not report cancer as a punishment from God, but rather as a force of nature that only God could eradicate. Future research could examine this question in relationship to cancer prevention to determine whether a sense of fatalism among Latinas reduces use of cancer-prevention measures.

Aspects of social structures, such as access to health information and financial resources, also have the potential to shape how members of the Latino community make sense of their cancer experiences (Dutta-Bergman, 2004). The participants in this study indicate that they tend to avoid gaining health information about their cancer experiences as a means of expressing the level of control they feel (or do not feel) about their cancer experience. They may feel that even if they cannot control the experience of cancer, they can control the amount of health information they acquire and choose to avoid this information. The participants also touched on the structural theme of control when discussing their lack of access to financial resources.

The struggle between *bienstar* and *fatalismo* suggests that Latinos believe that they have some level of control in the prevention, treatment, and survivorship of cancer, but they tend to attribute control of only survivorship to fate, or God. This indicates confusion about the level of control and agency they feel from a larger picture of their cancer experience. Other tensions revealed in their communication may indicate attempts by the participants to gain control in other aspects of their cancer experiences.

Conclusion

These findings have important implications for future research in health and cancer communication. Rather than taking a more general focus on improving communication between patients and providers, health communication research should explore ways that culture and discourse enhance or diminish patients' perceived agency in the health-care setting. The findings about how the patients use communication and culture to interpret their cancer experiences in the context of a privileged biological/technological ideology reveals specific areas for future research from a patient-centered perspective. Future projects could look for similar results in Latinas with differing types of cancer or different serious medical conditions. Research questions that build on the findings of this project include: how communication creates the construct of control, how low-income Latino patients act as agents for themselves during the cancer care process, and how discourse in health-care settings privileges the biological/technical paradigm.

References

Antshel, K.L. (2002). Integrating culture as a means of improving treatment adherence in the Latino population. *Psychology, Health and Medicine, 7*, 435–449.

Ashton, C.M., Haldet, P., Paterniti, D.A., Collins, T.C., Gordon, H.S., O'Malley, K., Petersen, L.A., Sharf, B., Suarez-Almazor, M.E., Wray, N., & Street, R. (2003). Racial and ethnic disparities in the use of health services. *Journal of General Internal Medicine, 18*, 148–152.

Bach, P.B., Cramer, L., Warren, J.L. & Begg, C.B. (1999). Racial differences in the treatment of early stage lung cancer. *New England Journal of Medicine, 341*, 1198–1205.

Baquet, C.R., & Hunter, C.P. (1995). Patterns in minority and special populations. In P. Greenwald, B. Kramer, & D.L. Weed (eds), *Cancer Prevention and Control.* New York: Marcel Dekker, pp. 23–36.

Beck, C. (2001). *Communicating for Better Health: A Guide Through the Medical Mazes.* Boston: Allyn and Bacon.

Bowker, J. (1996). Cancer, individual process, and control: A case study in metaphor analysis. *Health Communication, 8*, 91–104.

Brashers, D.E., Goldsmith, D.J., & Hsieh, E. (2002). Information seeking and avoiding in health contexts. *Human Communication Research, 28*, 258–271.

Cora-Bramble, D., & Williams, L. (2000) Explaining illness to Latinos: Cultural foundations and messages. In B.B. Whaley (ed.), *Explaining Illness: Research, Theory, and Structure.* Mahwah, NJ: Erlbaum, pp. 259–279.

Dutta-Bergman, M. (2004). The unheard voices of Santalis: Communicating about health from the margins of India. *Communication Theory, 14*, 237–263.

Dutta Bergman, M. (2005). Theory and practice in health communication campaigns: A critical interrogation. *Health Communication, 18*, 103–122.

Ellingson, L.L., & Buzzanell, P.M. (1999). Listening to women's narratives of breast cancer treatment: A feminist approach to patient satisfaction with physician/patient communication. *Health Communication, 11*, 153–183.

Gibbs, R.W., & Franks, H. (2002). Embodied metaphor in women's narratives about their experiences with breast cancer. *Health Communication, 14*, 139–165.

Grenier, L.M. (1995). Cancer information and resources for Hispanic populations. *Cancer Practice, 3*, 317–319.

Guarnaccia, P.J., Parra, P.A., Deschamps, A., Milstein, G., & Nuri, A. (1992). Si Dios quiere [God Willing]: Hispanic families experiences' of caring for a seriously mentally ill family member. *Culture, Medicine, & Psychiatry, 16*, 187–215.

Gudykunst, W.B., Matsumoto, Y., Ting-Toomey, S., Nishida, T., Kim, K., & Heyman, S. (1996). The influence of cultural individualism-collectivism, self construals, and individual values on communication styles across cultures. *Human Communication Research, 22*, 510–543.

Hargraves, J.L., Stoddard, J.J., & Trude, S. (2001). Minority physicians' experiences obtaining referrals to specialists and hospital admissions. *Medscape General Medicine, 3*, 10.

Kakai, H., Maskarinec, G., Shumay, D.M., Tatsumura, Y., & Tasaki, K. (2003). Ethnic differences in choices of health information by cancer patients using complementary and alternative medicine: An exploratory study with correspondence analysis. *Social Science and Medicine, 56*, 851–862.

Keeley, M.P. (1996). Social support and breast cancer: Why do we talk and to whom do we talk? In R L. Parrot, & C.M. Condit (eds), *Evaluating Women's Health Messages: A Resource Book*. Thousand Oaks, CA: Sage, pp. 293–306.

Kreps, G. (2006). Communication and racial inequities in health care. *American Behavioral Scientist, 49*, 1–15.

Lara, M., Gamboa, C., Kahramanian, M.I., Morales, L.S., & Bautista, D.E. (2005). Acculturation and Latino health in the United States: A review of literature and its socio-political context. *Annual Review of Public Health, 26*, 367–397.

Leydon, G.M. (2000). Faith, hope, and charity: An in-depth interview study of cancer patients' information needs and information seeking behavior. *Western Journal of Medicine, 173*, 26–31.

Lu, L., & Flores, G. (2005). Pay now or pay later: Providing interpreter services in health care. *Health Affairs, 24*, 435–444.

Lupton, D. (1994). Toward the development of critical health communication praxis. *Health Communication, 6*, 55–67.

Maduro, R. (1983). Curandismo and latino views of disease and curing. *The Western Journal of Medicine, 139*, 868–874.

Martin, J.N., Nakayama, T.K., & Flores, L.A. (1997). A dialectical approach to intercultural communication. In J.N. Martin (ed.), *Readings in Cultural Contexts*. Mountain View, CA: Mayfield, pp. 5–12.

McGorry, S.Y. (1999). An investigation of expectations and perceptions of health-care services with a Latino population. *Journal of Health Care Quality Assurance, 12*, 190–197.

National Institutes of Health (n.d.) Addressing health disparities: The NIH program of action. http://healthdisparities.nih.gov/whatare.html. Retrieved February 23, 2005.

Neff, J.A. (2001). A confirmatory factor analysis of a measure of "machismo" among Anglo, African American and Mexican American male drinkers. *Hispanic Journal of Behavioral Sciences, 23*, 171–188.

Office of Minority Health, US Department of Health and Human Services (2003). National study of culturally and linguistically appropriate services in managed care organizations. www.omhrc.gov/cultural/MCOCLAS-1%20Final%20Report%20 Main1.pdf. Retrieved August 9, 2005.

O'Hair, D., Villagran, M.M., Wittenberg, E., Brown, K., Ferguson, M., Hall, H.T., & Doty, T. (2003). Cancer survivorship and agency model: Implications for patient choice, decision making, and influence. *Health Communication, 15*, 193–202.

Pargament, K.I. (1997). *The Psychology of Religion and Coping: Theory, Research, and Practice*. New York: Guilford Press.

Rees, C.E., & Bath, P.A. (2001). Information seeking behaviors of women with breast cancer. *Oncology Nursing Forum, 28*, 691–698.

Ross, C.E., Mirowski, J., & Cockerham, W.C. (1983). Social class, Mexican culture, and fatalism: their effects on psychological distress. *American Journal of Community Psychology, 11*, 383–399.

Sabogal, F., Marin, G., Otero-Sabogal, R., Marin, B.V., & Perez-Stable, E.J. (1987). Hispanic familism and acculturation: What changes and what doesn't? *Hispanic Journal of Behavioral Sciences, 4*, 397–412.

Smedley, B.D., Stith, A.Y., & Nelson, A.R. (2003). *Unequal Treatment: Confronting Racial and Ethnic Disparities in Health Care*. Washington, DC: National Academics Press.

Solis, H.L. (2003). Health disparities: A growing challenge in the Latino community. *Harvard Journal of Public Policy, 16*, 53–68.

Strayhorn, C.K. (1998). Window on state government website. "Colonias: A Symptom, Not the Problem." Bordering the Future. www.window.state.tx.us/border/border.html. Retrieved September 5, 2005.

Stevens, E. (1973). Machismo and marianismo. *Society, 10*, 57–63.

Sullivan, M.C. (2001). Lost in translation: How Latinos view end-of-life care. *Plastic Surgical Nursing, 21*, 90–91.

Thomas, S.B., Fine, M.J., & Ibrahim, S.A. (2004) Health disparities: The importance of culture and health. *American Journal of Public Health, 94*, 9–36.

Trevino, F., Moyer, M., Valdez, R., & Stroup-Benham, C. (1991). Utilization of health services by Mexican-American, Mainland Puerto-Ricans and Cuban-Americans. *Journal of the American Medical Association, 265*, 233–237.

U.S. Cancer Statistics (2003). Incidence and mortality. Department of Health and Human Services, Centers for Disease Control and Prevention, and National Cancer Institute. http://apps.nccd.cdc.gov/uscs/. Retrieved September 30, 2005.

U.S. Census (2000). www.census.gov/. Retrieved October 25, 2005.

Villagran, M.M., Bains, Y.S., Guajardo, J., Munoz, O., & Thomas, C.R. (2005) Preliminary investigation of preferred mediated and interpersonal sources of health information among low-income Hispanic program women receiving mammograms: The Laredo NCI U56 Health Care Disparities Navigator. Paper prepared for the 2005 American Society of Therapeutic Radiation and Oncology Conference, Denver, CO.

Villagran, M., & Hoffman, M. (2006). Creating culturally appropriate organizational communication messages to combat health disparities in cancer care. In L. Sparks, H.D. O'Hair, & G.L. Kreps, (eds), *Cancer Communication and Aging*. Cresskill, NJ: Hampton Press.

Wilson, R.H., & Guajardo, M. (n.d.) Capacity building and governance in El Cenizo. www.utexas.edu/academic/uip/inside/cyprojects/copcyrs/cscape.html. Retrieved September 10, 2005.

Wood, M.L., & Price, P. (1997). Machismo and marianismo: Implications for HIV/AIDS reduction and education. *American Journal of Health Studies, 13*, 44–53.

Chapter 10

El Poder y la Fuerza de la Pasión[1]

Toward a model of HIV/AIDS education and service delivery from the "bottom-up"

Ariana Ochoa Camacho, Gust A. Yep,
Prado Y. Gomez, and Elissa Velez

> If the diverse and heterogeneous Latino populations in the United States are to successfully fight AIDS in their communities, then *todo* [everything]—not just Anglo domination—"tiene que cambiar" [needs to change].[2]
>
> David Román (1998, p. 183)

Latino communities disproportionately have been affected—and devastated—by HIV/AIDS since the beginning of the epidemic in th United States (Arend, 2005; Díaz, 1998; Greene et al., 2003; Román, 1998; Yep, 1992). The severity of these effects is directly related to individual and group locations in current U.S. race, class, gender, and sexuality hierarchies (Ford & Yep, 2003; Minkler, 1998; Robert & House, 2000). For example, people at the bottom of these hierarchies (e.g., poor, transgender women of color) lack access to medical and social services, have fewer social, cultural, and political resources, and die younger and more quickly once they contract HIV when compared to individuals at higher locations in these hierarchies (e.g., white, middle-class gay men) (Arend, 2005; Nemoto et al., 2005). Latinas/os living with HIV/AIDS frequently experience some combination of racial and gender discrimination, poverty, homophobia, and AIDS-phobia and discrimination, often from within and outside of their own communities (Díaz, 1998; Román, 1998; Roque Ramírez, 2005). Calling our attention to the daily realities of Latino gay and bisexual men with HIV/AIDS, Alice Villalobos (as cited in Román, 1998, p. 184) writes:

> [These men] are usually forced to live within the homophobic Latino/a community because of poverty and oppression. Not only are they rejected by their own people, but they also have to deal with a white, Anglo culture that categorizes them as second-class citizens merely because of the color of their skin.

For HIV/AIDS education and service delivery programs to be effective, they must attend to the complex social and cultural realities that Latinos currently face in the United States (Díaz, 1998; Yep, 1992).

Traditional health education and service delivery programs, including HIV/AIDS work, tend to be designed by "experts" in the medical and health-care establishment. Communication, in this model, is

> largely regarded as a "top-down" and somewhat paternalistic exercise, in which those with the medical or public health knowledge, whether they be physicians, other health care professionals, or health educators, perceive their role as disseminating the "right" message to the masses for their own good. [These masses] are often regarded . . . as apathetic and ignorant, needful of persuasion to change their behavior, resistant to change, obstinate, recalcitrant, lacking self-efficacy, chronically uninformed, and "hard to reach."
>
> (Lupton, 1994, p. 56)

Recognizing that this approach reproduces and reinforces current social inequities and heeding Dorsey's (2003) observation that in the field of health communication "there has been an emerging recognition, particularly within underserved and hard-to-reach areas, that *perhaps the most helpful health interventions are those planned and executed by communities themselves*" (p. 205, our emphasis) and Prohaska et al.'s (2000) call for "direct involvement in collaborative partnerships and a mutual exchange of information" (p. 371), this chapter articulates a community-generated and culturally and historically specific "living theory" of wellness, health behavior, and HIV/AIDS education that Proyecto ContraSIDA Por Vida (PCPV or Proyecto) created, designed, delivered, and assessed in the Latino communities[3] in San Francisco, California. To accomplish this, our chapter is divided into four sections. First, we discuss our approach to this project. Our commitments are based on the ideals of a critical health communication praxis, "third-order" research, and collaborative community dialogue. Next, we provide a description of PCPV, the community organization that enabled and exemplified the creation of a HIV/AIDS education and service delivery model from the "bottom-up." Third, we describe this model and provide specific examples based on Proyecto's work with community members. We conclude by discussing the implications of the project for future theory, research, and praxis.

Toward a critical health communication praxis: "third-order" research and community dialogue

> [Critical health communication focuses] attention on discourse and the ways in which the use of language in the [health-care] setting acts to perpetuate the interests of some groups over others. Questions to be asked

include: In whose interests is the discourse operating? What (and whose) values, beliefs, and concepts are espoused, and what others are neglected? What preestablished knowledge or belief systems are drawn upon to create meaning? What types of social differences are established or perpetuated?

Deborah Lupton (1994, p. 55)

In response to the growing social inequities and health disparities in contemporary society, critical health communication emerged in recent years (e.g., Airhihenbuwa, 1995; Airhihenbuwa & Ludwig, 1997; Ford & Yep, 2003; Lupton, 1994; Mokros & Deetz, 1996; Ray, 1996). This approach highlights the importance of power, ideology, and hegemony in health-care contexts. According to Foucault (1978), power is a network of relations that circulates through all social relationships—including health-care interactions and medical encounters—and all levels of society. This network is not simply constraining and limiting (power-over) but also productive and enabling (power-to). Critical health communication scholars recognize that power is ever present in all aspects of health care ranging from health-care provider–patient interactions to health policies and cultural beliefs about health, wellness, and illness. Ideology generally refers to attempts to fix meaning to maintain and support the worldviews of the powerful. For example, the medical establishment attempts to provide meanings associated with health and illness that are presented as universal and taken-for-granted truths while obscuring how such meanings are used to maintain the power of medical professionals and the profit margins for health-care industries. The power of ideology is to naturalize certain meanings—the way health is or should be—by making them beyond question. Finally, hegemony is a temporary closure of meaning to support the interests and beliefs of the powerful. This is accomplished by the winning of consent in which historically powerful groups—for example, health policy makers and pharmaceutical companies—exercise social authority, control, and leadership over the general population. Critical health communication scholars and practitioners call for an ongoing attention to and analysis of how power, ideology, and hegemony operate in health-care contexts, and explore ways in which health disparities may be reduced or eradicated in society.

According to Lupton (1994), critical health communication is characterized by four fundamental commitments. First, it recognizes and unpacks the role of ideology in health communication theory, research, and practice. For example, much of current health promotion work, with such an emphasis on individualism, personal choice, cost effectiveness, and the evaluation of measurable effects, adheres to the dominant ideology of the state and its funding agencies. Second, it proposes a broader conceptualization of culture that includes both a) values, beliefs, attitudes, language, institutions, and structures of power and b) a variety of cultural practices such as eating habits, daily activities, artistic forms, media products, mass-produced commodities, and consumption patterns. In this sense, health, disease, and illness are products of a range of cultural practices and norms. Third, it highlights the role of power at all levels of health-care delivery, design, and implementation. For example, a health-care provider–patient relationship takes place in a field of inequality and struggle that is supported by larger social discourses about health, illness, and the body and enacted and negotiated by the individuals in a health-care relationship. Finally, it emphasizes the importance of advocacy in critical health communication work. It calls for health communicators to refrain from becoming representatives of medical hegemony and to intervene in multiple ways to resist oppressive discourses and improve quality of life and health environments for everyone. These commitments also suggest a distinct approach to research.

Conscious of the ever-present danger of research and knowledge production to recreate and perpetuate relations of inequality and injustice in society, Santiago-Valles (2003) suggests "third-order, praxis, or participatory action research" in which the researcher(s) and community being researched are working as collaborative partners in "conversation across cultures" (p. 60). This type of practice is set apart from first- and second-order research. First-order research, such as many types of surveys characteristic of etic research techniques, reproduce unequal relations where one side (the researcher) interrogates and the other side (the subject) is interrogated. The subject is expected to answer the questions and the researcher is authorized to make sense of the subject's answers; in other words, the subject is relatively passive. In second-order research, such as discussion groups typical of emic research techniques, the roles of interrogator and respondent are exchanged and information is produced in conversation. However, the researcher maintains the power to set the agenda for the exchange and the authority to extract information. Although the respondent is more active, unequal relations between the researcher and researched remain. Third-order research, such as socioanalysis that incorporates both etic and emic research techniques, is driven by the need to understand unequal power relations and the impulse to follow such understanding with action. This approach to research is culture-centered.

In health communication, the works of Collins Airhihenbuwa and Mohan Dutta-Bergman stand out as culture-centered. Airhihenbuwa and associates (e.g., Airhihenbuwa, 1990–1991, 1993, 1995; Airhihenbuwa et al., 1992) insist that health communication messages and programs should be sensitive to and consistent with the cultural framework of the targeted audience, or to put it differently, they argue for the centrality of the cultural realities and experiences of the individuals and community members deemed to be the recipients of such messages and programs. If culturally sensitive health intervention programs are developed, implemented, and evaluated, no "cultural barriers" exist. These barriers often result when dominant and hegemonic social and cultural standards are applied to less privileged groups—for example, the application and imposition of male, middle-class, English-speaking, European American values and beliefs about health, wellness, and illness on female, poor, non-English speaking, people of color (Airhihenbuwa & Obregon, 2000). Instead of imposition of dominant cultural values and its accompanying processes of erasure, devaluation, and annihilation of the values and culture of less privileged communities, Airhihenbuwa (1995) warns us that "empowerment of and participation by the people a program is intended to benefit must take into account the degree to which individual decisions are mediated by power, politics, class, and cultural understanding of the meaning of participation and empowerment" (pp. 123–124) and challenges health communication professionals to interrogate their own social locations before adopting any strategy for improving health conditions.

Dutta-Bergman's (2004a) work moves away from a focus on successful message transmission to emphasize the cultural and structural contexts of health. This approach is based on a critique of the underlying preset individualistic cultural bias of the dominant health communication approach. Such a bias largely ignores the role of context and structure in addition to being cognitively biased (Dutta-Bergman, 2005). Cognitive approaches are only able to account for individual behavioral choices that result from an active process of information evaluation, attitude formation, and then "rational" choice based on this process. Notably, even many individualistic health-based behaviors such as affective-laden choices, habitual behavior, and spur of the moment choices cannot be understood with such an approach. For example, in their hierarchical prioritization of "at-risk behavior" these models essentially fragment communities into categories that treat "risk" behavior as if it were distinct and separate from relationships—relationships between people, regardless of age, gender, ethnicity; and even draw distinctions between different aspects of one's self—spiritual wellness, physical health and psychological well-being. A health and wellness intervention would be rooted at the level of the collective rather than the individual (Dutta-Bergman, 2005). By understanding community health-related behavior as more than just an unconnected series of individuals behaving, Dutta-Bergman locates the collective at the core of health behavior.

This approach to research calls for the expansion of the locus of change from the individual to the collective and requires attentiveness to capacities, structures, and community. First, dealing with basic life issues is an important aspect of understanding this health communication work. Dutta-Bergman (2004a) urges health communication theorists and practitioners to "locate poverty and the lack of basic resources at the center of human behavior and communicative choice" (p. 114). For example, we cannot expect a sex worker to demand a client to use condoms and risk losing business when he is worried about feeding himself or his partner. Second, we should be attentive to structures as another relevant factor for health. For example, socioeconomic barriers can play an important role in early detection of many diseases because of the costs involved in screenings and clinic visits. Finally, understanding the community as the center of a bottom-up approach is crucial. Together with community members, critical health communication works to identify the structural impediments to health and acts as a team with community members to mobilize around these issues. This calls for understanding the experience of health or dis-ease from the perspective of community members. To be more explicit, such a critical health communication approach also engages with the agency of its clients or participants where community members can contribute to creating conditions that support (and sustain) healthy living by addressing social inequities that contribute to health inequities and moves toward health justice (Dutta-Bergman, 2004b).

Committed to understanding, listening, and negotiating our worldviews and driven by the impulse to articulate the dense particularities of the actions, ideals, and wisdom of the guiding principles and the everyday work of a culturally affirming, holistic, grassroots, and "alternative" HIV/AIDS community organization, our team[4] came together in February 2004. Other than these commitments, our collective goal was emergent rather than definitive. We met on a regular basis—sometimes several times a month—to discuss the nature of Proyecto's work, current theories and models of health behavior, recent research findings, and critical issues in HIV/AIDS work in the Latino communities in San Francisco. In these discussions, it became apparent that while PCPV's work is influenced by health behavior theories and models (e.g., health beliefs, theory of reasoned action, ecological model, the political economy of health, among others), it is ultimately guided by a unique—and valuable—perspective that is conspicuously absent in the current health communication literature. We started working toward the articulation of Proyecto's approach to HIV/AIDS and wellness between June 2004 and October 2005. Our approach to the work as a team was characterized by connectedness, respect, trust, openness, and multiplicity—all features of dialogic relations (Kristiansen & Bloch-Poulsen, 2000; Zoller, 2000). Together, we co-constructed a model that guides Proyecto's work while recognizing that such a model is always emerging, shifting, and changing as it interacts with social and environmental constraints and possibilities.

PCPV: a site of theory, a site of action

Proyecto ContraSIDA Por Vida is a nonprofit community organization in San Francisco's Mission district "guided by a vision of a healthy community capable of resisting/responding to HIV and other dis-ease with creativity, strength and faith." Proyecto describes its primary objective as "to provide a safe space, programs and services that invigorate Latina/o bisexual, lesbian, transgender and gay gente [people] in the San Francisco Bay Area with debate and desire, intellectual thought, erotic imagination and heartfelt passion" (PCPV, 2005). In this section, we provide a historical context for Proyecto's development and community work.

In 1993, PCPV was founded by members of the queer Latino community in response to a lack of services after the dissolution of San Francisco's first gay Latino HIV agency, CURAS (Communidad Unida en Respuesta al AIDS/SIDA/Community United in Response to AIDS/SIDA). CURAS was formed in the late 1980s in response to racial and sexual dynamics that resulted in the institutionalized lack of concern for queer Latinos from Latino agencies and larger AIDS organizations. Proyecto arose from residual CURAS funding and support from LLEGO (the National Latino/a Lesbian and Gay Organization). National focus on HIV prevention for gay men of color and black men through the National Task Force on AIDS Prevention (NTFAP) was an important structural component that also made Proyecto possible. NTFAP was formed in response to gay men of color organizing to address their own needs with respect to AIDS (Roque Ramírez, 2006). While continuing CURAS' emphasis on queer Latinos, Proyecto took off in new directions with an agenda to bring further visibility to this community (Roque Ramírez, 2001).

Since its foundation, Proyecto has been dedicated to the recognition, celebration, and continuation of local queer (gay, lesbian, bisexual, and transgender) Latina/o life and history. Some of this work has been documented in academic research conducted at PCPV. In addition, Proyecto has also shaped a creative community of intellectuals[5] and artists[6] whose work consistently offers insightful work on a broad range of issues concerning the extended queer Latino community. Propelled into existence by an activist vision (Roque Ramírez, 2001), the ideological forces guiding Proyecto from its inception have included multigender organizing, sex-positive programming, neighborhood-based and harm reduction strategies (Rodríguez, 2003). Rodríguez further elaborates:

> Underlying Proyecto's prevention agenda is the belief that giving people a reason to want to live, survive, and resist erasure is imperative if we are to combat the spread of HIV and promote health in our diverse communities. Its work challenges basic assumptions that have guided much of mainstream AIDS prevention, namely, that all people want to live, that all of us are equally capable of negotiating sexual contracts, and that all of us benefit equally from health maintenance.
>
> (2003, p. 54)

As a program of Mobilization Against AIDS International, Proyecto strives to provide inspirational, relevant, and responsive services shaped by a complex and diverse Latina/o experience and based in a harm reduction philosophy. Committed to a holistic approach to wellness, Proyecto aims to address the various human needs of queer Latina/os with the understanding that the improvement of quality of life has a direct impact on the level of risk someone has of becoming infected with HIV and/or how someone experiences HIV if s/he becomes infected.

Varying aspects of our identities as well as our communities are both independent and interdependent. The term holistic in the context of PCPVs work is intended to honor the complex wholeness of people and their relationship to their environment, including others. This philosophy of health and wellness contrasts the individualistic bias of dominant disease-based models often used by government (Choi et al., 1998). Although PCPV includes opportunities for peer support to people-based shared identities (transgender specific, men only, women only, youth specific), the organization also recognizes that knowledge and support is shared across many different segments of our communities. People do not always limit or define their social support networks by these differences. Proyecto provides opportunities for socializing and learning in "mixed" settings that allows the community to work toward health and wellness in existing and familiar structures. In working toward optimum health and wellness both as individuals and as a whole community, this approach concomitantly creates other openings by emphasizing shared and differing needs. These openings allow members to speak from experience in addressing biases and ignorance that may exist among community members. Specifically, PCPV attempts to provide a space that honors the complexity of these relations—even as it continues to be a place where community members can access and share accurate, non-judgmental information and tools for improving health and wellness across racial, gender, generational and sexual identities. For example, this holistic perspective allows PCPV to recognize the equal importance of creating programs for artistic expression as well as providing free condoms. One meets the need for emotional and spiritual nourishment within a community setting and the other supports safer sexual expression.

Another important frame for Proyecto's work is a non-essentialized understanding of identity. Identities are in constant formation as we revise them in response to our changing social conditions (Hall, 1992, 1996). Identity is fluid and fluctuating in relation to the heterogeneous fields of power of our social environments. This approach foregrounds political questions about the contested nature of identities and their relation to power. We are in constant contact with these external forces as we find and define forms of subject expression (Fusco, 1995). In this sense, identity is not about an essence or essential way of being but an ongoing process of making claims within a contested field of social relations. While PCPV recognizes that people's health needs may indeed differ depending on individual differences and along different identity categories, the organization does not place people into the identity boxes that they might check on a survey form. PCPV recognizes identities are constantly changing, relational, and contextual. For example, PCPV is able to work with a person who identifies with one sexual identity at a club and another in other settings without an overwhelming conflict with regard to community programming, access to services, and participating in community relations. PCPV does not work to resolve these different tensions between differing identifications because the organization understands the constant tensions of identity as ever shifting and contextual. Programming and information work to encourage community members to express their identities in positive environments and analyze the contexts in which they create those identifications. The person and all of their multiple identities are able to participate within the space created by PCPV. The organization provides a space for difference and identity to come together in the creation of a vibrant and diverse community.

Critical to this approach is the high appreciation for agency. Agency is an important foundational concept in Proyecto's work and is respected as central to all engagements with individuals. Subaltern studies work has identified agency as central to understanding the voices of marginalized people. Spivak (1999) notes the powerful silencing of subaltern subjects in dominant modern Western discourses. By highlighting subaltern classes as victims, dominant discourses silence subaltern voice. In her famous question, "Can the subaltern speak?" Spivak asks us to reconsider the complex process of silencing the subaltern. Women of color have taken up this question to highlight agency as bounded and stressed the need to understand choices within the material and ideological contexts of daily life (Mohanty, 2003). Although Spivak (1999) emphatically states that the subaltern cannot fully participate in the production of hegemonic speech (and have no such political investment), she notes that the subaltern can and do speak. In this sense, a subaltern studies approach to agency demands attention to voice. Dominant approaches to health communication that do not foreground marginalized community members' voices are thus potentially complicit in such silencings. By addressing the question of agency as an ongoing process, Proyecto offers one approach for prioritizing subaltern voice in critical health communication.

Proyecto serves a diverse Latino community that is multiracial, multiethnic and represents at least twenty-three countries in the Western hemisphere. While the Latina/o population in the Bay Area is predominantly of Mexican and Central American heritage, PCPV opens its doors to a wide range of people in this community. Proyecto has reached bilingual and monolingual queer Latinos aged 15–65, many of whom share the realities of being immigrants and sex workers with limited English-speaking skills.

During 2005, Proyecto offered programs for men-who-have-sex-with-men (MSM), transgender people, and youth. In other years programs for women and other members of the community were offered from time to time, including Tetatud and Las Diablitas, when financial support was available. While the MSM and transgender programs are often funded by population-specific support, programs for other segments of the queer Latino community are often under-funded. This strategic funding of single-population-based programs often undermines PCPV's holistic approach to healthy communities. For example, in San Francisco, most of the HIV funding in 2004 was allocated to men-who-have-sex-with-men (MSM) and male-to-female (MTF) transgender populations while virtually ignoring the education and prevention needs of other Latino groups including young women or the partners of transgender individuals (HIV Prevention Council, 2004).

The community's ability and potential to address dis-ease can be undercut by these funding strategies. Selectively funding portions of this work while simultaneously under-funding others encourages community fragmentation, and a weaker overall community. These barriers to honoring a holistic approach to HIV/AIDS work indicate the need to rethink how we approach communities, program evaluation, and assessment. By expanding our under-standing of health communication to include holistic approaches, we can envision a model for addressing HIV that leverages the strength of the community. Despite these limitations, Proyecto has offered innovative and effective programs for these populations.

Proyecto is caught between state-defined models for HIV work that leverage essentialized identity categories while understanding the dynamic nature of such identities (Rodríguez, 2003). The agency has always been "wary of the limits of the agency as an HIV institution that is part of the larger AIDS industry or infrastructure" often dependent on Centers for Disease Control (CDC), state government, city, and/or philanthropic individuals (Roque Ramírez, 2001, p. 400). While PCPV is more than just a health service agency and tries to move *beyond* service provision, the core of recent funding has been from sources that do not take a broader vision of a holistic community agency that embraces all of its community members. With decreasing financial support, PCPV has been slowly strangled by the mandates of governmental agencies and their limited understanding of holistic, culturally specific health work. Optimistically, these unmet needs also offer an opportunity to make an entire community strong and healthy to deal with the presence of HIV/AIDS. Specifically, this project provides others undertaking this work with a model for understanding HIV/AIDS and health education programs on the broader terms of queer/LGBT familia, community survival, and cultural work.

The RICCA model: "living theory" in action

The RICCA model was developed to capture the complex interrelationships and interactions of dynamic elements implicated in community health work from the "bottom-up." RICCA reflects an extended engagement with the staff of Proyecto focused on an effort to articulate the model in-practice that informs their work with community. The name reflects the agency's tradition of employing bilingual/bicultural, sex-positive acronyms. RICCA[7] (meaning rich, productive, and desirable) is a culturally positive emphasis on quality of life for queer Latinos. Specifically, it emphasizes a further move away from the dis-ease model often employed by health service provision work, particularly with HIV/AIDS. The model consists of five interrelated components:

Recipiente/Receptacle, Individual/Individual, Communidad/Community,
Cruces/Crossings, Ambiente/Atmosphere.

Larger political and global forces affect the lives of the queer Latino
community, as well as the institutional landscape Proyecto navigates. Recognizing that multiple forces impact communication between Proyecto's staff
and their community of clients, different levels of engagement are represented
in the RICCA model. In particular, we have tried to articulate the ways in
which intrapersonal, interpersonal, family, and community float within a larger
sociocultural context that impacts communication about health. In the
following sections, we describe each of these elements in detail and how they
interact within the communication system that Proyecto conducts its work.

Recipiente/Receptacle

The communication system of the organization and its extended network of
contacts throughout the local community are represented by a flexible frame
or "receptacle" composed of living, breathing cultural fabric. Consisting of
living cultural material, the flexible frame, never static, offers an organizing
structure to interactions. Importantly, the receptacle does not restrict
interaction, but rather describes Proyecto's work as dynamically engaging with
it. The specific cultural elements that compose it are diverse and vary
depending on what the individuals involved bring to it. While variable and
changing, the receptacle provides a structural reference for engagements
between staff and community members.

The container's shape is formed by the push and pull of sociocultural forces
against its walls that sometimes resist or draw its edges in. Orbiting the flexible
receptacle are social and cultural forces that shape it. Specifically, attitudes,
beliefs, values, and spirituality flow through the structure to contour the terrain
in which communication occurs. Attitudes toward sex, desire, queerness, race,
gender, and religion impact the receptacle in different ways. They flow through
all local levels of interaction and are influenced by—and influence—the larger
contexts in which they occur. Further, they are interconnected and affect each
other. These forces offer a multifaceted landscape containing openings and
closures for health-related intervention. For example, religious and cultural
attitudes toward queer sexual contact circumscribe all interactions about
sexuality and health at PCPV. At times, these forces can tightly constrict the
bounds of work. Outreach work outside its walls and communication with
community members is conducted with a careful understanding of the norms
of conduct in the greater heteronormative Latino community. This is
exemplified by the Corazón in Proyecto's lounge mural. The Corazón, or sacred
heart with thorns, appears to reflect a cultural engagement with Catholicism.
However, the Corazón has been transformed to a queer-positive symbol to talk
about desire in a queer-positive way. The design has come to be a central
element of Proyecto's visual work. In this sense, culture is not a barrier, but an

element of the landscape for health work that also offers openings and possibilities.

Individual/Individual

Within the flexible receptacle, the individual and the community are engaged in a dynamic dance that also influences the system. Committed to meeting individuals "where they are at," PCPV's work is sensitive to the sociocultural terrain queer Latinos navigate, and recognizes that individuals bring different talents, abilities, and challenges to their interactions with others. In this sense, Proyecto is considerate of the specific intra- and interpersonal abilities of each person the organization comes into contact with. The organization's staff is sensitive to the different ranges of abilities to engage in communication about sexual health issues within their community. Three principles guide much of Proyecto's work with individuals. Naming, agency, and visibility are all carefully considered when engaging individuals through programming and direct service.

First, individuals are accorded with *the power to name*. In the commitment to the diversity of its community, Proyecto offers individuals opportunities to engage in naming, but does not require it to receive support or services. Proyecto does not impose identity labels on the individuals that come through its doors. In this sense, Proyecto allows individuals to identify themselves and their realities in their own ways without imposing gender, sexuality, or substance-use labels. This allows the agency's services to be accessible to members connected with the queer Latino community that are not named within the laundry list of essentialized identities common to demographic analysis models.

Proyecto recognizes and engages with people that are not easily labeled, but are connected to the greater queer Latino community. For example, partners of transgenders are another such group that may not identify as particularly queer, but also have an investment within a queer Latino community. These people have casual sexual contact, pay for sex, or are in relationships with transgendered individuals. The partners of transgendered people vary greatly in terms of their self-ascribed sexual identities; however, they can and do benefit from Proyecto's services such as condom distribution, drug information, and negotiating relationships to stay healthy without the need to commit to identity categories.

Second, agency is also respected as central to all engagements with individuals. Proyecto understands that individuals can and do exercise agency (and also choose not to exercise it) in different situations. In this sense, Proyecto's work moves beyond the dis-ease model that conceptualizes people as passive in the course of managing their lives and health. At Proyecto, community members can and do have the power to make their own decisions. The organization provides a supportive environment and provides individuals with resources to make their decisions, but is always respectful of the decisions they choose.

Proyecto's work with sex workers is exemplary in this sense. Derived from a harm reduction philosophy, the services provided at PCPV seek to identify and address where sex workers are experiencing harm. Importantly, their strategy recognizes the need for sex workers to make a living. As a population of people that are often undocumented immigrants and socially marked, these workers often find few occupational choices available to them. The agency's focus in engaging this population is to support sex workers and teach them how to minimize risk in their work. While the organization is attentive to the structural issues such as the criminalization of sex work and the related activities that expose sex workers to harm, Proyecto is not focused on legalizing prostitution. Instead, the agency assists sex workers in reducing harm by significantly decreasing the occupational risks of violence and arrest, in addition to sexually transmitted diseases. Some strategies the organization offers to sex workers concentrate on finding ways to take work off the street such as web-based and periodical-based work to decrease their exposure to danger on the streets. Sex workers are also encouraged to express their agency and conduct work on their own terms and in safer spaces including their own homes.

For example, Proyecto teaches sex workers skills of negotiation necessary in asserting their agency to improve their working conditions. While these range from more standard HIV/AIDS practices such as playful condom use to English for negotiating business and relational transactions, the overarching goal is to work with sex workers in a way that respects their self-determination. Although most of this work usually occurs in the context of one-on-one service provision, the organization also has offered classes and group activities. One workshop offered sex workers a "how-to" web-based training for individuals who wish to facilitate their work online. Workshops and events also try to provide general information for insuring safer sex and safer drug use. Whereas most harm reduction strategies limit their focus to specific behaviors, PCPV also encourages sex workers to invest and manage their own financial resources. Proyecto moves beyond harm reduction to address harm in a more holistic way to help sex workers to live healthier lives.

Third, "yo existo" ("I exist") is also asserted as part of a greater dialogue on health. Many of the people that walk through Proyecto's doors come struggling with their own invisibility in the worlds around them. While its physical and programmatic presence provides a level of visibility to queer Latinos within the community, individuals are encouraged to assert their existence on their own terms despite their absence in white gay and Latino straight communities. In this sense, Proyecto engages its members in dialogues of visibility that are central to self-worth and positive mental health. Recognition of self and building a positive self-concept is central to work for an often-invisible group. The discourses of self-worth move queer Latinos toward spaces of self-care and away from spaces of self-neglect. Encouraging its community members to conceptualize health as an extension of asserting their existence moves the focus of health work from a fixation on self-destructive behaviors and toward a holistic self-concept that values life and living.

Some community members come to Proyecto with advanced intrapersonal and interpersonal skills to engage in personal development and growth around sexuality, identity, gender, and culture, but have not been so engaged in the course of their lives around these issues. Others arrive with considerable artistic talents and well-developed self-concepts, but with limited abilities to engage others with them around these issues. Still others arrive struggling to function and survive. Proyecto's programming has been able to address all of these audiences in different ways. While these differences sometimes require separate programming (e.g., youth focused), Proyecto has also been able to provide programming that reaches all of these audiences simultaneously.

While many community members come to Proyecto as clients and participants in programming and services, the organization also offers them the opportunities to provide services and encourages them to develop and leverage the different skills that they bring. People come through Proyecto's doors for support, services, or community, and then realize that they can also participate in providing services. In this sense, Proyecto encourages members of the community to take on agency to care for and build the queer Latino community.

Communidad/Community

While community has many different meanings at Proyecto, it is clear that it is central to the agency's work. However, it is in this area that existing models are incomplete for understanding this aspect of Proyecto's practices. This has often been a central area of tension in funding for the agency. By understanding individuals' very "being" as enmeshed within the greater networks around them, Proyecto is attentive to the geospatial, linguistic, activity-based, and identity-based communities to which individuals may claim belonging.

Proyecto's work is engaged with space in dynamic ways. PCPV constructs their space carefully to engage in dialogue and resistance with the forces working to—quite literally—make Latinos invisible. Space itself is an assertion of existence within the geopolitical spaces of international, national, state, and local spheres in which Proyecto works. With many anti-immigrant initiatives in recent years, questions of belonging often come up and are expressed in the cultural geographies of the immediate community. Staking out a geographic claim is a response to these attacks and narratives that work to erase queer Latinos both within and outside the Latino community. Located in an area that has experienced recent gentrification, the agency has staked its claim of belonging within a specific geopolitical space where the belonging of Latinos is constantly under local attack from a young white professional middle class. San Francisco's internet boom brought significant change to the area including raising property values and, subsequently, rents. This jump in housing prices forced many to move away from the heart of the Mission into other areas of San Francisco and the greater Bay Area. Proyecto represents resistance to efforts that literally push Latinos into the fringes. With an awareness of the immediate neighborhood and local community, Proyecto engages in important geographic work in establishing a *queer* Latino space in the heart of the Mission.

The agency also moves through space with its community. This mobility is central to understanding how Proyecto's work simultaneously navigates a variety of spatial locations. By following the community through the street, club, living room, dark room, cyberspace, among the many in which its members move, Proyecto demonstrates its continuing commitment to meeting its community where they are at.

The language of programming at Proyecto moves fluidly through a group with a diversity of Spanish, Spanglish, and English abilities and uses language as a point of intervention. Rather than looking to get past a linguistic barrier often associated with monolingual Spanish speakers, Proyecto discards these presumptions of linguistic deficiency and leverages Spanish, Spanglish and English in playful ways to enrich its interaction with community members. By moving through the three languages playfully, Proyecto works in a space of richness where it can leverage English, Spanglish, and Spanish that not only respond to the needs of its community members but also stake a claim of cultural resistance.

Moving away from sterile English health terminology of "outreach" or "condom distribution," Proyecto used "La Condonera" to distribute condoms to queer Latinos in clubs (Roque Ramírez, 2001). Playfully using the Spanish "-era" grammatical structure, Proyecto staff turned the Spanish word for condom (which sounds much like the English) into a full personality of "La Condonera," a condom fairy giving condoms to club patrons. Proyecto leverages terms with negative connotations in other contexts, and often turns these meanings on their heads to describe different kinds of queers and different kinds of gente (people). In this sense, all three languages are resources to describe and recognize the value of queer Latinos.

Youth programming is where language intersections are most prevalent. Programs at Proyecto describe identity possibilities to youth in English, Spanglish, and Spanish. While the organization is committed to a Latino cultural frame, African American and youth from other communities of color join the mostly U.S.-born Latinos. PCPV fosters an environment that is affirming to realities of a broad range of people of color. Language in posters and postcards used to describe themselves addresses youth in all languages. Although the focus was for queer Latinos, at the youth poetry slam and open mike, playful talk captured an audience of young gay men, transwomen, and young straight women through the use of language that opened to all identities.

Rather than offering rigid, essentialized identity categories, activity-based communities provide Proyecto with the opportunity to interact with community members on different terms while recognizing the health risks of specific activities. Activity-based communities allow Proyecto to provide services to individuals who engage in specific high-risk activities such as IDU (intravenous drug use), prostitution, and MSM sex without affixing identity labels to them.

However, activity-based communities are not limited to risk behaviors. Through Proyecto's Las Diablitas soccer team, the agency formed a queer-positive space for women under 25. By increasing the number of queer positive spaces for Latinas, who are often limited to a monthly/bi-monthly club or a house party scene where drug and alcohol use are common, *El Colegio* class offered the Latinas participating (and spectators) the opportunity to form a positive self-image as queer women in an environment emphasizing health and sport. This activity-based community moved Latinas toward practicing healthy habits for self-care while building self-esteem and offering them the opportunity to form community with other queer women.

While activity-based communities are one level of intervention, identity-based communities are also another level for engagement. Proyecto offers programming for youth, men who identify as gay, transgendered-specific programming, women, and questioning individuals. Although the staff and agency recognize the fluidity of categories, they are also able to leverage them for their work. Proyecto's work with transgendered individuals addresses the specific needs that they deal with as unique and different. One event offered through the agency was a trip that took twenty-five transgendered women to Reno over the weekend. The bus ride there and back was used to talk about histories, drug use, make-up tips, cosmetics, HIV/AIDS education, and exchange personal stories of survival. An illuminating by-product of this program was that the bus driver said that he had learned a lot, that his "eyes and world [have] opened up." By interrogating transgender as an identity category, women discussed the diversity of experiences as well as formed common understandings of what it means to be a queer male-to-female (MTF) Latina.

The cultural programming at Proyecto moves it well beyond simply being a health agency. Serving as a queer Latino community center, the organization encourages the production of artistic work not only to establish a visible community presence, but also as a call for social justice. This activist call is a demand to address issues of race, class, gender, sexuality, and immigration that impact queer Latinos. Proyecto advances the health of its entire community with an artist-activist vision that includes addressing the greater sociological issues that create disease. The event *Día de Los Muertos* is an example of Proyecto's work that calls attention to structural/sociological issues that impact the queer Latino community. The event honors those from the Proyecto community who have been lost to HIV, drug overdose, and violence. As part of an artistic endeavor, the lounge at the agency is filled with pictures, candles, and decorations that overflow on top of an altar to lost loved ones. Open to a greater community, the event offers the opportunity to claim the culturally specific holiday within a Latino queer context. This event calls the community to observe the injustices the queer Latino community faces.

Cruces/Crossings

Proyecto works at the intersections of these many forces that affect queer Latinos. However, these intersections are heterogeneous points informed by values, beliefs, attitudes, and spirituality. These elements often conflict and offer sites that must be creatively negotiated by the agency. For example, Proyecto's commitment to a multigendered, queer-positive environment is in direct dialogue with larger cultural attitudes toward gender prescription for women and men. In previous years, Proyecto offered beauty courses for MTF women and drag queens that brought a hard-to-reach population enthusiastically to its doors. Las Diablitas challenged cultural norms of gender prescription, particularly for a sport such as soccer associated with masculinity, while offering alternative spaces outside the club for queer and questioning women. In addition to creative programming, artistic expression is a methodology often employed in this negotiation. Filmmaking, photography, theater, and creative writing have all been courses offered through El Colegio.

By reading these forces from sites within the queer Latino community, Proyecto's staff identifies and creates spaces of intervention where these elements converge. Throughout the talk of staff about their work, "where they are at" articulates this commitment and awareness navigating and leveraging the cultural forces that shape their work. PCPV also goes to "meet their clients where they are at" by conducting outreach in local clubs, sex spots, etc. as well as through networks of friends and lovers. Rather than serving as "cultural barriers," Proyecto transforms the terrain most other HIV/AIDS models define as inhospitable into a rich site of intervention and productive cultural work. Through the methodology of reading the terrain from within, Proyecto deals with and recognizes the many forces that push in on the community. However, their work also mobilizes queer Latinos to push back by and respond to these forces artistically, intellectually, and through their every daily practices that include recognition, resistance, and survival.

Ambiente/Atmosphere

Ambiente focuses on the cultural and political contexts of Proyecto's work. As the atmosphere in which Proyecto conducts its work, ambiente provides life sustaining, nourishing elements for its work, but can also be toxic. Ahogar (to drown) and desahogar (to un-drown) are often used to describe the struggle with these forces. The environment can be oppressive in ways that limit the possibilities for work. However, it can also provide resources for work. Public policy and institutions are an intrinsic element of Proyecto's environment as an agency. These policies can range from immigration law to educational institutions through the structure of health insurance. While Proyecto does not have the institutional resources to address many of these, the work that it conducts is always in dialogue with these forces.

Funding priorities, opportunities, and models are the most forceful factors in the day-to-day operations of the agency. The CDC model for HIV work is one such powerful element of the environment. The evaluative model of the CDC forces staff to focus on quantitative measures for the success of their work. However, the philosophy of the organization also addresses qualitative factors that go unrecognized in these measurements. This tension affects the functioning of the organization substantially, often constraining its work. In this sense, CDC policy and governmental funding priorities are formative environmental forces for Proyecto.

Notably, history and power are understood as formative to the realities of queer Latinos. Proyecto's staff and community recognize queer Latinos as entangled in a web of living histories including those of colonialism in Latin American *and* California, as well as within neighborhood tensions. In this way, the impact of Proyecto's work should also be understood as important within a national and transnational context. While these forces may manifest differently in each personal history, the understanding that queer Latinos are influenced by these histories is central to Proyecto's analysis of community health. Colonization of the Americas is a reality of the environment in which queer Latino health work is conducted. For example, the forces that drive and propel immigration are recognized throughout its engagement with community members. Proyecto addresses the recent immigrant and the Chicano (who might descend from pre-treaty of Guadalupe of Hidalgo Mestizo ancestry) as intrinsically connected in its community through the colonization and domination of the Americas by U.S., Spanish, and Latin American nations. In this sense, the community of people impacted by Proyecto's work extends through these networks and histories in transnational ways to families in Latin America and across the *familia* (family) of queer Latinos in the United States. While locally focused on the San Francisco Bay Area, Proyecto's work leverages the ties with these histories.

Implications and conclusions

The devastating effects of HIV/AIDS on Latino communities are startling and we began urging health communication program planners to take into account the social and cultural realities faced by Latinas/os in the United States today. Consistent with Dutta-Bergman's (2004c) observation that health "interventions need to address structural, cultural, and individual-level factors that limit individual action" and the belief that "a homogenized 'one size fits all' approach" (p. 406) is of limited effectiveness, we proposed a model of

HIV/AIDS education and service delivery that emerged from work with community members. After several months of engagement with Proyecto's staff, we decided that the primary aim of the project was to articulate this model using "third-order" research techniques by creating a space for sustained dialogue between the researchers and community members that comprised our team. Through this engagement, we became even more conscious of the role of ideology and power, conceptions of culture, and the importance of advocacy in PCPV's work—all of which led to the emergence of the RICCA model. This model is fluid, elastic, and responsive as different forces push and pull on the different components—receptacle, individual, community, crossings, and atmosphere—creating an ongoing struggle for balance and wellness in a larger social, cultural, and political system that sustains, expands, and constrains life chances for Latinas/os facing the challenges of HIV/AIDS. Using examples from Proyecto's work, we described the RICCA model as a living and breathing entity. We conclude this chapter by exploring some of the theoretical and community implications of our work.

Theoretically, our work calls attention to the need to engage with ideology, power, history, and culture that shape, create, and perpetuate social inequities along with health disparities in contemporary society. This critical health communication project urges researchers and practitioners to engage in self-reflexivity about their work in serious, profound, and consistent ways. It calls for an intimate and ongoing engagement with the community and its members. To reflect on their work, HIV/AIDS researchers and educators might ask some of these questions. What is the dominant ideology related to their HIV/AIDS work? Is it sex-positive? Is it identity-affirming? Is it victim-blaming? Is it sensitive to the lifeworlds of the people it targets? Is it culturally affirming? Is it respectful of social differences? Is it linguistically appropriate? Is it supportive of the interconnections between mind, body, and spirit? Is it wellness-driven as opposed to disease-focused? How does power function to reinforce current social hierarchies based on race, class, gender, sexuality, ability, and nationality? How can researchers and community members resist these arrangements and reclaim their agency? Is it sensitive to communities and group histories? Does it respect the interconnected nature of the community? Whose version of history is recognized? Whose version is ignored and discredited? Whose culture is assumed in HIV/AIDS work? Whose culture is ignored, marked, pathologized, or deemed problematic? Although these are challenging questions, their answers might provide researchers and practitioners with a more socially conscious approach to their work.

This project also points to the promise of collaboration between academic researchers and community members to produce engaged action research. In spite of numerous differences—social, cultural, educational, political, linguistic, to name only a few—and potential obstacles—misunderstandings, differences in expectations, stereotyping, structural and institutional barriers, among others—individuals committed to a dialogic process and common goals can come together to bridge the theory–practitioner divide. In the end, it benefits everyone particularly those affected by HIV/AIDS.

Culture offers openings and possibilities in the landscape for health work (Airhihenbuwa, 1995). We urge researchers and providers to forge and enter into an ongoing dialogue with communities as way to find and leverage openings to improve the health of all our communities. Our project, in many ways, represents one attempt to answer Román's (1998, p. 183) plea, at the beginning of this chapter, that HIV interventions "tiene que cambiar" (need to change) by offering a culturally specific and historically situated intervention model from the "bottom-up." In closing, we offer to add to Román's remark "y siempre está cambiando" (and it is always changing) to adopt to the constantly evolving and shifting social, cultural, economic, political, and material conditions that affect the lives, health, and wellness of Latinas/os in the United States. With passion, strength, and power, we can respond to the injustices of health disparities in productive and healthy ways.

Notes

1   The phrase means "the power and strength of passion" in Spanish. In spite of multiple and simultaneous forms of oppression experienced by Latino community members at both microscopic and macroscopic levels, we use this phrase to highlight the power of individual and collective agency to survive and to move away from totalizing conceptions of victimhood.
2   All members of our research team are fluent in both English and Spanish and the translations are ours. They are presented in brackets immediately following the word(s) or phrases in Spanish.
3   We use the plural to call attention to the diversity and heterogeneity of Latina/os in the San Francisco Bay Area and beyond. This diversity is characterized by differences in immigration histories, geography, language use, social class, gender, sexuality, and nationality, among others.
4   We thank Gerianne Merrigan, Karen Lovaas, Carla Clynes, and Rafael Canadas, for participating in some of our original discussions.
5   This research has been published in both English and Spanish. For examples see (Ochoa, 2004; Rodríguez, 2003; Roque Ramírez, 2005). These are just some examples of a growing body of scholarly research that has been inspired by the work of PCPV.
6   For examples of artists producing work see (Cortez, 1999; Cortez & Herbert, 2004; Majano, 1998).
7   The referent here is the Spanish word "rica." RICCA, with two c's, is a play on this word.

References

Airhihenbuwa, C.O. (1990–1991). A conceptual model for culturally appropriate health education programs in developing countries. *International Quarterly of Community Health Education, 11*, 53–62.

Airhihenbuwa, C.O. (1993). Health promotion for child survival in Africa: Implications for cultural appropriateness. *International Journal of Health Education, 12*(3), 10–15.

Airhihenbuwa, C.O. (1995). *Health and Culture: Beyond the Western Paradigm.* Thousand Oaks, CA: Sage.

Airhihenbuwa, C.O., DiClemente, R.J., Wingood, G.M., & Lowe, A. (1992). HIV/AIDS education and prevention among African Americans: A focus on culture. *AIDS Education and Prevention, 4*, 267–276.

Airhihenbuwa, C.O., & Ludwig, M.J. (1997). Remembering Paolo Freire's legacy of hope and possibility as it relates to health education/promotion. *Journal of Health Education, 28*, 317–319.

Airhihenbuwa, C.O., & Obregon, R. (2000). A critical assessment of theories/models used in health communication for HIV/AIDS. *Journal of Health Communication, 5*(Suppl), 5–15.

Arend, E.D. (2005). The politics of invisibility: Homophobia and low-income HIV-positive women who have sex with women. *Journal of Homosexuality, 49*(1), 97–122.

Choi, K.H., Yep, G.A., & Kumekawa, E. (1998). HIV prevention among Asian and Pacific Islander men who have sex with men: A critical review of theoretical models and directions for future research. *AIDS Education and Prevention, 10*(Suppl A), 19–30.

Cortez, J. (ed.) (1999). *Virgins, Guerrillas y Locas: Gay Latinos Writing about Love.* San Francisco, CA: Cleis Press.

Cortez, J., & Herbert, P. (2004). *Sexilio/Sexile.* Los Angeles: The Institute for Gay Men's Health.

Díaz, R.M. (1998). *Latino Gay Men and HIV: Culture, Sexuality, and Risk Behavior.* New York: Routledge.

Dorsey, A.M. (2003). Social and community health issues. In T.L. Thompson, A.M. Dorsey, K.I. Miller, & R. Parrott (eds), *Handbook of Health Communication.* Mahwah, NJ: Lawrence Erlbaum, pp. 205–206.

Dutta-Bergman, M.J. (2004a). The unheard voice of Santalis: Communicating about health from the margins of India. *Communication Theory, 14*(3), 237–263.

Dutta-Bergman, M.J. (2004b). Poverty, structural barriers, and health: A Santali narrative of health communication. *Qualitative Health Research, 14*(8), 1107–1122.

Dutta-Bergman, M.J. (2004c). An alternative approach to social capital: Exploring the linkage between health consciousness and community participation. *Health Communication, 16*, 393–409.

Dutta-Bergman, M.J. (2005). Theory and practice in health communication campaigns: A critical interrogation. *Health Communication, 182*, 103–122.

Ford, L.A., & Yep, G.A. (2003). Working along the margins: Developing community-based strategies for communicating about health with marginalized groups. In T.L. Thompson, A.M. Dorsey, K.I. Miller, & R. Parrott (eds), *Handbook of Health Communication.* Mahwah, NJ: Lawrence Erlbaum, pp. 241–261.

Foucault, M. (1978). *The History of Sexuality, Volume 1: An Introduction.* (R. Hurley, trans.) New York: Vintage.

Fusco, C. (1995). *English is Broken Here: Notes on Cultural Fusion in the Americas.* New York: The New Press.

Greene, K., Derlega, V.J., Yep, G.A., & Petronio, S. (2003). *Privacy and Disclosure of HIV in Interpersonal Relationships: A Sourcebook for Researchers and Practitioners.* Mahwah, NJ: Lawrence Erlbaum.

Hall, S. (1992). The question of cultural identity. In S. Hall, D. Held, & T. McGrew (eds), *Modernity and its Futures.* Cambridge: Polity Press, pp. 273–326.

Hall, S. (1996). Introduction: Who needs identity? In S. Hall & P.D. Gay (eds), *Questions of Cultural Identity*. Thousand Oaks, CA: Sage, pp. 1–17.

HIV Prevention Planning Council. (2004). *San Francisco HIV Prevention Plan*. San Francisco, CA: SF Department of Public Health/AIDS Office. Retrieved on August 29, 2006 from www.dph.sf.ca.us/HIVPrevPlan/hppchome.html.

Kristiansen, M., & Bloch-Poulsen, J. (2000). The challenge of the unspoken in organizations: Caring container as a dialogic answer? *Southern Communication Journal*, 65, 176–190.

Lupton, D. (1994). Toward the development of critical health communication praxis. *Health Communication*, 6, 55–67.

Majano, V. (1998). *Calle Chula*. Independent documentary film. For ordering information go to: http://subcine.com/gone-majano.html

Minkler, M. (1998). Introduction and overview. In M. Minkler (ed.), *Community Organizing and Community Building for Health*. New Brunswick, NJ: Rutgers University Press, pp. 1–19.

Mohanty, C.T. (2003). *Feminism without Borders: Decolonializng Theory, Practicing Solidarity*. Durham, NC: Duke University Press.

Mokros, H.B., & Deetz, S. (1996). What counts as real? A constitutive view of communication and the disenfranchised in the context of health. In E.B. Ray (ed.), *Communication and Disenfranchisement: Social Health Issues and Implications*. Mahwah, NJ: Lawrence Erlbaum, pp. 29–44.

Nemoto, T., Operario, D., & Keatley, J. (2005). Health and social services for male-to-female transgender persons of color in San Francisco. *International Journal of Transgenderism*, 8(2/3), 5–19.

Ochoa, M. (2004). Ciudadanía perversa: Divas, marginación y participación en la 'localización. In D. Mato (coord.), *Políticas de Ciudadanía y Sociedad Civil en Tiempos de Globalización*. Caracas, Venezuela: FACES, Universidad Central de Venezuela, pp. 239–254.

Prohaska, T.R., Peters, K.E., & Warren, J.S. (2000). Health behavior: From research to community practice. In G.L. Albrecht, R. Fitzpatrick, & S.C. Scrimshaw (eds), *Handbook of Social Studies in Health and Medicine*. London: Sage, pp. 359–373.

PCPV (Proyecto ContraSIDA Por Vida). (2005). Organizational website. Retrieved on March 12, 2004 from www.pcpv.org/e/index.html.

Ray. E.B. (ed.) (1996). *Communication and Disenfranchisement: Social Health Issues and Implications*. Mahwah, NJ: Lawrence Erlbaum.

Robert, S.A., & House, J.S. (2000). Socioeconomic inequalities in health: Integrating individual-, community-, and societal-level theory and research. In G. L. Albrecht, R. Fitzpatrick, & S.C. Scrimshaw (eds), *Handbook of Social Studies in Health and Medicine*. London: Sage, pp. 115–135.

Rodríguez, J.M. (2003). *Queer Latinidad: Identity Practices, Discursive Spaces*. New York: New York University Press.

Román, D. (1998). *Acts of Intervention: Performance, Gay Culture, and AIDS*. Bloomington, IN: Indiana University Press.

Roque Ramírez, H.N. (2001). Communities of desire: Queer Latina/Latino history and memory, San Francisco Bay Area, 1960s–1990s. *Digital Dissertations*, 63(02), 636. (UMI No. 3044657)

Roque Ramírez, H.N. (2005). Claiming queer cultural citizenship: Gay Latino (im)migrant acts in San Francisco. In E. Luibhéid, & L. Cantú (eds), *Queer*

Migrations: Sexuality, U.S. Citizenship, and Border Crossings. Minneapolis, MN: University of Minnesota Press, pp. 161–188.

Roque Ramírez, H.N. (2006). Praxes of desire: Remaking queer Latino geographies and community health through Proyecto ContraSIDA por Vida. Paper presented at Case Western Reserve University.

Santiago-Valles, W.F. (2003). Intercultural communication as a social problem in a globalized context: Ethics of praxis research techniques. *International and Intercultural Communication Annual, 26*, 57–90.

Spivak, G.C. (1999). *A Critique of Postcolonial Reason: Toward a History of the Vanishing Present*. Cambridge, MA: Harvard University Press.

Yep, G.A. (1992). Communicating the HIV/AIDS risk to Hispanic populations: A review and integration. *Hispanic Journal of Behavioral Sciences, 14*, 403–420.

Zoller, H.M. (2000). "A place you haven't visited before": Creating the conditions for community dialogue. *Southern Communication Journal, 65*, 191–207.

Chapter 11

Interrogating the Radio Communication Project in Nepal

The participatory framing of colonization

Mohan J. Dutta and Iccha Basnyat

The use of entertainment platforms such as popular music, radio, and television programming to diffuse information, attitudes, and behaviors has received considerable attention in recent years (Singhal & Rogers, 2001, 2002; Storey et al., 1999; Storey et al., 1996). Of particular relevance is the growth of participatory communication techniques in entertainment education (E-E) programs. The Radio Communication Project (RCP) in Nepal has been cited widely in the E-E literature to demonstrate the effectiveness of the participatory E-E approach and to delineate E-E from the more top-down diffusion of innovations models (Boulay et al., 2002; Storey et al., 1996, 1999). In this project, we critically analyze the published scholarship on the RCP to closely examine the claims of participation made by the developers and evaluators of the programs in the backdrop of the participatory communication techniques that are actually used in the program. This exploration is necessary because claims of participatory communication by mainstream civil society organizations often co-opt the true participatory potential of marginalized communities (Dutta-Bergman, 2004a, 2005). Also, programs such as the RCP that emphasize family planning centralize the consumption of health by the individual, shifting the locus of responsibility on the individual and typically leaving out the culture and context within which the behavior is embedded. In doing so, these programs continue to marginalize those individuals and groups that they propose to help by ignoring the structural elements that fundamentally impede access to basic health care. Our critical review in this chapter is informed by the culture-centered approach to health communication because it provides a theoretical lens to examine a) the interplay of structure and culture in health communication programs, and b) the participatory processes among subaltern groups (Airhihenbuwa, 1995).

Contrary to the evaluation-based perspective that simply measures health communication programs in terms of their effectiveness in the backdrop of a certain set of predetermined objectives set up by funding agencies and campaign planners, we explore the ideology underlying E-E interventions through the case of RCP in Nepal. An ideological interrogation digs beneath the taken-for-granted assumptions that drive the objectives of interventions, and asks questions such as: Who is privileged by the campaign objectives? Who has voice in setting up the objectives? Whose agendas are served by these objectives? It is important to examine the underlying ideology of participatory E-E programs because they claim to be democratic and dialogical. The case of RCP provides a discursive space for the exploration of the ways in which ideology is played out via E-E interventions, particularly in the backdrop of the participatory claims of RCP (Boulay et al., 2002; Storey et al., 1999). The investigation of RCP is illuminating, given the widespread use of the program as an exemplar of participatory E-E (Jacobson & Storey, 2004; Storey & Jacobson, 2004). In discussing the ideologies that are played out via the E-E programs, we examine the published scholarship on the RCP in Nepal, the annual reports regarding the RCP published by Johns Hopkins University/ Center for Communication Programs (JHU/CCP) and the tactical materials used for the RCP. In the following sections we will describe the participatory communication approaches in E-E, the context of Nepal, and the background of RCP. This descriptive information will provide the platform for the critical interrogation of the RCP using the culture-centered approach. Culture-centered health communication envisions culture as transformative, constantly metamorphosing, and constitutive in the realm of health meanings (Airhihenbuwa, 1995; Dutta-Bergman, 2004a, 2004b, 2005). Foregrounding the agency of cultural participants, the approach foregrounds the agency of cultural participants in actively defining problems and developing solutions that are meaningful to them (Dutta-Bergman, 2004a, 2004b, 2005). As depicted in Figure 11.1, in the culture-centered approach to health communication, culture

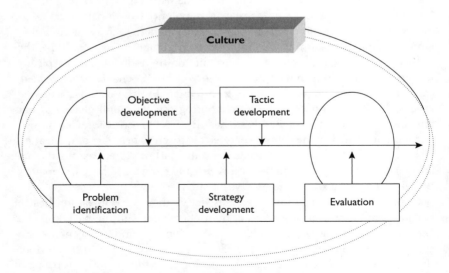

Figure 11.1 A culture-centered model of health communication

envelops the communicative processes, and provides the entry point for problem identification, objective development, strategy development, development and implementation of tactics, and evaluation of the campaign. Culture, then, is the core of praxis such that cultural participatory communication also becomes centralized in campaign design, implementation, and evaluation.

Participatory communication in E-E

As stated in the introduction, participatory communication has recently been used in a plethora of E-E programs in communities across the globe (Singhal & Rogers, 1999; Storey & Jacobson, 2004; Jacobson, 2003). Recent years have witnessed a growth in scholarship on E-E programs that seek to employ the participatory technique or that position themselves as participatory E-E campaigns. Journal articles published on the topic celebrate the emancipatory power of participation invoked by E-E programs (Jacobson & Storey, 2004; Rogers & Singhal, 2003; Storey & Jacobson, 2004). The growing popularity of participatory techniques in E-E is attested by the recognition of participatory communication as a theme for the 2004 E-E annual conference held in Cape Town, South Africa.

An increasing number of articles on E-E characterize E-E programs in terms of their participatory nature. For instance, articles written about the E-E radio soap opera *Tinkha Tinkha Sukh* discuss the community participation generated by the radio soap opera (Rogers & Singhal, 2003). Voices of listeners are presented as representations of participation and are cited within the articles to demonstrate the emancipatory power of E-E (Papa et al., 2000; Singhal & Rogers, 2002). The articles often cite a 20-by-24-inch poster letter pledge that was mailed by the residents of a village named Lutsaan to All India Radio which was broadcasting the program *Tinkha Tinkha Sukh* (Papa et al., 2000; Singhal & Rogers, 1999, 2002). This pledge is cited by the campaign developers and evaluators as an example of collective action and audience participation. Similarly, letters written to the All India Radio by the listeners are depicted as examples of the participatory nature of the E-E program. The voices of letter writers have also been used with reference to programs such as *Humlog* to articulate the role of participation in E-E. In this context, audience response to the program is used as an example of participation.

Rogers and Singhal (2003) discuss another E-E radio soap opera *Taru* as an example of participatory E-E, articulating that the program integrates traditional mass media techniques with community-based activities such as wall paintings, posters, stickers, folk media performances, and listener groups. *Taru* was developed as a fifty-two-episode E-E radio soap opera that would promote small family size, reproductive health, gender equality, caste and community harmony, and communal development (Singhal and Rogers, 1999). The use of community-based activities such as wall paintings, folk performances and listener groups in *Taru* is used to support the participatory claim of the program.

The program collaborated with *Janani*, a nongovernmental organization that focused on training 20,000 rural medical practitioners and their spouses in reproductive health. Folk performances were deployed to publicize the program, distribute publicity materials, and establish listening groups for the radio program. Also, in line with *Taru's* participatory focus, audience responses are reported in participatory formats such as reports of community members.

Similarly, a campaign in Nepal on population control has been the topic of much discussion in the realm of participatory E-E campaigns (Jacobson & Storey, 2004; Storey & Jacobson, 2004). The Radio Communication Project (RCP) has been presented as an exemplar of the shift from one-way communication to more participatory forms of communication that involve dialogue and community involvement. Designed to promote contraception, RCP has been used as a poster child of participatory E-E in much of the recently published scholarship on the topic. For example, Jacobson and Storey (2004) discuss the aspects of participation involved in the interpersonal communication counseling component, the mass media campaign, and the community-based grassroots level health activities of the population control program. According to the authors, the program not only employed mass media, interpersonal communication and community channels as tactical tools but also with the goal of broadening the communication opportunities for community members. In doing so, the program used participatory communication "both as a means to behavior change and a cherished end-state of its own" (p. 111). In this instance, the very tactical adoption of communication channels such as the mass media, community organizations, and interpersonal channels is considered participatory communication. As this section demonstrates, published scholarship on participatory E-E programs has taken a crucial turn in emphasizing the role of participation in E-E and have positioned participatory E-E as an alternative to the traditional one-way diffusion of innovations model by adopting participatory techniques. In this project, we seek to examine the participatory processes embodied in E-E by interrogating the discursive space in the widely cited RCP in Nepal.

The context

Backdrop of Nepal

The kingdom of Nepal is landlocked between India and China and is only about 500 miles long and 110 miles wide. Nevertheless, this small country is home to sixty ethnic groups, who speak more than twenty different languages, according to the 1991 Census. Bista (2000), the first anthropologist of Nepal explains that, geographically, the country can be divided into four major regions: (1) Himalayan highlands with the snow mountains and glacial valleys; (2) Lower Himalayan ranges (hill regions) with the green forest and long slopes leading to fertile valleys, which is the most developed part of the country and is home to 45 percent of the population; (3) forest areas of the inner Terai, the low river valleys and the foothills; (4) the flat and fertile land of the Terai, the north edge of the Gangetic plain—the flat lands covers 23 percent of the land but is home to 47 percent of the population. Politically, Nepal is divided into five developmental regions, seventy-five districts and 3,913 Village Development Committees (VDC) and each is further subdivided into nine wards (the smallest administrative unit).

In 1990, Nepal became a constitutional monarchy. It is the only Hindu nation, though it is also the birthplace of Buddhism. Muslim and Christianity are also part of the culture. Despite of Nepal's rich heritage, 80 percent of Nepal is inaccessible. Today, many people in the rural areas still live without basic services such as electricity, mostly due to lack of transportation and communication. This inaccessibility has also dampened the endeavor to educate all, such that the literacy rate for women is only 27 percent and 57 percent for men. Nepal, despite its rich culture and tradition, is among one of the poorest countries with a per capita income of US $210 and estimated 42 percent of the population living in poverty.

In addition, inaccessibility to many parts of Nepal has also hindered proper health care being provided or accessed by all Nepalese. For example, a 1999 Asian Development Bank (ADB) report indicates that diarrhea, acute respiratory infection (ARI), vitamin A and other micronutrient deficiencies and measles are the major causes of death among children under five. All of these can be prevented. Nepal also has the highest maternal mortality rate in Asia with 539 deaths per 100,000 live births.

Background of RCP

Due to the limitation of access to health care, a Radio Communication Project (RCP) was started in Nepal through Johns Hopkins University/Population Communication Service (JHU/PCS) or what is now referred to as Center for Communication Programs (CCP) with the goal of diffusing contraceptive use and family planning in Nepal. Funded by the United States Agency for International Development (USAID), the RCP was developed through the collaboration among JHU/PCS, the Nepal Ministry of Health's National Health Education, Information and Communication Centre (NHEICC), the National Health Training Center (NHTC), and the Family Health Division (FHD). The RCP was designed to achieve three objectives: a) to satisfy the large unmet need for contraception in Nepal; b) to improve the quality of services and service delivery, especially the interpersonal communication and counseling (IPC/C) skills of clinic-based health workers; and c) to increase service utilization and contraceptive use by enhancing the image and expectations of health workers and service of clients (Storey et. al., 1999). The agenda of RCP fitted within the broader agenda of USAID to support population control based on the ideology that population growth is the primary barrier to global stability and the primary cause of world food shortage (see Dutta-Bergman, 2004a, 2004b).

Targeted toward the general public and broadcast nationally on the government's Radio Nepal channel, the radio drama *Cut Your Coat According to Your Cloth* was aired weekly for a year between December 1995 and December 1996, aimed, "at improving public perceptions of health-service providers and repositioning contraception away from its historical focus on sterilization toward a broader notion of 'the well-planned family.'" The program aired under the Nepali name of *Ghaanti Heri Haad Nilaun*—a more literal translation being "bite only what you can swallow." The story of the radio program revolved around the lives of Harke and Putali, a young couple in the fictional village of Salghari who struggled with tradition and with each other to create a happy and healthy family. The program included specific messages about contraceptives, pregnancy, birth spacing, and contraceptive decision making. In addition, community-based events such as display exhibitions, games, street theater, and song competitions were created around the theme of the well-planned family to provide a platform for community-wide diffusion of the program. According to Storey and Jacobson (2004), this use of community platforms makes RCP participatory because the proposed behaviors are subject to review under democratic conditions. During this phase, another radio drama called *Service Brings Reward* geared toward health workers was also being pilot tested. This six-month drama was aired twice a week in the Midwestern region of Nepal. The program was designed to be interactive, where "print materials such as discussion guides and pre-printed feedback aerograms (pre-stamped, airmail letter-writing paper) were provided to the health workers who had registered with the project" (Storey & Boulay, 2000).

Implementation of RCP

JHU/CCP, in partnership with His Majesty's Government of Nepal's Ministry of Health (HMG/MH) and United States Agency for International Development (USAID), aired RCP phase I in December 1995 to December 1996. This drama serial had phases I to IV, each fifty-two episodes long, with the story continuing. However, each of phases I to IV has its own design document. Phase V took the story from phase I, revisited the content, made slight edits, updated the messages and the information was re-broadcasted. Then phase VI took the content from phase II and the same thing for phase VII, which revisited from phase III, with only phase IV left to be re-broadcasted in phase VIII.

Cut Your Coat According to Your Cloth June 1995, phase I was (re)broadcasted in phase V with minor edits, changes and updates. The drama was aired with the objective of "measurable increase" in behavioral interventions. The objectives can be classified into the following themes: individual responsibility, social responsibility, lack of communication skills, incompetent individuals, and roles of husband/wife—all of which are geared toward skills building for better contraceptive choices, offered under the rubric of entertainment education. The next section offers a critical interrogation of the phase I of RCP, drawing from the underpinnings of the culture-centered approach.

Critical interrogation of the RCP

The critical interrogation of the RCP presented here is informed by the culture-centered approach (Dutta-Bergman, 2004a, 2004b, 2004c, 2005; Dutta-Bergman & Basnyat, 2006). Central to the culture-centered approach is the idea that cultural members are active participants in meaning communities, and therefore, have a key role to play in the definition of problems, formulation of theories, and the application of solutions. In this realm, health communication solutions emerge from within the community through the active engagement of community members in problem definition and solution development. Foregrounding the relevance of opening up legitimate discursive spaces that are open to the voices of members of marginalized cultural groups, the culture-centered approach to health communication builds on the two key concepts of agency and context. Agency taps into the inherent capacity of cultural members to develop meaningful understanding of the conditions within which they live their lives and the day-to-day struggles that are built around negotiating these structural constraints. Agency in the realm of identifying key problems and corresponding solutions is enacted through the day-to-day lived experiences of cultural members, and, therefore, becomes meaningful when articulated with respect to the context within which cultural members live their lives. Voices of cultural members are central to the articulation of problems and the identification of solutions and cultural members develop solutions that are meaningful to them through the process of dialogue. It is in the backdrop of these two ideas of agency and context that we provide an analysis of the RCP in Nepal. The juxtaposition of the culture-centered approach in the backdrop of the RCP is critical because it provides a theoretical lens for examining the claims of democracy and participation made by the developers and evaluators of RCP. In the following section, we articulate the ways in which the objectives of the RCP and the constructions of Nepalese people in the RCP discourse undermine the agency of the Nepalese people, and, therefore, fundamentally contradict the participatory claims of the RCP.

Objectives: the lacking body

The objectives of the RCP dictated the design and development of the program. Therefore, it is critical to examine these objectives from a culture-centered perspective, and interrogate them in the backdrop of the participatory rhetoric adopted in the published literature about the RCP (Jacobson & Storey, 2004; Storey & Jacobson, 2004). One of the key elements in the formulation of objectives was the assumption of incompetence among the Nepalese people. For example, a key objective of the program was to attain a "measurable increase" in "inter-spousal communication and intra-family communication." This assumes that there is a lack of communication skills among the general population of Nepal, thus there needs to be an increase in building their skills for the proper way of inter-spousal and intra-family communication.

The objective stated above assumes that there is one best way to communicate in inter-spousal and intra-family settings. Also, what this leaves out from the discursive space is the context in which such conversations occur and the cultural location of conversations and skills within relational spaces. For instance, an inter-spousal communication strategy that works well in the United States might not really be the most suitable inter-spousal communication strategy in the Nepalese context. What this example demonstrates is the one-way top-down nature of E-E programs in spite of the participatory or dialogical rhetoric adopted in E-E scholarship that presents the RCP as a poster child of participation (Dutta-Bergman, 2004a, 2004b, 2005).

Further, the objective embodies a colonialist assumption regarding the lack of adequate communication skills among the Nepalese, a trait that is perhaps more reflective of the modern sender, who, as an embodiment of these skills, is in a position to teach the Nepalese people. It embodies the presumption that if "they" can be "taught to communicate properly," then there will be increase in health outcomes. Identities of the target audiences are constructed in terms of absences, in terms of those characteristics that are lacking. The traditional construction of the receiver exists in a dialectical relationship with the modern identity of the sender of the message.

Episodes 2–5 dealt with developing the story line for the drama, where the emphasis was on "learning some interesting things, especially in relation to family life and the new modern approach to the well-planned family." This can be observed in the script, which begins with two children playing and chatting—the script paints a picture that because they go to school the children are happy and do not fight and quarrel among themselves.

SANU: Father, Father! They say quarreling takes place in the absence of knowledge. Harke Uncle's place lacks knowledge.
GYANU: Don't you know even that, you dumb fool. Harke Uncle and Putali Aunty always quarrel. This is because they lack knowledge, is it not so father?

As the discussion continues among the children and their father, there is an addition of two other characters: mother and a school teacher. They further emphasize that ignorance of the other couple, who constantly argue (due to lack of education, which leads to un-planned family and unhappy marriage and hinders the ability of husband/wife to communicate compared to neighbors).

BELI: (mother of Sanu/Gyanu) Teacher, if we compare that he has more land than us but the productivity is less, there will always being a quarrel. Their children do not go to school like ours. Only the number of eating mouths increases.

BIRE: You don't have to carry the burden of providing the basic needs, anyway.

BELI: Look how you talk about your friend! There is always disease and problems in his house. They say Putali is pregnant again.

Another example: episodes 6–8 dealt with new approach to well-planned family. The purpose of these episodes was to:

> Stress on all aspects of the well-planned family. Address the idea that traditional beliefs being somewhat outdated. The belief in the importance of sons over daughters can be addressed with the proverb "chhora ra chorri dui aankhaka nani" (A son is the pupil of one eye and the daughter pupil of the other eye) . . . Explain how the modern approach to a well-planned family can lead to "improved quality of life."
>
> (JHU/CCP, 1998)

This notion that a *new* approach that requires usage of modern medicine and modern medical options is better than traditional methods lends to the degradation of traditional cultural systems juxtaposed in the backdrop of the celebration of the modern contraception technique. The negative construction of traditional practices leads to dehumanization of subaltern Nepalese classes who are often not able to afford or have access to the "well-planned family" through contraceptives usage. The message might be framed differently but the core is the same that family planning needs to be done and done through modern techniques. This can be noted, for example, in episode 6 where the purpose and the objectives were "to encourage the target audience to understand that the *new* focus is on the well-planned family rather than family planning." Here a campaign tells mothers to buy condoms, and yet does not address issues such as if she can afford to buy one, or why she keeps having children and, more importantly, whether she even has a choice in making this decision about not only purchasing the contraceptive technology, but also negotiating the use of it within the relationship. In focusing on individual choices, such campaigns become functions of institutional and social forces that construct the production of health at an individual level (Airhinhenbuwa, 1995, p. 114), thus perpetuating the notion of acquiring health through consumption. Given that 80 percent of Nepal is inaccessible and has a per capita income of $US 210, transportation and lack of basic resources need to be investigated, and policy makers first need to ensure that people in these marginalized sectors have access to basic health care (see Dutta-Bergman & Basnyat, 2006, for a detailed discussion). Simply asking one to engage in a behavior without addressing the social and economic conditions surrounding the behavior only leaves those who cannot participate in the decision-making process isolated and marginalized.

Further, the construction of the receiver in terms of absences homogenizes human experiences in subaltern spaces, reducing such experiences to those forms that are acceptable to and supportive of the sender's position. This imposition of a dominant ideology on the receiver culture participates in the oppression of the culture by seeking to transform its practices through the construction of such practices and the underlying beliefs as undesirable (Dutta-Bergman, 2004a, 2004b). The objectives further assume that there is a certain way a husband/wife should interact as well as communicate in order to have a well-planned family.

Further examples can be seen in episode 10 where the discussion of conception and contraception is started. The purpose of this episode was to explain the male role in conception and how conception can be prevented. The objective of the program is to make sure the audience knows:

1. To share information with their families about reproductive growth and health with their children.
2. How to share this information with their children.
3. How to explain male reproductive growth.
4. That it is the male sperm alone that determines the sex of the child—not to blame the women.
5. That infertility is sometimes a problem with the male (not always the female).

The design document suggests that the way to achieve these goals is by creating content in the script that "demonstrates for the audience how husbands and wives talk together and talk with the Health Worker about planning their families and making their contraceptive choices" (JHU/CCP, 1998). Clearly, the assumptions guiding the objectives are that the Nepalese people are incompetent and are not aware of their individual and/or social responsibilities. The solution to the problem, therefore, is in teaching conversational strategies between husband and wife. What does not get presented in the discourse is that patriarchy is deeply rooted in the cultural practices and the information provided not only needs to address the context within which patriarchal practices occur but also ways in which the underlying causes can be changed. What is left out of the discursive space is the lack of resources and infrastructures that would be instrumental in negotiating better health. Airhihenbuwa (1995) states that, "it is critical to establish a balance between the behavior the individual is capable of changing and the socio-political factors in the environment that must be managed before those changes are meaningful and sustainable" (p. 91). For instance, in discussing the negotiation of contraception, the document emphasizes that, this is an area of difficulty because of the long held taboos about discussing sexual matter between husband and wife. The program should provide clear suggestions of how a husband or a wife can initiate such discussion, and let them see the real advantage of moving into this modern approach to the well-planned family.

(JHU/CCP, 1998)

In simplistically providing solutions about initiating discussions between husbands and wives, the program fails to recognize and meaningfully engage with sociocultural practices that would provide entry points for social change. Also worth noting here is the presentation of the program within the dichotomy of tradition versus modernity where the well-planned family being proposed by the program represents modernity.

Here's another example of a program description from the RCP design document that stigmatizes the traditional way of life in Nepal and creates the binary of tradition–modernity: "She asks them to change their old ways of thinking." Or note the excerpt describing a character: "Shersingh's oldest son Gopi is not educated; he is ignorant of the well-planned family. Because he is old fashioned he does not practice planning the family and keeps on having daughters in the hope of getting a son . . . His children are suffering from malnutrition and a lot of diseases" (ibid.). The culturally embedded decision to not practice family planning is considered a barrier, one that must be refuted in order to carry out the population control agenda of the funding agency. In order to do so, the culture of Nepal is marked as traditional and undesirable, and juxtaposed in the backdrop of the desirable modern. This desirability of modernity serves as the colonial logic for introducing the program, thus supporting the political economy of RCP. In yet another instance, the first program that was aired on March 13, 1998 started off asking the listeners, over the course of the fifty-two episodes to "consider change as with the change of time, and to please change yourself, your family, by examining incorrect beliefs and traditions" (JHU/CCP, 1998, p. 88)—nowhere is there a discussion of why such beliefs and traditions came into existence or how "new belief" can be incorporated into the "old." Furthermore, inherent in the discourse of this so-called participatory program are the devaluation of the Nepalese culture, and the deployment of categorizing schemes based on the notion of Western superiority. The discourse emphasizes the need to replace the incorrect beliefs of the traditional Nepalese culture with the "correct" beliefs of the modern senders of the messages. Furthermore, there is no examination of what cultural and structural barriers prevent the individuals from incorporating the new beliefs; instead it is assumed that people will enact new behaviors once they have the information. What good will the information do if the structural changes also do not occur simultaneously to allow for these behavior changes to happen?

Not practicing family planning is old fashioned and ignorant. It is this assumption of inability and ignorance amidst the receiver population that drives the logic of E-E campaigns. Hence, the portrayal of the Nepalese people as devoid of agency and in terms of absences justifies the economic logic of the E-E campaigns. Also worth noting in the above excerpt is the articulation of causality of malnutrition and poverty; poverty is located in the realm of individual choice to have a large family. Therefore, another aspect of the objectives of the RCP is the location of the problem at the individual level, thus shifting the potential for blame and the onus of responsibility on the subaltern subject without taking into account his/her situation and the structural forces that encompass his/her life. For example, missing from this discussion in the RCP (with suggestions for procuring clean water, promoting smokeless rooms and building latrines) are questions such as: How are the villagers to access clean water if there is no system for water supply such that they either rely on their wells and/or lake/rivers? How are the cultural participants to promote smokeless rooms if they rely on wood burning stoves to cook? How are the cultural members to build latrines if there is no proper drainage system? Fundamentally missing from the RCP discourse is the context of the day-to-day lives of subaltern Nepalese groups.

Objectives: individual-level responsibility

In addition to constructing the third world subject in terms of critical absences, the objectives of the RCP propose solutions that are focused on changes at the individual level. Such individual-level emphasis creates situations for stigma by blaming the subaltern classes in Nepal for the poverty they experience. The solutions advocated mostly included change in individual level beliefs, attitudes, and behaviors, implicitly assuming that such individual-level changes would address the health problems of the target audience. This assumption of individual-level responsibility and the teaching of skills as a solution to health problems can also be seen in the objectives of the RCP described below:

1. Husbands' and wives' knowledge about planning the family and seeking advice and counseling.
2. Knowledge of husbands and wives about the source of all contraceptive methods (including spacing and limiting).
3. Knowledge of husbands and wives to postpone the age of the first birth until the wife is at least 20 years old.
4. The willingness of husbands and wives to visit the health post together.
5. The knowledge of the benefits of the well-planned family.
6. The attitudes and behaviors with regard to family life that reflect a positive understanding of the benefits of a well-planned family.

These "measurable" objectives lack the impetus to initiate and engage in changing the structural factors that surround behavioral acts. Also, they fail to acknowledge the context within which knowledge and behavior are located. The knowledge and motivation goals defined as objectives of the campaign do not take into account the role of structure, and in doing so, place the onus of the subaltern condition of the receiver. Extant research documents that individual agency is often severely constrained by the lack of availability of resources (Dutta-Bergman, 2004a). The objectives suggest that a well-planned family is the ultimate solution to the poverty and malnutrition experienced by subaltern classes in Nepal, without much regard to personal and environmental beliefs of what compromises a well-planned family. The location of the solution to poverty in the realm of the well-planned family also ignores cultural values and beliefs in the context of the intervention being proposed. Note that the location of the problem at the individual level is accompanied by the stigmatization of the Nepalese culture as primitive for not engaging in family planning. Moreover, it is noted that the script should stress that the well-planned family takes into account:

- Number of children
- Timing of birth
- Comfortable communication between husband and wife on all topics
- Comfortable communication among family members (in-laws, etc.)
- Improved living standard for all family members
- Equal responsibility and opportunity between husband and wife, improved quality of life.

For the radio drama, there is a presumption that there is a lack of communication skills, especially between married couples, and this is the cause of unplanned families. Without engaging in dialogue through participatory platforms, the RCP assumes that communication (or lack thereof) lies at the heart of unplanned families. The underlying assumption inherent in the episodes is that—"If we can train them into taking on their 'proper' roles and responsibilities, then all 'problems' with families will be eliminated." The alleviation of hunger and poverty is shifted again to the individual—who is only fueling the cycle and as soon as they limit their reproductive health, then adequate food and health of their family will be restored and thus also benefiting their community. The design document points out that the well-planned family gains improved quality of life by having:

- Equal opportunities for good health for all family members
- Access to clean water
- Comfortable housing
- Adequate food and clothing

- Education (as far as it is available)
- Literacy
- Leisure time for women
- Sharing family duties
- Possibility of family savings.

(JHU/CCP, 1998)

Therefore, access is obtained through the proper planning of family, not through the redistribution of resources. Proper family planning, the document suggests, leads to equal opportunities for good health, and access to clean water, naively ignoring the limited structural constraints within which subaltern participants carry on their day-to-day lives.

The objectives assume that lack of knowledge prevents people from becoming competent family planners. In other words, the objectives demonstrate the cognitive orientation of the campaign messages that assume that information is the key to change. This, once again, shifts the burden and locus of responsibility to the individual, who becomes responsible for himself and his community and removes the burden from the government and the donors to provide/improve infrastructures and barriers to health outcomes. Questions of poverty get located in the realm of individual choice, and are distanced from issues of economic capability building and redistributive justice. By locating health problems in the realm of individually modifiable behaviors, the entertainment education model ignores the responsibility of national governments in supplying their citizens with fundamental resources of life (Dutta-Bergman, 2004a, 2004b). Further, the one-way modes of transmission of population control messages create spaces of violence where the subaltern subject is acted upon, and limit the possibilities for dialogue.

One-way objectives: minimizing dialogue

Although scholars working on E-E use the RCP in Nepal as an example of the participatory approach in E-E, the analysis provided above suggests that the E-E program constructs the Nepalese people in terms of absences, imposes a set of beliefs regarding the Nepalese culture, and shifts blame on the individual without taking into account the structural and cultural contexts surrounding family planning. In this section, we will demonstrate that the RCP propagates violence by conducting one-way campaigns without creating spaces of dialogue, inherently contradicting the participatory claim of the E-E scholars. Note the one-way embodiment in the following objectives of the RCP:

7. The credibility of the radio as a reliable source of information on planning the family.
8. The satisfaction of clients with service (especially, counseling received at the health posts).

This assumes the power of the sender, such that the "positionality" of the sender is credible and correct and things should be fixed according to the sender's access to power. The discussion of the radio as a credible source of information delivery demonstrates the emphasis on carrying out the RCP agenda through the use of mass media channels that are credible. The problem is solely articulated by the sender and not determined in dialogue with the receiver population. Instead of creating a space of dialogue with the intended audience, it is assumed that what is needed is understood by the sender.

Essential to E-E programs is the imposition of the value system of the sender of the message on the receiver with the goal of changing the receiver. It is desired that the receiver will ultimately accept the value system espoused by the sender (Dutta-Bergman, 2004a, 2004b). This can be further seen throughout the design document, where the fifty-five episodes are divided into five episodes of introduction and story establishment, six episodes of well-planned family, two episodes of conception and contraception, two episodes of infertility, twenty-two episodes of modern contraceptive methods, five episodes of summary and inter-activity programs, three episodes of roles of health worker in your life and ten episodes of entertainment through stories.

Each content group of episodes has specific program purpose and objectives, which provides guidelines for the script writers as to what needs to be achieved through each episode. For example, one of the objectives defined the potential knowledge gain by the target audience at the end of the program. It states that at the end of the campaign, the audience will understand "What is meant by 'well-planned family' and its components," and "What is meant by 'quality of life' and how planning the family can contribute to a better quality of life." The intention of this episode is for the listeners to 1) begin to adopt and use the phrase "the well-planned family" instead of family planning; 2) become more concerned about the benefits of well-planned family; and 3) feel happy and confident about being someone who knows the concept. The program assumes that the people will appreciate the information being presented to them without exploring possibilities through dialogue with participants. The materials diffused through the mass media are predetermined, not arrived at through a dialogical process with community members. In the absence of dialogue, what is left out of the discursive space is the lack of resources, lack of infrastructure and, more importantly, the context in which the "well-planned" family is located. This is accompanied by lack of empathy for the underlying causes of poverty based on the assumption that subaltern classes make the volitional decision to live their life in hunger and poverty.

Discussion

Due to Nepal's geographical, social, political, and economical composition, programs such as *Cut Your Coat According to Your Cloth* play an important role in connecting with hard to reach sectors of the country. The investigating of the RCP in Nepal is particularly important, given the strategic use of the program as an example of participatory E-E by campaign developers and evaluators (Jacobson & Storey, 2004). An investigation of the program demonstrates that the RCP is anything but participatory. It co-opts the participatory rhetoric to push the one-way diffusion agenda of U.S. actors (primarily USAID, the funding agency that sponsors RCP) to promote population control as the solution to problems of global resource inequity, simultaneously backgrounding critical questions of resource redistribution and redistributive justice that underlie issues of poverty and global health inequality (see Dutta-Bergman 2004a, b for detailed discussion of the USAID agenda served by programs such as the RCP). In pushing the agenda of population control, it embodies the one-way diffusion framework of early development communication work, and uses participation of subaltern Nepalese people to reach the objectives of USAID. Dutta-Bergman (2004a) argues that such one-way diffusion of predetermined solutions (primarily population control) perpetuates violence on subaltern spaces by not taking into account the agency of subaltern people, and by fundamentally co-opting the participatory openings of social change initiatives in subaltern sectors of the world. Furthermore, the academic presentation of programs such as RCP as exemplars of participatory programs serves the dominant power structures, simultaneously backgrounding the one-way diffusion of communication that is actually embodied in such programs.

The problem identification, message design, and evaluation strategies of the RCP lack the basic premise of culture-centeredness, in which case, cultural values, norms, and attitudes are taken into account in creating and facilitating dialogical spaces for the articulation of problems and solutions in subaltern spaces. By not taking people's voices into account and by pushing dominant values without considering the cultural context, the RCP seeks to colonize the subaltern spaces of Nepal with its modernist agenda and the dichotomizing rhetoric of tradition versus modernity. The use of participatory rhetoric seeks to obscure this colonizing agenda, and simultaneously present programs such as RCP as new alternatives that are distinct and different from the old one-way models of diffusion of innovations embodied in early development campaigns. Our analysis presented here suggests the relevance of interrogating the very claims of participation that are made by so-called participatory programs funded by agencies such as USAID. The programs are inherently the same, but have developed new ways of spinning themselves as more participatory and democratic as compared to the earlier programs of development that were critiqued by subaltern studies scholars for their one-way flow.

Furthermore, this analysis points out that there must be an attempt made to modify the underlying causes of behaviors the RCP attempts to change. RCP's six goals cannot be addressed without addressing education, literacy, transportation, electricity, and communication tools—the basic needs of survival. These basic resources for survival are articulated in much of the published scholarship that uses the culture-centered approach in marginalized spaces (Dutta-Bergman, 2004a, 2004b). However, addressing the basic structural resources is not enough; the ways in which such structural resources are addressed ought to gel with the values of a culture and the meanings that circulate within the cultural community. Essential to this is the foregrounding of the agency of the cultural participants and the creation of dialogical spaces that are open to alternative epistemologies articulated from within marginalized spaces. The emphasis of the researcher shifts from one of the expert problem solver to one of the listener who is open to arriving at meaningful understandings of problems and solutions based on dialogue. Essential to this dialogical process is the role of mutual respect; it is only by adopting a stance of respect and valuing fundamental human dignity that the researcher could perhaps arrive at the position of the listener who learns to value alternative ways of knowing and being in the world. Without listening to the voices of the subaltern people and without working with them to secure the necessary tools, programs such as RCP cannot alone lead to behavior change. Instead, such programs stand the risk of stigmatizing and marginalizing members of target communities by not making available the means of achieving behavior change. Moreover, the evaluation of programs such as RCP need to take into account the cultural context and engage in dialogue with members of the community and identify critical indicators that make sense to community members. This process of dialogue via the culture-centered approach is more likely to generate meaningful measures of the health-care intervention.

Although Storey and Boulay (2000) emphasize the use of the theories of reasoned action (Ajzen & Fishbein, 1975), planned behavior (Ajzen, 2005), and observational learning (Bandura, 1986) to take into account the role of environmental constraints and efficacy in seeking to change behavior, our analysis demonstrates the absence of the context in informing the nature of the strategic and tactical materials in RCP. Thoroughly absent from the RCP documents are the day-to-day lived experiences of cultural members in interactive relationships with social, cultural, and political processes. The objectives of RCP Cut Your Coat According to Your Cloth operate under the premise that behavior is rational, and cognition plays a central role in informing the behavior of the participants. There is a lack of understanding of norms and cultural values that lead to certain attitudes and behaviors, which must be understood in the realm of the social and cultural contexts that surround the behavior. Also missing from the strategic and tactical materials is an understanding of the economic context in the ways in which it constrains human behavior and limits the human ability to achieve changes in behavior at the individual level (see for instance the example of building latrines).

The need for RCP in Nepal is taken for granted without taking into consideration where the need arises from and how best the need can be addressed. The program is not really built on the basis of dialogue that engages cultural participants to arrive at meaningful problem articulations and solution configurations. The participation of the Nepalese people garnered through community channels such as folk theaters and song competitions is enlisted to diffuse the agenda of USAID, and not to create spaces for addressing basic issues as envisioned by subaltern Nepalese people. In this realm, participation is included in the campaign process at the tactical stage, thus serving as a tactical tool for the E-E interventionists. From a culture-centered standpoint, the campaign continues to be top-down by pushing solution configurations that make sense to community members. This generates conditions under which organizations such as USAID, JHU/CCP and NHEICC can operate, create, and implement RCP programs to seemingly address superficial behaviors without needing to address the underlying conditions for those behaviors and social, cultural, and economic contexts that surround them. What this analysis demonstrates is the need for dialogue as a tool for listening to the voices of members of marginalized communities. What it also demonstrates is the relevance of interrogating the claims of participation that are made by programs such as the RCP. Ultimately, it is only by listening to subaltern voices that academics and practitioners develop meaningful health interventions that respond to the needs of the community and the culture.

References

Airhihenbuwa, C. (1995). *Health and Culture: Beyond the Western Paradigm*. Thousand Oaks, CA: Sage Publications.

Ajzen, I. (2005). *Attitudes, Personality, and Behavior*. 2nd edn. Milton Keynes, UK: Open University Press/McGraw-Hill.

Bandura, Albert. (1986). *Social Foundations of Thought and Action: A Social Cognitive theory*. Englewood Cliffs, NJ: Prentice Hall.

Bista, D. (2000). *People of Nepal*. Botahity, Kathmandu Nepal: Ratna Pustak Bhandar.

Boulay, M., Storey, J.D., & Sood, S. (2002). Indirect exposure to a family planning mass media campaign in Nepal. *Journal of Health Communication, 7*, 379–399.

Dutta–Bergman, M. (2004a). The unheard voices of Santalis: Communicating about health from the margins of India. *Communication Theory, 14*, 237–263.

Dutta-Bergman, M. (2004b). Poverty, structural barriers and health: A Santali narrative of health communication. *Qualitative Health Research, 14*, 1–16.

Dutta-Bergman, M. (2005). Theoretical approaches to international health communication campaigns: A critical viewpoint from a marginalized space. *Health Communication, 14*, 237–263.

Dutta-Bergman, M.J., & Basnyat, I. (2006). The Radio Communication Project in Nepal: A culture-centered approach to participation. *Health Education and Behavior, 20*, 1–13.

Fishbein, M., & Ajzen, I. (1975). *Belief, Attitude, Intention, and Behavior: An Introduction to Theory and research*. Reading, MA: Addison-Wesley.

Jacobson, T.L., & Storey, J.D. (2004). Development communication and particiation: Applying Habermas to a case study of population programs in Nepal. *Communication Theory, 14*, 99–121.

Jacobson, T.L. (2003). Participatory communication for social change: The relevance of the theory of communicative action. In P. Kalbfleisch (ed.), *Communication Yearbook 27*. Mahwah, NJ: Erlbaum, pp. 87–124.

Johns Hopkins University/Center for Communication Programs (JHU/CCP). (1998). *Design Document: Cut Your Coat According to Your Cloth*. Radio drama serial phase III for the General Audience. NHEIC, NHTC, DHS/MH, JHU/CCP and USAID.

Papa, M.J., Singhal, A., Law, S., Pant, S., Sood, S., Rogers, E.M., & Shefner-Rogers, C.L. (2000). Entertainment-education and social change: An analysis of parasocial interaction, social learning, collective efficacy, and paradoxical communication. *Journal of Communication*, 50(4), 31–55.

Singhal, A., & Rogers, E.M. (1999). *Entertainment-education: A Communication Strategy for Social Change*. Mahwah, NJ: Lawrence Erlbaum Associates.

Singhal, A., & Rogers, E.M. (2001). The entertainment-education strategy in communication campaigns. In R.E. Rice & C.K. Atkin (eds), *Public Communication Campaigns*. Thousand Oaks, CA: Sage, pp. 343–356.

Singhal, A., & Rogers, E.M. (2002). A theoretical agenda for entertainment-education. *Communication Theory*, 12, 117–135.

Storey, D., & Jacobson, T. (2004). Entertainment-education and participation: Applying Habermas to a population program in Nepal. In A. Singhal, M. Cody, E. Rogers, & M. Sabido (eds), *Entertainment Education and Social Change*. Mahwah, NJ: Lawrence Erlbaum, pp. 377–397.

Storey, D., Karki, Y., Heckert, K., & McCoskrie, M. (1996). *Nepal Family Planning Communication Survey, 1994: Key Findings Report*. Kathmandu, Nepal: National Health Education, Information, and Communication Center, Department of Health Services, Ministry of Nepal.

Storey, D., Boulay, M., Karchi, Y., Heckert, K., & Karmacharya, D. (1999). Impact of the integrated radio communication project in Nepal: 1994–1997. *Journal of Health Communication*, 4, 271–294.

Part III

Medical communication

Introduction

Heather M. Zoller and Mohan J. Dutta

Part III focuses on communication and medical care, and approaches questions of medical communication through explorations of the intersections among meaning, culture, and power. These chapters represent emerging interest in the variety of contexts in which medical communication occurs. These settings include an emergency room, a dialysis clinic, and a mobile health clinic, as well as the "virtual" setting of a commercial website representing the interests of pharmaceutical companies. In this introduction, we describe the genesis of interpretive, cultural and critical perspectives in medical communication, and note important directions for continued research.

Brown et al. (2003) describe the primary concerns of extant post-positivist research in provider–patient communication. Patient outcomes of interest include satisfaction, adherence to treatment and directives, and health outcomes. Reflecting a bias toward the needs of providers, the outcomes studied include malpractice protection and time management. Gillotti's (2003) review of the literature adds complexity by noting problems of disclosure, truth telling, and informed consent in interaction. Still, despite well-known works in sociology and communication that address the relationship among medical interactions, culture, and social power (Geist & Dreyer, 1993; Sharf, 1990; Stein, 1990; Waitzkin, 1991), this literature rarely focuses in depth on questions about whose agendas dominate discussions and whose values are promoted through interactions. The interpretive methodologies used by the authors in this book (ethnography, observation, rhetorical analysis), and the critical orientation they adopt, thus expand the literature by investigating meaning, everyday experiences, and power relationships in medical settings. These works draw from some early innovations in communication research.

In the field of health communication, Sharf (1990) introduced the insight that physician–patient interactions can be understood in terms of rhetoric and persuasion, as both patient and physician frame their discourse in order to achieve cooperation from the other. Geist and Dreyer (1993) proposed a dialogic perspective as a lens for understanding the relational constitution of meaning in these interactions, significantly challenging theories that reflect medical paternalism.

Howard Waitzkin (1991), a physician and sociologist, famously introduced critical and poststructural theories to analyze the micro-politics of doctor–patient interactions. His analysis found that physicians' approaches to patients' contextualized social problems reinforce physician social control and reflect white, upper-middle-class, and masculine ideologies. While acknowledging the insights resulting from quantitative doctor–patient research, he argued that such studies "do not help very much in understanding the social, political, economic and historical context in which micro-level encounters occur" (p. 51).

Interpretive perspectives in health communication have helped to formulate and advance patient-centered theories by exploring the meanings constituted through texts and interactions. For example, Vanderford et al. (1997) encouraged us to revise theories of patients as passive recipients and reactors to others' messages to understand patients as active interpreters of their health care. The authors recommended that narrative perspectives, garnered through ethnographic and interview research, be used to capture patients' experiences and social contexts. Sharf's personal narrative "How I fired my surgeon and embraced an alternative narrative" (2005) exemplifies this call by sharing her experiences of moving toward a more active role as a patient. Interpretive research facilitates a wider range of perspectives on medical interactions, as we see with feminist researchers Ellingson and Buzzanell (1999), who found that women's medical narratives problematize traditional communication satisfaction research. Women's narratives reflected a dialectic negotiation involving preferences for respect and caring within systems of expertise.

Critical and cultural perspectives, less common in medical communication research, promote attention to how culture and power are intertwined in medical practice. For example, Johnson et. al (2004) investigate discriminatory medical treatment. Through in-depth interviews and focus group discussions with South Asian immigrant women, the authors uncover how othering (as a practice of constructing identities in opposition and magnifying differences) takes places in the form of essentialist, culturalist, and racialized medical explanations, and describe women's experiences of these practices. The research highlights the importance of treating culture as a network of meanings tied to sociopolitical processes, and the need for physicians to address the individual as well as their knowledge of the culture, because "cultural sensitivity" approaches to provider communication can encourage static and stereotypical views of the individual.

Research into the everyday experience of medical care and provider–patient communication adds insight into how issues of illness, identity, and compliance are accomplished in contextualized interaction. This research addresses effectiveness, but because it does not privilege provider perspectives, it also introduces other concerns such as whose agenda prevails, how risk communication is interpreted, and how patients' life contexts are accounted for in interactions. Critical and cultural research also broadens the scope beyond interpersonal interaction by attending to the personal, social, and political contexts that influence medical care. For example, Japp and Japp (2005) described one woman's quest for legitimacy (both moral and medical) as she dealt with the biomedically invisible disease of chronic fatigue, and the accompanying shame and stigma that constituted her experience. They theorize her efforts as resistance to the metanarrative of biomedicine. Nadesan (2005) expands on the political context through a genealogy of autism, examining how multiple historical and contemporary professional discourses (psychiatric, psychological, and biogenetic) have constituted autism as a diagnosable "disorder," and their implications for the autistic self. Nadesan described the challenge of theorizing illness as a confluence of materiality/biology, cultural interpretive frameworks, and culture without reifying these complex concepts. This insight helps to set the agenda for social constructionist research into illness categorization.

In the last ten years, we have seen emerging interest in the organizational contexts of medical care, with an emphasis on hospital, health maintenance organizations, and hospice settings (Lammers et al., 2003), as well as communication in health-care teams (Poole & Real, 2003). These studies highlight the complex organizational relationships that influence health communication. Interpretive organizational research has broadened theorizing to include less powerful participants in the medical process (for example Noland & Carl, 2006; Orbe & King, 2000). Ellingson (2003) used Goffman's theory of dramaturgy to research the "backstage" teamwork of an interdisciplinary geriatric oncology team at a cancer center. The author concluded that studies of interdisciplinary health teams fail to account for informal interaction by focusing on formal meetings (thereby privileging public, "masculine" forms of communication). Backstage communication about patients influenced caregiver perceptions of patients before they meet them, which at times facilitated helpful interventions by increasing knowledge of patients' situations, but at other times acted as a barrier to care by stereotyping patients.

Organizational research attends to structural issues, such as Lammers and Geist's (1997) description of how managed care has transformed caring as it treats patients as consumers and hospitals as factories and bureaucracies. They encourage us to question the implications for patients when biotechnical language substitutes for human knowledge. This essay is a significant start toward addressing the context of business, and the communicative implications of capitalist systems on health-care communication. We need to attend to emerging issues related to the changing organization of for-profit medicine. For instance, the rise in power of the pharmaceutical industry has transformed our understanding of medical care (Blech, 2006), as had the proliferation of medically related internet sites, although in potentially very different ways.

The chapters in this section of the book illustrate the theoretical contribution of ethnographic participant observation of everyday experiences of health care as well as textual analysis of important sources of medical information for the public. Often drawing from Foucault (1973; 1980), they illustrate that issues of power, knowledge, and identity are inextricably linked with medical care. Through their accounts of the interpenetrations of power, culture, and meaning in health-care interactions, the chapters open up new avenues for exploring the structurally situated nature of medical communication processes.

In Chapter 12, "Streams of action: power and deference in emergency medicine," Alexandra G. Murphy, Eric Eisenberg, Robert Wears, and Shawna J. Perry get rare access to the everyday interactions between physicians, nurses, staff, and patients in an emergency room. The authors describe the erosion of medical authority and growing awareness of medical mistakes as they investigate how medical knowledge is produced and sustained through medical staff and patient interactions. These authors provide unique insight by examining emergency departments as political settings, seeking to understand how power relationships among physicians, nurses, and other staff members influence sense making and negotiation processes in diagnoses and treatment. The authors note that "It is these political relationships that determine who speaks, who listens, who defers, and who is deferred to" (p. 278). The chapter notes the role that discursive closure plays in what are typically thought of as rational interactions. Discursive closure occurs when certain voices are excluded from participation, or certain positions are marginalized (Deetz, 1992; Habermas, 1970). Yet the authors also note that power, understood in disciplinary terms (Foucault, 1979) is both enabling and constraining as it guides the routinization of actions in a chaotic and stressful environment. By presenting key in-depth examples, the chapter allows readers to understand how decision making unfolds among multiple actors over time, and the problems that can develop as a result of taken-for-granted roles and structures. The authors use this analysis to suggest interventions in emergency departments that can prevent discursive closure and promote more open communication even in situations of intense time pressure.

Laura Ellingson also addresses how medical communication shapes and reflects systems of power and knowledge that influence patient experiences in Chapter 13, "Changing realities and entrenched norms in dialysis: a case study of power, knowledge, and communication in health-care delivery." Ellingson investigates how macro-level issues—the acute care model of health and its problematic application to the treatment of chronic illness, and continued traditional professional hierarchies in the face of rising reliance on para-professionals—influence everyday interaction in health-care settings. The author draws from Foucault's work on power, knowledge, and surveillance to "explore dialysis care as an exemplar of how power manifests itself in daily, seemingly unremarkable communication in health care" (p. 294). Ellingson's chapter demonstrates how health workers actively draw from existing medical power relationships to manage their daily interaction with patients, even when these undercut the needs of both paraprofessionals and patients. These findings encourage health communication scholars to challenge the tenets of the biomedical model and to create normative models of communication that promote patient-centered collaboration that is more egalitarian than hierarchical. She notes in the conclusion that the very objections to such models (e.g., impossible, too expensive, too difficult) reinforce problematic structures.

Chapter 14 is called "Changing lanes and changing lives: the *shifting* scenes and *continuity* of care of a mobile health clinic," by the authors Lynn M. Harter, Karen Deardorff, Pamela Kenniston, Heather Carmack, and Elizabeth Rattine-Flaherty. This narrative ethnography draws our attention to the multiple ways that health care is experienced in the United States, particularly in marginalized communities. The research investigates how mobile clinic staff members address the communicative problems that arise from the material limitations of a mobile health clinic. Reflecting an interpretive perspective, these authors emphasize the active agency of these workers, showing how they improvise with existing resources to deliver the best care possible under the circumstances. Thus the paper investigates how marginalized groups and the professionals that serve them create ways of managing within systems of inequality. Their methodology allows readers to engage with both participant narratives and the experiences of the authors themselves. The authors call for additional work that addresses how groups may actively resist and transform the macro-level inequalities that structure experience in the mobile clinic.

Finally, Ashli Quesinberry Stokes examines the increasingly important role of electronic communication and corporate marketing by rhetorically analyzing the discourse of *Healthology*, a producer of electronic direct to consumer (eDTC) pharmaceutical public relations in Chapter 15, "The paradox of pharmaceutical empowerment: Healthology and online health public relations." The author describes how techniques of third-party endorsements and the rhetoric of empowerment serve the marketing goals of the pharmaceutical industry, while shaping audience identities and communicative behaviors in sometimes paradoxical ways. The paper highlights the importance of linking theories of rhetoric, public relations, and organizational discourse with health communication scholarship.

Interpretive, critical, and cultural perspectives have played a key role in denaturalizing the biomedical model and the communicative authority of the physician that is embedded within it, at least within the discipline. Murphy et al. (this book, Chapter 12) illustrate its continuing dominance in U.S. health care, and the problematic consequences that ensue for both patients and medical workers. These works offer alternative models for medical staff communication that focus on collaboration and dialogue. Given structures of physician authority, dialogic models entail significant revision to the existing system, encouraging open questioning of standard orders and valuing the perspectives of those workers with less formal education, but more contact with patients. Moving forward, these studies provide a rich grounding for additional research that develops these models at the level of theory and practice. Of course, influencing medical practice is difficult. Yet the kind of access represented by these chapters shows us that academic–public partnerships can be built, and can be used as a basis to influence communication in medical settings.

"Alternative" research perspectives also bring our attention to how marginalized groups actually experience health care, such as through mobile health clinics and on the internet. Harter et al. (this book, Chapter 14) make clear that these experiences require the modification of provider–patient communication models. Moving forward, health communication researchers can continue to develop these models, building theories around marginalized experiences. On the other hand, health communication researchers also should pursue more passionately advocacy and activist efforts to reduce inequalities in medical care.

Critical perspectives also expand health communication theorizing by locating medical communication within capitalist relations of profit. The field must take the "business" of health care more seriously, investigating how profit motives shape health-care practices and distort healing relationships. For instance, in Chapter 15, Stokes shows us how the pharmaceutical industry uses promotional communication to construct knowledge about health and illness in ways that promote pharmaceutical intervention. A communication perspective marks the failure to identify the sponsors of communication and their motives as an ethical lapse. If the field of communication is to achieve the advocacy role recommended by Sharf (1999), we must articulate the values and ethics of genuinely equitable and open communication to the public at large, and encourage productive deliberations about issues of culture, power, and profit in medicine.

References

Blech, J. (2006). *Inventing Disease and Pushing Pills. Pharmaceutical Companies and the Medicalisation of Normal Life.* London: Routledge.

Brown, J., Stewart, M., & Ryan, B. (2003). Outcomes of patient-provider communication. In T.L. Thompson, A.M. Dorsey, K.I. Miller, & R. Parrott (eds), *Handbook of Health Communication.* Mahwah, NJ: Lawrence Erlbaum, pp. 141–162.

Deetz, S.A. (1992). *Democracy in an Age of Corporate Colonization: Developments in Communication and the Politics of Everyday Life.* New York: State University of New York Press.

Ellingson, L. (2003). Interdisciplinary health care teamwork in the clinic backstage. *Journal of Applied Communication Research, 31*(2), 93–117.

Ellingson, L.L., & Buzzanell, P.M. (1999). Listening to women's narratives of breast cancer treatment: A feminist approach to patient communication. *Health Communication, 11*(2).

Foucault, M. (1973). *Birth of the Clinic.* New York: Pantheon Press.

Foucault, M. (1979). *Discipline and Punish: The Birth of the Prison* (A. Sheridan, trans.). New York: Vintage.

Foucault, M. (1980). *The History of Sexuality: An Introduction* (R. Hurley, trans. Vol. 1). New York: Vintage.

Geist, P., & Dreyer, J. (1993). The demise of dialogue: A critique of medical encounter ideology. *Western Journal of Communication, 57*(Spring), 233–246.

Gilloti, C. (2003). Medical disclosure and decision-making: Excavating the complexities of physician-patient information exchange. In T.L. Thompson, A.M. Dorsey, K.I. Miller, & R. Parrott (eds), *Handbook of Health Communication.* Mahwah, NJ: Lawrence Erlbaum, pp. 163–182.

Habermas, J. (1970). On systematically distorted communication. *Inquiry, 13,* 205–218.

Japp, P., & Japp, D. (2005). Desperately seeking legitimacy: Narratives of a biomedically invisible disease. In L.M. Harter, P.M. Japp, & C. Beck (eds), *Narratives, Health, and Healing.* Mahwah, NJ: Lawrence Erlbaum, pp. 107–130.

Johnson, J., Bottorff, J., & Browne, A. (2004). Othering and being othered in the context of health care services. *Health Communication, 16*(2), 253–271.

Lammers, J.C., Duggan, A.P., & Barbour, J.B. (2003). Organizational forms and the provision of health care. In T.L. Thompson, A.M. Dorsey, K.I. Miller, R. Parrott (eds), *Handbook of Health Communication.* Mahwah, NJ: Lawrence Erlbaum, pp. 319–346.

Lammers, J.C., & Geist, P. (1997). The transformation of caring in the light and shadow of "managed care." *Health Communication, 9*(1), 45–60.

Nadesan, M.H. (2005). *Constructing Autism: Unravelling the 'Truth' and Understanding the Social.* London: Routledge.

Noland, C., & Carl, W. (2006). "It's not our ass": Medical resident sense-making regarding lawsuits. *Health Communication, 20*(1), 81–89.

Orbe, M., & King, G. (2000). Negotiating the tension between policy and reality: Exploring nurses' communication about organizational wrongdoing. *Health Communication, 12*(1), 41–61.

Poole, M.S., & Real, K. (2003). Groups and teams in health care: Communication and effectiveness. In T.L. Thompson, A.M. Dorsey, K.I. Miller, & R. Parrot (eds), *Handbook of Health Communication.* Mahwah, NJ: Lawrence Erlbaum, pp. 369–402.

Sharf, B.F. (1990). Physician-patient communication as interpersonal rhetoric: A narrative approach. *Health Communication, 2*(4), 217–231.

Sharf, B.F. (1999). The present and future of health communication scholarship: Overlooked opportunities. *Health Communication, 11*(2), 195–199.

Sharf, B.F. (2005). How I fired my surgeon and embraced an alternative narrative. In L.M. Harter, P.M. Japp, & C.S. Beck (eds), *Narratives, Health, and Healing: Communication Theory, Research, and Practice.* Mahwah, NJ: Lawrence Erlbaum, pp. 325–342.

Stein, H.F. (1990). *American Medicine as Culture.* Boulder, CO: Westview Press.

Vanderford, M.L., Jenks, E.B., & Sharf, B.F. (1997). Exploring patients' experiences as a primary source of meaning. *Health Communication, 9*(1).

Waitzkin, H. (1991). *The Politics of Medical Encounters.* New Haven: Yale University Press.

Chapter 12

Contested streams of action
Power and deference in emergency medicine

Alexandra G. Murphy, Eric M. Eisenberg,
Robert Wears, and Shawna J. Perry

Over the past decade, significant interdisciplinary attention has been paid to the conduct of health care in the United States, and in particular to the status of medical knowledge. In many academic fields—but mainly in anthropology, sociology, and communication—the prevailing image of medical knowledge as "unassailable 'God's Truth' has shifted to something socially produced and symbolically mediated bringing forth questions of power and authority in the negotiation and control of that knowledge" (Kuipers, 1989, p. 100). An emerging critical consciousness regarding medical expertise has coincided with myriad practical frustrations with the delivery of care. Widespread medical error, difficulties in navigating managed care and hospital bureaucracies, increased patient access to health information on the web, and the availability of various forms of alternative medicine all contribute to a growing skepticism among health-care consumers (Andrews et al., 1997; Leape, 1994; Leape et al., 1993).

In this context, it is important to seek a deeper understanding of the factors that shape how medical knowledge is produced and sustained through medical staff and patient interactions. Atkinson (1988) noted that most research on medical discourse limits its focus to doctor–patient communication. Recently, however, the scope of this work has begun to expand. For example, Bosk (1979) followed a surgical teaching service for a year and studied how what he dubbed the "tribe of surgeons" communicated the norms and mores of medical practice. Andrews et al. (1997) conducted an ethnographic study of hospital-wide communication and culture, and Schryer et al. (2005) analyzed case presentations by medical and optometry students. There have also been a series of studies on physician communication and patient safety in the Intensive Care Unit by Albolino and Cook (2005), Kowalsky et al. (2004), and Nemeth et al. (2005).

Close analyses of communication such as these are especially warranted in emergency care, where how issues are framed and interpreted have literal life or death implications (e.g., Eisenberg et al., 2005). Behara et al. (2005) performed an in-depth study of communication during handovers in emergency departments (ED). While a relatively new area of specialization, emergency medicine has become a central part of health care in North America. For most hospitals, more than half of admitted patients come through the ED. But ED activity is in many ways different from care delivered elsewhere in a hospital. Unlike specialized care administered on the hospital floors, emergency medicine providers are faced on a daily basis with a high volume of patients with a wide range of complaints and diseases, all with varying degrees of urgency. Under these pressures, ED personnel must negotiate patient care and seek to create a sense of order and certainty in a chaotic environment (Eisenberg et al., 2005; Schenkel, 2000).

Drawing on extensive observations of EDs and interviews with ED personnel, this study explored hospital EDs as *political* environments. By characterizing them in this way, our explicit focus was on the interplay of individual and professional interests as it is manifest in communication and behavior. We began by looking at how medical knowledge is constituted in the ED through discursive relationships based on power and authority. Next, we examined the impact of this knowledge on the medical decisions that were made, and how these decisions both enable and constrain certain specific streams of action. We do this through a series of examples from our fieldwork that feature considered communicative relationships among patients, family members, nurses, interns, residents, and attending physicians. In these examples, we highlight how particular communicative exchanges established, reinforced, or challenged particular streams of action. Finally, we identify two communicative dialectics that emerged in our data: 1) Certainty/Vulnerability, and 2) Deference/ Challenge. We close by offering specific recommendations for how to encourage medical personnel to keep multiple perspectives in play even when a stream of action has been clearly established.

Knowledge/Politics

French social theorist Michel Foucault (1980) established an important link between knowledge and power in social life. For Foucault, power relations between institutions, groups, and individuals are both accomplished and revealed through discourse, with privilege afforded to those who claim specialized knowledge, such as lawyers and physicians. Moreover, in highly specialized fields actions are governed by the constituents of the power structures themselves, that is, there cannot be criminology without prisons, forensic DNA without police, nor institutionalized medicine without hospitals.

Foucault's work has seen rich application to research in medical settings (e.g. Ceci, 2003, 2004; Gibson, 2001; Heartfield, 1996; Henderson, 1994; Huntington & Gilmour, 2001; Lynch, 2004; Riley & Manias, 2002; Sullivan, 1986) and "provides for insightful analysis of unacknowledged assumptions and metaphors in health care practice" (Henderson, 1994, p. 935). For example, Foucault (1980) exposes the power of the "gaze" in defining and normalizing the patient as a body; as an object of inquiry (Henderson, 1994). Sullivan (1986) notes the implications of viewing the human body as a "pathological object" by saying that "it allowed the eye of the physician to replace the words of the patient as the measure of similarity and difference between diseases . . . thus disease begins to be autonomous from patients' experienced sense of disability" (p. 333).

Foucault's concepts of power and knowledge have been fruitfully applied to the analysis of the behavior of medical professionals. For example, Lynch (2004) used Foucault's concepts of power and discipline to examine the changes in behavior in an A&E department (Accidents and Emergency—the UK equivalent to EDs in North America) during a week-long audit by the National Health Service (NHS). The NHS had reorganized and refined its requirements for hospital stays including requiring that 90 percent of all patients admitted to A&E must be "seen and sorted" within four hours (p. 1). Prior to the audit, the hospital was not even close to the 90 percent target. During the audit, however, additional medical and nursing staff was added, senior management roamed the wards, and the management style was autocratic and at times even dictatorial. Ninety-five percent of all patients were "completed A&E episodes within four hours" (p. 2). For Lynch, the gaze normally reserved for patients was turned on the medical staff themselves, constructing them as compliant subjects in pursuit of these temporal targets. In this case, "the production of knowledge and the exercise of administrative power intertwine, and each begins to enhance the other" (Allen, 1999, p. 70).

Foucault has also been applied extensively in studies of nursing. A common theme in the nursing literature is the expression or suppression of nursing knowledge and power (Huntington & Gilmour, 2001). Riley and Manias (2002), for example, argue that discipline "informs the professional activities of operating room nursing and shapes nursing practices by imposing set ways of behaving" (p. 322). Heartfield (1996) uses Foucault to show that the role of nurses is more complex than simply carrying out the knowledge disciplines of others. She explains that routine practices such as the daily written nursing documentation of patient events result from "hegemonic influences that construct a knowledge and therefore a practice of nursing" that place limits on how the role of nursing is perceived by others and the nurses themselves (p. 98).

Ceci (2004) analyzed how the deaths of twelve children during cardiac surgeries could be linked to the lack of credibility afforded to nurses who voiced concerns about the behavior and expertise of a surgeon. She found that the hospital-based inquiries disregarded the nurses concerns and the physician was not defined as at fault until an independent judge reviewed the case and gave credence to the nurses' knowledge claims. According to Foucault, when someone asserts a statement, it becomes "power" when someone else (the other) takes the statement as "true." For example, Allen (1999) explains when a media text asserts to an audience that a certain fact is "true," the statement becomes powerful when it is transmitted and carried through the economy of discourse. Similarly, when one physician asserts a certain "fact" about a patient, it becomes powerful when accepted by another as "true." While, as Ceci (2004) showed, when the nurses asserted a "fact" about a physician, it did not become power until the independent judge accepted it as true.

From this perspective, knowledge is established through argument and justification, there is no de-contextualized, transcendent truth, and to "know" means to be able to give reasons for one's beliefs that are accepted by practical communities as valid (Ceci, 2004, p. 1881; May, 1993). That is, knowledge is justified relative to claims a community is willing to take seriously (Anderson, 1995). Truth, as Shapin (1994) argued, becomes a matter of collective judgment, collective activity: "truth consists of the actions taken by practical communities to make the idea true, to make it agree with reality" (p. 6). Knowledge then is a "thoroughly social affair" (Ceci, 2004, p. 1881). Our problem becomes not distinguishing truth from fiction, in any particular situation, but seeing how the effects of truth are accomplished, how "truth" is produced and administered, and the behavioral consequences that follow from the ratification of any knowledge (Ceci, 2004, p. 1881).

It is therefore important to pay attention to the social context within which medical decisions are made—to understand how knowledge is determined, by whom, and in what situations. To put it simply, "what one believes crucially depends on whom one believes" (Anderson, 1995, p. 189). Medical communication practices should be recognized as *political* and studied as such. It is these political relationships that determine who speaks, who listens, who defers, and who is deferred to. Furthermore, these established relationships function in accordance with social norms and background beliefs that tell us who can be trusted, whose words are credible or authoritative and why.

Deetz (1991) calls the privileging of certain discourses—and the marginalization of others—"discursive closure." The most common form of discursive closure is disqualification, or the "denial of the right of expression, denying access to speaking forums, the assertion of the need for certain expertise in order to speak, or through rendering the other unable to speak adequately" (p. 187). Discursive closure suppresses potential conflicts as it normalizes who is authorized to speak and when. Individuals who violate the norms of discursive closure are socially sanctioned by their peers. For example, a low-level resident who "acts" as though he or she has more standing or voice in a situation will be ignored and disliked. On the other hand, a high-level resident or attending physician will be expected to take a stand in a situation and may be marked as incompetent if he or she does not.

While emergency medicine is a highly uncertain and high-risk environment (given the sheer number of patients and their wide variety of conditions), much of the action that takes place is routine behavior based on recurrent interpretations and actions. While the United States does not (yet!) have a national target rate of "sorting and sending" patients out of the ED within four hours, the organizational structure does not allow for a patient to have extensive care in the ED. The staff is disciplined to work from an established template for categorizing patient symptoms ("triage") that also sorts patients into categories of severity. In triage, if a patient appears to meet the criteria of a routine event—for example, heart attack or stroke—the orders are pre-printed and the medical staff starts treatment immediately.

In a related study, we explored how a patient's original story given upon arrival in the ED is translated into a technical list. Based on that established template we found that narrative rationality, or the patient's story, was consistently subjugated to technical rationality, or actionable lists (Eisenberg et al., 2005). The technical list became both the medium and the outcome of the patient plan of action. How a patient is talked about during the initial triage phase influences the next conversation and creates a stream of action (e.g. tests ordered, medications given) that both enables and constrains how the patient is seen and described. The technical list reinforces how that patient is talked about during the course of their stay in the ED and directs the stream of actions related to the patient's care. The process, as seen in other high-risk industries, helps individuals reduce the amount of possibilities to a manageable number of choices (Weick, 1995).

Once underway, these streams of action are difficult to stop because the process tends to be driven by *plausibility rather than accuracy*. Once people have found an answer to a problem or question, they tend to stop searching for alternative explanations. A plausible explanation is enough to offer the sense of certainty that the medical staff seek in this very uncertain environment characterized by limited information, competing goals, and institutional and community pressures. These explanations become what Giddens (1979) calls practical consciousness or common-sense behavior that is no longer discussed or questioned. He distinguishes this from discursive consciousness where behavior is not rote, but knowingly reflected and accounted for. This reflection is the first step toward a possible change in knowledge; it is not plausible for humans to always exist at a level of discursive consciousness. What appears to be key is the ability to access both levels of consciousness at least some of the time.

The most significant danger in all of this is that health-care providers may pay too much attention to cues that match normalized expectations for a patient. Once they have the plausible diagnosis and action plan established and collectively agreed upon, it becomes "truth" and they are not likely to question it. This is not so much out of individual reluctance, but more due to the rigid disciplinary social structure of the health-care environment in which knowledge is expected to come from a perceived credible source based on hierarchy (organizational or occupational roles) and a history of institutional and industry-wide discursive closure.

Our earlier work focused on the vulnerability of key communication processes in EDs over time and called for a heightened awareness of the bias for technical over narrative rationality in emergency medicine as an important first step toward anticipating potential failures and better ensuring patient safety (Eisenberg et al., 2005). This project focuses more specifically on the political cues for coordination such as hierarchy, stereotypes, and occupational roles; to reveal how socially based power relations permeate the content of knowledge and have become equally as taken-for-granted and unquestioned as the technical rationality of the list. With this in mind, we pose several questions concerning power, knowledge and decision-making in hospital emergency departments:

- How is medical knowledge of a patient determined, by whom, and in what situations?
- Who has the power to question and/or redirect an ongoing stream of action?
- What conditions are most likely to lead people to challenge accepted knowledge about a patient?

Method

The data for this study was drawn from a larger analysis of communicative transitions of patient care in six North American EDs over a period of about six months. The interdisciplinary research team included two communication scholars, two emergency medicine physicians, and one ED registered nurse. There were also medical staff contacts at each hospital that sponsored the study and joined in discussions at their respective hospitals. The participating EDs were located in different regions of the United States and included two hospitals in Canada with a cumulative annual patient volume of 325,000. The main observers were the two communication scholars and the registered nurse who functioned as a medical consultant. Each emergency room was observed for a period of four days with observation rounds lasting approximately eight hours each day for a total of 135 hours of observation. Informal interviews were also conducted during the observation periods and more formal discussions occurred with physicians and the registered nurse who comprised the research team during and after the observation periods.

What follows are three extended examples that demonstrate the communicative and power relationships among nurses, interns, residents, attending physicians, and patients. These examples focus on signovers, those moments when patient care is being transferred from one member of the medical staff to another. These transitions in care not only transfer authority and responsibility for patient care, but also reveal how medical knowledge is constituted and demonstrate how streams of action are established, reinforced, or at times challenged.

Findings

We have chosen to organize our findings through key extended examples that represent the ways in which medical knowledge and subsequent courses of action were discursively constituted, negotiated, and at times resisted, manifesting various power relationships in the ED. The findings are followed by an analysis in which we discuss key dialectical tensions in these cases. This is followed by a discussion of the implications for practice.

A potential paralysis

A male patient was brought into the trauma section of the ED with a serious injury to his neck with a complaint of mild tingling to his arms and legs. Accepted medical protocol states that he should be placed in a cervical collar (c-collar) to protect his neck from further movement during medical evaluation. The junior resident (male) and two nurses (female) assigned to the patient had trouble getting the collar on because it was painful to the patient and decided to forgo further attempts as they did not want to risk further injury. After the ED evaluation was completed, the junior resident called a more senior resident in orthopedics to come to the ED and consult on the patient. This is a common procedure in the ED. A physician must call and "consult" the medical service to which they want to admit the patient.

Upon his arrival, the orthopedic resident (male) immediately yelled at the nurses for not having the patient in the c-collar. To show his displeasure, he kicked over some medical supplies sitting in a bucket on the floor. The consultant then went over to the patient and immediately and firmly "manipulated" him to fit in the collar resulting in worsening of the patient's numbness, potentially worsening a presumed neurological injury. This stream of action was being investigated at the hospital while we were there.

The manipulation event speaks directly to tensions involving various definitions of knowledge, power, and voice. Two levels of knowledge were operating in this case. The first was the practical consciousness of clinical protocol: when a patient comes in with neck pain or injury, he/she is automatically placed in a c-collar. This is the level from which the orthopedic resident was operating when he arrived in the trauma room. He was not made aware that the ED staff had moved beyond this level of clinical action with this individual patient because they had tried to put the c-collar on, discussed that it was not working, and decided it was not worth the risk of trying again. This conversation and its conclusion were not, however, ever shared with the orthopedic resident. So, a critical question in this case is why would people who had critical knowledge in this case—the junior resident, the nurses, and even the patient, himself—not speak up to tell the orthopedic resident not to force the cervical collar on as directed by protocol? A partial explanation is that there was not time. The orthopedic resident moved very quickly and did not offer an opportunity for a conversation. Still, the ED staff did not attempt to confront his actions. Alternatively, why did not the orthopedic resident take a moment to ask if there was anything more he needed to know before he took action?

The initial explanations at the time of this example, focused almost exclusively on the behavior and attitude of the orthopedic resident. One physician explained, "this guy is really an asshole; he is kind of setting himself up for this and not matching well with our [ED] culture." The perception was that the orthopedic resident bullied the ED staff, was not interested in anything they had to say, and did not allow them the opportunity to speak. In fact, it appeared that medical mishap was being built around the orthopedic resident as a difficult person to work with as if this were a unique event determined mainly by the personality of the individual physician consultant.

There are other possible explanations. One consideration is the relationship between power and role status and authority. Emergency physicians are well versed in a wide range of medical specialties from trauma to toxicology, from pediatrics to psychiatry, making them the consummate "generalists." ED physicians must also be able to determine life-threatening from nonlife-threatening conditions and involve other sub-specialties when necessary to address a patient's clinical needs. When a medical "consult" comes into the ED, the ED physicians are often deferential to their expertise. Adding to this is the status of the two physicians as residents. The orthopedic resident was a more senior physician than the ED resident. Typically, in a case like this, the ED attending (board certified supervising physician) would be more actively involved. His/her authority as an attending physician could offset the status of the orthopedic resident. In this case, however, the ED attending was working another case in a different part of the ED. He was not aware that the situation was out of hand.

In fact, according to hospital authority chains, neither resident is ultimately responsible in this case. The attending physicians have the primary authority and responsibility for all the actions their residents take. As noted earlier, the ED attending was busy in another trauma area. The orthopedic attending does not routinely accompany the orthopedic residents on consults and would not be directly involved until after the perceived error happened. This is more likely because both attendings were too busy to be involved and not because they were unwilling. Workload pressures add to occupational stress, and when in stressful situations, people revert to their first-learned responses (Weick, 1995). In this case, the orthopedic resident relied heavily on learned protocols (both clinical in putting the patient in the c-collar and relational in his communication with the ED staff) and did not take the time to explore contextual information or alternative options for action.

The nurses also had knowledge about this incident but did not speak up. Even if they had, it may not have made a difference; when nurses do speak up, they are often ignored (Ceci, 2004). Again, we can see how role status relates to issues of authority and voice in health care. Nurses are commonly seen as the executors of physician orders rather than conveyors of medical knowledge. They are not meant or trained to directly challenge a physician's orders. In fact, we witnessed a new nurse being told by a more senior nurse that, "you never tell a physician that he/she is wrong; instead, you say, 'are you sure you want to do that?'" In this case, even if the nurses had asked if the orthopedic resident was "sure he wanted to do that," his response would have been "yes" based on the knowledge he had of the patient and protocol.

Finally, the patient himself had more knowledge than the orthopedic resident as to why the c-collar was not in place. He did not tell the resident, nor did he speak up to stop manipulating his neck when he was uncomfortable. This is not an uncommon experience for patient relationships with doctors. Most patients willingly concede total authority to a physician in the conscious or unconscious hope that they have the knowledge to help them get better.

In the end, the patient's neck pain was the result of an abscess along his spine. Had the orthopedic resident left him in his original position, the abscess would not have compressed his spinal cord resulting in possible long-term neurologic injury. The reasons for this event go beyond a simple explanation of a "difficult" physician who does not listen to anyone. Individuals had knowledge in this case, but because of an authoritarian climate and culture, the right questions were not asked nor answered or considered.

A disruptive patient

One of the difficulties/dangers of the practice of emergency medicine is the lack of information about a patient or access to methods for verifying the information available when the patient arrives at the ED. This leaves room for the introduction of incorrect or biased information from which the stream of action of clinical care begins. The way a patient is initially "marked" when arriving in the ED can significantly influence how that patient is viewed and the treatment decisions that follow. In another case, a patient was brought into the ED by the rescue paramedics. The patient was white, male, about 22 years old. He was strapped to the gurney and was wearing a plastic face mask because he was violent, spitting and shouting at the staff. The paramedics told the triage nurse that the patient was "a drug overdose that was found knocked out on the ground." This type of patient is not unusual at this ED as it is located in a community-based hospital that serves an economically depressed neighborhood. The triage nurse recorded this information and it was passed along to the resident assigned to his case. Several hours later, the patient was sleepy and subdued. The resident's shift was over and he was transitioning the patient to incoming physicians. At this hospital, the transition of patients happens in a large group with incoming and outgoing attendings and residents altogether. When it was this resident's turn to transition his patient he said, "[he] is a drug overdose found down."

Because the patient appeared groggy and incoherent, one of the incoming residents and the incoming attending asked what kind of tests had been run and then suggested running an additional test on the patient to rule out an internal head bleed. The resident who had been taking care of him insisted that this was not needed. He made a show about going over and thumping on the patient's chest saying, "You hear me? You remember what happened earlier." The patient said, "No." The resident said, "See, he's awake and alert. I rest my case." The conversation quickly escalated as each doctor demonstrated a need to be right. The outgoing resident was relying on his knowledge of the patient from the rescue paramedics and his earlier erratic behavior. The incoming physicians were relying on their knowledge of the patient as he appeared at that time. In the end, the outgoing resident left and the additional test (a head CT) was performed. When the test returned, the patient did shown signs of an internal brain bleed. This new information led to a re-evaluation of the entire case including a conversation with the patient's family who stated that there was little reason to suspect drug overdose as a potential reason for the patient's violent behavior.

The knowledge the resident had for this patient was greatly influenced by the initial statements made by the rescue paramedics. Any new information he might have gotten on the patient was filtered through this early knowledge. This filtering will typically continue when the physicians and nurses pass the information on to the next physician shift taking over the case. Given this, the outgoing physicians have significant power in shaping the way information about a patient is communicated and in shaping the diagnostic direction of the case. And as we have argued in related work, the outgoing physicians have significant ego invested in presenting their cases as resolved, even when they are not (Eisenberg et al., 2005). In this case, although he did not appreciate it, the outgoing physician was challenged and the participants argued over the best direction to take the case. The decision became a communal event, with multiple parties invested in the outcome. When the certainty of the outgoing diagnosis is publicly and communally questioned, the incoming physicians are granted permission to consider alternative directions of patient care. While we saw more of these public challenges happening in this ED, most likely because of the communal transition process, it was certainly not the norm in this ED and definitely not the norm in other EDs where the patient transitions happened more dyadically (between the two ingoing and outgoing physicians).

An interrupted plan of action

In this situation, an ED resident was assigned to a patient who was brought to the ED by his family for erratic behavior and psychiatric evaluation. The resident's shift was ending and he was transitioning his other patients because he thought the situation was resolved and that the patient was being admitted. But, the psychiatry consult, on her way out of the ED, casually mentioned that she did not believe that a patient should be admitted. She explained that the patient's family called for the ambulance, and the patient shows no evidence of being confused at the present time. The resident disagreed and insisted that the patient should be admitted. He explained that the patient has been in the ED twice that week already, something the psychiatry consult did not know.

Both these physicians had forms of knowledge in this case. The psychiatry consult was relying on her clinical expertise and the manner of the patient at the current time. The ED resident was relying on knowledge of the patient's pattern of behavior. Ultimately, at this hospital, the attending physicians make the final decision. So, the ED resident and psychiatry consult walked over to the patient area just as the attending who was leaving for the day was transitioning the patient over to the incoming attending. At this site, rather than the communal transition described in the earlier example, the outgoing residents transition their specific patients to the incoming residents assigned to their patient beds. There is just one ED attending on duty who supervises the entire area. When that attending is ready to leave, a new one comes in and they have a separate transition of all the patients without any residents present. The outgoing ED attending, who had just listened to the psychiatry consult, was telling the incoming ED attending that there is "nothing wrong with the guy" and he could be sent home. When the incoming asked what brought the patient to the ED in the first place, the outgoing attending "normalized" the patient conduct as he told the patient's story to the incoming who agreed with him. He said, "He got frustrated when he couldn't get the door open, and so he knocked it down." The incoming responded, "I know I have felt like doing that at times."

The ED resident interrupted them and said, "There has never been anything wrong with him. It's his family who thinks so and if you send him home, they will just call rescue and send him back." Hearing this, the outgoing attending started to change his mind and said, "That is a good enough reason to keep him." With the conversation more open, and the plan of action for this patient challenged, a nurse joined in the conversation and offered even more knowledge. She said, "He [the patient] is in denial. He is totally out of it. He had a machete and knocked down a door because his wife changed the locks." The nurse had been present when the patient had first come in very agitated and violent. After he had been sedated for several hours, he woke up and appeared quite normal. None of the physicians, including the psychiatry consult, were aware that a machete had been used to knock down the door or that the door would not open because the patient's wife had changed the lock because she was afraid of him. This is not surprising since in the ED, patient stories are not as a rule documented in their charts. In related work, we draw on Browning (1992) to show how much of the context of patient stories are lost when they are translated and documented as technical lists of symptoms and behaviors (Eisenberg et al., 2005). In this case, the narrative was only communicated orally and was reduced to "a frustrated man whose family overreacted when he kicked down a door that would not unlock." The key decision makers, therefore, did not have complete information and were attempting to construct a plausible story in the absence of credible information.

The picture of the patient significantly shifted with the new knowledge. Furthermore, the nurse had spent much more time with the patient and had witnessed several other periods of agitation and confusion, while during the physician encounters, the patient had appeared coherent.

As a result of the discursive interruptions by the resident and the nurse, the stream of action for this patient changed substantially from a decision to discharge to one to admit. This could easily, however, not have happened. Had the psychiatric consult not alerted the outgoing resident of her decision, the resident would not have gotten reinvolved in the case as the attendings were discussing it. Also, it is important to note that the nurse was not formally "invited" into the conversation; her knowledge was not solicited; yet, it was critical to the decision. She just happened to be walking by and heard the physicians discussing the case and spoke up.

Analysis: communicative dialectics

We identified two important, and related, dialectical tensions that emerged when medical professionals engaged in conversation. The first dialectic involves the degree of certainty (the correct diagnosis or plan of action) versus vulnerability (an openness to multiple possibilities) that an individual expresses—or is expected to express—when participating in a patient discussion. The second dialectic refers to the degree of deference or challenge an individual expresses or is expected to express when participating in a patient discussion. Both the expectation and expression of behavior are critical components in these dialectics as it is not only how the individual perceives his or her role, but how others perceive his or her role in a given situation that can guide whether or not a person speaks up or even if he or she does speak up, whether or not anyone pays attention.

For example, in the case of the potentially paralyzed patient, all parties expressed a high level of certainty and little vulnerability (or openness to other options). Given his occupational role as a "consultant" the orthopedic resident behaved with a high level of certainty when he arrived in the ED. Given their experience with the patient, the ED resident and nurses were equally certain that he should not be moved to fit into the neck brace. In terms of the second dialectic, the orthopedic resident immediately challenged the position of the ED staff when he arrived and moved the patient. Though equally certain, the ED staff, on the other hand, did not challenge his position, but deferred to his authority. In this case, there was no discussion across the authority gradient of the risks and benefits for forcing the cervical collar on the patient.

In the case of the suspected drug overdose, the initial resident presented the case from a position of certainty: that the patient *was* a drug overdose. The incoming physicians, including an attending physician, expressed a desire to remain more open to other possibilities and vulnerable in the diagnosis. The initial resident continued to challenge their desire for openness and defend his certainty. With neither party willing to defer to the other, the case was settled simply because the initial resident left the ED at the end of his shift. There was, therefore, no collective knowledge gained in this situation (Weick & Sutcliffe, 2003) with the decision for more testing occurring after the resident had left therein allowing him to save face but ultimately not learning from his experience.

The case of the psychiatric patient provided the most potential for collective knowledge since the plan of action actually shifted as a result of the discussion. While all parties demonstrated a level of certainty, the overt challenges to each other's perspectives inadvertently invited the nurse to come forward with knowledge that helped clarify the case. This caused a disruption in the "norm" of patient discussions (that typically only include the physicians) and allowed the physicians to move to a more vulnerable place in their deliberations.

Random disruptions such as this are not common. In emergency medicine a medical staff relies on previously established protocols and patient cues to reduce the amount of diagnostic possibilities to a manageable number of choices. Physicians will mark this kind of patient as a "good story," meaning that their account corresponds to both their symptoms and available diagnostic categories. For example, if a 65-year-old, overweight man complains of chest pain, protocol dictates a very clear path of doing chest X-rays and EKG. To some extent, this must happen to expedite the process and allow the patient to move through the hospital system, being discharged or admitted. Because not a lot of conversation would be needed to decide this route, the information is passed along to other medical staff through an efficient monologue and in most cases without incident. The danger, however, as shown in the examples above, is a failure to recognize that *choices* are being made; that initial cues are selected and a patient diagnosis is created, not discovered. Participants remain certain, vulnerable, deferential, or challenging according to the expected patterns of their occupational and organizational roles; nurses remain quiet, residents defer to attendings or overly assert themselves to prove their worth, and outside ED consultants are treated as the final authority. Also at play are extra-organizational issues such as cultural and social assumptions of patient background and behavior. For example, a young, white male from a depressed economic background is assumed a drug overdose while a middle-aged, white male from a middle-class background is assumed safe to send home to his family even though he used a machete to get into his house. As we saw, reliance on these expected patterns of behavior may set a clinical stream of actions in motion that could cause significant risk to the patients involved.

Implications for practice: deliberate disruptions

We believe that a *deliberate disruption* has a place in patient diagnosis for several important reasons. First, as we have seen, the rote passage of patient information must be interrupted to move participants out of practical consciousness to a more reflective discursive consciousness where they are required to be accountable for their ideas and actions. Time pressures mitigate against this kind of pause, hence this disruption must be deliberate in the sense that it is planned and on purpose.

Second, a deliberate disruption can create room for a more open exchange of ideas, working against the risks of discursive closure. As we saw in the case of the assumed drug overdose, a discussion can acknowledge that there are multiple ways to view a patient case, forcing participants to offer and account for their perspectives. The main risk, of course, is that the person with the most persuasive position may not be the person with the most complete knowledge of the case. Given differences in power and authority, not all participants will have an equal stance in the discussion, or even be present for the conversation. And, like the first resident who declared the patient a drug overdose, individuals may stubbornly stick to their initial diagnosis in an effort to prove themselves "right" and establish their power and credibility over the present case as well as for future cases and decisions. Of course, in the case of the drug overdose, that resident lost the debate because he left the hospital and the incoming physicians took over. Because he was unwilling to examine his assumptions and his position was found inaccurate, he will have less credibility and authority in future cases when he might have the better perspective.

Therefore, during a deliberate disruption, participants must be willing to "hang their assumptions" out in plain view for others to consider, question, and engage (Senge, 1991). They must not only question their own positions on a patient case, but also their positionality in terms of the dialectical tensions. In other words, are they remaining silent because they are expected to be deferential or are they expressing more certainty than they feel because of their occupational roles? This requires a level of discursive consciousness, self-awareness, and reflexivity of their occupational positionality and voice.

Participants may mistakenly treat the dialectical tensions as "either/or" rather than "both/and." In other words, in a given situation, a nurse may believe he/she must be *either* deferential or challenging. Or, a resident may believe he/she must be either vulnerable or certain. Dialectical tensions, however, must allow for the opposing positions to exist simultaneously. A nurse must recognize both deference and challenge; and a resident must recognize both vulnerability and certainty. Someone could express both vulnerability and certainty by saying, "Well, I'm not sure why I feel this way, but there is something else going on here." In an environment of discursive closure, people are going to hold their tongues deferring to the organizationally recognized authorities who are empowered to have a voice. The risk then, is premature closure, of shortchanging or skipping the needed discourse/conversation because it takes time and always opens a possibility of another perspective.

In the face of competing goals in the ED (move patients quickly, stabilize the critically ill, patient education, documentation for billing), entertaining other perspectives through deliberate disruptions may be perceived as costly and unwelcome—but in the end, may provide for better patient care. Therefore, it is important to consider some practical ways such changes can be introduced and encouraged. In that vein, we offer several suggestions for practical implementation of deliberate disruptions that we have learned from our work.

First, we recommend redesigning physician and nursing rounds to better support group dialogue and make deliberate disruptions an expectation rather than an exception to the group norms. Even in teaching hospitals, we found rounds to primarily focus on transferring patient information and if and when someone questioned that information, it was viewed as a challenge rather than an invitation for conversation. Following the model of hospital surgical teams incorporating "stop and pause" step as part of their routine during surgeries, EDs should integrate the deliberate disruption as a required practice during rounds.

Second, we recommend that nurses and physicians "round" together for at least part of the conversation. When we began our research, we were told that nurses and physicians did not round together because the information they were exchanging was not really relevant for each other (e.g. nurses wouldn't be interested in the overall diagnosis—just what orders had been filled or needed to be filled). After our observations, however, we learned that the nurses and physicians have very similar types of conversation, just not together. Granted, nurses do not need to go "round" with all the patients, they should just join during the discussion of their assigned patients. Having nurses explicitly participate in the conversation may be an effective way to empower nurses to challenge physician judgment as they can offer their expert knowledge of the patient which may include more contextual cues since nurses spend so much more time with the patients.

Third, the communication between ED physicians and consulting physicians should be standardized to help reduce the effects of the power dynamics. The deliberate disruption must happen at the beginning of the interaction to allow each part to clarify their understandings of the patient condition. It must be acceptable for each party to express vulnerability and at the same time challenge the other's perceptions. This is likely the most difficult recommendation to implement because unlike ED rounds, the interactions are random and much more variable, making them much harder to control. It also requires buy-in by hospital staff beyond the ED and for the ED to be recognized as an area of expertise—not just a holding area for patients until the "expert" doctors can see them. Therefore, the intervention must take place at a hospital level, not just a departmental level.

Finally, to encourage these changes, it is important for the participants to understand that the changes are a result of careful observation and critical analysis and to engage them in the process as much as possible. Not only was our research team multidisciplinary, including communication experts, physicians, and nurses, we also worked closely with contacts at each hospital we observed to report key learnings and to discuss options for interventions. In this way, we could offer general recommendations based on all of our research and also tailor suggestions according to individual needs. As noted earlier, to understand emergency medicine within the context of knowledge and power is to pay attention to social cues for coordination such as hierarchy, stereotypes, and occupational roles, and to reveal how socially based power relations permeate the content of knowledge. It is the social and political relations that determines who speaks, who listens, who defers, and who is deferred to, and further, establishes these relations in accordance with social norms and background beliefs that tell us who can be trusted, whose words are credible or authoritative and why. It is important to be mindful of these discursive practices, to move beyond the monologic protocol and practical consciousness to more open conversations that allow a reflective, discursive consciousness, where decisions and actions are no longer rote, but knowingly and deliberately considered.

References

Albolino, S., & Cook, R.I. (2005). Making sense of risks: A field study in an intensive care unit. In R. Tartaglia, S. Bagnara, R. Bellandi, & S. Albolino (eds), *Healthcare Systems, Ergonomics and Patient Safety*. Leiden, NE: Taylor and Francis, pp. 208–214.

Allen, B. (1999). Power/Knowledge. In K. Racevskis (ed.), *Critical Essays on Michel Foucault*. New York: G.K. Hall & Co.

Anderson, E. (1995). The democratic university: The role of justice in the production of knowledge. *Social and Political Philosophy, 12*(2), 189–219.

Andrews, L.B., Stocking, C., Krizek, T. Gottlieb, L., Kvizek, C., Vargish, T., and Siegler, M. (1997). An alternative strategy for studying adverse events in medical care. *Lancet, 349*, 309–13.

Atkinson, P. (1988). Review of *The Discourse of Medicine*, by Elliot Mishler. *Culture Medicine and Psychiatry, 12*, 249–256.

Behara, R., Wears, R.L., Perry, S.J., Eisenberg, E., Murphy, A.G., Vanderhoef, M., et al. (2005). Conceptual framework for the safety of handovers. In K. Henriksen (ed.), *Advances in Patient Safety*, vol. 2. Rockville, MD: Agency for Healthcare Research and Quality/Department of Defense, pp. 309–321.

Browning, L. (1992). Lists and stories in organizational communication. *Communication Theory, 2*, 281–302.

Bosk, C.L. (1979). *Forgive and Remember: Managing Medical Error*. London: University of Chicago Press.

Ceci, C. (2003). Midnight reckonings: On a question of knowledge and nursing. *Nursing Philosophy, 4*, 61–76.

Ceci, C. (2004). Nursing, knowledge and power: A case analysis. *Social Science and Medicine, 59*, 1879–1889.

Deetz, S.A. (1991). *Democracy in An Age of Corporate Colonization*. Albany, NY: SUNY Press.

Eisenberg, E., Murphy, A., Sutcliffe, K., Wears, R., Schenkel, S., Perry, S., & Vanderhoef, M. (2005). Communication in emergency medicine: Implications for patient safety. *Communication Monographs, 72*(4), 390–413.

Foucault, M. (1980). *Power/Knowledge: Selected Interviews & Other Writings 1972, 1977*. Ed. C. Gordon. New York: Pantheon Books.

Gibson, T. (2001). Nurses and medication error: A discursive reading of the literature. *Nursing Inquiry*, 8, 108–117.

Giddens, A. (1979). *Central Problems in Social Theory*. London: Hutchinson.

Heartfield, M. (1996). Nursing documentation and nursing practice: A discourse analysis. *Journal of Advanced Nursing, 24*, 98–103.

Henderson, A. (1994). Power and knowledge in nursing practice: The contribution of Foucault. *Journal of Advanced Nursing, 20*, 935–939.

Huntington, A.D., & Gilmour, J.A. (2001). Re-thinking representations, re-writing nursing texts: Possibilities through feminist and Foucauldian thought. *Journal of Advanced Nursing, 35*(6), 902–908.

Kowalsky, J., Nemeth, C.P., Brandwijk, M. & Cook, R.I. (2004). Understanding sign outs: Conversation analysis reveals ICU handoff content and form. Retrieved November 7, 2005, from www.ctlab.org/documents/Sccm2005 percent20POSTER. pdf.

Kuipers, J. (1989). "Medical discourse" in anthropological context: Views of language and power. *Medical Anthropology Quarterly, 3*(2), 99–123.

Leape, L.L. (1994). Error in medicine. *Journal of the American Medical Association, 272*, 1851–1857.

Leape, L.L., Lawthers, A.G., Brennan, T.A., & Johnson, W.G. (1993). Preventing medical injury. *QRB Quality Review Bulletin, 19*, 144–149

Lynch, J. (2004). Comment section: Foucault on targets. *Journal of Health Organization & Management, 19*(2/3), 128–135.

May, T. (1993). *Between Genealogy and Epistemology: Psychology, Politics and Knowledge in the Thought of Michel Foucault*. University Park, PA: Pennsylvania State University.

Nemeth, C.P., O'Connor, M., Nunnally, M., Klock, P.A., & Cook, R.I. (2005). Distributed cognition: How hand-of communication actually works. Retrieved November 7, 2005, from www.ctlab.org/documents/2005%20Distributed%20 Cognition.pdf.

Riley, R., & Manias, E. (2002). Foucault could have been an operating nurse. *Journal of Advanced Nursing, 39*(4), 316–324.

Schenkel, S. (2000). Promoting patient safety and preventing medical error in emergency departments. *Academic Emergency Medicine, 7*, 1204–1222.

Schryer, C., Lingard, L., & Spafford, M. (2005). Techne or artful science and the genre of case presentations in healthcare settings. *Communication Monographs, 72*, 234–260.

Senge, P. (1991). *The Fifth Discipline: The Art and Practice of the Learning Organization*. New York: Doubleday/Currency.

Shapin (1994). A social history of truth: Civility and science in seventeenth-century England. Chicago: University of Chicago Press.

Sullivan (1986). In what sense is contemporary medicine dualistic? *Culture, Medicine, and Society*, 10(4), 331–350.

Weick, K. (1995). *The Social Psychology of Organizing*, 2nd edn. Reading, MA: Addison-Wesley.

Weick, K., & Sutcliffe, K. (2003). *Managing the Unexpected: Assuring High Performance in An Age of Complexity*. San Francisco: Jossey-Bass.

Chapter 13

Changing realities and entrenched norms in dialysis
A case study of power, knowledge, and communication in health-care delivery

Laura L. Ellingson

The more things change, the more they stay the same. The U.S. health-care system has undergone enormous technological and organizational change over the past few decades (Geist-Martin et al., 2003) and yet remains remarkably inflexible and static in terms of its disciplinary hierarchies, organizational power structures, and day-to-day communication practices that both arise from and perpetuate those hierarchies and structures (Ellingson, 2005). The current U.S. medical system is neither natural nor neutral; it is the result of specific historical events, and it perpetuates a rigid hierarchy among health-care providers and between providers and patients (Ehrenreich & English, 1973; Foucault, 1973). Power in the medical establishment involves complex contemporary and historical intersections of race, gender, class, sexuality, educational level, and able-bodied privileges and oppressions (Wear, 1997). Historical inequities have engendered communication norms within health care that often serve neither patients nor health-care providers effectively. Such ineffectual norms persist despite important changes in health-care delivery and in the populations who are served.

In this chapter, I explore two macro-level trends in health care in order to demonstrate how they manifest themselves through mundane daily communication in a particular health-care setting. First, health-care communication norms developed based upon an acute care model and poorly serve health-care providers who face an ever-increasing need to manage ongoing treatment for people living with multiple chronic illnesses. Second, traditional professional disciplinary hierarchies and boundaries persist in the face of a changing workforce and enormous reliance on skilled but not formally educated paraprofessionals (e.g., technicians, nursing assistants) to provide the vast majority of hands-on patient care. By examining how these systemic trends play out on a micro level, this chapter proposes that the U.S. health-care system perpetuates a hegemonic power structure that makes superficial stylistic changes to adapt to consumer demands while reinscribing the norms of biomedical power.

The negotiation of power and expertise among collaborating health-care providers and between health-care providers and patients directly impacts the quality of patients' care. Moreover, this case study points to the central role of "unbounded" (i.e., brief, unscheduled, collaborative) communication as constitutive of medical work, countering the scholarly bias toward bounded physician–patient interactions (e.g., Atkinson, 1995; Ellingson, 2003, 2005). Hence this investigation of dialysis care functions as a microcosm for understanding the manifestation of communication and power in health-care delivery in the United States more broadly; simply put, dialysis is only the tip of the health-care iceberg. In scrutinizing the communicative norms of this space, I intend to promote dialogue and hopefully to inspire productive change.

I will explore power, knowledge, and communication surrounding these two health-care trends by using an outpatient dialysis unit as a case study. I will suggest that some of the difficulties in providing and receiving dialysis care are due in part to the inability and/or unwillingness of patients and health-care providers to adapt their communication and practice norms and expectations to keep pace with drastic changes in the health-care system and instead reinforce traditional hierarchies. Drawing upon Foucault's work on power, knowledge, and surveillance as a critical lens, I will explore dialysis care as an exemplar of how power manifests itself in daily, seemingly unremarkable communication in health care. Following a brief introduction to dialysis treatment, I will discuss two of Foucault's philosophical concepts as a framework for an interpretive study of a dialysis treatment unit. I then provide a description of my methodology. Next I explore patients and paraprofessionals in the daily world of dialysis care. Finally I offer several implications of this case study for patients and providers in dialysis, for health-care administrators and policy makers, and for further research.

Dialysis

The advent of dialysis treatment in the 1960s and its wide availability following the 1972 passage of the Medicare ESRD Program legislation by the U.S. Congress were heralded as a miracle that saved people from certain death due to end-stage renal disease (ESRD, i.e., kidney failure). More than 250,00 ESRD patients in the United States rely on outpatient treatment units that provide dialysis care to patients in a clinical setting (National Kidney and Urologic Diseases Information Clearinghouse (NKUDIC), 2003). Dialysis technology has improved dramatically over the last few decades. At the same time, the number of people suffering from diabetes and high blood pressure (the leading causes of ESRD) has skyrocketed, and dialysis is being made available to a much broader array of patients than previously (Beckett-Tharp & Schatell, 2001). Increasing the scope of care given to ill people is a laudable goal, of course, but there are some drawbacks. Dialysis care has become increasingly expensive, problematic (particularly with the growing nursing shortage), and in some cases, of questionable benefit (Moss, 2003).

Dialysis treats people with ESRD by using machines to filter the blood, removing excess fluid and waste materials. Dialysis treatment is life sustaining, but also a demanding process accompanied by strict monitoring of diet, fluid intake, and other lifestyle factors (NKUDIC, 2003). At best, dialysis replaces only 10 percent of normal kidney function; as a result, patients receiving dialysis have numerous health problems and complications (Loghman-Adham, 2003). Outpatient dialysis treatments typically occur three times per week, for three to four hours per session. Many high-functioning patients (often younger) are able to have dialysis at home and enjoy a high quality of life. In outpatient units, patients typically have co-morbidities (other illnesses and conditions), often are frail elderly, and may not have people available to help with home dialysis (NKUDIC, 2003). Treatment involves several steps: at each session, patients go through an initial review of current weight, blood pressure, and other standardized assessments with a patient care technician (PCT). Once those checks and the checks on the dialysis machine are complete, the PCT places the needle, the "fistula" (surgical graft that functions as an access site), and then starts the machine cycle. After monitoring the treatment, the patient's blood is returned, the needles are removed, either clamps or a patient's fingers are used to put pressure on the access site to encourage clotting, a final blood pressure measurement is taken, and patients weigh themselves to determine the amount of fluid removed. Patients are socialized to expect and accept routine violation of their bodies (Bevan, 2000); huge blocks of time are spent traveling to dialysis, waiting, undergoing dialysis, waiting to recover, traveling home, and resting in response to the fatigue engendered by dialysis (Kierans & Maynooth, 2001).

Direct care is administered by a nephrology care team including a nephrologist (M.D.), registered nurses, a registered dietitian, a clinical social worker, and the clinical nurse manager (Stoner, 1999). Nephrologists monitor patients but are not part of everyday dialysis care, instead seeing patients in office visits or during very brief rounds. Studies in dialysis have focused on communication between nurses and patients. Faber (2000) found that despite the lengthy treatment times, "very little social interaction occurred . . . between the people on dialysis and the health care practitioners" (p. 28). Perceptions of atmosphere in the dialysis unit varied significantly between patients and nurses (Vitri et al., 2001). Patients report difficulty dealing with some health-care practitioners (Faber, 2000), while nurses express frustration with trying to help noncompliant patients (Friedman, 2001). Mediation has been found to be an effective approach to resolving conflicts between nurse and patients (Johnstone et al., 1997), and at times, appropriate use of humor can assist in alleviating tension between nurses and patients (Leibovitz, 1998). Hines et al. explored communication between nephrologists and dialysis patients (which occurs primarily in office visits) regarding informed consent for treatment and the complexities of end-of-life decision making (e.g., Hines et al., 1997).

A limited amount of previous work has explored explicitly power within the renal nurse–dialysis patient relationship (see Bevan, 1998, 2000; Polaschek, 2003), but little has been done to articulate how power over patients is set within a larger hierarchy, that of the Western medical system, with its ever-increasing pool of paraprofessional health-care providers. With spiraling medical costs, more and more direct care is now delivered by low-status, low-paid workers with little education who operate sophisticated technology and equipment and bear the responsibility for patients' well-being, but whose judgment is not accepted by those who are culturally authorized as knowledge producers (i.e., administrators and physicians). Illuminating the naturalized power relations in which dialysis care is provided is central to critiquing health-care norms and to developing ways to improve health-care delivery for both recipients and providers through effective communicative practices (Giacchino et al., 2000).

Theoretical framework

Foucault articulated two elements of the manifestations of modern power that are useful in describing communication and knowledge production in the dialysis unit. First, Foucault suggests the inseparability and mutuality of power and knowledge:

> power produces knowledge . . . power and knowledge directly imply one another . . . there is no power relation without the correlative constitution of a field of knowledge, nor any knowledge that does not presuppose and constitute at the same time power relations.
>
> (Foucault, 1977, p. 27)

That power and knowledge are mutually productive is nowhere more apparent than in the contemporary U.S. medical establishment (e.g., Wear, 1997).

Second, Foucault argued that power is not something that a group has or holds, but instead a force that circulates in and among people. Thus, the power of the medical gaze is not embodied by physicians or other personnel, nor by the patients; instead, exaltation of the biomedical codes and standards is a discourse participated in by all parties and the structures within which they operate. Invoking the architectural figure of Bentham's panopticon, Foucault suggests that like prisoners who never know when they are being observed from a central observation post and hence internalize the gaze of the guards, citizens internalize social rules and restrictions (in this case, of biomedicine) and practice self-surveillance.

The efficiency of power, its constraining force have, in a sense, passed over to the other side—to the side of its surface of application. He [sic] who is subjected to a field of visibility, and who knows it, assumes responsibility for the constraints of power; he makes them play spontaneously upon himself; he inscribes in himself the power relation in which he simultaneously plays both roles; he becomes the principle of his own subjection. By this very fact, the external power may throw off its physical weight; it tends to the non-corporeal; and, the more it approaches this limit, the more constant, profound and permanent are its effects.

(Foucault, 1977, pp. 202–203)

Circulating throughout hospitals, clinics, and other medical settings, the constraining discourse of biomedical expertise no longer resides in an authoritarian, material physician body, but circulates among staff of a variety of disciplines and patients, internalized in the form of self-surveillance that relieves the physicians from the need to exert power directly, or even to represent the discourse of biomedicine. Instead, all participate in its circulation, whether by conformity or resistance, as both service to naturalize the norm.

Method

This case study is part of a larger ethnographic study of communication within an outpatient dialysis (Ellingson, in press). Western Valley Dialysis (a pseudonym) owns and operates fourteen units in the Western United States. I secured entry to one unit through the organization's director of social work services, with the consent of the unit's nurse manager. The unit employed about twenty-five people, including registered nurses, licensed vocational nurses, patient-care technicians (PCTs), technical aides (TAs), clinical social worker, registered dietitian, head technician, unit secretary, and nurse manager, with per diem nurses and PCTs augmenting the staff. The dialysis unit operated from 6:30am to roughly 6:30pm, with three staggered shifts of three hours each, plus time for patient turnover. The facility had one isolation unit; the other twenty-four chairs were arranged around the perimeter of an open room, with a nurses' station in the middle.

Data collection

I engaged in participant observation for two to three hours per session, approximately twice per week, from October 2003 to June 2004, culminating in over 100 hours of observation. I adopted the observer-as-participant role (Lindolf & Taylor, 2002). That is, both staff and patients were aware of my identity as a researcher, and I observed and conversed with patients and staff, while assisting in minor tasks (e.g., lowering patients' recliner position). When time permitted, I asked staff members questions in informal interviews. While in the treatment room, I took notes and transcribed brief conversations on a palmtop computer; these notes were expanded into fieldnotes, for a total of 191 single-spaced, typed pages. From June to August 2004, I conducted semi-structured interviews with seventeen staff members. Interviews were audio-recorded and transcribed, yielding 226 single-spaced, typed pages of transcription. Next, I recruited twenty patients to participate in a structured oral questionnaire on perceptions of staff communication. Questions and responses were transcribed, totaling sixty-eight typed pages.

As a feminist ethnographer, I was highly cognizant during my fieldwork of power—who had it, how they got it, how it was invoked and resisted, what it did, how it was revealed and obscured in discourse, and how I, as a researcher, both participated in and resisted it (see Ellingson, 2005; Reinharz, 1992). Documenting evidence of power intersecting with knowledge and communication practices in my fieldnotes was a conscious and deliberate choice. Research on health communication and readings in critical theory guided my sense of what power dynamics formed the context for outpatient health-care delivery, and my case study analysis of fieldnotes, interviews, and organizational documents from the dialysis unit focused on describing micro practices of communication through which power was manifested.

Power in the dialysis unit

Despite the advent of dramatic changes such as the prevalence of managed care organizations and recent trends toward a more consumerist mindset on the part of some patients, physicians remain highly respected, well paid (albeit less so than before managed care), and very powerful both within health-care organizations and society at large (e.g., Frank, 2004). Physician knowledge is the most prestigious form of biomedical expertise; other medical staff enjoy less credibility as knowledge producers, and patients are positioned as recipients of knowledge only. Of nonphysician health-care professionals, those closest to a physician role (physician assistants and nurse practitioners) typically occupy higher levels on the hierarchy, while those dealing with nurturing and less biomedical care-giving tasks, such as clinical social workers, and those providing hands-on care of patients' bodies (e.g., nursing assistants) occupy the lowest rungs of power (Wear, 1997). Patients are widely regarded by health-care professionals as unreliable sources of information and poor judgment (Polaschek, 2003). This hierarchical medical system context is not merely the background in which the dialysis staff and patients communicated; on the contrary, the present (and historic) conditions of the medical system greatly influenced the communicative processes and were enacted through language in dialysis staff members' daily communication with each other (Barge &

Kenton, 1994). Thus professional discipline, patient status, and other factors significantly impacted how knowledge was (and was not) constructed, acknowledged, and acted upon.

Patients

Despite some critique (e.g., Thorne, 1990), communication between dialysis providers and patients emphasizes health-care provider's knowledge and expertise while reinforcing patient's passive role. In an acute care model where illness is a crisis that interrupts normal life with a significant, even life-threatening problem, patients' respectful cooperation and compliance with physicians' orders appears a logical, reasonable expectation. After all, the physician is the one with the necessary knowledge for addressing a heart attack or other serious illness. However, with advances in technology, patients now survive what used to be acute illnesses that in the past were either cured or terminal. Now, the majority of patients need ongoing management for noncurative but treatable chronic illnesses (Charmaz, 1991). The expectations of unquestioning compliance with physicians' orders are no longer (if they ever were) appropriate or reasonable. Yet, the subtext of communication in health-care delivery retains the very real, if more indirectly expressed, expectation that patients should not question, disobey, or negotiate with health-care providers. Patient self-reports of behavior are viewed with suspicion and often hold little credibility for health-care providers, particularly when such reports appear to conflict with medical evidence such as test results (Polaschek, 2003).

Certain historical factors led to the expectation of compliant, successful dialysis patients. Because early studies of dialysis' effectiveness were highly selective of candidates for dialysis, otherwise healthy ESRD patients enjoyed extremely high success rates. With wider availability of the technology and legislation that guaranteed federal funding for dialysis, criteria for candidacy was changed radically, allowing people with many other chronic illnesses and the very old to receive dialysis (Bevan, 2000). Because such patients would have previously been excluded from the selective patient pool, their inclusion has led to much lower rates of success with patient outcomes. Yet, this early success led to the institutionalization of a perception of normative success that remains firmly in place, despite the fact that with present population of dialysis patients, it is unrealistic to maintain this supposed "norm." Currently,

whilst the individual should not be held to account for the limitations of dialysis and its fabricated life, more often than not this may be the case. The individual can be held responsible because the individual is an extraneous variable, an uncontrollable element . . . To view the individual as a whole requires the individual to be open with nursing or medical staff . . . this openness is the very crux of the control of the dialysis patient. Every nook and cranny is explored by the nurse, doctor and associates, to expose any frailties that may provide a basis for the failure of the [dialysis] experiment.

(Bevan, 2000, p. 440)

Dialysis patients are subject to relentless surveillance in the form of the biomedical gaze. Dialysis patients are positioned as objects to be scrutinized by the medical gaze; they are not viewed as knowledge producers or even as necessarily capable of receiving knowledge. The patient is "one who is seen but does not see, he is an object of information, never a subject of communication" (Foucault, 1977, p. 200). The gaze manifests itself in medical personnel, blood and urine tests, and the scale (patients are weighed before and after each dialysis treatment). Patients who are perceived of as failing to conform to the rigid, complex, and demanding regimens for diet, fluid intake, and medications that accompany dialysis treatment are labeled noncompliant. Noncompliance encompasses a range of biomedically undesirable behaviors such as being late for or skipping dialysis treatments, gaining too much weight between treatments, elevated blood levels of certain minerals, omitting doses of prescribed medications, illicit drug use, and significant failure to follow dietary and fluid restrictions (Friedman, 2001). In addition, behaving in a physically or verbally hostile manner to staff also is often included in definitions of noncompliance. While not an official policy, it is nonetheless well documented that patients who are perceived of as compliant and suffering from circumstances beyond their control often are given preferential treatment by healthcare providers (e.g., Morgan-Witte, 2005).

Issues of power, knowledge, and compliance were prevalent in daily interactions within the dialysis unit. One well-loved patient was a handsome 80-year-old man, Mr. Mitchell, who was an avid gardener, drove himself to his dialysis treatments (which was unusual among the unit's patients), and diligently followed medical regimens and dietary restrictions with good humor. Staff members frequently engaged in small talk with the patient, whom they all addressed informally using his nickname. One day when the dietitian came to speak to him about his monthly blood test results, she tugged up his pant leg to take a look and revealed a deep laceration with thick scabs. Mr. Mitchell and the dietitian discussed the wound, which had resulted from calcium and phosphorus build up in his leg, but through no fault of his own. She gently asked how bad the pain was, and he replied, "Severe. I don't mean to be asking for sympathy, but it is bad. I need pain medication and it is still really bad at times; it really hurts." The dietitian nodded sympathetically, expressed her concern for him, and then gave him some news about a new medication about to receive FDA approval for which she had been promised early sample doses to give to him. She was making every effort to help her patient, who was suffering despite ample evidence of his compliance with his recommended regimen.

However, many patients refuse to submit as "docile bodies" to the surveillance of the dialysis staff. Consider the example of a relatively young (mid-
40s) male patient who was not well liked by the dialysis staff. Mr. Ortega was
a double-amputee, a sad-looking man whose body was ravaged by a deadly
combination of poorly regulated diabetes, erratic dialysis treatment, and illicit
drug abuse. His appearance was unkempt, and he frustrated staff since he would
not perform the niceties of small talk in which most patients engaged. Mr.
Ortega was noncompliant with his regimen to the extent that the unit had a
policy of not setting up his dialysis machine in advance of his arrival because
he skipped treatments a lot, and the wasted supplies used to prepare the
machine were not reimbursable from Medicaid. Mr. Ortega died during my
fieldwork, and the note in the unit's communication (log) book simply stated
that the patient had "expired" and noted the date. When I inquired about the
terse description, the social worker explained that Mr. Ortega went to the
hospital after his last dialysis treatment, where he was found to be overloaded
with fluid and his diabetes and blood pressure out of control. The emergency
room staff treated and released him, and his sister took him to her home,
where he died suddenly. The dialysis unit was not informed as to the exact
cause of his death. The social worker added with resignation, "He has been a
frustrating patient all along." The staff's tepid reaction to Mr. Ortega's
"expiration" contrasted sharply to their verbal and nonverbal emotional
expressions of grief over the death of other, more pleasant and compliant
patients.

Patients' choices to not comply with medical advice directly affect staff
members: "Coping with the stress inducted by ESRD patient noncompliance
is a time consuming, nonproductive, demoralizing undertaking that is unavoidable" and "disrupts unit function and frustrates well-meaning staff" (Friedman,
2001, pp. 23–24). For example, patients regularly arrived for treatment
overloaded with fluid due to excessive intake, and they needed longer
treatments to remove the fluid. Many times lengthening treatment time for a
patient was difficult or impossible, since a precise schedule of patients often had
to be maintained for each machine to enable all patients to receive their
required treatments during the facility's operating hours. Other patients
frequently and vigorously complained about symptoms but resisted staff
members' suggestions on how to improve those symptoms through changes in
their diet or fluid intake. Staff members in the dialysis unit frequently expressed
frustration with patients' choices.

Adding further complexity to this discussion of compliance is the myth that
compliant patients will necessarily be healthier than noncompliant dialysis
patients. Research clearly documents that following the prescribed regimens
often does *not* correlate with successful outcomes for dialysis patients. That is,
the patients can do precisely as they are instructed in regards to activity level,
diet, fluid intake, medication dosage, and dialysis treatment, and still face
declining health, complications, and poor quality of life (Polaschek, 2003;

Sensky et al., 1996). Yet because health-care providers enjoy significantly more power and authority than patients (e.g., Opie, 1998), discussions of patients' noncompliance in the renal literature are "almost always according to the professional premise of its 'irrationality' from health care providers' point of view (Polaschek, 2003, p. 358). But patients also have legitimate perspectives that need to be acknowledged and respected. Not complying with extremely limiting, frustrating, and often unpleasant regimens may make more sense when one considers patients' quality of life; it seems reasonable for health-care providers to accept thoughtfully chosen variations in patients' regimen's when they constitute a "covert caring for the self," a way of negotiating daily life with symptoms of chronic illnesses that the medical profession often cannot adequately address (Ellingson, 2004; Lindsay, 1997).

Patient care technicians

PCTs, who spend the most time with dialysis patients of any health-care providers, are also mired in outdated expectations and power systems in which they both participate and practice resistance. Antiquated system of medicine assumes all knowledge is held and created by physicians, that nurses simply carry out physicians' orders, and that PCTs perform purely technical tasks to keep machines operating. These historical arrangements led to power dynamics that do not function well anymore, if they ever did. The privileging of physicians' biomedical expertise remains characteristic of the U.S. medical system, and physicians' knowledge claims carry more weight in decision making than those of other (historically femininized) disciplines (e.g., nursing) (Ellingson, 2005). The medical establishment, like all bureaucracies, obscures its socially constructed nature, making it appear natural, inevitable, and normal; it produces standards for evaluation and then justifies itself according to those standards (Foucault, 1975). Such systems privilege particular groups (and their values, language, and modes of behavior) over others, while obscuring that privilege as inevitable and normative. Multidisciplinary care teams—such as those in dialysis—are intended to promote more egalitarian interactions among health-care providers; however, they generally maintain professional hierarchies far more than they subvert them (Ellingson, 2005; Opie, 2000).

Stein's (1967) classic rendering of the "doctor-nurse game" depicted dominating doctors to whom nurses made diagnostic and treatment recommendations in a submissive manner, such that the recommendation appeared to have been initiated by the physician. This pervasive pattern served to reinforce the existing hierarchy that framed nurses as "handmaidens" to physicians (Prescott & Bowen, 1985). The fact that nursing still is overwhelmingly female and medicine was almost exclusively a male province until the last twenty-five years reinforced this dynamic. The addition of more female physicians has not brought about rapid change in the nurse–physician relationship (e.g., Wear, 1997). What has changed is the role of nurses shifting from direct care providers to often supervising numerous paraprofessionals who provide most of the direct care. PCTs do much of what used to be done by nurses before that became economically unfeasible (Polaschek, 2003). Advances in biomedical technology both make the trend toward paraprofessionals providing care to patients possible (even necessary), and at the same time makes it conceptually aberrant within the traditional hierarchy and philosophical underpinnings of U.S. health care. PCTs are required to have either a high school diploma or an equivalency. Although the details vary by state, ten weeks of training in classroom, a licensing exam, and on the job training are typical requirements. According to the National Kidney Foundation, a patient care technician is the "primary direct care giver" for dialysis patients and works with registered nurses "as an important member of the patient care team" (www.kidney.org).

Unlike most other forms of invasive, life-sustaining medical treatment, routine outpatient dialysis care does not directly involve physicians, who see and evaluate patients monthly outside of the clinic but are present in the dialysis unit only for periodic, very brief (less than a minute per patient) clinical rounds. In extensive fieldwork, I encountered only three physicians, and they were present in the unit for less than 10 minutes each. The dialysis unit managers are virtually always nurses or nurse practitioners, and a charge nurse runs each shift. Physicians are medical directors of the unit, but they exert that control via periodic meetings, never by actually engaging in the management of the unit or the provision of dialysis treatment. Their absence was most notable by the changes that occurred during their rare appearances: physicians were addressed formally as "Doctor" while everyone else was addressed by first name only; all staff deferred to physicians physically by making room at counters, offering seats, and moving aside to allow physicians to pass; any requests from physicians were immediately addressed; and banter among staff all but disappeared while the physician was present. Staff members' verbal and nonverbal communication reflected an intent to seem more business-like, efficient, and serious. While no staff expressed fear of physicians or indicated anxiety about their visits, staff nonetheless were quieter than normal and behaved submissively toward physicians.

Because physicians are not present to gather information on their patients first hand, PCTs act as an intermediary between professionals—physicians and to a lesser extent nurses—and those over whom the professionals are supposed to be most knowledgeable. This reflects a partial decoupling of expertise and knowledge from authority: "technicians did much more than produce data: they buffered the professionals who used the data from the very empirical phenomena over which the latter were reputed to have mastery" (Barley, 1996, p. 420).

Yet despite their physical absence, nephrology physicians' presence is inscribed throughout the unit via discourses of power that circulate among the dialysis staff and patients. Physicians give orders, monitor outcomes, and receive a steady flow of detailed information on each of their patients and, by implication, the performance of the nurses and technicians who care for those patients. Statements such as "I'll ask the doctor," "I don't have doctor's orders on that," "I've left a message with the doctor about the problem," and "When did you last see your doctor?" were constant in the dialysis unit. Physicians also functioned as medical directors of the organization, and were referred to indirectly but frequently as "management" in terms of policies and procedures. More generally, biomedical knowledge and perspectives dominated the communication climate in the organization (Geist-Martin et al., 2003). Despite sincere efforts by staff to treat patients holistically and humanely, communication in the unit largely concerned results of blood, urine, and other medical tests, functioning of dialysis machinery, accessibility of fistulas, medication regimens, physical assessment of patients (e.g., temperature, blood pressure), and treatment requirements, all of which reflected highly technological approaches to medicine.

Despite their clear differentiation from the knowledgeable physicians and nurses, PCTs are told repeatedly that it is their duty to be professionals. For instance, the training manual used at Western Valley Dialysis (produced by a pharmaceutical company and widely used nationally) establishes early on the importance of presenting a professional demeanor.

> One of the most important skills to learn is how to behave in a *professional* manner. Professionalism is hard to define, and thus hard to teach. It comes from within, and can be thought of, in part, as the desire to behave in a manner that carries a core value of compassion, as well as skill and competency in technical procedures. . . . Remember that knowledge is power, and power is confidence. It takes time and discipline to acquire the knowledge you will need, but the rewards will be shown in many ways. Knowledge can be seen in the positive outcomes of patients, and felt as the result of your discipline and commitment.
>
> (Beckett-Tharp & Schatell, 2001, Module 1, p. 18)

In addition, the manual described a number of behaviors from which PCTS must abstain such as getting "too close" emotionally to patients and using profanity or telling crude jokes, abstinence from which was considered integral to professionalism. In my interview with the training coordinator for the organization, she stressed the importance of instilling a sense of professionalism in the PCTs; her comments largely equated professionalism with a sense of responsibility for patient welfare, of taking seriously the need to care for them properly, efficiently, and with a pleasant demeanor.

The language of professionalism was used regularly in daily communication within the unit to reprimand PCTs for undesirable behavior. For example, a note in the unit's communication book from the nurse manager criticized several PCTs about behaving "unprofessionally"—leering, joking, and making inappropriate comments of sexual nature—when an attractive and provocatively dressed young woman arrived to pick up her grandmother. Likewise, teamwork was linked to professionalism when the nurse manager reprimanded some PCTs for sitting and/or chatting while others worked; she said it was unprofessional to be relaxing when others were working hard either to care for patients or to prepare materials for incoming patients. PCTs echoed the same language in our interviews: "I try to communicate professionally, but I don't want to be looking like an uptight [person] so I try to mix up the professionalism with, you know, being a friend."

In addition, PCTs were marked as nonprofessionals through many elements of daily practice. PCTs' working conditions treat them as tightly controlled, not even semi-autonomous service employees. The nurse manager explained her supervisory role to me by saying that "part of my job is being their mother." She and the charge nurses regularly (usually quite gently) scolded PCTs who were not pitching in to help others (Ellingson, in press), urged them to adhere to unit schedules as precisely as possible, and reminded them not to waste supplies. For example, one day as a group of PCTs were having a social discussion, the nurse manager approached them, smiled, and said with mild sarcasm, "I hate to break up the party, but. . . ." Also, regulations limit the sphere of PCTs' practice, requiring them to ask nurses for assistance on many tasks, including accessing catheters for patients who did not have fistulas, administering medications, etc. Moreover, PCTs were not allowed to call physicians when problems arose, but reported them to nurses who then contacted a physician if necessary. I am not arguing that such practice restrictions are necessarily inappropriate, only that the constant need for PCTs to request assistance communicated their lower position in the unit.

PCTs also had many organizational reminders of their low status as well. For instance, they were given "Western Valley Bucks" that they could save up and redeem for a variety of items in a company catalogue (like green stamps) as rewards for completing perfect time sheets and performing other basic tasks; it is hard to imagine physicians being patronized in such a manner. The reward system did not appreciably add to PCTs' standard of living and being rewarded with tokens for good behavior was definitely not a mark of professionalism. Accountability requirements were another way in which they were not treated as professionals: if PCTs wanted to swap assigned shifts among themselves, they had to complete and sign a form that had to be given to the nurse manager well ahead of the date involved, rather than being trusted to negotiate such changes independently. Like many service workers, several of the PCTs moonlighted at other local dialysis units in order to make more money, a trend perhaps more pronounced given the very high cost of living in the area in which the unit was located. I, too, was complicit as an ethnographer in marking them as nonprofessionals of low status; while I treated them warmly and respectfully and always answered their questions, I did not require or seek their permission for my fieldwork. The nurse manager gave it on their behalf (although interviews were voluntary), and neither the management nor I gave them an authentic opportunity to object to my presence, an opportunity that physicians surely would have been granted.

Moreover, PCTs clearly were not considered knowledge producers within the organization. Health-care organizations typically exclude PCTs from formal definitions (and meetings of) the care team (Stoner, 1999). Western Valley Dialysis disenfranchised its PCTs by not allowing them to attend patient-care team meetings, monthly meetings to which every other discipline is invited: management, nursing, social work, nutrition, and medicine. When the voice of the PCTs is left out of discussions of patient care, vital insights may be omitted in the pool of patient information, and opportunities for improved quality of care missed. In addition, researchers produce little knowledge about PCTs, who are all but absent from the nephrology literature. Since the powerful generate knowledge, research on communication in dialysis focuses on physicians and nurses. The scarcity of work that takes seriously the role of the PCT in patients' care reflects their low status in the field (for studies of paraprofessionals, albeit unrelated to dialysis, see Anderson et al., 2005; Colon-Emeric et al., 2006).

Technicians in many organizations do have expertise; they lack disciplinary prestige and educational attainment, but possess a great deal of contextual, hands-on knowledge of processes, equipment, and patients (Barley, 1996). An underclass of technicians has emerged that occupies a paradoxical organizational position: they are experts in operating and maintaining technologically sophisticated machinery and are responsible for performing risky procedures on which patients' lives depend, but hold no authority. Physicians are experts but few of them could operate a dialysis machine properly; the technology changes often, and PCTs often had the most knowledge of the machines, the quirks of patients' fistulas, and other idiosyncrasies of patient care. PCTs claim their expertise, explaining in our interviews that "you have to know patient habits . . . especially know their accesses" and "you know your people, you know how they react—their bodies—you can see your patients' bodies and how much fluid they can handle . . . you just know the look on their face." A PCT articulated PCTs' proficiency with the clinical gaze and asserted that they actually saw more than the nephrologists: "The only thing [doctors] look at is lab [reports]. That's it. They're not in here looking, they're not in here twelve hours a day . . . We're the ones watching them." PCTs expressed frustration when physicians did not take their advice seriously. For example, a PCT noticed a problem with a patient's fistula and asked the nurse to report it to the physician. The physician replied that the problem was not severe and could wait until the patient's next scheduled appointment. The PCT then had to struggle to complete the patient's treatment, which required frequent fiddling with the access and resetting of the machine. Technicians describe themselves as experts at what they do (Curtis, 1996), and I certainly concur with their judgment of their value. Their place in the organizational hierarchy, however, remained firmly at the bottom.

Despite their resistance to its constraints, PCTs also co-opted physician power to deal with conflicts with patients or pass on troublesome problems to nurses, social worker, dietitian, or the nurse manager. Strategic essentialism is the use of stereotypes of a group (in this case PCTs) in order to achieve a goal (Spivak, 1988). PCTs both resisted the medical gaze directed at them, but also co-opted that same gaze in order to assert control over patients by denying their own ability to resist physicians' orders. This enabled them to diffuse confrontations with patients by aligning themselves with the patients as powerless in the face of the absent but all-knowing and controlling physicians. For example, a PCT I will call Tim was asked by his patient, Mrs. Albright, to increase the amount of weight removed during her treatment one day. Although she did not explain why, her motivation was a misguided attempt to lose weight. Tim looked at her blankly and turned to check the display screen of her dialysis machine to ensure that it accurately reflected the prescribed amount. Seeing that it was correct, he told her he could not make that change without a physician's order. The patient continued to argue with him, and Tim brought in a nurse to handle the conflict. The nurse repeated the same thing that the PCT had said—that they were not authorized to make a change without a physician's prescription—and promised to call and leave a message for her physician. The patient continued to insist that the physician had given her permission, but both the PCT and the nurse repeated their explanation. In this way, the PCT and nurse claim powerlessness to solve the patient's complaint, since that was much easier than persuading her that dialysis is not the weight loss method the patient perceived it to be. In addition, they reduce antagonism (or at least try to) but disavowing any responsibility for the failure to do as the patient requested. Hence, the PCT's ability to accomplish his goal may be an act of power and control, but it also further entrenches the discourse of physician power and delegitimizes his own expertise.

Thus, PCTs face complex power and knowledge relations that do not fit static norms for reinforcing hierarchy. Thus far, the ambiguity has not led to significant changes in hierarchical communication among dialysis care providers.

Implications

Using a dialysis unit as a case study, I have explored some of the ways in which the U.S. health-care system remains entrenched in hierarchies that directly impact communication within a dialysis unit. The pitfalls of hierarchical notions of patient "compliance" and the limitations imposed by organizational marginalization of PCTs both suggest that new models of the relationships among medical technology, professional expertise, patient autonomy, and communication are needed. Despite changes in patient needs and the types of health-care providers meeting those needs, communication remains locked within repressive cycles that reinforce hierarchy of providers over patients and professionals over paraprofessionals. New models should acknowledges different kinds of expertise and de-center physicians from our theorizing to be inclusive of both patients and a broad range of health-care workers (see Opie, 2000). While it may not be realistic that hierarchies will be abolished any time soon (see Ellingson, 2005), casting a critical eye upon taken-for-granted power relations is a necessary first step toward promoting awareness and inspiring change.

Of course, challenging assumptions of power tends to generate enormous resistance, even from well-meaning people and those who are disenfranchised by the system. As a health communication ethnographer and a cancer survivor, I am well schooled in the self-justifying logic of the medical system. Proposed changes—or even just questioning why things are the way they are—sound impractical, even impossible, because we are so well trained in the system (Foucault, 1977). We can think easily of how chaos would ensue if PCTs were paid more, physicians were required to collaborate more directly with paraprofessionals, or nurses were given sufficient time in their schedules to engage PCTs in informal case-based education in the midst of providing patient care. Steeped in the biomedical model, we can immediately object to such far-fetched ideas—they are too expensive, no one would support them, this would be impractical to implement with the current nursing shortage. Financial and other constraints do exist and must be addressed, of course. However, some imagination is also called for. Health communication scholars' thinking too often reflects the logic of biomedicine and fails to push its boundaries. If we cannot even question the taken-for-granted assumptions of the system, we limit our ability to formulate alternatives. Open dialogue is needed that does not begin with the assumption that disciplinary hierarchies are natural and inevitable. In addition to my call for more dialogue among health communication scholars, I offer several specific suggestions for dialysis practice.

First, we must move beyond paying lip service to the idea of patients as members of the care team. Given the extent of chronically ill patients who require illness management rather than curing, new models of communicating expertise and conflicting goals between health-care providers and patients are needed that do not merely label patients as "noncompliant" (Friedman, 2001) or "nonadherent" (Lundin, 1995), as were the patients in the dialysis unit studied. Such labels reinforce the power of health-care providers by indicating that health-care providers rightfully have the knowledge and the power to give orders to patients, whose only acceptable choice is compliance. Some researchers have sought more positive, patient-centered models, such as "constructive noncompliance" (Thorne, 1990) and "negotiated care" (Polaschek, 2003). Changing labels will not be enough to change the power dynamics, but they could be an effective communication tool that brings those persistent (yet often ignored or trivialized) ways of reinforcing power into a more prominent level of awareness.

One way to move past compliance and toward partnership is for units to make every effort to invite and facilitate the attendance of patients at their periodic case review conferences with their interdisciplinary care team. Patients' voices are essential to decision making (Opie, 1998). By being welcomed into the meetings, patients may take more ownership and responsibility for their own choices and decision making regarding their treatments, diet, etc. Open discussions of treatment, lifestyle restrictions, and patients' needs and desires could take place, and ideally negotiation could result in more realistic standards for compliance and hence better patient satisfaction and perhaps better clinical outcomes.

Second, representatives of the unit's PCTs should also attend patient case review conferences as members of the interdisciplinary care team. Participation in patient care conferences with professionals can help PCTs learn about clinical reasoning while also helping to establish relationships between PCTs and professionals, relationships that could improve subsequent collaboration about patients. Professionals can also gain important insights into individual patients by hearing about PCTs' daily experiences with caring directly for patients.

Third, organizational efforts should be made to foster open and regular interactions among PCTs, nurses, physicians, and other staff. Research on certified nursing assistants in nursing homes who, like PCTs, deliver most frontline care while supervised by registered nurses, revealed a lack of communication channels between professionals and nursing assistants (Anderson et al., 2005). In dialysis units, nurses to whom PCTs bring patient problems could return to the PCTs and briefly explain how they addressed the problem, and what factors led to their (and/or the physicians') decision. Such informal educational practices could gradually increase PCTs' ability to contribute to patients' care. Physicians doing Medicare-mandated monthly rounds could set aside several minutes to discuss a selected patient with a PCT or two and receive information from the PCT on machine functioning or other technical topics. Such informal interactions could help increase shared knowledge and improve relationships.

Finally, the scholarly bias toward studying the "important" health-care providers (those with high levels of education and status) must be corrected. Of course we need research on how physicians and nurses communicate with patients. But since PCTs spend many magnitudes more time with patients than these professionals, health communication scholars must critically attend to the roles and communication practices of paraprofessionals such as PCTs. Health communication scholars could partner with the National Association of Nephrology Technicians, the National Kidney Foundation, or some of the

nursing and medical associations within the field of nephrology to conduct research on PCTs and their interactions with patients and other staff.
Of course, the ideas presented herein are based on case-study methodology that focused in-depth on a single dialysis unit. Nonetheless, this investigation points to the persistence of hierarchy and its influences on day-to-day communication. Raising awareness of how structural inequalities are continually reinforced as normative is a good first step toward change.

References

Anderson, R.A., Ammarell, N., Bailey, Jr., D., Colon-Emeric, C., Corazzini, K.N., Lillie, M. et al. (2005). Nurse assistant mental models, sensemaking, care actions, and consequences for nursing home residents. *Qualitative Health Research*, 15, 1006–1021.

Atkinson, P. (1995). *Medical Talk and Medical Work*. Thousand Oaks, CA: Sage.

Barge, J.K., & Keyton, J. (1994). Contextualizing power and social influence in groups. In L.R. Frey (ed.), *Group communication in Context: Studies of Natural Groups*. Hillsdale, NJ: Lawrence Erlbaum Associates, pp. 85–106.

Barley, S.R. (1996). Technicians in the workplace: Ethnographic evidence for bringing work into organization studies. *Administrative Science Quarterly*, 41, 404–441.

Beckett-Tharp, D., & Schatell, D. (2001). Today's dialysis environment: An overview. In C. Latham, & J. Curtis (eds), *Core Curriculum for the Dialysis Technician*, 2nd edn, Amgen, Inc, Module I, pp. 1–26.

Bevan, M.T. (1998). Nursing in the dialysis unit: Technological enframing and a declining art, or an imperative for caring. *Journal of Advanced Nursing*, 27, 730–736.

Bevan, M.T. (2000). Dialysis as "*deus ex machina*": A critical analysis of haemodialysis. *Journal of Advanced Nursing*, 31, 437–443.

Charmaz, K. (1991). *Good Days, Bad Days: The Self in Chronic Illness and Time*. New Brunswick, NJ: Rutgers University Press.

Colon-Emeric, C.S., Ammarell, N., Bailey, D., Corazzini, K., Lekan-Rutledge, D., Piven, M.L., et al. (2006). Patterns of medical and nursing staff communication in nursing homes: Implications and insights from complexity science. *Qualitative Health Research*, 16, 173–188.

Curtis, J. (1996). Technicians in the renal care environment; Part II: A model for the patient care technician. *Nephrology News & Issues*, 10(8), 34–35.

Ehrenreich, B., & English, D. (1973). *Witches, Midwives, and Nurses: A History of Women Healers*. New York: Feminist Press.

Ellingson, L.L. (2003). Interdisciplinary health care teamwork in the clinic backstage. *Journal of Applied Communication Research*, 31, 93–117.

Ellingson, L.L. (2004). Women cancer survivors: Making meaning of chronic illness and alternative medical practices. In P.M. Buzzanell, H. Sterk, & L. Turner (eds), *Gender in Applied Communication Research*. Thousand Oaks, CA: Sage, pp. 79–98.

Ellingson, L.L. (2005). *Communicating in the Clinic: Negotiating Frontstage and Backstage Teamwork*. Cresskill, NJ: Hampton Press.

Ellingson, L.L. (in press). The performance of dialysis care: Routinization and adaptation on the floor. *Health Communication*.

Faber, S. (2000). An investigation of life with end stage renal disease: Sociocultural case studies analysis. *CANNT (Canadian Association of Nephrology Nurses and Technologists) Journal*, 10(3), 24–34.

Foucault, M. (1973). *The Birth of the Clinic: An Archaeology of Medical Perception* (A.M.S. Smith trans.). New York: Vintage Books.

Foucault, M. (1975), *Discipline and Punish: The Birth of the Prison* (A. Sheridan trans.). New York: Vintage Books.

Foucault, M. (1977). Nietzsche, genealogy, history (D. Bouchard & S. Simon trans.). In L.E. Cahoone (ed.), *From Modernism to Postmodernism: An Anthology*. Cambridge, MA: Blackwell, pp. 360–381.

Frank, A.W. (2004). *The Renewal of Generosity: Illness, Medicine, and How to Live*. Chicago: University of Chicago Press.

Friedman, E.A. (2001). Must we treat noncompliant ESRD patients? *Seminars in Dialysis*, 14, 23–27.

Geist-Martin, P., Ray, E.B., & Sharf, B.F. (2003). *Communicating health: Personal, Cultural, and Political Complexities*. Belmont, CA: Wadsworth.

Giacchino, F., Manzato, A., De Piccoli, N., & Ponzetti, C. (2000). Patient's needs in substitutive dialysis treatment: Some psychosocial and organizational considerations. *Panminerva Medica*, 42, 207–201.

Hines, S.C., Babrow, A. S., Badzek, L., & Moss, A.H. (1997). Communication and problematic integration theory in end-of-life decisions: Dialysis decisions among the elderly. *Health Communication*, 9, 199–217.

Johnstone, S., Seamon, V.J., Halshaw, D., Molinari, J., & Longknife, K. (1997). The use of mediation to manage patient–staff conflict in the dialysis clinic. *Advances in Renal Replacement Therapy*, 4, 359–371.

Kierans, C.M., & Maynooth, N.U.I. (2001). Sensory and narrative identity: The narration of illness process among chronic renal sufferers in Ireland. *Anthropology & Medicine*, 8, 237–253.

Leibovitz, Z. (1998). Humour and dialysis. *EDTNA/ERCA Journal*, 24(4), 17–18.

Lindlof, T.R., & Taylor, B.C. (2002). *Qualitative Communication Research Methods*. 2nd edn. Thousand Oaks, CA: Sage.

Lindsay, E. (1997). Experiences of the chronically ill: A covert caring for the self. *Journal of Holistic Nursing*, 15, 227–242.

Loghman-Adham, M. (2003). Medication noncompliance in patients with chronic disease: Issues in dialysis and renal transplantation. *American Journal of Managed Care*, 9, 155–171.

Lundin, A.P. (1995). Causes of non-compliance in dialysis patients. *Dialysis and Transplantation*, 24, 176 & 202.

Morgan-Witte, J. (2005). Narrative knowledge development among caregivers: Stories from the nurses' station. In L.M. Harter, P.M. Japp., & C.S. Beck (eds), *Narratives, Health, and Healing: Communication Theory, Research, and Practice*. Mahwah, NJ: Lawrence Erlbaum, pp. 217–236.

Moss, A.H. (2003). Too many patients who are too sick to benefit start chronic dialysis: Nephrologists need to learn to "just say no." *American Journal of Kidney Disease*, 41, 723–732.

National Kidney and Urologic Diseases Information Clearinghouse. (2003). Kidney failure: Choosing a treatment that's right for you. NIH Publication No. 03-2412.

Retrieved October 28 from http://kidney.niddk.nih.gov/kudiseases/pubs/choosing treatment/.

Opie, A. (1998). "Nobody's asked me for my view": Users' empowerment by multidisciplinary health teams. *Qualitative Health Research, 8*, 188–206.

Opie, A. (2000). *Thinking Teams/Thinking Clients: Knowledge-based Teamwork*. NY: Columbia University Press.

Polaschek, N. (2003). Negotiated care: A model for nursing work in the renal setting. *Journal of Advanced Nursing, 42*, 355–363.

Prescott, P.A., & Bowen, S.A. (1985). Physician-nurse relationships. *Annals of Internal Medicine, 103*, 127–133.

Reinharz, S. (1992). *Feminist Methods in Social Research*. New York: Oxford University Press.

Sensky, T., Leger, C., & Gilmour, S. (1996). Psychosocial and cognitive factors associated with adherence to dietary and fluid restriction regimens by people on chronic dialysis. *Psychotherapy and Psychosomatics, 65*, 36–42.

Spivak, G.C. (1988). Can the subaltern speak? In C. Nelson, & L. Grossberg (eds), *Marxism and the Interpretation of Culture*. London: Macmillan, pp. 271–313.

Stein, L.I. (1967). The doctor–nurse game. *Archives of General Psychiatry, 16*, 699–703.

Stoner, M.H. (1999). The hemodialysis team. In C.F. Gutch, M.H. Stoner, & A.L. Corea (eds), *Review of Hemodialysis for Nurses and Dialysis Personnel*. St. Louis, MO: Mosby, pp. 1–9.

Thorne, S.E. (1990). Constructive noncompliance in chronic illness. *Holistic Nursing Practice, 5*, 62–69.

Vitri, N., Attlas, M., Elharrat, K., & Hener, T. (2001). The social climate in chronic haemodialysis units. *EDTNA/ERCA Journal, 27*, 178–180.

Wear, D. (1997). *Privilege in the Medical Academy: A Feminist Examines Gender, Race, and Power*. New York: Teachers College Press.

Chapter 14

Changing lanes and changing lives

The *shifting scenes* and *continuity* of care of a mobile health clinic

Lynn M. Harter, Karen Deardorff, Pamela Kenniston, Heather Carmack, and Elizabeth Rattine-Flaherty

It was a sultry June morning in southeastern Ohio. The mobile van was parked in the lot of a volunteer fire and rescue as Linda and Janet prepared and administered vaccines for children and adults alike. Twelve-year-old Sarah stood outside the clinic as her mom, Joyce, completed the intake forms provided by Rick (another staff member of the clinic). Many of Sarah's peers from school had come and gone as she remained outside. While outside and in anticipation of the "doom" that immunizations represented to her, Sarah wrote her will on a paper napkin. "I will my fish and my bike to my brother Andrew," wrote Sarah. Joyce reminded Sarah that she could not start seventh grade until her immunizations were up to date and that it would be impossible for her to take off work to travel with Sarah the forty miles to their family physician's office for the vaccination. Moreover, they did not have insurance coverage to cover the complete costs of the vaccination. Sarah nodded that she understood but continued to cry. Linda came down the stairs of the van and welcomed Sarah and Joyce to the clinic. Once inside the exam room, Linda talked to Sarah and Joyce about the importance of the immunization Sarah would receive, described potential side effects, swabbed Sarah's arm with alcohol and encouraged her to let her arm hang loose like a wet noodle. "OK, I'm ready, go ahead and give me the shot," Sarah finally said as tears continued to stream down her face. "It's already done," shared Linda. "No way, this is the first time I've got a shot that didn't hurt!" exclaimed Sarah. Joyce gently told Sarah she could tear up her will. Throughout the morning, Linda, Janet, and Rick worked in tandem to ease the tensions that naturally arise when youth, like Sarah, get immunizations. As the van traveled back home, one of the authors, Lynn, a participant observer of the mobile clinic's activities, reflected on a billboard advertising a new state of the art medical complex constructed of metal, glass, cement and human suffering. "While you are changing lanes, we are changing lives," read the billboard. In the case of the mobile clinic, the staff are changing lanes and changing lives.

(Fieldnotes)

Mobile health clinics represent an alternative way of organizing health-care resources for traditionally underserved populations. This chapter provides a narrative ethnographic account of a mobile health clinic that provides a variety of free or low-cost services to residents of twenty-one Appalachian counties in southeastern Ohio. Like the broader region of Appalachia, residents served by the clinic generally have less access to health care due to fewer material resources (Smith & Tessaro, 2005), experience geographic isolation from mainstream medical infrastructures and a lack of transportation (Schell & Tudiver, 2004), and face uneven distribution of health-care providers across rural and urban settings and disparities in the availability of health-care services (McKinley, 2005). By the very nature of how it provides services (e.g., curbside care), the mobile health clinic enacts fluid and shifting spatial boundaries and disrupts otherwise fixed barriers to health care including isolation and separation through geography, inability to miss work or school, and lack of financial resources. By changing lanes in order to change lives, the mobile health clinic provides twenty-first-century "house calls" and offers a hopeful vision for community-based health care.

Over the past two decades mobile health clinics have emerged to address unmet needs among underserved populations including the identification and treatment of sexually transmitted diseases (Liebman et al., 2002), osteoporosis (Newman et al., 2004), and even HIV and AIDS (Zabos & Trinh, 2001). Although scholars and practitioners in health-related fields have explored design and implementation considerations for mobile clinics (e.g., Cummings et al., 2002), communication scholars have remained notably silent about the organizing of health care in such non-traditional settings. In critiquing communication theory for its lack of attention to diverse contexts, Sharf (1993) argued, "It is insufficient and perhaps misleading to examine clinical communication as if all doctors, patients, and settings are essentially comparable. Taking account of contextual variability will sharpen the utility of our work and clarify which findings transcend these distinctions" (p. 37). In similar fashion, Ford and Yep (2003) urged communication scholars to enlarge their scholarly reach to include community-based health organizing (see also Zoller, 2005). Because narrative theorizing generally draws our attention to relationships between scenes, acts, agents, agency, and purpose (see Burke, 1969), it provides a rich perspective for understanding how context matters. Burke, for example, emphasized the importance of scene as he argued that, "terrains determine tactics" (p. 12). This maxim of narrative theory is particularly salient given the ever-evolving settings of mobile health. Fluid and shifting situations impact how mobile clinic providers and patients alike perform their roles.

We present a narrative ethnographic portrait of a multifaceted mobile clinic that: 1) provides primary care to uninsured individuals living at or below 150 percent of the poverty level through a free clinic; 2) sponsors a child and adult immunization program available to anyone irrespective of socioeconomic status; 3) conducts glucose, blood pressure, and cholesterol screenings for at-risk individuals; and 4) offers breast and cervical cancer screenings and education for uninsured women. Formed in 1996 to attend to the ongoing health-care needs in its host region, the clinic is sponsored by the Community Service Program (CSP) affiliated with an osteopathic college of medicine at a Midwestern university and travels over 14,000 miles per year to provide health-care services. We draw on participant observations and narratives collected through in-depth interviews with staff to explore how *space* shapes and is shaped by the enactment of cultural rituals, and as such has important implications for thinking about the *continuity* of care amidst *shifting* scenes of health care. Guided by narrative theory, we situate the practices and patterns of the clinic amidst larger, historically contingent, and shifting discursive and material fields. Like other scholars (e.g., Massey, 1994), we view space as both material and symbolic, and work to reveal how participants engage in role improvisation and maintain traditional privacy scripts of mainstream medicine in light of environmental and social constraints and changing cultural scenes.

Narrative as theory and praxis

Individuals, in both mundane and extraordinary moments, draw on and mobilize a variety of storytelling resources from their surround to understand and define relationships and events. In outlining the epistemological importance of narrative, Burke (1941) described the human condition using the metaphor of a "parlor" that we enter upon birth. The stories we encounter in the parlor offer cultural idioms including archetypal characters, plots, and settings. We make sense of our experience in light of hegemonic scripts, constructing our knowledge using prior experiences and socially sanctioned norms and interpretations that are interwoven (and sometimes resisted) in stories about who we are and how we got here. In and through these cultural idioms we build ourselves, our roles, and our dramas.

Narrative endows human experience with meaning by connecting characters in a web of relationships composed of symbolic, institutional, and material practices. *Narrating* as *emplotting* refers to how characters and actions are organized in time and space in ways that imply movement or action—characters situated in the complexities of lived moments of struggle, maintaining or restoring continuity in their lives amidst disruption (Ricouer, 1984). Narratives, thus, represent "equipment for living" (Burke, 1954/1984), sense-making structures that allow us to size up situations in various ways, craft livable truths, and offer frameworks for "possible worlds" (Bruner, 1986). Different storied imaginings, then, offer different possibilities for being.

Thus, we approach narratives as constituting knowledge of self and other, as well as the lived sociocultural and political contexts in which individuals (re)create and perform stories.

Narrative sensibilities provide a robust lens for exploring how organizations of all sorts, including the mobile clinic, take shape in and through symbolic interactions. Burke, for instance, was interested in the symbolic processes through which *orientations* develop (i.e., worldviews, accumulation of plotlines, and relations among characters), how orientations necessarily give rise to partial perspectives that result in *trained incapacities* (i.e., one's training results in one's incapacities), and how trained incapacities can lead to *fossilized institutions*. In sum, Burke was interested in "How society's ways of life affect its modes of thinking, by giving rise to partial perspectives or 'occupational psychoses'" (1954/1984, p. 4). Goffman (1959), too, focused on the institutionalization of particular scripts and the "bureaucratization of the spirit" (p. 56) needed to carry out routine performances in front and back regions. Yet, like other discursive formations, narratives emerge as contested terrains—dynamic, situated, and indeterminate processes of sense making. Indeed, in advancing a poetic metaphor for human action, Burke (1954/1984) argued that "though the materials of experience are established, we are poetic in our rearrangement of them" (p. 218).

An increasing number of scholars across disciplines envision narrative sensibilities as promising for advancing health-related theory and practice (e.g., Harter et al., 2005; Frank, 1995; Hunter, 1991). If, as Frank argued, illness is a call for stories, then the provision of health care would be impossible were it not for our human capacity to organize and embody lived experience in narrative form (Hunter, 1991). Morgan-Witte (2005) empirically located the narrative structure of medical knowledge through an ethnographic portrayal of nurses' stations as storytelling hubs even as Ellingson (2005) connected the frontstage and backstage of clinical care in narrative fashion. Through dialogue with his father, Dr. Jack Rawlins, Rawlins (2005) poignantly situated health-care providers as characters within and co-authors of patients' autobiographies. The biomedical model, too, can be understood as a grand narrative, an ongoing structure of values and beliefs including a hierarchy of characters, sacred scripts and spaces (Morris, 1998). From a narrative perspective, then, health organizations such as the mobile clinic are not merely the repositories or settings of stories but constitute stories themselves.

A narrative perspective, however, ought not deny the nonsymbolic aspects of storied experience, and in fact loses strength when it fails to acknowledge corporeality and materiality. "Foregrounding intersections between the physiological, material, environmental, and symbolic," argued Beck et al., (2005), "would be a welcome development in narrative theorizing specifically and communication research more generally" (p. 440). In similar fashion, Cheney (2000) argued that interpretive communication scholars too often have suffered from a case of "symbol worship," and suggested, "interpretive scholarship needs to *come to terms with the material world*" (Cheney, 2000, p. 44, emphasis in original). Cloud (1994), too, urged communication scholars to recognize that symbols are not the only things that matter. Of course, symbols do matter—they have material consequences and serve material interests in the world. Narrative scholars enjoy a repertoire of tools for understanding how political and even economic power is symbolically (re)produced and disrupted. Even so, material practices and environmental conditions intermingle with and shape symbolic interactions.

We seek to consider material and symbolic experiences as they mutually inform one another, and in so doing recognize "the material parameters for symbolic maneuverings" (Cheney, 2000, p. 45). Like Ashcraft and Mumby (2004), we approach discourse and materiality as mutually constitutive and dialectically related. Symbolic interactions certainly render the world meaningful, and we are keenly interested in the processes through which certain frames or definitions translate into lived consequences for individuals, organizations, and communities. Yet, we also recognize that the material world gives rise to certain communication practices and rituals. It is the concrete circumstances, the materiality, of "settings," "scenes," or "contexts" that too often fade from view in narrative analyses. Our ethnographic portrait of the mobile health clinic bears witness to the symbolic and material nature of storied health care.

The curbside care offered by the clinic by its very nature defies contemporary and social understandings of health-care settings. The material scenes of health care literally shift to homes, community centers, churches, and parking lots as such settings are redefined through performance. We did not enter the field with a specific vision of understanding the *continuity* of care amidst *shifting* scenes (although a narrative perspective remains particularly robust for understanding relations between scene, act, agents, agency, and purpose). These foci emerged through the constant comparative process of discourse collection and analysis beginning with our ethnographic observations. In the remainder of this chapter, we work to understand how staff members provide routinized and quality care amidst shifting scenes and in light of the material and social exigencies of people's lives. We shed insight into tensions that emerge when providers bring health care to the primary scenes of people's lives and with limited environmental resources. In this chapter, we address the following research question: How do staff members provide continuity of care amidst shifting scenes?

Research practices

While engaged in ethnographic fieldwork for this project, we took on the role of *observers as participants*. Indeed, while observing the interactions between and among the Community Service Program (CSP) staff and their patients, we assisted with patient registration, helped hold and entertain children who were getting immunizations, loaded and unloaded supplies, and assisted with the set-up of clinics and health fairs. We ate lunch with staff members and with health fair participants. A few of us even became patients ourselves, receiving tetanus shots and undergoing blood pressure, glucose, and cholesterol screenings.

Setting

Formed in 1996 to help meet the growing health-care needs that existed in their twenty-one county service area (eleven of which are considered Appalachia counties), the Community Service Program (CSP) is affiliated with the College of Osteopathic Medicine at Ohio University (OUCOM). Although childhood immunizations are offered two half days a week at a small fixed clinic within (OUCOM), most of the CSP clinics are conducted in two 40-foot mobile units in various outreach sites that have been established throughout their service area. The outreach sites are often no more than the parking lot of a community or senior citizens' center, a local elementary school or a gas station. When serving especially rural or Amish communities, it is not unusual to find a mobile unit parked in a field or in the driveway of someone's farm. Depending on the community being served or the nature of the clinic being held, the CSP mobile unit often utilizes additional space inside a near-by facility. For example, when conducting bus driver physicals at an elementary school, patients were sent inside for vaccinations and vision, hearing and blood screenings before boarding the mobile unit for the actual physical examination.

The primary CSP staff consists of one director, one administrative assistant, one full-time and one part-time van driver, one nurse practitioner, one certified medical assistant, six registered nurses, and an occasional rotating physician (primarily at the monthly free clinic). Often a university student in the AmeriCorps program will assist with patient intake, with updating patient records on the computer, or with loading and unloading supplies to set up a clinic or health fair. As indicated earlier, the clinic offers glucose and cholesterol screenings, immunizations, physicals, breast and cervical cancer screenings, a well-child and well-family program for pregnant women and children, and a referral system for other services. Most of these services, which are offered free of charge or for a small fee, are provided in cooperation with the Centers for Disease Control and Prevention, the Ohio Department of Health, county health departments, community agencies, area hospitals and businesses.

Discourse collection procedures

Upon receiving approval from our Institutional Review Board, we collected discourses from three sources: 1) participant observations; 2) in-depth interviews with staff members; and, 3) documents produced by the CSP.

Participant observations

Over a period of 12 months, the research team traveled over 900 miles and spent more than 200 hours observing the interactions between and among the CSP staff and clients at various clinics, health fairs, and staff meetings. Each member of the team engaged in participant observations; each observation period ranged in length from one to ten hours depending on the location and nature of the services being provided. During observations, we each took handwritten field notes and attempted to document key phrases of conversation verbatim. Throughout observations, we reflexively tried to account for how we as participant observers potentially affected the performances including what was observed and how it was interpreted. Before observing an examination, either the researcher or a nurse talked about the nature of our project and asked the patient for permission to engage in participant observation. When granted permission to observe, we tried to be as unobtrusive as possible by sitting or standing in a corner of the exam room. When asked by a nurse, we participated in the process by fetching materials, making phone calls, organizing materials, and even holding the hands of children receiving immunizations. The observation hours resulted in 175 single-spaced pages of field notes.

In-depth interviews

After having been in the field for three months, we conducted on-site, in-depth interviews with eight staff members (four RNs, two bus drivers, one certified medical assistant, and one nurse practitioner).[1] The interviews, which were audio-taped and transcribed, lasted approximately 60 minutes each. We developed a tentative interview protocol, which included open-ended questions about the core values that guided members' work, rural health in the context of Appalachia, personal and professional issues resulting from the performance of emotion work, and the challenges and opportunities resulting from the fluidity of space encountered in the mobile-clinic setting. The interview sessions were semi-structured to allow participants to talk about their individual experiences and insights. In addition to the formal interviews, throughout our fieldwork we engaged in informal playback sessions or member-checking interviews in which we talked with staff about patterns we were observing. These informal dialogues allowed us to reflexively pay attention to our own interpretations and directed our attention to things we might be missing while in the field.

Discourse analysis procedures

Generally, we relied on a constant comparative method (Glaser & Strauss, 1967) to conduct a thematic analysis of the discourses. This process begins with data "reduction" and "interpretation." After reading all the transcripts and fieldnotes and gaining a holistic sense of the discourses, we started the actual analysis. The constant comparative method allowed us to identify recurring patterns of behavior and meaning in the participants' accounts and performances. The process began by manually coding the data on the actual transcripts and fieldnotes. We made note of both patterned regularities in the way participants' accounted for their experiences as well as counter-evidence and alternative viewpoints. Originally, we identified three broad themes in the discourses. As we delved deeper, we realized that two of the themes were inter-related with a broader issue: how to provide continuity in care amidst shifting scenes. It is this over-arching dilemma and how it is accomplished through role improvisation and while (mostly) maintaining the script of provider–patient confidentiality that became the focus of this chapter.

Importantly, narrative theory shaped how we collected and analyzed the discourses and wrote about them. We understand narrative from an explicitly broad vantage point, casting a wide net that incorporated autobiographical stories, performed scripts, and institutional plots that surround an issue or idea over time. We approached narratives as texts—the topics, characters, content, style, functions served, context and telling of narratives by participants during interviews and in the course of their daily work routines. Yet, epistemologically and methodologically, we also understood narratives as performances that shape and are shaped by material circumstances (see also Cortazzi, 2001). Clinic staff performed social scripts; likewise, we became co-performers through our retrospective sense making.

We now present a co-constructed account that privileges the voices of participants but also recognizes our position (and power) in identifying, framing, and understanding participants' experiences. We weave between the discourses of participants and philosophical fragments authored by the research team based on our theoretical sensibilities. As argued by Alvesson and Skoldberg (2000), the "interplay between philosophical ideas and empirical work marks high-quality social research. While philosophical sophistication is certainly not the principal task of social science, social research without philosophically informed reflection grows so unreflective that the label 'research' becomes questionable" (p. 7). Throughout the results, we identify how existing theory shaped our meaning-making process. Meanwhile, we recognize that no textual (re)production of experiences, including this one, is value-free. Our narrative sensibilities and personal experiences, for instance, drew out some interpretive possibilities while suppressing others. The lead authors, Lynn and Karen, for instance, grew up in poverty. Of particular interest in their research agendas and praxis is the identification of resources that allow people to be resilient in the face of what others might consider to be inhospitable conditions. Their standpoint no doubt influenced how the research team as a whole approached the mobile clinic as a boundary-spanning organization that works within the parameters of mainstream society to serve those typically relegated to the margins.

Shifting scenes and continuity of care

> Our van broke down at one point and to make sure that we did service the location that we were supposed to go to, Janet went and called and got a van from over at the motor pool. Umm, it was a van that the back doors opened up and there were two seats. So she then proceeded to go and get like a beach chair so we could set it up in the back. And strangely enough the location was in Jackson. It was outside in the parking lot of Foodland but right in back of us was the police department and so there were no markings on this van that said we were a mobile clinic offering immunizations. So I would stand out and kind of wave to people to let them know and every now and then a person would come in and we would open the doors to the van, close the door because it was cold, and Janet would proceed to give the immunizations and the child would get out and we'd get to laughing and wondering if the police were wondering what exactly we were selling out of this van. Opening and closing the doors and having these people come in. It was very primitive but the vaccines were the same. The procedure was similar. We still provided the service. But, we are flexible, we have to be. There is no reason not to be.
>
> (Interview transcript, Linda)

The mobile clinic's curbside care functions to disrupt material and geographic barriers to health-care access as it shifts the settings in which the provision of services unfold. As revealed by Linda's narrative, although the scenes of health care *shift*, staff members work to be *consistent*—to provide reliable and quality care. One of the clinic nurses, Janet, stressed, "We really hate to cancel a clinic, and one of the things that we have to be with the mobile unit is reliable. So we work hard at that." Another nurse, Angela, explained, "I just think that, you know, a lot of it is that it takes a lot to get that patient there. So, just up and canceling it, we may not have that opportunity to get that patient there again." The staff of the mobile clinic coordinates with county health departments, school nurses, local physicians, and other community stakeholders to ensure that they provide dependable and quality services in convenient settings and at times that are least disruptive to patients' lives.

The populations served by the clinic have salient concerns that often prohibit them from taking full advantage of traditional health care including the inability to pay for services, geographic isolation and separation from health-care resources, and inability to leave work for appointments. The mobile clinic answers this call for care by using traditional space in a fixed clinic and a movable space in the mobile clinic van. Jackie, a nurse, shared, "We *reach* of lot of uninsured people and we target *places* that reach the uninsured like the food pantries. . . . Sometimes just by some of the locations we go to we know we're going to reach the low income and uninsured." The mobile clinic alleviates the pressures of finding the time, money, and transportation needed to visit a clinic by 1) providing most services free of charge to qualified individuals, and 2) bringing care to the places where people live and work. Wes, a driver, shared:

> Well, you know, we do take health care to the community. And that is a good thing. Some of these folks wouldn't have health care. They wouldn't get flu shots, they wouldn't get, umm, blood pressure testing, their kids might not get immunizations. So, the van, we bring everything to them.

The clinic works to ensure that people have the opportunity to receive consistent care by expanding the traditional scenes of health care. "I think the best thing is that we do bring the services to the people. A lot of people can't travel into other locations to get their medical care. So, we bring it to them," shared Denise, a nurse, "Some of the folks just walk here. You don't need transportation. Especially with gas prices and everything, it's a lot easier, a lot more convenient for people. I think that is the best thing—that we bring the service to the people."

How does the staff provide what one nurse, Melissa, described as a "medical home," (i.e., quality and consistent care) because of and amidst shifting settings and in light of the material and social exigencies of people's lives? What tensions and contradictions arise when providers bring care to the primary scenes of people's lives: churches, community centers, grocery stores, and even the lawns of their homes? In order to answer these questions, we analyze the 1) improvisational nature of organizing, and 2) the disruption and maintenance of privacy scripts.

Improvisation and organizing

> We departed at 7:15am for a breast and cervical cancer screening program in Waverly. Upon arrival, the nurses worked to arrange intake forms in the waiting area and materials in the exam rooms including speculums, KY jelly, paper gowns and lap coverings. Soon after the first patient, Erin, was escorted into one of the exam rooms, the lights on the van flickered off. As Rick checked on the generator, Angela took a small flashlight off her key chain in order for Melissa to continue with the pelvic exam and pap smear, which she did! As the third patient was escorted to an exam room, the nurses were still working with makeshift lighting, and due to the increasing temperature outside, the van was stifling hot. Jackie went in search of an alternative setting in which to see the remaining patients. The van happened to be parked by the county health department and a doctor's office, the latter of which agreed to provide an examination room for the rest of the day as well as part of an office for an intake area. The setting for the clinic shifted mid-morning, yet the nurses' performances seemed

quite fluid, the disruption barely noticeable in terms of its impact on how the nurses provided care.

(Fieldnotes)

Because health care is provided in community settings and away from the nurses' home base, the nurses often "go with the flow," according to Angela, and figure out how to do their job based on available resources. On numerous occasions, we observed the staff improvising *how* to provide consistent care based on the nature of the physical space, the (un)availability of phone services, the weather, the van's generator, and other material and social exigencies. Linda shared:

> There was a death in the driver's family, we had a big clinic down in Wheelersburg. So, we called up the Kroger store and said listen we don't have the van is there any way we could do it in your building. And they set us up with a card table and some chairs in front of the pharmacy. And, we did quite a few that day as they lined up through the aisles of Krogers. And we've found that because of good working relationships with communities, we usually haven't had problems finding locations. If it is an emergency, people understand that. Vans break down. And they know the benefits to the community.

Improvisation allows nurses to provide continuity in care amidst the shifting scenes of care.

Many nurses use a vacation metaphor to describe how they "pack" for various trips, often forgetting some supplies. Jackie shared:

> You do have to pack up, like I keep that little gray box, that's what I take on all my B&C clinics. It's got my paperwork. And then when I go into Parks Hall I take that blue tub cause that has all our supplies, our gowns and specs and everything that we use so we don't have to use theirs. So you pack it all, you pack it around a lot.

While one of the researchers was observing a HAP screening, the staff realized the batteries on one of the glucometers had died and they did not have back-up machines or batteries with them. Melissa exclaimed, "It's like going on vacation, you always forget something!" On another occasion, the Childhood Immunization Program (CHIP) nurses realized that they had short supply of needles for immunizations. Finding themselves two hours away from their office and not wanting to cancel the day's clinics, Linda contacted the county health department who was able to provide more needles. Jackie, admitted, "You know you've got to pack so much stuff. Making sure that you have all your supplies you need, that's a tough one I think. I always forget something." The shifting nature of care settings often demands creativity on the part of staff in order to provide uninterrupted care. Such imagination is critical given that the mobile clinic's services remain the most reliable care many of its stakeholders receive. Ironically, many of the clinic's patients previously received very little continuity in overall health care from mainstream medicine.

Problems that emerge in relation to the scenes of health care often demand abrupt shifts to other settings and call nurses to *account* for such changes and comfort patients. Consider the following story shared by Angela:

> We were out doing physicals in Vinton County one day on the mobile van and the electricity went out again. At that time we had an awning, and we set up chairs outside for people to sit, because it was cooler outside than it was inside. And, we used the flashlights that we had . . . These were little kids, and [we] just brought on board and kind of told them that is was, you know, kind of like Halloween, it's a little dark, but it's going to be fun, and kind of got 'em interested in everything, did as much as we could off of the van. Melissa kind of made do . . . parents seemed to be okay with that.

As captured by Angela, the material exigencies shape the nature of communication between the nurses and children. Meanwhile, the material and symbolic dimensions of scenes are inseparable from the improvisational nature of how roles are performed by providers. Staff members reframe how settings are understood through performance: grocery stores become examination or procedure rooms, doctors offices usually accessible only to those who can pay become sites for free care, unmarked vans serve as immunization posts. The practices of staff members reveal how communication practices can literally invent, not only recreate or respond to, material conditions. A case in point: staff claim, mark, and redefine material space through visual images, colors, logos, blood pressure cuffs and glucometers. In doing so, they shift communal understandings of scripts that ought to guide interactions in those scenes.

Staff members we observed generally seem to flourish amidst the indeterminate symbolic and material redefinition of "scene." Janet shared, "Linda and I are both change agents and we both thrive on it and we sort of like having to work out little problems, and the big problems." Importantly, the staff of the mobile clinic story their experiences in particular ways (e.g., we are engaged in creative work that requires improvisation) in lieu of other narratives that could be told (e.g., we are surrounded by sub-standard resources that cause stress and burnout). Such stories represent equipment for living, stories that engender edifying dwellings for staff and patients alike. As such, nurses propose a possible world where the work they perform and the ways they do so are bearable—even noble.

Of course, not all disruptions related to the shifting settings can be addressed by role improvisation. During interviews, staff consistently identified weather as the biggest threat to mobile health care, a threat they generally remain unable to address. Wes shared:

Last year, during flu season, we had about twenty people lined up and waiting outside in the rain for shots. And we were running low, and several people, I'd say about five people, they never got shots. But they were standing out in the cold because we didn't have enough room. It was cold. Then finally we had to tell them we didn't have any shots left.

Another driver, Rick, emphasized that weather also influences whether or not people come to a clinic, "We can usually get there, but a lot of times people won't come like they would when the weather is decent. Weather does have a bearing."

The geographic, material, and social exigencies of people's lives also influence if and how consistent care can be provided. Linda stressed:

There are hills in Appalachia and with those hills, mobile phone service is not always reliable. If the only location where we can park the van is a church parking lot and it is located in the hallow, then there is no phone service. We just have to deal with it. We try to bring our computer with us now that has records of all the children who we've seen. But that doesn't help if the child's parents comes in with no immunization records and we can't call the physician to find out what the shots were.

Given that most clients served by the various clinics live at or below 150 percent of the poverty level, the staff also has had to rely on alternative methods to advertise their services. "I think in the beginning, advertising in the *Messenger*, they did advertise quite a bit but the people that we are serving don't buy the *Messenger*, they can't afford it," stressed Denise, "so I think we are now turning to radio and things like that. I've taken flyers and actually gone to a couple of churches and the library where we are more apt to reach the populations that we aim to serve."

Organizational communication scholars generally have neglected coordinated action amidst ambiguous conditions (see critiques by Eisenberg, 1984, 2001). Role performances by the clinic staff unfold in turbulent and unpredictable settings, and reveal the saliency of adaptation and improvisation. Like the jamming sessions among musicians described by Eisenberg, the role performances of the clinic staff remain rule-governed and characterized by fluid behavioral coordination yet the options for individual moves are unlimited—there is great latitude for characters to shift performances within otherwise fairly structured experiences. Of course, improvisational freedom is called into being by the shifting settings of the mobile clinic juxtaposed with well-defined rules and roles in health care more generally (see also Miller et al., 2000). Improvisation is inherently embroiled in what staff members do— in the texture and practices of their daily lives. Indeed, staff describe improvisation as a key to providing consistent (i.e., ritualized) care amidst shifting scenes. As such, the mobile clinic provides us with a vision for how to *structure* for *surrender*, or "learn more about surrender, in order to better live within the flow" (Eisenberg, 1990, p. 156). Indeed, the "resources of ambiguity" (Burke, 1969) allow participants to further individual and organizational goals as they negotiate their roles and routine organizational tasks amidst "shifting scenes," and turbulent environments.

The disruption and maintenance of privacy scripts

Upon our arrival at the community center, the HAP staff quickly worked to set up a four-table station for glucose, blood pressure, and cholesterol screening. Due to spatial constraints, the tables were four to five feet apart—at most. Participants would complete the intake survey at the first table and sign the HIPA/patient privacy form. Rick would guarantee that the staff would keep their information confidential (including test results) and not share the information with other providers without the patient's permission. The individual would then either proceed to one of the screening tables or take a chair in the makeshift "waiting area." The screening and intake tables were close enough that individuals, if they so desired, could overhear conversations that ensued among other providers and clients. The very nature of this space rendered impotent the privacy disclosure policy. I (Lynn) could not help but wonder if service provision in this context defies the privacy/confidentiality script that Americans have come to expect in provider–patient interactions. Is this a tradeoff that those who otherwise remain underserved must live with in order to access services? Is it a tradeoff of curbside care? Staff members seem dependent on available (if even inadequate) space in parking lots, schools, and community centers. How do they manage traditional privacy scripts in light of sociospatial dynamics?

(Fieldnotes)

Traditional codes of ethical conduct among health professionals assume that providers will do their patients "no harm" in part by maintaining a "duty of silence" with respect to patients' private information (Everstine et al., 1980). The mobile health clinic is no exception. Melissa shared, "I really respect privacy. It's nobody's business what goes on and of course the nurses and myself, we all work here, we've all had to sign confidentiality forms. It's a given being a professional." Sharing information about patients is expected and often demanded in health-care contexts as providers (and usually funding agencies) work interdependently to address patients' health-care needs. Even still, the broadening of access to patients' personal health information is supposed to be done with patients' permission. Although privacy policies are in place at the mobile clinic and staff sign confidentiality agreements upon being hired, practices of confidentiality can become strained in part due to the material and social nature of the settings. Staff members have developed sophisticated strategies for trying to maintain the often taken-for-granted script of provider–patient confidentiality in spite of shifting material and social exigencies that call it into question.

Realities exist beyond text—experience cannot be reduced solely to the symbolic (Ashcraft & Mumby, 2004; Cloud, 1994). The material contexts of the staffs' health-care performances (including the van itself as well as other community spaces that staff members use to provide services) shape discursive practices and patterns in critical ways. The amount of space available is often limited, especially on a 40-foot van. Each van is organized with two examination rooms and a waiting area that also serves as a place for staff to organize materials including computer equipment, information brochures, the landline telephone, etc. The spatial dimensions make it difficult, if not impossible, to protect patients' privacy. Jackie emphasized, "We try to be as confidential as we can . . . we're smaller so it is harder with patient confidentiality, that's more of a challenge. It's just smaller." In addition, one of the vans does not have metal doors, making it difficult to establish clear boundaries between "frontstage" and "backstage" areas of health care. Permeable and paper-thin doors pose formidable material barriers for staff who seek to sustain privacy for patients. In fact, due to the materiality of the scenes, the disclosure of private information may occur beyond the knowledge or control of the primary interactants.

The social dimensions of community-based health care also pose unique challenges for the mobile clinic staff. Consider the following story shared by Angela:

> And meeting them in their own environment, in their own community, having them come on the van with, even though it is supposed to be confidential, it's hard to not, to sometimes keep it confidential because they'll sit down and it will be their neighbor that's sitting behind them. Or, their cousin or somebody else that's sitting beside them, especially in a small community.

In short, the discursive struggle to maintain the script of patient privacy occurs within the parameters of material and social environments.

The privileging of certain practices on the part of staff members translates into lived consequences for participants. Like the gynecologists described by Emerson (1970), staff members deliberately act in ways that work to sustain appropriate frames or definitions for encounters (e.g., provider–patient encounters ought to be private ones). To begin, staff members create makeshift "backstage areas" in which they can interact with other clinic staff and connect with providers in the broader medical community. In many cases, some patients are relocated from the "waiting area" in order for nurses to reclaim that space as a clinical backstage or nurses wait until the setting allows for privacy. "You don't want to make a phone call to make an appointment and say I have John Smith who has a hernia in front of six people waiting in that waiting room, so you need to wait and call the patient back and that is very challenging," shared Melissa. Of course, the lived material conditions of the patients also must be considered, as revealed by Angela:

> It's easier for us to schedule like mammographies on the van when the patients are there, because they may not have a phone. It's hard to play telephone tag back and forth. So if I have to schedule those, what we try to do is do it with the patient there in the waiting room and hopefully get the other patients in one of the other two rooms so that the information we're giving on the phone is in front of the patient and not in front of a whole group. That works out sometimes, but sometimes we can't do it that way. Or I'll walk outside on my cell phone or whatever.

We also observed nurses create backstage areas (e.g., use an examination room) to dialogue about a patient's case away from the patient and others in the waiting room.

Drawing on the work of Goffman (1959), Ellingson (2005) astutely observed that the clinic backstage remains intricately interwoven with the clinic frontstage. Ellingson's (auto)ethnographic portrayal of an inter-disciplinary cancer care unit revealed how backstage *communication* shapes and is shaped by frontstage *communication* (see also Morgan-Witte, 2005). We extend these arguments by revealing how the *material* dimensions of settings cannot be separated from the *symbolic* dimensions. Social realities are embodied in routines, reproduced in social interaction, and situated in material circumstances. On numerous occasions, we witnessed staff members creatively manipulating the environment and/or making strategic choices to carry off the performance of privacy. "We've turned radios up before so that people don't know what is going on between the walls," stressed Denise as she reflected on the fact that the waiting area is in close proximity to the examination rooms. Drapes were also installed in the exam rooms so that if an exam room door is open, people in the waiting area could not see who was in the exam room. Because the waiting area also functions as a "nurse's station," or what is traditionally understood as a clinical backstage, staff are challenged to protect data typically stored in this information hub. Jackie stressed, "Well we try not to leave any schedules out in the open, charts out in the open. We turn them down so people can't look and see who's coming in. We always shut the little doors when we are getting a patient ready or when we're talking to a patient." Angela shared, "we keep the charts upside down—it's really hard when you've got people filling out forms and sitting in this little van side by side." In short, concrete material exigencies represent substantial threats to nurses and challenge them to sustain the provider–patient confidentiality expected in traditional health-care contexts. The privacy script is taxed by the settings of the mobile clinic and created anew through ingenuous symbolic and material maneuverings of staff.

The routinized procedures and improvisational acts of nurses, however, do not always work to protect patients—breaches in privacy occur. Angela shared, "I know that we don't always protect their privacy and I wish that we could. It's just that space is an issue." Of course, patients are actively involved in the co-construction of privacy scripts, as alluded to by Anne:

> Sometimes I know that patients have started to ask questions when, like when Melanie has come out, in front of other patients. And sometimes if it starts to get too complicated, either I or Janice will pull them into another room because . . . you know they're okay about discussing it in front of other people. I still think it needs to be done in somewhat private.

In short, the coordination of privacy scripts becomes more complicated and contested in the material and social settings of mobile units that provide community-based health care.

Discussion

We undertook ethnographic fieldwork in a context that expands traditional understandings of clinical settings: the OUCOM mobile health clinic. The mobile clinic represents an alternative approach to organizing health-care resources by providing health care in the primary spaces of people's lives including schools, community centers, and grocery stores. Importantly, narrative sensibilities allowed us to situate the mobile clinic interactions within larger institutional and social contexts and highlight the intertextual dimensions of narrative activity (e.g., the performed stories of staff derive meaning in part from their relationship to other stories such as scripts of the biomedical model). As Goffman (1959) reminded us, the performance of a particular routine is modified to fit into the understanding and expectations of the society in which it is presented. Role performances of the clinic staff are no exception. We witnessed heroic efforts on the part of nurses to maintain and affirm a sacred script of modern Western medicine—privacy—amidst material and social circumstances that work to erode it.

Theoretically, this chapter reveals another heuristic potential of narrative ethnography—its ability to draw attention to the symbolic and material nature of storied lives. Participant observations revealed how contextual constraints (e.g., paper thin doors) give rise to communication patterns among staff (e.g., turning up the radio) as they try to maintain sacred scripts of Western medicine (e.g., provider–patient confidentiality). The settings of the clinic emerge as contested terrains as staff members conduct serious business in some spaces not originally designated as clinical areas. Nurses are ingenuous in their use of limited and shared spaces and privacy continues to be sought and privileged amidst conditions that threaten to disrupt it. In so doing, staff members reveal the interdependency between the symbolic and the material aspects of

330 L.M. Harter et al.

experience and provide a hopeful model for the delivery of health care in community-based settings.

The mobile clinic staff members also provide us with a vision of how to expand the reach of mainstream medicine to individuals who face persistent barriers to quality health care, including the stigma and shame of poverty. Johnson et al. (2004) urged communication scholars to unmask "othering" practices in health-care contexts, the dynamics through which lived differences (e.g., racial, gendered, classed) are magnified in such a way as to result in marginalization of individuals and groups and inequities in health care and health outcomes. Just as everyday and innocuous communicative practices can work to separate individuals (Burke, 1954/1984), the mobile clinic staff members reveal how rituals can create consubstantiality between individuals in lieu of the mystery that too often emerges from hierarchy (i.e., order/ organization of individuals and resources). Ultimately, our analysis bears witness to how staff members tirelessly work to ensure that underserved individuals are granted the same respect (e.g., provider–patient confidentiality) as those with wider access to mainstream medicine. Through improvisation, staff members provide *consistent* and quality care amidst *shifting* scenes.

Continuing the conversation

Alvesson and Skoldberg (2000) reminded interpretive researchers to remain reflexive throughout the knowledge production process, recognizing that any references to empirical discourses are the constructions and results of interpretations. As such, interpretive analyses are inherently ambiguous and pregnant with the possibility for alternative sense making. We do not argue that our storied reading of this mobile clinic at this point in time is the only, or even best, reading of the symbolic and material nature of health-care provision. In fact, we believe that a primary marker of insightful inquiry is its ability to stimulate the imagining of alternative readings. As argued by Alvesson and Skoldberg:

> Authorship is about increasing the opportunities for different readings. The reader becomes significant, not as a consumer of correct results—the right intended meaning from the text and its author(ity)—but in a more active and less predictable positioning, in which interesting readings may be divorced from the possible intentions of the author.
>
> (p. 171)

We offer our arguments as plausible, viable, and tentative—open to revision by others operating from different standpoints or with different theoretical underpinnings. We invite others into our textual (re)production in hopes of generating fruitful dialogue.

A primary reason why interpretive researchers engage in reflexivity about the inquiry process and textual products is to understand what the analysis is not capable of saying. In other words, any repertoire of interpretations necessarily limits the possibilities of advancing certain claims. What stakeholders and discourses must we turn to next, and for what theoretical and practical purposes? This chapter represents the initial phases of a longitudinal research project. During this phase, access was granted by the director of the CSP to engage in participant observations and interview staff. To the best of our ability, we included the voices of patients as embodied in their encounters with staff as observed and interpreted by us. As we continue to work with the CSP, our goal is to broaden the scope of data collection and interview patients of the clinic in order to further include their voices in the project and explore if, and how, they experience breaches of privacy and other rituals and relationships in a mobile clinic setting. For example, it is possible that at times the clinic inadvertently works to disincent people from accessing care. If patients wait for extended periods of time in inclement weather and do not receive shots, are they likely to return the next time the mobile clinic offers services? If patients repeatedly experience privacy breaches, not accessing care may be more "rational" than it is often treated in scholarly literature.

Meanwhile, we must shift our attention to the broader social domain where health care is provided and rendered meaningful. This mobile clinic, like any discursive and material formation, bears the imprints of ideologies, expresses power relations, and implies socially determined restrictions for experiencing the world. The nurses we interviewed overwhelmingly indicated that they generally thrive in a chaotic and under-resourced environment that demands their ingenuity in order to provide respectful and quality care to patients. Indeed, our analysis bears witness to the micro-level performances and strategies of staff who must cope with less than perfect and unpredictable sociospatial exigencies. Even so, staff recognized that this system is not ideal. As Angela shared, "Yeah, we absolutely need better, more universal health care for the folks we serve, state of the art care and facilities. But in the meantime, we are doing the best we can with what we have." In this moment, Angela articulated a critique of the system of which she is a part and recognized the need for longer-term fixes to the problems of unequal distribution of financial resources, health care, and life opportunities. Clearly, the health concerns and needs of those who depend on mobile clinics are positioned differently (in the social organization of health-care resources) than those with higher social class (see also Ford & Yep, 2003). In other words, the health-care system reproduces and reflects other systems of inequality that exist in the United States today—an issue that demands further consideration by communication scholars.

The mobile clinic served as a particularly rich context in which to observe improvisational organizing amidst complex and ambiguous conditions. Although this mobile clinic by design demands creativity and imagination in response to shifting scenes, mainstream medicine in Western contexts more generally is increasingly recognized as chaotic—"complex adaptive systems" that demand self-organizing for system regulation (see McDaniel, 1997). Yet, Miller (1998) cautioned that living on the edge of chaos, or in what Stacey (1996) discussed as the space for creativity, is not a pleasant place for some people to reside. In fact, the uncertainty and complexity of systems such as the mobile clinic have the potential to lead to burnout. In contexts in which the lives and livelihoods of individuals remain at stake, scholars and practitioners must explore the potential dark side of organizing by improvising.

We close by noting the oxymoronic character of "celebrating" an organization that exists because segments of society lack access to quality health care. Discourse, scholarly or otherwise, risks naturalizing such inequities. The microstrategies engaged by staff members, as powerful as they are, cannot completely counteract the many forces that affront the sensibilities of those living in poverty. We hope our analysis can inspire additional inquiry and interpretations about the possibilities and limits of mobile health clinics.

Note

1   Pseudonyms are used throughout this chapter in order to protect the identities of individual participants. We received permission from the Dean of the OUCOM to identify the clinic by name.

References

Alvesson, M., & Skoldberg, K. (2000). *Reflexive Methodology: New Vistas for Qualitative Research*. Thousand Oaks, CA: Sage.

Ashcraft, K.L., & Mumby, D.K. (2004). *Reworking Gender: A Feminist Communicology of Organization*. Thousand Oaks, CA: Sage.

Beck, C.S., Harter, L.M., & Japp, P.M. (2005). Continuing the conversation: Reflections on our emergent scholarly narratives. In L.M. Harter, P.M. Japp, & C.S. Beck (eds), *Narratives, Health, and Healing: Communication Theory, Research, and Practice*. Mahwah, NJ: Lawrence Erlbaum, pp. 433–444.

Bruner, J. (1986). *Actual Minds, Possible Worlds*. Cambridge, MA: Harvard University Press.

Burke, K. (1954/1984). *Permanence and Change*. Berkeley: University of California Press.

Burke, K. (1969). *A Grammar of Motives*. Berkeley: University of California Press.

Burke, K. (1941). *The philosophy of literary form*. Berkeley: University of California Press.

Cheney, G. (2000). Interpreting interpretive research: Toward perspectivalism without relativism. In S.R. Corman, & M.S. Poole (eds), *Perspectives on Organizational Communication: Finding Common Ground*. New York: The Guilford Press, pp. 17–45.

Cloud, D. (1994). The materiality of discourse as oxymoron: A challenge to critical rhetoric. *Western Journal of Communication*, 58, 141–162.

Cortazzi, M. (2001). Narrative analysis in ethnography. In P. Atkinson, A. Coffey, S. Delamont, J. Lofland, & L. Lofland (eds), *Handbook of Ethnography*. Thousand Oaks, CA: Sage, pp. 384–392.

Cummings, D.M., Whetstone, L.M., Earp, J.A., & Mayne, L. (2002). Disparities in mammography screening in rural areas: Analysis of county differences in North Carolina. *The Journal of Rural Health, 18,* 77–83.

Eisenberg, E.M. (1984). Ambiguity as strategy in organizational communication. *Communication Monographs, 51,* 227–242.

Eisenberg, E. (1990). Jamming: transcendence through organizing. *Communication Research, 17,* 139–164.

Eisenberg, E.M. (2001). Building a mystery: Toward a new theory of communication and identity. *Journal of Communication, 51,* 534–550.

Ellingson, L.L. (2005). *Communicating in the Clinic: Negotiating Frontstage and Backstage Teamwork.* Cresskill, NJ: Hampton Press, Inc.

Emerson, J.P. (1970). Behavior in private places: Sustaining definitions of reality in gynecological examinations. In H.P. Dreitzel (ed.), *Recent Sociology no 2: Patterns of Communicative Behavior.* New York: Macmillan Co, pp. 74–97.

Everstine, L., Everstine, D.S., Heyman, G.M., True, R.H., Frey, D.H., Johnson, H.G., & Seiden, R.H. (1980). Privacy and confidentiality in psychotherapy. *American Psychologist, 35,* 828–840.

Ford, L.A., & Yep, G.A. (2003). Working along the margins: Developing community-based strategies for communicating about health with marginalized groups. In T.L. Thompson, A.M. Dorsey, K.I. Miller, & R. Parrott (eds), *Handbook of Health Communication.* Mahwah, NJ: Lawrence Erlbaum, pp. 241–262.

Frank, A.W. (1995). *The Wounded Storyteller: Body, Illness, and Ethics.* Chicago: University of Chicago.

Goffman, E. (1959). *The Presentation of Self in Everyday Life.* New York: Anchor Books.

Glaser, B.G., & Strauss, A.L. (1967). *The Discovery of Grounded Theory.* Chicago: Aldine.

Harter, L.M., Japp, P.M., & Beck, C.S. (2005). Vital problematics of narrative theorizing about health and healing. In L.M. Harter, P.M. Japp, & C.S. Beck (eds), *Narratives, Health, and Healing: Communication Theory, Research, and Practice.* Mahwah, NJ: Lawrence Erlbaum, pp. 7–30.

Hunter, K.M. (1991). *Doctors' Stories: The Narrative Structure of Medical Knowledge.* Princeton, NJ: Princeton University Press.

Johnson, J.L., Bottorff, J.L., Browne, A.J., Grewal, S., Hilton, B.A., & Clarke, H. (2004). Othering and being othered in the context of health care services. *Health Communication, 16,* 253–271.

Liebman, J., Lamberti, M.P., & Altice, F. (2002). Effectiveness of a mobile medical van in providing screening services for STDs and HIV. *Public Health Nursing, 19*(5), 345–353.

Massey, D. (1994). *Space, Place, and Gender.* Minneapolis, MN: University of Minnesota Press.

McDaniel, Jr., R.R. (1997). Strategic leadership: A view from quantum and chaos theories. *Health Care Management Review, 22,* 21–37.

McKinley, A. (2005). Promoting access and care in rural and underserved areas. (Electronic version). *Healthcare Financial Management, 59,* 6–17.

Miller, K., Joseph, L., & Apker, J. (2000). Strategic ambiguity in the role development process. *Journal of Applied Communication Research, 28,* 193–214.

Miller, K. (1998). Nurses at the edge of chaos: The application of "new science" concepts to organizational systems. *Management Communication Quarterly, 12,* 112–127.

Morgan-Witte, J. (2005). Narrative knowledge development among caregivers: stories from the nurses' station. In L.M. Harter, P.M. Japp, & C.S. Beck (eds), *Narratives, Health, and Healing: Communication Theory, Research, and Practice*. Mahwah, NJ: Lawrence Erlbaum, pp. 237–258.

Morris, D.B. (1998). *Illness and Culture in the Postmodern Age*. Berkeley: University of California Press.

Newman, E.D., Olenginski, T.P., Perruquet, J.L., Hummel, J., Indeck, C., & Wood, G.C. (2004). Using mobile DXA to improve access to osteoporosis care. *Journal of Clinical Densitometry, 7*, 71–75.

Rawlins, W.K. (2005). Our family's physican. In L.M. Harter, P.M. Japp, & C.S. Beck (eds), *Narratives, Health, and Healing: Communication Theory, Research, and Practice*. Mahwah, NJ: Lawrence Erlbaum, pp. 197–216.

Ricoeur, P. (1984). Narrative time. *Critical Inquiry, 7*, 169–190.

Schell, R., & Tudiver, F. (2004). Barriers to cancer screening by rural Appalachian primary care providers. *The Journal of Rural Health, 20*, 368–373.

Sharf, B.F. (1993). Reading the vital signs: Research in health care communication. *Communication Monographs, 60*, 35–41.

Smith, S.L., & Tessaro, I.A. (2005). Cultural perspectives on diabetes in an Appalachian population. *American Journal of Health Behavior, 29*, 291–301.

Stacy, R.D. (1996). *Complexity and Creativity in Organizations*. San Francisco: Berrett-Koehler.

Zabos, G.P., & Trinh, C. (2001). Bringing the mountain to Mohammed: A mobile dental team serves a community-based program for people with HIV/AIDS. *American Journal of Public Health, 91*, 1187–1189.

Zoller, H.M. (2005). Health activism: Communication theory and action for social change. *Communication Theory, 15*, 341–364.

Chapter 15

The paradox of pharmaceutical empowerment

Healthology and online health public relations[1]

Ashli Quesinberry Stokes

A spoonful of public relations helps the medicine go down.
(*British Medical Journal*, May 2003)

Today public relations plays an increasingly important role in promoting the products of the pharmaceutical industry. Many are familiar with pharmaceutical advertising, which attempts to create a positive emotional connection with consumers by buying space in a medium to directly connect a product with a specific company. Public relations, however, creates a positive relationship between a corporation and consumer in a more indirect manner. It frequently employs the "third-party technique" to engage in its media relations practices. Here someone outside of a pharmaceutical company, typically a journalist or medical professional, reviews a product or service. The external, hopefully positive, review helps to give drug companies credibility, as a promotional message is separated from the promoter in a variety of newsmedia. That is, if a pharmaceutical company either defends or promotes one if its own products, it "would have much less credibility than if an opinion leader or a prescriber said it" (Burton & Rowell, 2003. p. 1205). With the more subtle influence of public relations, news stories about a particular drug or issue "just seem to emerge spontaneously, usually with no obvious connection to a commercial source" (Abramson, 2004, p. 159). Indeed, these techniques are becoming popular ways of influencing both public opinion and health policy, earning health-care public relations firms more than $300 million in 2002.

There are dangers in using a third party source to carry a corporation's message. Journalistic and medical gatekeepers may ignore important information when publishing news about a particular product. Given that consumers are more likely to find information received through media gatekeepers more credible, the reliance on the third-party technique thus carries potentially negative implications for consumers making health decisions, obscuring the promotional intent underlying the seemingly credible health information (Catlett, 2003). Abramson (2004) cautions about public relations' covert commercial influence, pointing out that "at least with advertising, the fundamentally commercial purpose of the message is clear" (p. 159). This subtlety means that public relations' own role in supporting particular health-care interests has been overlooked. The omission is significant, as up to 90 percent of health and medical news originates from third-party techniques (Corbett & Mori, 1999).

This chapter investigates the important role public relations plays in shaping health beliefs and behaviors by examining Healthology, a leading third-party health website content provider sponsored by a variety of pharmaceutical companies. Healthology supplies physician-generated health and wellness information to approximately 4,000 websites (Healthology.com). Its clients include Pfizer, Bristol Myers Squibb, Inamed, Schering Plough, Novartis, and Astra-Zeneca. Although Healthology's websites may provide consumers with valuable information, I argue that their simultaneous use of empowering language for promotional purposes may help shape a more pharmaceutically empowered audience identity, or perception of the self, that carries negative implications in terms of health citizenship. Paradoxically, consumers may use Healthology to empower themselves, but they receive information that stresses certain products, treatments, and worldviews over others. The very information that helps to empower may simultaneously commodify them. To illustrate the emergence of this paradoxical identity, I first explain the relationship between pharmaceutical promotion, constitutive approaches to public relations, and empowerment, thereby theoretically grounding the chapter. I then describe my rhetorical methodology and Healthology's websites. By analyzing their textual components, I show how they draw on empowerment rhetoric to craft this pharmaceutically influenced identity. I consider finally the implications of online pharmaceutical public relations, arguing that its empowerment discourse commodifies conceptions of identity when it comes to health.

Theorizing health on "empowerment.com"

Pharmaceutical promotion

Pharmaceutical promotion has become more sophisticated and pervasive over the last decade. As a result of a 1997 landmark guidance by the Food and Drug Administration (FDA), pharmaceutical marketers could more directly target the public through a variety of media. Once only able to target physicians, the approval of direct to consumer (DTC) prescription drug marketing allowed television, print, radio, and the web to offer product-specific, prescription-drug advertising. These ads are ubiquitous, with consumers learning that Zyrtec, to use a familiar example, can help them deal with their seasonal allergies. Proponents of DTC advertising argue that consumers have easy access to information about new treatments and are more likely to comply with current treatments and make better-informed decisions as a result of the practice (Bradley & Zito, 1997; Holmer, 2001). Proponents also claim that such a site "empowers the patients, addresses the problems of underdiagnosis and undertreatment, and increases the dialogue between doctors and patients" (in Teinowitz, 1999, p. 55). Critics argue the practice drives up medical costs, increases reliance on prescription drugs, and disempowers the patient–physician relationship (Hoffman & Wilkes, 1999; Wilkes et al., 2000; Abramson, 2004). As DTC has been given a green light for the foreseeable future by the FDA in 2004, these debates are likely to continue.

In fact, arguments about product-specific advertising may increase because of "eDTC," the online component of DTC advertising. Eight out of ten U.S. citizens with internet access use the Web to get health information and 70 percent of consumers report that online health information influences their health decisions. As a result, pharmaceutical marketing's promotional Web presence can potentially figure prominently in how consumers manage their health (Fox, 2005; Horrigan & Rainie, 2002). Indeed, two of the four main ways consumers can find health information online potentially involve commercial interests. Patients can visit websites sponsored by the pharmaceutical industry; for example, lipitor.com, disease society sites such as the American Heart Association, the FDA itself, and third-party medical information sites, such as WedMD, RxList, and Healthology (Goldhammer, 2004). The FDA has not created specific guidelines for online promotion, except to state that pharmaceutical companies *can* partner with third-party "content" producers to offer consumers more information about different illnesses and treatments. As a result, Healthology's eDTC campaigns adapt the classic public relations' third-party technique to the information age environment. As opposed to ads that openly tout a particular drug for dealing with a health problem, Healthology's focus on a physician's discussion of a condition, its symptoms, and available treatment information distinguishes it from traditional DTC advertising. Its subtle public relations techniques perhaps more strongly shape consumer identities that support a pharmaceutical, corporate orientation toward health.

Constitutive theoretical approaches

Although scholars explore the impact of both DTC and eDTC on consumer purchasing decisions, they are just now beginning to examine how such corporate discourse influences individual identities by constituting and constraining such identities (Bradley & Zito, 1997; Teinowitz, 1999). Public health is socially and culturally constructed and is influenced by political, economic, and social forces (Lupton, 1995). As a result, pharmaceutical campaigns can shape how audiences think and talk about a variety of issues. They deserve a theoretical perspective that recognizes that they offer a "way of seeing, a method of ordering or judging, or a means of selection and preference" that encourages, but not dictates, the way consumers may begin to think about health (Lupton, 1995; Sholle, 1989; Stokes, 2005; Cheney & Vibbert, 1987; German, 1995). Just as the medical profession provides certain socially accepted ways of thinking about illness and health, public relations' promotional economic discourses also "serve as routes through which we understand, think and talk about, and live our bodies" (Lupton, 1995, p. 6). Indeed, promotional public relations language, like other types of discourse, has a taken for granted quality where people may "define themselves and their beliefs without realizing that the words they use are not necessarily their own" (Elwood, 1995, p. 7). As Deetz (1992) explains, organizational messages broadly produce personal identity, values, knowledge, and reasoning by shaping our subjectivities, or our senses of self. Scholars should therefore examine how health public relations texts are not value free or neutral but instead privilege certain corporate values, interests, and types of knowledge (Lupton, 1995).

One way to understand this process is through the use of a constitutive theoretical perspective. Scholars employing a constitutive framework are particularly interested in this process of how people are, in effect, created by and utilize the discourse with which they identify, or relate. Burke (1950) begins these constitutive lines of inquiry by arguing that identification is more important in rhetorical discourse than persuasion. Charland (1987), along with Burke, argues that it is incorrect to assume that a person's identity is extrarhetorical, existing as a given before one encounters forms of persuasion. People are called into being by rhetorical documents; indeed, they are not only persuaded by rhetoric but find their subjectivities and language shaped by its influence (Jasinski, 1998; Duquette Smith, 2000; Stein, 2002). Healthology's health information websites draw on a variety of tropes and particular idioms to allow people to conceive of health issues and decisions in a particular way (Jasinski, 1997, 1998). So, if "treating illness" is construed repeatedly as "taking prescription drugs," or engaging in "medical treatments," alternative understandings may be constrained. Constitutive criticism can thus help examine how online public relations discourse frames perceptions, as well as expectations, about healthcare.

Constitutive theoretical approaches thus reveal and critique the impact of public relations on the creation of identities. Although we are subject to many conflicting discourses today, promotional corporate discourse is a major productive text (Deetz, 1992). The subtle influence of promotional corporate discourse, particularly in terms of "below the radar" public relations messages, can make it less likely that people question corporate motives. And, although public interaction with a variety of texts cannot guarantee the creation of a particular corporate, or other type, of identity, texts do make it "easier" for audiences to read a particular meaning over another (Condit 1994). Audiences may not necessarily critically examine the messages they consume. With constitutive rhetorical criticism, "we are concerned not simply with the text . . . but with what that text is saying in the culture. Also, what kind of culture are we creating by that particular text?" (Mickey, 1997, p. 282). Public relations helps develop a culture in which corporations play a more central role in helping patients manage, maintain, or achieve health.

Constituting the empowered patient

Understanding public relations' ability to create a particular health culture is particularly important in light of the societal trend of lauding the empowered patient and celebrating information access as empowering. Relying on empowering rhetoric for promotional purposes conflicts with the idea of patient empowerment that has become a key principle in the field of public health (Masi et al., 2003). Healthology's websites are paradoxical because consumer empowerment may objectify or commodify rather than empower patients (Pires et al., 2006). The concept of patient empowerment in the health communication literature contrasts with its discussion in the marketing literature, and creates a tension in claiming that Healthology's websites are empowering.

In the health communication literature, empowered health consumers achieve health citizenship, thereby increasingly involving themselves in individual and collective decision making about health-care decisions (Dutta-Bergman, 2005, p. 1; Dutta-Bergman, 2004b; Rimal et al., 1997; Zoller, 2005). These responsible, active, and motivated individuals seek out information and resources to enhance health, sometimes seeking information beyond a doctor and engaging in healthy behaviors (Dutta-Bergman, 2005; Rimal et al., 1997). In essence, empowered individuals are likely to have "high levels of control over their everyday lives" and are more likely to "take control of their health" (Dutta-Bergman, 2004b, p. 395; Campbell & Jovchelovitch, 2000, p. 262). Empowered health citizens are given, or take, the tools to exercise more control over their lives (Pacanowsky, 1988). To do so, they need increased information access, which is necessary for developing new partnership relationships between health-care providers and patients (Henwood et al., 2003; Masi et al., 2003). Empowered patients use information to redistribute medical power and accept responsibility for increased knowledge, adequately cope with health situations, and move beyond beliefs of self-efficacy to actively participating in the decision-making process (Gutierrez, 1990; Pacanowsky, 1988; Conger & Kanugo, 1988; Roberts, 1999; Masi et al., 2003). In terms of individual public health, feelings of empowerment are crucial, that is, patients who are empowered combine increased knowledge of a condition with the confidence to act (Gutierrez, 1990; Pacanowsky, 1998; Conger & Kanugo, 1988; Roberts, 1999; Masi et al., 2003).

The internet's array of information is considered to be a promising source for boosting empowered health citizenship, but can be co-opted by commercial interests (Ferguson, 1997; Eysenbach, 2000). On the one hand, internet use leads to greater health consciousness, which is in turn positively associated with health information seeking (Dutta-Bergman, 2005). Further, since the internet provides consumers with information sources beyond the doctor, it can reach the health-active segment of the population and inform health conscious individuals about different preventions and treatments (Dutta-Bergman,

2004a). Access to online health information has been shown to empower low-income community members, HIV-positive individuals, and women interested in hormone replacement therapy (Masi et al., 2003; Henwood et al., 2003; Reeves, 2000).

Pharmaceutical marketing, however, also capitalizes on the tendency for the health active segment of the population to utilize the internet. Marketers view consumer empowerment as a business structural change that they cannot afford to ignore because its popularity is beneficial toward improved business results (Wright et al., 2006). In marketing, consumer empowerment is viewed as "cutting edge" because it anticipates customer wants and expectations (ibid.). Consumer empowerment involves helping consumers "choose what they want, when they want it, on their own terms" (Turquist, 2004, p. 939). Although marketing's adoption of an empowering approach does not necessarily exploit customers, a paradox emerges. Consumers are offered more control over their health but their decisions and choices are delimited or restricted by corporate rhetorical devices. That is, "while cited as consumer empowerment, what consumers are allowed to do is determined, regulated, and controlled by the supplier" (Pires et al., 2006, p. 939). Further, as consumers interact with these marketing practices, they may construct and reconstruct their identities accordingly (Markus & Nurius, 1986). As a result, the industry's power over health decisions may increase in ways that rhetorical criticism helps examine.

Healthology

Healthology cannot be seen as *just* a consumer health-care information resource. It generates revenue primarily from sponsorship and production by charging its customers, most of which are pharmaceutical and health-care companies, for the creation, production, and distribution of health-related content and streaming media (McCormick, 2005). Additionally, Healthology derives revenue through the electronic distribution of its newsletters that help drive traffic to client sites (ibid.). According to its CEO, Healthology's websites are positioned as primarily educational, and not promotional, resources as the information is targeted to medical professionals and consumers for educational purposes (ibid.). McCormick emphasizes the educational goal of Healthology by noting that the content is "mostly" generated by physicians and/or accredited medical societies. As a result, the company claims these sites offer consumers quality, trustworthy health programs while offering a unique marketing solution because its content is produced in consultation with more than 20,000 licensed, practicing physicians.[2] The company takes pains to notify potential "sponsors" (i.e. pharmaceutical companies) that acceptance of "educational grants" (i.e. sponsorships) in no way indicates Healthology's endorsement of a company's products or services. Healthology also argues that its peer-review process creates content that is used on more websites that any other source. In essence, Healthology capitalizes on the third-party technique because although its sites may discuss a particular product more than others or suggest a client's particular treatment, doctors, not pharmaceutical companies, suggest ways to deal with a condition. Healthology's peer-review stamp, however, does not allow it to escape negative evaluation (Arnold, 2005). The company, like some other users of the third-party technique, has been criticized for blurring the line between promotion and education because consumers may or may not realize the source of the information (Arnold, 2005; Pear, 2004).

On any of its websites, consumers choose from a content library offering 1,200 streaming videos and 2,000 articles and transcripts featuring journalists interviewing doctors about a particular health issue. Consumers can also sign up for health newsletters through email, participate in chat rooms, and access other editorial features. Healthology is available through search engines such as Yahoo or Google, is linked to the websites of many large newspapers such as *Miami Herald* and the *Los Angeles Times*, and is available through web portals such as Ivillage.com. Using any of these methods, if a Web user is interested in arthritis or cancer treatment, for example, they can visit sites such as "arthritisanswers.org" or "cancerinfo.com."

Healthology websites address a wide spectrum of diseases and conditions, including men's and women's health, a variety of types of cancer, gastro-intestinal, mental, cardio, skin, and sexual health. The websites also address various other illnesses and conditions. Particular topic sites are created through a process where doctors decide what areas need to be covered, then confer with pharmaceutical advertisers who might have an interest in making sure there is particular information available, and then Healthology's network of roughly 20,000 physicians create the content (McCormick, 2005).

Methodology: analyzing Healthology through rhetorical criticism

The rhetorical criticism offered here investigates how empowerment rhetoric functions paradoxically on Healthology's websites. The method helps describe, analyze, interpret, and evaluate the persuasive, and sometimes subtle, uses of its constitutive language (Hart, 1990; Campbell & Burkholder, 1997). By examining the order and preference of some interpretations of Healthology's information, I examined how the sites help shape knowledge about health care and subject positions that correspond to that domain (Sholle 1989). I explored what some of the unintended consequences of these online texts might be and what types of audience identities their language choices encouraged. The *key words, metaphors, themes, narratives*, and *images* were identified among a set of Healthology websites (Berkowitz, 2003; Condit, 1994). In doing so, I explored the major themes, hidden contradictions, and ways that commercial interests are served by this particular discourse (Condit, 1994).

Since it appears that different levels of corporate sponsorship exist in Healthology, only those websites marked as sponsored through "unrestricted educational grants" were examined. These sites practice the third-party technique and offer textual evidence of doctors subtly supporting the particular client sponsor's treatments over others. Indeed, on many, the website would contain a link to the particular pharmaceutical company sponsoring the website, with the product discussed on the Healthology website also featured on the client site. I analyzed sponsored Healthology webcasts addressing a variety of types of cancer, irritable bowel syndrome, overactive bladder, allergies, and weight loss on sites named: TargetTumors.com, IBS-help.com, advancesinoncology.com, oabrelief.com, breastcancer-answers.com, and weightfocus.com. I thus explored discourse about diseases and conditions with varying levels of severity and duration (although "unrestricted educational grant" websites are found within most of Healthology's topic libraries).

Analyzing Healthology's pharmaceutically supported websites

The websites' content fell under three major themes that support the creation of a more pharmaceutically empowered, not patient empowered, identity. The websites 1) used scientific/medical language for promotional purposes, 2) favored particular pharmaceutical treatments, and 3) encouraged a commercial worldview in approaching health. Examining each of the three themes shows how empowering discourse employed by the sites acts in specifically commercial ways. Although each theme performs specifically, the rhetoric's strength comes from the way in which the themes interact, because if support for one theme is granted, approval for the dominant, overarching theme of pharmaceutical consumer empowerment can result (Perelman & Olbrechts Tyteca, 2000, p. 81). Since empowerment is a flexible concept, it performs as a type of condensation symbol, subsuming each of these themes within it (Graber, 1976; Hales, 1999). Although Healthology visitors can interact with lifestyle, condition, and treatment information on these sites, the prevalence of each of these three themes may empower audiences to begin to view prescriptions and pharmaceutical companies as primary in managing health instead of seeing them as part of an overall health-care philosophy. We should ask where this more privileged identity might take us in terms of overall patient empowerment. One way to begin is by exploring how the websites rely on medical/scientific authority to promote products.

Promoting products through medical/scientific authority

To capitalize on consumers' desire for health education, Healthology's websites incorporate medical/scientific authority language that may help consumers feel more in control of their disease or condition because they can "learn from the experts" about their symptoms and possible treatments. The language of medical/scientific authority increases the websites' credibility. Examining two sub-themes shows how this reliance on medical authority also helps subtly promote products.

Promoting through medical novelty

Pharmaceutical empowerment rhetoric focuses on providing visitors with the newest, most innovative information regarding treatment options and research. This language emphasizing novelty, however, may suggest that traditional treatments are inadequate and privilege newer and costlier prescription treatments over previous approaches. Here, consumers are encouraged to feel as if they have access to the same sort of information as health experts. On the TargetTumors.com site, for example, a specific type of drug treatment is discussed as being the newest option for treating cancer: "Targeted cancer therapies, which attack cancer cells in unique and precise ways, are an important part of oncology's *cutting edge*."[3] Similarly, the IBS-help.com (irritable bowel syndrome) site talks of how "researchers have *recently* made major advances" and the site "will keep you *up-to-date*" on the latest developments in treatment. Although it may be the case that consumers *are* learning about the newest treatments, this language does more than notify them of treatment developments. All of these language choices bring the audience closer to the inner "medical circle" and create a sense of being informed and current, just as they expect their doctors to be. As a result, readers may feel more confident asking their doctors for a particular treatment because they feel aware of the most current options available. The emphasis on novelty also may help consumers who think there is no help available feel more optimistic in seeking treatment options. For example, transcripts note that there are "a lot of solutions" to overactive bladder and tell audiences that, "you *can* find an effective medical therapy. There are lots of different types of medical therapies *now* and some that can just be given as a once a day formulation." Although this information may motivate consumers, it also suggests that treating illness means using the latest prescription treatment.

Promoting through scientific credibility

In addition to favoring newer, perhaps costlier products, consumers are assured they are being provided with quality scientific information to help make decisions. The scientific language in which the program transcripts are written conveys a feeling of authority that imparts credibility. These transcripts assume a level of familiarity and most contain a good deal of complexity, which seems to suggest that the content producers are targeting those consumers who already have a working knowledge of a disease. The reader would need to have some knowledge of the differing types of cancer for the following exchange to make sense:

SALLIE GLANER: Doctor, how are neuroendocrine tumors different from the more common types of cancer, say, breast cancer? LOWELL ANTHONY, MD: Well, neuroendocrine tumors overexpress, oversecrete hormonal products which are not common in breast cancer, lung cancer, or colon cancer. And these hormonal products may be related to serotonins or it could be peptides that are secreted.

Although the doctor's differentiation would probably be unclear to some visitors, these exchanges impart credibility because the doctors clearly demonstrate their expertise.

These sites also try to assure consumers by frequently mentioning many scientific studies but not discussing their status in credible medical research. For example, the IBS site says in a number of its transcripts, "Several good studies over the last few years have shown," and "research has shed light," without discussing the origin and credibility of this information. Similarly, statistics are often used in this way, with visitors encountering statements such as "anywhere between 7 and 30 percent of individuals with IBS will report they had previous proven bacterial gastroenteritis" (ibs-help.com). Visitors are offered the appearance of medical authority by the volume of these statements, rather than by their credibility within the medical field. Even the site names and URLs are designed to promote the websites as educational resources. For example, ibs-help.com, targettumors.org, and advancesinoncology.com all convey a place to learn about a condition, not one that is focused on sales. By using these naming strategies, the sites are differentiated from Healthology, their content producer, but more importantly, they are distanced from the companies who make the products discussed on the sites.

In addition, the websites are positioned as repositories of consumer health education that may boost their credibility with consumers. Each claims to be the primary education center on the Web for a particular condition. The IBS Help website, for example, bills itself as "your online destination for essential information on IBS." On targettumors.com, the homepage states, "Whether you are seeking information for yourself or a loved one, Target Tumors will provide you with the information you need." In all cases, sites are positioned as resources that individuals can use to find answers to their health questions. They are addressed specifically to those most interested in seeking help— either those afflicted with or affected by the disease. This ability helps to differentiate eDTC sites from traditional DTC commercials. Since consumer interest is already established, the educational, rather than promotional, nature of the site is maintained. Pharmaceutical empowerment rhetoric thus downplays the sales initiative and may help consumers trust the content. After all, studies have shown that consumers do not fully trust traditional DTC advertisements for completely and accurately conveying information because of its commercial basis (Henwood et al., 2003; Herzenstein et al., 2004; Wilkie, 2005). Healthology's educational third-party approach encourages consumer trust.

With both of these sub-themes at work, a more pharmaceutically empowered audience identity may develop as consumers educate themselves. The medical information received may be empowering, but it also strengthens the primacy of pharmaceutical companies in the medical structure. For example, on a site dedicated to breast cancer, visitors learn: "The survival rate for breast cancer has improved over the years, due in part to earlier detection, but also because of better treatments. See how hormonal treatments have helped women with certain types of breast cancer live longer with the disease." Women are encouraged to learn more about hormonal pharmaceutical treatments, rather than being empowered to learn about the causes of breast cancer or what they can do to reduce their chances of developing the disease. This site does not mention the controversial nature of hormonal treatments for breast cancer, and it does not discuss environmental and even pharmaceutical causes of breast cancer (Ehrenreich, 2001). As some scholars argue that interventions against breast cancer have done little to change the death rate since the 1930s, understanding environmental causes may be necessary to change this pattern (ibid.). However, because the field of information is delimited, audiences may become empowered to act with pharmaceutically based information more in mind and ignore this issue.

Promoting particular treatments or products

The sites rely on medical/scientific authority to subtly sell products and treatments, and their efforts to promote particular products build on this authority. Gobé (2002) suggests that as pharmaceutical companies move toward a more consumer-product mode more available to them as a result of the softening of FDA regulations, they need to be more sensitive and responsive to people's needs. By relying on subtle promotion that continues to emphasize the value of medical/scientific information, marketers can more easily create the perception of customer sensitivity in their promotional strategies. If a company presents product information to educate the consumer, it is not just trying to sell a pill. Indeed, as Gobé (2002) states, "The idea here is to create a relationship with the consumer through education, with the focus on consumers and their needs and experiences—as opposed to pushing the product itself" (p. 66). This strategy is realized on Healthology's eDTC sites in two ways.

Promoting particular products

A common, if subtle, practice on the sites finds physicians favoring drugs produced by the sponsor of a particular health website topic. For example, doctors will discuss a variety of treatments and rely on a particular drug as representative of that option. There are exchanges like the following:

BRETT SCOTT: Dr. Connors, there are a number of different types of targeted therapies for cancer? What are they? And how do they work? JOSEPH CONNORS, MD: I think of them in two broad types . . . (goes on to explain in detail what the types are) . . . BRETT SCOTT: Dr. Druker, *Gleevec* has received a lot of press lately. What class does it fall into and how does it work?

In these exchanges, the doctor featured in the webcast will go on to explain why the featured drug works in treating the discussed disease.

Doctors also will discuss an entire class of treatments as being effective, yet highlight one by noting its performance in patient trials or touting its advantages over the other treatments. When Claritin became available over the counter in 2002, Schering Plough's educationally sponsored allergy site offered:

ANNOUNCER: Many consumers seek out the over the counter oral antihistamines like Benadryl, Chlor-Trimeton, and Dimetapp. MARION RICHMAN, MD: Over the counter antihistamines are effective, probably just as effective as the prescription ones, *but they have that very serious side effect of making people sleepy.* ANNOUNCER: Some physicians caution their patients against using these sedating medications for their potential safety risks they pose. *But recently, a non-sedating antihistamine, Claritin, has become available over the counter.*

By introducing specific products or treatments within the context of a more generalized exchange about treatments, the doctors remain authoritative, rather than overtly promotional, while simultaneously promoting a specific pharmaceutical product. This technique has advanced beyond a commercial declaring, "four out of five doctors choose product X."

Promoting through subtle product comparison

Interestingly, doctors will support two different drugs if both are made by pharmaceutical companies who rely on Healthology to produce Webcasts featuring journalists interviewing doctors about their particular products or health issues. For example, Femara is made by Novartis while Arimidex is made by Astra-Zeneca, both Healthology clients. In these cases, after the relative merits of both are discussed, consumers see the following:

HYMAN MUSS, MD: I think, by and large, all these compounds are extremely well tolerated . . . I would say that there probably aren't any convincing studies to me of patient preferences that I would use to select one over the other.

In general, this subtly promotional tactic helps Webcasts to not appear overly self-interested. Another example of this practice is seen in a discussion of leukemia drugs. Although Gleevec is produced by Novartis, a Healthology client, doctors also discuss the potential of a newer, potentially competing drug in other leukemia programs. For patients who develop resistance to Gleevec, we find this exchange about another option, produced by another "educational grant" supporter, Bristol Myers Squibb:

> ANNOUNCER: It was a Phase II trial, testing high doses of Gleevec against a new drug called dasatinib . . . Betty was randomly assigned to the new drug, and the initial results were quite good. NEIL SHAH, MD, PhD: . . . And she subsequently has had bone marrow biopsies which have shown a complete cytogenetic remission, which is *really very exciting*, that we can take patients who otherwise have very few options to control their disease and get it back into a remission state *that's pretty much as good as anything Gleevec could accomplish.*

This practice is seen on several of the educationally sponsored websites, though the product-specific promotion described previously is more common. Both themes demonstrate that consumers are exposed to seemingly objective information that favors certain products over others.

Promoting a pharmaceutical worldview

With the previous themes at work, consumers may learn the names of particular products and ask their physicians for a particular treatment. These sites also generally support a more pharmaceutically based worldview where consumers may consider pharmaceutical companies' information to be the most important in how they understand their health. Instead of viewing health as comprised of many elements and/or choosing to achieve health in non-pharmaceutical ways, consumers may see pharmaceuticals as the primary way they should achieve empowered health citizenship.

Reassuring consumers to confront conditions

Webcasts focus on reassuring consumers that they should feel confident in confronting an illness or condition that is empowering to the patient; however, they are empowered in a commercial direction. Encouraging words, along with providing a supportive and trusting group atmosphere, empower individuals and reassure them they are not alone (Pacanowsky, 1988). This technique is found on the IBS site and others:

> They're scared to see a doctor. They're worried they're going to get bad news; many of these patients are very concerned their symptoms represent

cancer. They're embarrassed to talk about their symptoms. They're worried that there won't be any treatment for their symptoms. And so, many of these patients kind of remain hidden and remain undiagnosed.

By showing users that their fears of confronting the illness are common, these emotional statements reassure users that they should address the problem.

Transcripts are also interspersed with personal stories to retain user interest and identification, or common ground, between consumer and webcast presenters. This tactic works in two ways. Visitors will encounter a typical patient's experience with the drug or they will learn how a professional dealt with the disease. Either way, seeing how others benefit from beginning treatment may reduce anxiety. After discussing how he used to treat cancer patients before he became afflicted with the disease, a doctor on a cancer site notes,

> And since then, I've dealt with hundreds, and hundreds of people with cancer. And I understand what they're going through now. I didn't at the time. It's just not easy to describe the feeling you have, of fear and helplessness, and that you have to deal with it.

When "Bill" offers his support for bisphosphonates drugs, his enthusiasm, but in particular, his experience with a particular treatment, is then more persuasive. By treating the disease in human terms, consumers are reassured again that their anxiety over an illness is expected. These strategies are particularly powerful when they draw on a fellow sufferer's experience. In an overactive bladder transcript, for example, one woman says,

> THERESA ROCHE: If I was going to be out in the park walking, I knew I had to wear a Depends. And if I was going some place to the supermarket, I knew every bathroom in every supermarket. I thought it was the normal part of aging. (oabrelief.com)

These statements legitimize conversation about a subject. As Gobé (2002) notes about their use in discussing men's health issues, for example, these types of statements "gives [sic] men who are often reluctant to address this issue permission to do so" (p. 66).

Encouraging words also reassure visitors to act on the knowledge received from the sites. In most webcasts, the announcer and the featured doctor work together to encourage users to visit a doctor and get the reward of better health. On the IBS site, for example, consumers see or listen to the following exchange:

> ANNOUNCER: While the causes of IBS remain unknown, doctors can provide a great deal of help. In fact, one of their key messages to people

suffering from gastrointestinal disorders is: don't try to go it alone. BRIAN LACY, MD: As a physician, one of the frustrating things I find about IBS is that oftentimes patients with chronic symptoms don't see a doctor. And I think that we need to educate patients better about that to get them to come in so we can reassure them. And to let them know there are now medications available that can improve their symptoms and improve their quality of life.

This language allows the doctor's expertise to motivate the user and is not the same as the advertising practice of showing a product and saying "ask your doctor." These exchanges focus more on the doctor serving as a counselor positioned on the healthcare team. By creating a team discourse among doctors, patients, and products, pharmaceutical empowerment rhetoric encourages a "we" attitude between patients and health-care providers (Pacanowksy, 1988). Pharmaceutical empowerment rhetoric thus reduces the distance between health-care participants. Note, however, that the doctor emphasizes medication rather than lifestyle changes to deal with the particular condition.

As a result, the pattern of reassuring language employed here may be cause for concern. The emphasis on these sites is to reassure consumers to do something, but most of the time, the "doing something" culminates in receiving pharmaceutical treatment. Healthology implies that treatment is not comprehensive unless a prescription undergirds behavioral or alternative methods.

Equating pharmaceutical treatments with "normalcy"

With reassurance in place, patients are ultimately encouraged to visit a doctor about their respective pharmaceutical treatment options. One way the sites try to encourage people is through playing on the desire to become "normal" again. For example, the IBS site states on the homepage, "Let IBS Help improve your ability to manage and cope with this condition—and get your life back." Meanwhile, an overactive bladder site's transcript encourages: "So if you're one of the many people who are suffering needlessly from overactive bladder, talk to your doctor today because regaining control means winning back your freedom." This tactic subtly suggests *not* acting to fix a health condition keeps one from becoming "normal" like everyone else. Relying on "I thought I had to put up with this" examples tells the visitor that putting up with the condition is *ab*normal. To suffer from creaking joints, sexual dysfunction, or frequent bathroom trips means that one is not empowered by knowledge like everyone else. This form of pressure shows how a person is lacking (here's how to fix that little sexual malfunction) but tells the consumer that they have access to numerous pharmaceutical sources to fix the problem. In fact, not seeking treatment results in a variety of unpleasant social consequences; for example, "IBS is a disease where not seeking treatment comes at a high cost, both in terms of the patient's quality of life and the pocketbook. There are patients who pass up promotions, because they can't travel. They pass up social events. They miss their kids' soccer games and things." Again, while this may be true, subtle pressure makes *medical* treatment almost an obligation of the consumer if he or she wants to be empowered. Pharmaceutical companies just make meeting that demand easier and/or more comfortable.

A large number of the educationally supported websites examined follow this pattern. Doctors discuss how a given condition makes a patient suffer abnormally, a patient then offers his/her story, and then the participants note that prescription, medical treatments regain normalcy. From IBD products, to allergy discussions, to even cancer treatments, doctors frequently reflect that before the product/surgery/medical treatment, their patients had "forgotten what normal life was all about. Now they have a normal life and they're so grateful for it." Variations of this program pattern are seen almost in every transcript. It thus becomes "normal" to think of the pharmaceutical industry when faced with a health issue; the pharmaceutical industry and its products are attributed the magical quality of restoring life to normalcy that was otherwise disrupted by the disease.

These language choices also emphasize undergoing medical treatments rather than engaging in health behaviors, which ironically may disempower consumers, particularly to the degree that patients do not "do something" but have something done to them. The sites may encourage audiences to become objects of treatment. Instead of changing their diet, or exercising more, these language choices suggest that acting to take charge of health correlates with acting to receive pharmaceutical treatment. Indeed, it is rare that the very powerful, but differently empowered, position of rejecting treatment is presented as an active choice; instead, the site treats this choice only as an avoidance mechanism. As Fuqua (2002) observes, such language "reinforces the already existing idea that the patient/consumer is in a state of need and that this need can be met through medical advice, and most importantly, consumption of a particular prescription drug" (p. 664). Overall, then, these texts pharmaceutically empower the consumer by helping them view health through a framework that stresses products and simultaneously disempowers them by locating them as subjects of the biomedical gaze. Each theme points to the next, and if they are accepted, there is really only one choice to be made: see a doctor for this particular treatment and take charge of your health.

Conclusion and implications

Analyzing Healthology's discourse reveals that using empowerment language for promotional purposes offers marketers several rhetorical advantages. Third-party eDTC provides the pharmaceutical industry with opportunities to supply consumers with potentially empowering experiences that concurrently support corporate objectives. From a constitutive theoretical perspective, however, these types of experiences may reinforce the *industry*'s power, rather than working to truly empower patients. A constitutive perspective allows us to reflect on the ways in which eDTC campaigns such as Healthology's subtly encourage paradoxical patient identities. The analysis offered here reveals the simultaneously disempowering role of seemingly empowering rhetoric.

First, pharmaceutical empowerment rhetoric helps produce consumers who may take control of illness by assuming responsibility for a particular pharmaceutical treatment. Pharmaceutical marketers claim that today's consumers are empowered because the power that previously resided in the doctor's realm of authority has been extended to the patient. But note that much of the content analyzed here suggests that consumers may act on this increased power by accepting that a treatment needs to be done *to* them, rather than doing something for themselves. It is paradoxical, then, that some consumers might be empowered to be more passive as subjects of the pharmaceutical industry.

In addition, Healthology's brand of empowerment rarely leaves the medical and corporate realms, demonstrating the intertwined nature of medical and corporate interests. To be pharmaceutically empowered means getting a particular medical treatment that is produced by a corporation. Although Healthology includes lifestyle and nonprescription treatment information, this content is lower in the discussion hierarchy. Scholars should continue to explore if and how pharmaceutically sponsored websites are helping to create a general culture that privileges pharmaceutical medical treatments. Fuqua (2002) argues, for example, that the United States is cultivating a culture that encourages a normative health practice and a "medical perception of the self and everyday life" (p. 651).

It is not that these sites offer necessarily inferior information or encourage poor health behaviors. Indeed, eDTC empowerment rhetoric may constitute parts of consumer patient identity in a positive way. Illnesses increase feelings of uncertainty and bring new responsibilities and the need for new skills and guidelines. Resolving feelings of powerlessness and helping the patient cope with and control these feelings, then, is empowering. When empowered, patients gain a "can do" attitude where they feel they can be effective in executing a desired behavior and believe they can control their decisions more effectively (Conger & Kanugo, 1988, p. 477).

Yet, full ownership of a disease or illness requires adequate resources to make informed choices and decisions. In addition to considering whether these sites prevent consumers from exploring fully their options, we should consider whether these information choices are even accessible to those with either limited health literacy or resources. Pharmaceutical empowerment rhetoric may further marginalize certain audiences in terms of health care. To even participate in online pharmaceutical empowerment rhetoric requires access to a computer. Those without may be left out because, "those individuals in society who have the most resources have the best chance of becoming empowered" (Roberts, 1999, p. 86). These sites may reinforce the consumerism that makes health a commodity sold to those with the ability to buy, and that creates the belief that we are free to choose our treatments (Fuqua, 2002, pp. 660–663). For some, this may not be the case. Reference to a person's economic status or cultural resistance to a particular treatment is absent in the discourse. Healthology does not mention how someone may afford such treatments or the potential problems they may encounter when trying to pursue them. Further, those with limited media literacy may not be able to access, understand and evaluate, or apply the information provided on Healthology appropriately (Bernhardt et al., 2002). These websites may help instantiate a particular media grammar consumers need to understand in order to even glean helpful information. Meyrowitz (1998) argues, for example, that comprehensive media literacy requires understanding and recognizing each medium's unique grammar. Health empowerment becomes a trickier challenge when we recognize that audiences visiting these sites may not possess all of the needed skills (Meyrowitz, 2002, p. 107). Indeed, they may not even want to "take charge" of their health, as "many patients do not want to take responsibility or seek out information for themselves" (Hoek & Gendall, 2002, p. 71).

Ultimately, then, pharmaceutical empowerment rhetoric may constitute elements of identity paradoxically, shaping how we feel and talk about health care. With the introduction of Prozac, for example, it became more acceptable in society to talk about treating depression, yet this potential benefit is undercut by overpromotion. For example, after Paxil promotions, media references to "social anxiety disorder" increased from fifty in 1998 to one billion in 1999 (in Gobé, 2002, p. 65). As people participate in the rhetoric of pharmaceutical empowerment, similar patterns emerge. Consumers are encouraged to consider health-care options from a corporate perspective.

Public audiences are not simple dupes, but they are influenced in varying degrees by the discourse that surrounds them (Condit, 2001). We are increasingly encircled by the vested interests of the pharmaceutical industry (Jack, 2006; Griffith & Wiegand, 2005). The industry creates campaigns like the Boomer Coalition, a phony organization created by Pfizer's public relations agency in support of its cholesterol drug. Ten out of twenty-three members of the National Sleep Foundations have financial ties to sleeping pill manufacturers. In 2002, drug firms spent nearly $9.4 billion on marketing to American doctors (*Economist*, 2003). Since 1998, drug makers have spent $800 million on direct lobbying of Congress (*New Scientist*, 2005). The industry has also spent millions of dollars trying to prevent any significant cost-control measures from passing, including rejecting provisions allowing Americans to legally import drugs from Canada and Europe where medications retail for as much as 75 percent less than in the United States (Connolly, 2003). Globally, evidence increasingly points to obstructing the sale of cheap generic drugs in poor countries, drug manufacturing human rights violations, and intimidation of governments with threats of trade sanctions (Cook, 2004).

eDTC campaigns provide the industry with yet another channel to share its commercial interests and maintain its global hegemony while touting "empowerment." Healthology's public relations, indeed, can help the medicine go down.

Notes

1 This chapter is an extended version of an article published in *Studies in Communication Sciences*. This book chapter contains more detailed discussion of concepts and provides new examples, but does contain some similar themes and textual evidence.
2 Physicians do receive honoraria for their consultations.
3 All text samples can be found on www.healthology.com.

References

Abramson, J. (2004). *Overdosed America: The Broken Promise of American Medicine*. New York: Harper Perennial.

Arnold, M. (2005). New channels in TV. *Medical Marketing and Media*, (June): 50–55.

Berkowitz, S. (2003). Originality, conversation and reviewing rhetorical criticism. *Communication Studies, 54*, 359–363.

Bernhardt, J., Laviscy, R.A.W., Parrott, R.L., Silk, K.J. & Felter, E.M. (2002). Perceived barriers to internet-based health communication on human genetics. *Journal of Health Communication, 7*, 325–340.

Bradley, L.R., & Zito, J.M. (1997). Direct-to-consumer prescription drug advertising. *Medical Care, 35*, 86–92.

Burke, K. (1950). *A Rhetoric of Motives*. Berkeley: University of California Press.

Burton, B., & Rowell, A. (2003). Unhealthy spin. *British Medical Journal, 326*, 1205–1207.

Campbell, K.K., & Burkholder, T.R. (eds) (1997). *Critiques of Contemporary Rhetoric*. Belmont: Wadsworth Publishing Company.

Campbell, C., & Jovchelovitch, S. (2000). Health, community, and development: Towards a social psychology of participation. *Journal of Community & Applied Social Psychology, 10*, 255–270.

Catlett, D. (2003). Public relations and its role in pharmaceutical brand building. In Blackett, T., & Robins, R. (eds), *Brand Medicine: The Role of Branding in the Pharmaceutical Industry*. New York: Palgrave.

Charland, M. (1987). Constitutive rhetoric: The case of the Peuple Quebecois. *Quarterly Journal of Speech, 73*, 133–150.

Cheney, G., & Vibbert, S. (1987). Corporate discourse: Public relations and issue management. In Jablin, F., Putnam, L., Roberts, K., & Porters, L. (eds)., *Handbook of Organizational Communication: An Interdisciplinary Perspective*. Thousand Oaks, CA: Sage, pp. 165–194.

Condit, C.M. (1994). Hegemony in a mass mediated society: Concordance about "reproductive technologies," *Critical Studies in Mass Communication, 11*, 205–230.

Condit, C.M. (2001). Rhetorical formations of genetics in science and society. *Rhetoric Review, 20*, 12–17.

Conger, J.A., & Kanungo, R.N. (1988). The empowerment process: Integrating theory and practice. *Academy of Management Review, 13*, 471–482.

Connolly, C. (2003). Drugmakers protect their turf. *Washington Post*. November 21. Retrieved on October 30, 2006, from www.washingtonpost.com.

Cook, M. (2004). Who can cure the pharmaceuticals? *New Statesman*. November 15. Retrieved on October 30, 2006, from www.newstatesman.com.

Corbett, J.B., & Mori, M. (1999). Medicine, media, and celebrities: News coverage of breast cancer, 1960–1995. *Journalism & Mass Communication Quarterly, 76*, 229–249.

Deetz, S.A. (1992). *Democracy in An Age of Corporate Colonization: Developments in Communication and the Politics of Everyday Life*. Albany, NY: State University of New York Press.

Duquette-Smith, C. (2000). Discipline—it's a "good thing:" Rhetorical constitution and Martha Stewart Living Omnimedia. *Women's Studies in Communication, 23*, 337–366.

Dutta-Bergman, M.J. (2004a). Primary sources of health information: comparisons in the domain of health attitudes, health cognitions, and health behaviors. *Health Communication, 16*(3), 273–288.

Dutta-Bergman, M.J. (2004b). An alternative approach to social capital: Exploring the linkage between health consciousness and community participation. *Health Communication, 16*, 393–409.

Dutta-Bergman, M.J. (2005). Developing a profile of consumer intention to seek out additional information beyond a doctor: The role of communicative and motivation variables. *Health Communication, 17*, 1–16.

Economist. (2003). Pushing pills: A new problem for the pharmaceutical industry. *Economist*. Retrieved on October 30, 2006, from www.economist.com.

Ehrenreich, B. (2001). Welcome to cancerland. *Harper's Magazine*, (November): 43–53.

Elwood, W. (1995). *Public Relations as Rhetorical Criticism*. Westport, CT: Praeger.

Eysenbach, G. (2000). Consumer health informatics. *British Medical Journal, 320*, 7251, 1713.

Ferguson, T. (1997). Health online and the empowered medical consumer. *Journal of Quality Improvement, 23*, 251–257.

Fox, S. (2005). *Health Information Online*. Washington, DC: Pew Internet & American Life Project.

Fuqua, J. (2002). "Ask your doctor about . . ." Direct to consumer prescription drug advertising and the HIV/AIDS medical marketplace. *Cultural Studies, 16*, 650–672.

German, K. (1995). Critical theory in public relations inquiry: Future directions for analysis in a public relations context. In W. Elwood (ed.), *Public Relations as Rhetorical Criticism*. Westport, CT: Praeger, pp. 279–294.

Gobé, M. (2002). *Citizen Brand*. New York: Allworth Press.

Goldhammer, P. (2004). The internet and useful patient information. Pharmaceutical research and manufacturers of America. PowerPoint presentation. Retrieved from www.phrma.org on July 23, 2005.

Graber, D.A. (1976). *Verbal Behavior and Politics*. Chicago, IL: University of Illinois Press.

Griffith, D., & Wiegand, S. (2005). Health groups' funding faulted. *Sacramento Bee*. June 26. Retrieved on May 10, 2006, from www.lexis-nexis.com.

Gutierrez, L.M. (1990). Working with women of color: An empowerment perspective. *Social Work, 35*, 149–153.

Hales, C.P. (1999). Embellishing empowerment: Ideologies of management, managerial ideologies and the divergence between the rhetoric and reality of empowerment programmes. Proceedings of the 17th International Labour Process Conference.

Hart, R. (1990). *Modern Rhetorical Criticism*. Glenview, IL: Scott, Foresman, and Company.

Henwood, F., Wyatt, S., Hart, A., & Smith, J. (2003). "Ignorance is bliss sometimes": constraints on the emergence of the "informed patient" in the changing landscapes of health information. *Sociology of Health & Illness, 25*, 589–607.

Herzenstein, M., Misra, S., & Posavac, S.S. (2004). How consumers' attitudes toward DTC advertising of prescription drugs influence ad effectiveness, and consumer and physician behavior. *Marketing Letters, 15*, 201–212.

Hoek, J., & Gendall, P. (2002). To have or not to have? Ethics and regulation of DTC advertising of prescription medicines. *Journal of Marketing Communications, 8*, 71–85.

Hoffman, J.R., & Wilkes, M. (1999). Direct to consumer advertising of prescription drugs. An idea whose time should not come. *British Medical Journal, 31*, 1301–1302.

Holmer, A.F. (2001). Direct-to-consumer advertising builds bridges between patients and physicians. *Journal of the American Medical Association, 281*, 380–382.

Horrigan, J.B., & Rainie, L. (2002). *Counting on the Internet*. Pew Internet Project. Retrieved April 13, 2004, from www.pewinternet.org.

Jack, A. (2006). Big pharma: How the world's biggest drug companies control illness. *Financial Times*. Retrieved on May 10, 2006, from http://global.lexisnexis.com/us.

Jasinski, J. (1997). Instrumentalism, contextualism, and interpretation in rhetorical criticism. In W. Keith, & A. Gross (eds), *Rhetorical hermeneutics*. Albany: SUNY Press, pp. 195–224.

Jasinski, J. (1998). A constitutive framework for rhetorical historiography: Toward an understanding of the discursive (re)constitution of "Constitution" in *The Federalist* Papers. In K.J. Turner (ed.), *Doing Rhetorical History: Concepts and Cases*. Tuscaloosa: University of Alabama Press, 72–92.

Lupton, D. (1995). *The Imperative of Health: Public Health and the Regulated Body*. London: Sage.

Markus, H., & Nurius, P. (1986). Possible selves. *American Psychologist, 41*, 954–69.

Masi, C.M., Suarez-Balcazar, Y., Cassey, M. Z., Kinney, L., & Piotrowski, H. (2003). Internet access and empowerment: A community-based health initiative. *Journal of General Internal Medicine, 18*, 525–530.

McCormick, S. (2005). Ivillage conference call to discuss its acquisition of Healthology, Inc. Transcript. January 10. Retrieved on May 7, 2006, from http://global.lexis nexis.com/us.

Meyrowitz. J. (1998). Multiple media literacies. *Journal of Communication, 48*, 96–107.

Mickey, T. (1997). A postmodern view of public relations: Sign and reality. *Public Relations Review, 23*, 271–284.

New Scientist. (2005). Hey, big pharma. *New Scientist*. July 2005. Retrieved on October 30, 2006, from www.newscientist.com.

Pacanowsky, M. (1988). Communication in the empowering organization. *Communication Yearbook, 11*, 356–379.

Pear, R. (2004). U.S. videos, for TV news, come under scrutiny. *New York Times*. Retrieved on March 11, 2004, from www.nytimes.com.

Perelman, C., & Olbrechts-Tyteca, L. (1969/2000). *The New Rhetoric: A Treatise on Argumentation*. Notre Dame, IN: University of Notre Dame Press.

Pires, G., Stanton, J., & Rita, P. (2006). The internet, consumer empowerment, and marketing strategies. *European Journal of Marketing, 40*, 936–949.

Rimal, R.N., Ratzan, S.C., Arntson, P., & Freimuth, V.S. (1997). Reconceptualizing the "patient": Health care promotion as increasing citizens' decision-making competencies. *Health Communication, 9*, 61–74.

Reeves, P. (2000). Coping in cyberspace: The impact of Internet use on the ability of HIV-positive individuals to deal with their illness. *Journal of Health Communication, 5*, 47–59.

Roberts, K. (1999). Patient empowerment in the United States: a critical commentary. *Health Expectations, 2*, 82–92.

Sholle, D.J. (1989). Critical studies: From the theory of ideology to power/knowledge. *Critical Studies in Mass Communication, 5*, 16–41.

Stein, S. (2002). The "1984" Macintosh ad: Cinematic icons and constitutive rhetoric in the launch of a new machine. *Quarterly Journal of Speech, 88*, 169–192.

Stokes, A.Q. (2005). Metabolife's meaning: A call for the constitutive study of public relations. *Public Relations Review, 31*, 556–565.

Teinowitz, I. (1999). Drug marketers challenge study chiding DTC ads. *Advertising Age, 70*, 55–60.

Turnquist, C. (2004). VP value chain services: Syntegra and San Elbaum, VP. *Strategic Solutions*. Aberdeen.

Wilkes, M.S., Bell, R.A., & Kravitz, R.L. (2000). Direct to consumer prescription advertising: trends, impact, and implications. *Health Affairs, 19*, 110–128.

Wright, L., Newman, A., & Dennis, C. (2006). Enhancing consumer empowerment. *European Journal of Marketing, 40*, 924–935.

Wilkie, D. (2005). Patient empowerment or pandora's box? *The Scientist* (May 23): 35–37.

Zoller, H.M. (2005). Health activism: Communication theory and action for social change. *Communication Theory, 15*, 341–364.

Part IV

Communication and health policy

Introduction

Heather M. Zoller and Mohan J. Dutta

The early development of the health communication discipline emphasized interpersonal and mediated communication (Thompson, 2003). Much of this research relied on a narrow definition of communiation as message production and reception, and focused primarily on individual levels of analysis. Perhaps, as a result, extant research emphasizes subjects such as interpersonal support, provider–patient communication, and health campaigns, whereas attention to helath policy making as a significant communication process has been slow to develop. Indeed, some work in the field such as Freimuth et al. (1993) distinguished between policy interventions and "communication approaches" such as promotional campaigns.

Yet clearly health policy has an enormous influence on public health, and its construction, implementation, and contestation are communicative processes. Government policies influence medical care access, health education content, the availability of food and water, sanitation, housing, and environmental standards to name just a few. Corporate policies including product health and safety, occupational health protections, and marketing also have significant influence on public health (Zoller, 2003). Describing this vital role of policy in the realm of health care processes, Barbara Sharf (1999) called for greater attention to health-care policy in our research, and encouraged the field to work to increase our influence over policy making. She noted the particular need to address managed care, bioethics, and health activism. Sharf argued that addressing these issues would help to anchor our scholarship in the "three Cs:" contextualization, complexity, and consequences.

We would add that a communication perspective contributes uniquely to theorizing in health policy by addressing the role of language 1) as expression in terms of the influence of rhetorical choices on public persuasion, and 2) as constitutive in terms of building social knowledge about health, identity, and culture. As interpretive, cultural, and critical scholars have begun to answer Sharf's call, they have drawn our attention to processes of interpretation and negotiation in the context of health-care policies, and to connections between macro-social processes and everyday experiences of health policy. Here, we review some of the contributions of meaning-centered approaches to health policy in communication. Then we preview the chapters in Part IV, noting the ways that they expand this literature by investigating contemporary social changes such as globalization and neoliberal economic policy.

Existing work illustrates the role of rhetoric in setting public policy agendas. For instance, Perez and Dionisopoulos' (1995) investigated the influence of the Surgeon General's report on AIDS on Reagan's rhetorical management of the AIDS crisis. Critically oriented research investigates the ideologies reflected in, and reinforced by these agendas. Dejong and Wallack (1999) criticized the U.S. Drug Czar's antidrug media campaign for promoting simplistic antidrug messages while failing to make drug treatment more available or create community-based interventions that address structural forces. Zoller (2005) used feminist analysis to examine how the U.S. Public Health Service's *Healthy People 2000* publication guides public health policies in ways that may reinforce inequities among marginalized groups by failing to prioritize their social and material circumstances.

In terms of policy construction, Conrad and McIntush (2003) provide a number of theories for understanding U.S. health-care policy making as a process marked by complex interactions among rhetoric, ideology, and structure. Drawing primarily from organizational theorizing, they note that functionalist presumptions of rationality and equitable participation in policy-making are problematic from a communication perspective. Their work draws our atten-tion to the key question of who is able to participate substantively in policy decisions. Sharf (2001) addressed this issue of participation in terms of activist methodologies, describing personal narratives about breast cancer as a significant technique to influence the agendas of legislators and other health-policy leaders. However, she also remarks on the political complexities of funding a broad array of health initiatives, some of which have yet to build compelling narratives. Murphy (2001) investigated actual policy-making processes at the micro-level through textual analysis of congressional policy debates. More work remains to be done investigating actual policy processes among elites.

In addition, there is a need for more critical and cultural perspectives that link policy constructions, power, and the lived experience of marginalization. One good example is Gillespie (2001), who examined relationships between policy and health-care experiences of people with asthma. She used feminist and postmodern lenses to examine symbolic struggles over health-care utilization in Medicaid's managed care system. The author described how the disciplinary practices constituting managed care encourage patient self-care and responsibility. Physician communication, reflecting these expectations, fails to address material, class-based barriers (such as lack of control over living conditions, transportation) as well as social issues (depression), leading to "noncompliance" classifications. The study addressed the political complexities of policy and illness management. Such work is critical in bringing the con-texts of social policy and patients' lives to the study of physician–patient communication, which so often focuses on communication only as it takes place in the doctor's office.

Significantly, critical and cultural perspectives have begun to broaden our conceptions of what constitutes health policy by addressing the linkages among illness, health disparity, and larger social policies, including wealth distribution, education, and the cultural status of marginalized groups (Airhihenbuwa, 1995; Dutta-Bergman, 2005). This trend is most evident in work addressing health in impoverished countries. For instance, Chay-Nemeth (1998) contextualized the spread of HIV/AIDS in Thailand and the spread of sex work to these macro-level issues. Melkote et al. (2000) note that, "In Asia and Africa, poverty, malnutrition, unemployment, illiteracy, lack of infrastructural and basic primary health care systems, rural-urban migration, unemployment, poor sanitation, cultural factors (such as the low status accorded to women), and war, among other factors, create a favorable setting for the large-scale spread of HIV" (p. 23). These perspectives look at the interplay of personal and public meanings as well as social structures in the formation and negotiation of policies that affect health status.

Existing research sets the stage for building health communication theory by investigating the unique discursive and material resources and barriers entailed in health policy versus other forms of policy making. The chapters in this book add to this body of knowledge by investigating how health politics are inextricably linked with contemporary social problems associated with economic globalization. Addressing global trade and economic agreements is an important agenda for health communication, given that these agreements influence health status at the symbolic level by influencing perceptions of what health is and how it should be achieved, and at the material level by influencing the social determinants of health including income levels and access to food, water, education, and medical care (Drager & Beaglehole, 2001; Kim et al., 2000; Navarro, 1999). The chapters in Part IV focus on the influence of transnational trade agreements on pharmaceutical policies, drug pricing, and availability; neoliberal trade agreements and their influence on the social circumstances and economic determinants of health status; and genetic engineering and the rise of transnational activism. The chapters are rooted in Sharf's "three Cs" of contextualization, complexity, and consequences.

In Chapter 16, "Dealing drugs on the border: power and policy in pharmaceutical reimportation debates," Charles Conrad and Denise Jodlowski rhetorically examine struggles over pharmaceutical drug reimportation policies between the United States and Canada. Drug reimportation, which would allow U.S. residents and government agencies to purchase drugs at lower Canadian costs, is a potential weapon in the fight to reign in drug pricing and corporate control of medicine. The authors embed their description of state-level policies within larger political systems, including economic globalization, the power of the pharmaceutical industry, and the rhetoric of the free market.

The chapter provides important avenues for critically theorizing health policy making by introducing de Certeau's (1984) concepts of strategic action and Michael Mann's (1986) discussion of "outflanking" to examine the ways in which elites can dominate policy processes to their advantage. Given the complex moves and countermoves from lawmakers, regulators, the pharmaceutical industry and citizens, the authors note that "the drug reimportation experience highlights the dialectical nature of the outflanking–counteroutflanking process, and the relationship between social/political structures and rhetorical action" (p. 380). Through rich contextualization, the chapter provides insight into the rhetoric of economics, the corporate context of medical care, and inequalities in access to, and even awareness of, health policy making. Each of these topics represents key issues for the development of critical health communication theory.

Heather Zoller's Chapter 17, "Technologies of neoliberal governmentality: the discursive influence of global economic policies on public health," encourages attention to policies that have immense influence on the social determinants of public health, but which might not be thought of as "health" policy because their primary focus is economic. Taking a critical and post-structural approach, the chapter examines the discursive influence of neoliberal global trade and development policy on public health. Drawing from Rose and Miller (Rose, 1996; Rose & Miller, 1992) to establish a framework for analyzing governmental discourse, the chapter examines three significant international trade policy mechanisms as governmental technology: structural adjustment policies, harmonization rules, and investor-to-state lawsuits. She argues that these technologies 1) materially increase rates of illness and disease by increasing poverty and reducing social investments and 2) discursively undermine the ability of public health agents to reduce these harms by redefining health from a social good to a private commodity, shifting the burden of proof for establishing risk in regulation, and disqualifying health as a counter-discourse. Analysis highlights avenues through which communication scholars and health activists may resist, or at least avoid complicity with, the underlying economic orthodoxy of neoliberal governmentality. As such, the chapter has implications for how a broad array of health researchers and activists conceptualize what counts as both health communication research and health-promotion practice by including multisectoral policy advocacy, resistance, and activism.

In Chapter 18, "The paradox of 'Fair Trade': the influence of neoliberal trade agreements on food security and health," Rebecca Desouza, Ambar Basu, Induk Kim, Iccha Basnyat, and Mohan Dutta extend this focus on how economic globalization policy, seemingly unconnected to health, influences one of the most fundamental determinants of health—access to adequate food and water. The authors note that social marketing campaigns focus on promoting healthy eating without addressing key issues of access and affordability. The chapter promotes attention to the ways that health advocates may target neoliberal trade policies that shape "food security" in marginalized communities, examining the influence of the General Agreement on Trade and Tariffs (GATT) on the banana trade in Latin America and the African-Caribbean regions; the Agreement on Agriculture (AoA) on sugar trade in the Pacific Islands, and the Agreement on Trade Related Aspects of Intellectual Property Rights (TRIPS) on the rice trade in South Asia. The chapter is a useful example of how cultural studies rooted in structural critique (critical modernism) can identify opportunity for communication interventions in policy making that would create vast improvements in health status (particularly in comparison with the limited returns of lifestyle promotion).

In Chapter 19, "Globalization, social justice movements, and the human genome diversity debates: a case study in health action," Rulon Wood, Damon M. Hull, and Marouf Hasian examine the implementation and contestation of the Human Genome Diversity Project (HGDP). This chapter also represents an important direction for health communication scholars. The work addresses emerging policy issues from a culture-centered perspective and highlights the role of activism and agency among subaltern groups in shaping the course of genetic policy. The HDGP, a seemingly straightforward attempt to accrue diverse genetic samples to create a more complete genetic map, comes under attack from scholars and activists who embed the discussion of genetic diversity within larger contexts such as participation and control in science, racism, colonialism, and Western exploitation. This chapter examines how the clash of epistemes (scientific and modern, postmodern and cultural) foments new social alliances to contest the top-down approach of the HDGP. Thus it provides insight into the complexities of agency and the difficulty of achieving dialogue in the realm of science, particularly for marginalized people.

Part IV provides the groundwork for greater attention to policy construction as a major component of the study and practice of health communication. These works encourage additional investigation of the cultural and economic issues associated with globalization and neoliberalism in their changing forms. Of course, "policy" is a broad term, and we need additional research to investigate multiple forms of policy and their influence on health, as well as to trace commonalities and differences across political processes. The chapters reflect a variety of theoretical perspectives that can be brought to bear on the study of policy, including rhetorical, interpretive, cultural, critical-modern, and critical-postmodern. Certainly, policy is not the domain of interpretive, critical, and cultural research alone, and quantitative and post-positivist research also should play a significant role in investigating health outcomes tied to policy. Our focus in this book, though, is to point out how "World View II" inquiries highlight the contested role of meaning in policy making, and the relationships between local and macro-level contexts and their influence on how policies are interpreted, implemented, and contested.

References

Airhihenbuwa, C. (1995). *Health and Culture: Beyond the Western Paradigm*. Thousand Oaks, CA: Sage.

Chay-Nemeth, C. (1998). Demystifying AIDS in Thailand: A dialectical analysis of the Thai sex industry. *Journal of Health Communication*, 3(3), 217–231.

Conrad, C., & McIntush, H.G. (2003). Organizational rhetoric and healthcare policymaking. In T.L. Thompson, A.M. Dorsey, K.I. Miller, & R. Parrott (eds), *Handbook of Health Communication*. Mahwah, NJ: Lawrence Erlbaum Associates, pp. 403–422.

De Certeau, M. (1984). *The Practice of Everyday Life* (S. Rendall, trans.). Berkeley: University of California Press.

Dejong, W., & Wallack, L. (1999). A critical perspective on the Drug Czar's antidrug media campaign. *Journal of Health Communication*, 4(2), 155–160.

Drager, N., & Beaglehole, R. (2001). Globalization: Changing the public health landscape. *Bulletin of the World Health Organization*, 79(9), 803–804.

Dutta-Bergman, M. (2005). Theory and practice in health communication campaigns: A critical interrogation. *Health Communication*, 18(2), 103–122.

Freimuth, V.S., Edgar, T., & Fitzpatrick, M.A. (1993). Introduction: The role of communication in health promotion. *Communication Research*, 20(4), 509–516.

Gillespie, S.R. (2001). The politics of breathing: Asthmatic Medicaid patients under managed care. *Journal of Applied Communication Research*, 29(2), 97–116.

Kim, J.Y., Millen, J.V., Irwin, A., & Gershman, J. (eds). (2000). *Dying for Growth: Global Inequality and the Health of the Poor*. Monroe, ME: Common Courage Press.

Mann, M. (1986). *The Sources of Social Power*. Vol. 1. New York: Cambridge Press.

Melkote, S., Muppidi, S., & Goswami, D. (2000). Social and economic factors in an integrated behavioral and societal approach to communications in HIV/AIDS. *Journal of Health Communication*, 5(3), 17–27.

Murphy, P. (2001). Framing the nicotine debate: A cultural approach to risk. *Health Communication*, 13(2), 119–140.

Navarro, V. (1999). Health and equity in the world in the era of "globalization." *International Journal of Health Services*, 29(2), 215–226.

Perez, T.L., & Dionisopoulos, G.N. (1995). Presidential silence, C. Everett Koop, and the Surgeon General's Report on AIDS. *Communication Studies*, 46 (Spring/Summer), 18–33.

Rose, N. (1996). Governing "advanced" liberal societies. In A. Barry, T. Osborne, & N. Rose (eds), *Foucault and Political Reason: Liberalism, Neo-liberalism and Rationalities of Government*. Chicago: University of Chicago Press, pp. 37–64.

Rose, N., & Miller, P. (1992). Political power beyond the state: Problematics of government. *British Journal of Sociology*, 43(2), 173–205.

Sharf, B.F. (1999). The present and future of Health Communication scholarship: Overlooked opportunities. *Health Communication*, 11(2), 195–199.

Sharf, B.F. (2001). Out of the closet and into the legislature: The impact of communicating breast cancer narratives on health policy. *Health Affairs*, 20(1), 213–218.

Thompson, T.L. (2003). Introduction. In T.L. Thompson, A.M. Dorsey, K.I. Miller, & R. Parrott (eds), *Handbook of Health Communication*. Mahwah, NJ: Lawrence Erlbaum Associates, pp. 1–8.

Zoller, H.M. (2003). Health on the line: Identity and disciplinary control in employee occupational health and safety discourse. *Journal of Applied Communication Research*, *31*(2), 118–139.

Zoller, H.M. (2005). Women caught in the multicausal web: A gendered analysis of Healthy People 2010. *Communication Studies*, *56*, 175–192.

Chapter 16

Dealing drugs on the border

Power and policy in pharmaceutical reimportation debates

Charles Conrad and Denise Jodlowski

Economic globalization is not a new phenomenon, but its most recent individuation involves an unprecedented relationship between multinational corporations and governments (McNeil, 1978; Goverde et al., 2000; also see the chapters by Zoller, Desouza et al., and Wood et al. in this book). In some cases, multinationals are able to dominate national governments, either directly through economic means or indirectly through NGOs such as the WTO and IMF. In other cases, multinationals are not able to dominate governments, but are still major power centers that policy makers simply cannot ignore. In still other cases, states are sufficiently powerful to dominate multinationals, but public policy-making processes create rhetorical, political, and economic spaces within which those organizations can still exercise significant influence. Reflecting an emerging consensus (Goverde et al. 2000) Canadian sociologist Joel Bakan (2004) concludes that overall, "economic globalization and deregulation have diminished the state's capacity to protect the public interest . . . [and] have strengthened its power to promote corporations' interests and facilitate their profit-seeking missions" while preserving the state's power (p. 154; also see Kain, 1974, pp. 231, 234).

When two countries share a border, have extensive economic relationships, and have different cultures and political systems, the relationship between multinationals and public policy making is more complex, and the space within which multinationals can operate is enlarged substantially. Each nation's policy makers must remain cognizant of the political and economic context imposed by the other nation and by multinational organizations' ability to move between them. A paradigm case of the complex relationships among multinational corporations and public policy making is the current traffic in prescription drugs between the United States and Canada. This chapter examines discourse on both sides of the border surrounding this issue.

The drug reimportation debate

Understanding the debate over drug reimportation requires a basic understanding of the economics of pharmaceutical pricing, and the rhetoric of the industry and its critics. While the economics are very different on the two sides of the 49th parallel, the rhetoric is similar and inter-related.

The economics of drug reimportation

Although there is a great deal of debate about the effectiveness of the U.S. health-care system relative to other developed (OECD) countries, there is no question that it is the world leader in one measure—health-care spending. The United States spends much more per capita on health care than any other country ($5711 USD), at least 24 percent higher than the next-highest spending country (Luxembourg, $4611 USD), and "over 90 percent higher than in many other countries that we would consider to be global competitors" (Kaiser Family Foundation, 2007).

U.S. spending for prescription drugs in 2006 was almost $275 billion USD, more that six times the $40.3 USD billion spent in 1990, and almost double the amount ($156 billion USD) that Americans spend for petroleum products (*AARP Bulletin*, 2007, p. 6). Pharmaceutical spending was still a smaller proportion of total spending than hospital and physician services (10 percent vs. 30 percent and 21 percent respectively), but was the fastest-growing component between 1980 and 1999, when it peaked at a 20 percent annual growth rate (Kaiser Family Foundation, 2006). The rate moderated to an 8.1 percent increase in 2003, 7.2 percent in 2004, and 5.8 percent in 2005, still more than double the overall inflation rate, but returned to the 8 percent level in 2006 (*AARP Bulletin*, 2007; Gardner, 2007).[1]

In contrast, Canada's total health-care spending per capita ranks sixth among OECD countries ($2900 per person per year, 41 percent of the U.S. expenditure of $7100 per person per year), and the share of its GDP allocated to health care ranks eighth (65 percent of the U.S. figure) with comparable or superior health outcomes.[2] Canada's growth in health-care spending as a proportion of GDP was 2.7 percent between 1980 and 2003 (less than half the U.S. figure of 6.4 percent); and between 1990 and 2003 its growth rate was 0.9 percent, less than one-third of the U.S. growth rate of 3.3 percent. These differences stem directly from differences in the health-care systems of the two countries. Canada's population is 12–13 percent of the United States. With the exception of a more rapid population growth in the United States, its demographics and epidemiology are comparable. The Canadian health-care system emerged over a long period of time, beginning at the end of World War II. Like the 1947 Hill–Burton Hospital Construction Act in the United States, the 1957 Hospital Insurance and Diagnosis Services Act (HIDS) provided federal grants and subsidies to support the construction of additional nonprofit hospitals and established a 50–50 federal-province cost sharing arrangement.[3] Provincial governments were granted a wide degree of latitude in developing their own systems, but funding was provided contingent on meeting the five "principles" of public (rather than private-sector) administration; comprehensive coverage of all hospital services; universal coverage of all residents; portability of coverage from one province to another; and accessibility of service to all citizens.

The Canada Medicare Act of 1966 (implemented in 1968) applied the same principles to outpatient physician care, although a number of types of care (e.g., chiropractic) were excluded from the mandate, including prescription drugs administered outside of a hospital. By 1971 all provinces had implemented systems that met the federal criteria. Over time, the provinces increased their coverage of prescription drug costs, usually starting with inexpensively treated communicable diseases (e.g., tuberculosis) and slowly broadening their coverage. The result has been a "patchwork quilt" of coverage composed of some combination of out-of-pocket costs, private supplemental insurance, and government coverage that varies widely across provinces (Lynx & Salmon, 2006; Rachlis, 2004). In 2002, 36 percent of the costs of prescription drugs were covered by the government, compared with 90 percent or more of hospital and physician costs, and 71 percent of the total bill (Rachlis, 2004). By 2005, both the average percentage and the variability across provinces had risen; public sector spending per capita ranged from $105CD in Prince Edward Island to $341CD in Quebec. By 2005 privately financed prescription drug expenditures were higher (an average of $346 CD per Canadian per year) than public expenditures ($295CD per person per year). Compared to the thirteen other OECD countries, Canada ranked eighth in public sector spending per capita, and eleventh in public share in drug costs (Munro, 2006).

Two additional events influenced prescription drug costs in Canada. In 1987, parliament created the Patented Medicines Price Review Board, a national quasi-judicial body that sets the maximum prices a manufacturer can charge for drugs sold in Canada (Gross, 2003). Unlike countries with national health insurance (e.g., Australia) or single-payer systems (e.g., the U.K.) the federal government does not purchase prescription drugs—it merely sets maximum prices and approves new drugs for sale in Canada. Two bills (passed in 1987 and 1993), now generally accepted as part of the negotiations connected to the North American Free Trade Act (NAFTA), significantly increased patent protection for name-brand drugs.[4] As a result, Canada's prescription drug costs, which once ranked lowest among OCED countries, now rank second, behind only the United States, while millions of Canadians have no coverage at all. Drug costs increased 11 percent from 2004 to 2005, making it the fastest-growing aspect of health spending (Munro, 2006). Public health professionals and liberal politicians pushed for the creation of a National Formulary through which Ottawa would negotiate directly with pharmaceutical firms for drugs sold in Canada. Estimates are that a national plan would cost between $7 billion and $12 billion CD, as compared to the current taxpayer outlays of $8 billion CD. Although the idea of a national formulary received strong support from most provincial premiers, it was deemed too expensive by

Paul Martin's Liberal Party government. The current Conservative government is unlikely to revive the idea.[5]

Still, nongeneric prescription drug prices are substantially lower in Canada than in the United States, regardless of which drugs are used in the comparisons or what methodology is used. Democratic Representative Rahm Emanuel's (Illinois) staff compared the prices of ten oft-prescribed drugs at Costco stores in Chicago and Toronto and found a $1500USD difference in a one-month's supply (CBC, 2007). Of the ten drugs, only one (Viagra) could be purchased for less in the United States. Walgreens, the largest U.S. pharmacy, sells 180 tablets of breast cancer treatment Tamoxifen for $380.97 USD; Manitoba-based internet pharmacy Rx1 sells it for 73 percent less ($287.07). Overall, Canadians spend between 50 and 70 percent less that U.S. residents for identical prescriptions, depending on the drug and the province where it is purchased.[6] When Congressman Emanuel and North Dakota senator Byron Dorgan introduced the Pharmaceutical Market Access and Drug Safety Act on January 10, 2007, they estimated the potential savings to U.S. consumers at $50 billion USD over the next decade (CBC, 2007). Current cross-border trade is estimated at more than $1 billion annually with U.S. residents receiving more than two million packages of prescription drugs each year from Canada (CBC, 2007).[7] It comes as no surprise that drug reimportation is strongly opposed by the pharmaceutical industry, trade groups representing local pharmacies, and the Bush administration.

The rhetoric of pharmaceutical pricing

Typically speaking through the industry's lobbying group, PhRMa, drug makers argue that the industry produces miracle drug after miracle drug, which have lengthened the lives of millions of patients, improved the quality of life of millions more, and reduced or controlled overall health-care costs by providing alternatives to surgery or hospitalization.[8] They argue that because of government "price controls" in countries other than the United States, industry profits there are too small to fund the research necessary to keep these miracles coming. For example, thirty years ago, France was second in the world in pharmaceutical innovation. But, because of French price controls, it now ranks ninth (Eli Lily CEO Sidney Taurel, quoted in "The Other Drug War," 2003).[9] They say that high profits on sales in the United States are necessary for research to continue, and since Americans use more prescription drugs than any other country, its citizens benefit most from that research. Drug development is expensive, time-consuming, and very risky. It takes 12–15 years for a research idea to reach market. Only one drug in fifty survives clinical trials with animals, only one in five of those that reach the human-trial stage will make it to market, and only one in three drugs introduced to the market will reach a break-even point. When drugs are designed for a specialized market, for example AIDS patients in advanced stages of the disease or septic shock, prices must be exceptionally high to warrant their development, and it is the profits firms make on other drugs that allow them to embark on the research that leads to such drugs.

Pharmaceutical firms recognize that risks are inherent in a capitalist market, but they are willing to incur those risks because of the potential payoffs that are possible only in a capitalist system unfettered by government intervention.[10] The industry's arguments vary somewhat in response to different legislative proposals, but its rhetoric consistently uses some variant of the "free market" and/or "miracle drug" ideology.

Critics generally accept the industry's assertion that firms must make *reasonable* profits in order to sustain risky research-and-development, but assert that the industry's rhetoric wildly overstates the case and ignores a wealth of disconfirming empirical evidence. First, the industry is incredibly profitable, maintaining annual profits in the 18–25 percent range per year for the past two decades. The median profit margin for the Fortune 500 as a whole is one-sixth that of the pharmaceutical industry (3.3 percent) and oil company profits, which average 5.9 percent per year, pale in comparison to pharmaceutical profits. Second, very few of the so-called "new, miracle drugs" that reach market actually have new active ingredients; most are "copycat" drugs that differ from their competitors only in terms of inert ingredients, or in some cases, packaging, and thus require trivial R&D expenditures. In addition, there does not seem to be a positive correlation between industry profits and R&D success. Of the twenty drugs approved by the U.S. FDA in 2005, only seven actually had new active ingredients, and *all* of those were developed by European firms, where drug costs (and pharmaceutical profits) are less than half that of the United States. In 2004 the figures included thirty-six approvals, ten involving new compounds, eight of which were developed in Europe (Agovino, 2006). Indeed, allowing companies to make massive profits on "me too" drugs actually reduces the likelihood of their creating new "miracle drugs" because it gives them financial incentives to allocate R&D funds toward low-risk products: "the more we spend on the latest overpriced, oversold, me-too drug, the more we encourage industry to concentrate resources on producing and plugging more of the same" (Greider, 2004, p. B9). Third, the financial burden imposed by *industry* research and development spending is exaggerated. Industry figures extrapolate the most expensive form of drug research—new chemical compounds developed entirely inhouse—to all drugs, including "me too" compounds, and fail to factor in the massive tax breaks given by the federal government for R&D (Abramson, 2004; Angell, 2004). Even using the industry's misleading data, R&D costs average only about 15 percent of spending, less than profits, administrative overhead, or advertising. Furthermore, a sizeable percentage of R&D spending comes from federal taxpayers through NIH and NSF grants. About 80 percent of the drugs developed in the United States are supported by federal grants and between 25 percent and 40 percent of all R&D spending comes from the U.S. taxpayers (Angell, 2004).

Currently, most of those funds are spent on background research, which is made available to all companies. The federal government could recoup these costs when funded research leads to highly profitable drugs, but it has never done so.[11]

Finally, while the industry's "free market" arguments are symbolically appealing to a U.S. audience deeply suspicious of government activity, they distort the nature of health-care economics. The sector as a whole neither fulfills the requirements necessary for "free market" principles to apply nor operates in accord with the predictions of free market economics (Kuttner, 1997). The pharmaceutical market is a case in point. Customers with private sector insurance are isolated from the costs of their care, and lack the information necessary to make informed market choices. Almost half of the drugs consumed in the United States are purchased by government agencies, and protectionist trade provisions and patent protections grant drug companies virtual monopolies over the U.S. market (Abramson, 2004). The industry's success in undercutting legislation has resulted much more from the size of their campaign contributions and their ability to manipulate the policy-making system. Consistently ranking near the top of political contributions, the industry's total doubled from a little over $13 million USD in 1996 and 1998 to more than $26 million in the 2000 and 2002 federal election cycles. Of the $88.6 million USD donated between 2000 and 2006, $62.16 million USD went to Republicans (Center for Responsive Politics, 2007). In fiscal year 2004, PhRMA's budget included $17.5 million USD to influence policies of nonU.S. countries and trade negotiations, $1 million USD to "change the Canadian health care system", and $450,000 to stem reimportation of prescription drugs from online Canadian pharmacies. It also planned to spend $1 million USD to create an "intellectual echo chamber of economists—a standing network of economists and thought leaders to speak against federal price control regulations through articles and testimony" (Pear, 2003, p. 1).[12] When it became clear that Democrats would experience significant gains in the 2006 mid-term elections, the industry quickly moved to shore up its donations to candidates from that party (Pear, 2006). The combination of "regulatory capture" (Wilson, 1974), direct political influence through campaign contributions, active lobbying, and an abstract and overly generalized "free market/miracle drug" rhetoric has transformed government oversight/control into an industry-government alliance.[13] As Cornell economics professor Frank concludes, "There are compelling economic reasons for delegating the activities [ensuring access to health care, regulating environmental quality, and supporting basic scientific research] to national, rather than state or local governments. Yet in each arena, the federal government has failed to act" (2006).[14]

Using the reimportation debate as a case study, our goal in the remainder of this chapter is to examine the *processes* through which the pharmaceutical industry and its critics influence the development and implementation of public policy.

Multinationals, governments, rhetoric and strategic outflanking

Interest in organizational rhetoric has mushroomed during the past two decades (Cheney et al., 2004). Past research has focused on the communicative strategies that organizational rhetors use to create positive images and reputations, and/or to manage threats to those reputations. Early work was rather atheoretical (Cheney et al., 2004), or operated from a rationalistic neoAristotelian perspective (Conrad & Abbott, 2007). Both strains of research assume that organizational rhetors draw upon the core values of a culture and/or exploit the core beliefs of various stakeholder groups in an effort to legitimize their activities and social effects. In the process, they revise or reinforce those core values and beliefs. Similarly, advocacy groups draw on the same *topoi* in an effort to pressure organizations to adopt desired policies and practices (Manheim, 2001; May et al., 2007). In capitalist democracies, an important site for these conflicting pressures is the making and implementation of public policy. However, the public policy "playing field" is not level (Clegg et al., 2006).

Economic elites, outflanking, and public policymaking

Although all members of a society have influence strategies (*topoi*) available to them, the range and power of those strategies is asymmetrically distributed (Giddens, 1984). Elites are able to engage in what Michel de Certeau has called "strategic" practices—those in which "a subject of will and power (a proprietor, an enterprise, a city, a scientific institution)" employs force grounded in control of spaces in which relationships can be "managed/dominated relationships" (de Certeau, 1984, p. 36). Strategic action reflects a "*triumph of place over time*. It allows one to capitalize acquired advantages, to prepare future expansions, and thus to give oneself a certain independence with respect to the variability of circumstances" (de Certeau, 1984, p. 35). It relies on surveillance (what de Certeau calls, after Foucault, "panoptic practices") and the ability to "define the *power of knowledge* by this ability to transform the uncertainties of history into readable spaces" (p. 36). It underlies, and reproduces, a "sovereign" conception of power; one that Stewart Clegg (1989) argues was re-invigorated in Hobbes' *Leviathan* and introduced to modern social theory by Robert Dahl and his successors. Of course, the advantages built into strategic practices do not guarantee positive outcomes for elites; the possibility of resistance always is present.

Michael Mann (1986) has argued that, historically, elites have been able to "outflank" resistance by influencing "the laws and norms of the social group in which both [elites and the masses] operate" (p. 6).[15] Elites have three advantages that nonelites lack, all of which are grounded in the ability to form alliances with governments. First, elites can move among circuits of power—from one political or legal venue to another—in a search for the optimal configuration in particular cases. If workers strike, the army (or Pinkerton agents) can be called in to "restore order" or take over air traffic control (military circuit); corporations can hire "permanent replacements" to return idled plants to operation (economic circuit); evangelists can be hired to persuade workers that their pain is the result of their own sins (ideological circuit); the courts can be used to jail or execute resistance leaders, bankrupt union treasuries, or strictly regulate the conditions under which resistance takes place (e.g., the U.S. National Labor Relations Act; political circuit). Armed with superior resources and more responsive organizational structures, elites also can move more efficiently across time and space, from local to state to national levels and back again, or across national borders.[16]

Second, elites can strategically alter the institutional configurations themselves—the proverbial English gentlemen *can* always change the rules of the game. Ironically, elites are able to identify desired institutional changes by monitoring and interpreting successful *tactical* action by nonelites—without resistance, structural strategizing is impossible. Some of the elites' adaptations will fail—there is no reason to attribute either omniscience or omnipotence to them—and in other cases nonelites will quickly create/learn tactics that exploit the new institutional arrangements. But, tacticians will always be "playing catch up" and elites will always be modifying the rules of the game. Finally, elites also can engage in *tactical* action themselves by acting within and among existing circuits of praxis.[17]

Rhetoric and privatizing public policy making

Traditionally, rhetorical scholars, including those who focus on organizational rhetoric, have treated the social/political role of rhetoric as not especially problematic. After all, *public* debate about *public* policies is the essence of democracy. However, for organizations, some of the most potent political strategies involve privatizing public policy making, thereby eliminating the need to engage in public rhetoric. Open public policy debates are risky. They can lead to the formation of coalitions among low-power actors which may upset political power balances, and can even undermine the psychological processes that generate deference to elites (Vogel, 1989). Of course, the simplest means of privatizing public policy making is to press for the creation of structures that allow corporate elites to hide information about their operations. This can be done directly through legislation or regulations that allow corporations to obscure their operations in the guise of protecting "trade secrets" (Gormley, 2006). It also can be done indirectly, by reaching negotiated settlements with regulators, or out-of-court settlements with plaintiffs in which information gathered during legal proceedings is sealed from public view.

Perhaps the most potent form of privatizing public policy making is through the activities of professional lobbyists.[18] The number of registered lobbyists in

Washington, D.C., has exploded—up by a factor of ten since Ronald Regan's election, and a factor of two since George W. Bush became President. Many (250) are former Congresspersons or their aides. In 2006, the pharmaceutical industry spent $172 million USD on lobbying in Washington (Gorham, 2007). Comparable growth has occurred in the capitals of the largest U.S. states. Secrecy rules make it difficult to assess the scope of state-level lobbying, but in 2004 more than $1 billion was spent in the forty-two states that require detailed reporting; the pharmaceutical industry alone spent more than $48 million on state lobbying (Broder, 2006; Saul, 2006a). Almost all represent the interests of corporations or collections of corporations. Although press coverage of lobbyists and popular impressions of their activities focus on their influence over legislators, their greatest impact comes from constant contact with the career bureaucrats who implement public policies.[19]

Nonelite groups also can lobby legislators and bureaucrats (Kingdon, 1995; Redford, 1969). But pro-business and groups representing the interests of upper-class citizens generally are more effective. They are more tightly organized than groups that represent other interests, have greater money and prestige, are better able to exploit the decision processes of legislative bodies and administrative agencies, are better equipped to obtain and use private information provided by politicians, and are able to exaggerate their political power in the minds of policy makers (Schattschneider, 1935; Wilson, 1974). When elites' interests are threatened, they are able to quickly mobilize these resources to keep undesirable proposals off of the public agenda. In short, "when interests are well-mobilized on one side of an issue and poorly organized on the other, conflict and political debate are unlikely" (Baumgartner & Jones, 1993, p. 190; also see Stone, 1988; Wilson, 1973, 1974).

If elites do fail to keep a problem off of the public agenda, they have a number of strategies available to: 1) keep it from being placed on the *policy* agenda, 2) prevent unwanted policies from being enacted in a form that threatens the organization, and 3) prevent enacted policies from being implemented.[20] The first two goals are achieved through public discourse designed to: 1) influence the way in which "problems" are defined and policy questions are framed; 2) influence public opinion on the issue; and 3) define the terms of the public policy debate (Baumgartner & Jones, 1993; Cobb & Ross, 1997. In the United States, a common organizational strategy is to define a "problem" as a "private sector" concern, not a matter for public policy (Hall & Jones, 1997). Elites also can raise public fears about the impact of a policy proposal. The astonishing success of the "Harry and Louise" ads during the debate over the Clinton health-care plan in 1993–1994 made it abundantly clear that organizational rhetors, in the guise of "public interest" campaigns, can significantly influence the development of public policy by using media buys to directly mold public opinion (Beauchamp, 1996; Hacker, 1997; Skocpol, 1996). The process itself is conceptually quite simple—organizational rhetors draw on culturally sanctioned assumptions (*topoi*) to frame policy proposals in ways that make them seem objectionable. Some *topoi* are grounded in assumptions held by the populace in general; for example, the inherent superiority of free market capitalism over any other economic system, and the inevitable futility and perversity of government "interference" in the free market system (Aune, 1994, 2001). Other *topoi* are situation or industry specific. For example, health-care reformers have long been confronted with claims that the United States has the best health-care system in the world, a claim that can be supported only by a very careful definition of "best" and very selective presentation of the available evidence.

In the event that elites' policy-blocking strategies fail, their attention turns to the implementation process, which takes place in private where organizational actors have their greatest advantages. In some cases, implementation blocking involves persuading government officials to simply not enforce policies, or to do so in a way that minimizes their impact. In other cases, regulators can be persuaded to implement policies, but to do so in ways that undermine their intent. Finally, the executive branch can be persuaded to not provide the funds necessary to implement objectionable policies. In August 2005, New York's (Republican) governor George Pataki signed a law requiring the state to create an easily used website that consumers could use to compare prescription drug prices across the state. The pharmaceutical industry had tried to block the bill, but because the notions of rational choice based on accurate information is central to free market ideology, it was difficult for them to develop a persuasive public rhetoric. They were not even able to complain about the costs of the system because the state had sufficient funds on hand as the result of successful litigation against a drug company for price-fixing. The bill passed both houses of the New York legislature unanimously. Five months later, Pataki inserted a provision that would repeal the law "deep in one of the budget bills" that he proposed. When the reversal became public, the governor's office quickly backed off, but the outcome is still in doubt and the website still does not exist (Cooper, 2006).

All social actors have access to the same "rules and resources" (Giddens, 1984), the same political systems, rhetorical strategies, and social structures. But, elites, including organizations, are in positions to better exploit and manipulate sociopolitical rules, and to develop compelling rhetorical strategies. In short, all of the advocates are equal, but some are more equal than others.

Rhetoric and strategic outflanking in the reimportation debate

Health-care policy in general, and prescription drug costs in particular, are paradigm cases of "hot topics" that appear on the media and/or public agendas, only to disappear as attention wanes or shifts to other concerns (Iyengar, 1993). This is not to suggest that the issues are unimportant or that the general public is not interested in them. Americans have had serious concerns about the economic viability of the U.S. health-care system for decades, and seniors in particular, who consume most prescription drugs, have been angry about inflation since prices started to accelerate rapidly during the early 1990s. In some cases, media events captured public attention, as in Peter Jenning's 2002 ABC News broadcast, "Bitter Medicine," or the 2003 PBS *Frontline* episode entitled "The Other Drug War." In other cases, election campaigns or legislative proposals briefly capture public attention. This interest sometimes leads to political action. Bills were introduced in Congress to deal with drug costs for seniors in 1990, 1994, 1999, and 2000. None were passed; indeed, almost all quietly died in committee.

By the end of 2000, seniors with no or inadequate prescription drug coverage were giving up hope that the federal government would ever act ("The Other Drug War," 2003) and many states had tired of waiting for federal action to stem skyrocketing drug costs. The most visible was Maine. The state's senior citizens had long crossed the Canadian border to purchase prescriptions; indeed, an entire industry of drug bus tours had developed. On May 11, Chellie Pingree, the majority leader of the state Senate, introduced a bill that instructed the state's Commissioner of Human Services to negotiate reduced prices for senior citizens, who use one-third of the drugs sold in the state. The Commissioner was to use the state's Medicaid program, which purchases one-quarter of all the drugs sold in Maine, as a bargaining chip. Although Maine is too small a state to be financially important to the industry, its actions were symbolically very important because of the precedent the bill might set. PhRMa lobbyists descended on the state capital. In spite of its efforts, the bill passed by a unanimous vote in the Senate and a near-unanimous vote in the House. On October 25, 2000 the bill went into effect; the next day PhRMA successfully sued in federal court to stop its implementation. Maine appealed the decision, and on May 5, 2001, the first U.S. Circuit Court lifted the injunction. The industry appealed, but also redoubled its lobbying efforts to persuade the FDA to enforce existing bans on drug reimportation, to obtain federal legislation that would ban providing a prescription drug benefit on favorable terms, and to pressure Canadian governments and pharmacies to restrict cross-border sales.

Influencing national governments

Simultaneously, the industry started to pressure the Canadian government to restrict reimportation. In a few cases, drug companies such as GlaxoSmithKline reduced or eliminated shipments to Canadian pharmacies (Harris, 2003; Porter, 2004). At least one state, Minnesota, responded by filing suit in state courts (Barry, 2004). By early 2005, some members of Canada's Liberal government threatened to enact legal restrictions "in a bid to win trade favors from the Bush administration" (Krauss, 2005, p. 1; also see Canada.com, 2005 and McClelland, 2005). However, before any new legislation was passed, the

Liberal government was swept from office and its Conservative replacement has not continued the threats (Krauss, 2006).[21] More importantly, the industry diversified, setting up networks of suppliers and warehouses in Australia, New Zealand, Europe, and Asia (where most pharmaceutical drugs are produced) (Krauss, 2005, 2006).

During early 2003 the industry enlisted the FDA as an ally in its anti-reimportation campaign. FDA rhetors argued that it could not guarantee the safety of reimported drugs, and could not afford to set up an adequate safety-monitoring system (*Houston Chronicle*, 2003b, 2003c; Barry, 2004). From the outset, the agency's rhetoric was not credible. By early 2004 it admitted that it could produce no examples of a U.S. resident being harmed by reimported drugs (a position supported by Health Canada). It also admitted that it had never done any systematic research on the issue, and that each of the countries involved in the reimportation trade have drug safety systems that are at least as rigorous as the FDA's (*Houston Chronicle*, 2003b; Barry, 2004).[22] As UC-Berkeley economics professor J. Bradford DeLong concludes, "the safety issue is a made-up story" (2004, p. 1E), one that did little to reduce the cross-border trade (*Houston Chronicle*, 2003b).[23] In early 2004 the agency escalated its campaign by seizing an occasional shipment of drugs from Canada, a practice that accelerated in late 2005 (Girion, 2006).

Back to the states

In May, 2003, the U.S. Supreme Court upheld the Maine Rx program, and the "domino effect" that the industry feared started to materialize. Each effort was different, but all of them were carefully structured to undermine the industry/administration's safety claims.[24] By mid-2004, two dozen states and a number of cities had enacted reimportation programs or were considering them. Minnnesota, New Hampshire, North Dakota, Wisconsin, Nevada, and the District of Columbia set up websites linking their residents to approved Canadian pharmacies. New Hampshire also passed a bill reimporting drugs for its prisoners, retired state employees, and Medicaid patients. Illinois, however, appeared to receive the brunt of the attacks leveled by drug reimportation opponents.

In September 2003, Illinois governor Rod Blagojevich announced a new prescription drug plan, which he hoped would inspire other states experiencing similar frustrations with prescription drug prices and budget crunches. The Illinois plan constituted the greatest state threat that the FDA/industry alliance had faced, in part because of the economic power of the state, and in part because the proposal was carefully structured to undermine anti-reimportation rhetoric. It involved establishing an agreement with approved Canadian (and, later, New Zealand, Australia, and the United Kingdom) drug warehouses to re-sell prescription drugs to citizens of Illinois. The state government sent a panel of medical experts to each country that was being considered for the program, and it reported that each of those regulatory systems was at least as effective as the FDA, and that most were superior. The plan was described by Philadelphia's Action Alliance of Senior Citizens as "one of the best government responses" and Steve Hahn, spokesman for AARP, said that "All eyes will be on Illinois to see if they can get this tactic through" (Harper, 2003, p. A1). Blagojevich's plan violated FDA policy regarding drug importation, and he made several failed attempts to convince the FDA to reconsider. Despite the FDA, the reimportation website, www.I-SaveRx.com, opened for business and was also made available to citizens in Kansas, Wisconsin, Missouri, and Vermont.[25] It attracted significant criticism, most of which focused on the safety concerns. The FDA, according to the *New York Times*, disapproved: "Federal officials say drugs from Canada carry numerous potential risks: false labeling, counterfeiting and more" (Davey, 2003, p. A27).

Immediately following Blagojevich's 2003 announcement, the Illinois Policy Institute (2003), a conservative think tank operating out of Springfield, issued a policy brief that lambasted the governor for his decision. The Institute cited the plethora of agencies that saw the potential dangers in drug reimportation (e.g., the FDA and, incorrectly, the American Medical Association (see Choudhry and Detsky, 2005)). Their report also cited a *Wall Street Journal* summary of a Canadian report that found that "more than one third of Internet drug sites claiming to operate in Canada are actually located in shipping from other countries including Mexico, Thailand, and India" (Illinois Policy Institute, 2003, p. 2). A few months after the 2003 announcement, parroting the safety issues outlined by the FDA, the president of the Illinois Pharmacists Association wrote a letter published in the *Chicago Sun-Times*, condemning the governor's policy: "Illinois should not be putting the health of its state employees and retirees on the line by experimenting with a drug importation plan that poses serious safety hazards. There are no safeguards in place to ensure the quality, purity or efficacy of medications purchased from Canada. . . . Drug importation is not a risk Illinois should be taking. It's that simple" (Drabant, 2003, p. 46). Conservative groups and others with pharmaceutical ties perpetuated the safety rhetoric for years after the launch of I-SaveRx.

The fear of terrorism, especially, lent an emotional charge to the questions about safety. Undoubtedly, the pharmaceutical corporations exploited what Americans feared most: terrorists who might strike again in some frightening and surprising fashion. Recapping a public session in Washington, D.C., devoted to investigating drug importation programs cropping up around the country, the *Washington Post* noted that Bernard Kerik, the former New York police commissioner during 9/11, and thus a particularly symbolic figure, testified that "We are very concerned if wholesale importing is permitted, it will make this country's medicine supply extremely vulnerable to terrorist intervention" (Connolly, 2004, p. A3). Kerik also admitted that his investigation was conducted with the financial help of PhRMA. Poll data indicated that, like U.S. citizens as a whole, residents of Illinois have not been persuaded that reimported drugs are unsafe. By spring of 2007, the site also offered lower prescription drug costs and either reduced or eliminated copays for state employees.[26] In a letter written from Blagojevich to President Bush in October of 2006, the governor also continues to emphasize the need for federal officials to relax their laws on drug importation (Office of Gov. Rod Blagojevich, 2006).

In addition to failed safety rhetoric, the FDA's drug seizures also failed. Between 2001 and 2005, less than 1 percent of shipments were seized, and Canadian pharmacies absorbed the costs of replacing the seized drugs (Girion, 2006). No shipments from Mexico were seized, even though the possibility of counterfeit drugs moving across that border is generally seen as greater than it is with imports from Canada or Europe (Bernstein, 2003; Burns, 2005). Seizures angered senior citizens, who typically vote Republican, and spurred Congress to act.

Washington beckons, again

Buoyed by state successes, advocates persuaded Congresspersons to introduce two bills in Congress which would allow reimportation, create a federal system through which U.S. citizens would be linked to approved pharmacies in Canada and Europe, and ensure against the importation of counterfeit drugs.[27] Under heavy industry pressure, Senate majority leader Bill Frist (R-TN) kept both bills from reaching the floor of the Senate for debate because he knew that "if it was up [for vote] it would pass 75 to 25" (Sen. Charles Grassley (R-Iowa), cited in Barry, 2004, p. 11; also see Barry & Basler, 2004). By 2006, polls indicated that less than 20 percent of Americans believed that the reimportation ban/seizures were motivated by safety concerns, and more than half felt that they were the result of industry lobbying motivated by efforts to maintain high profit margins. In October, 2006, the Bush administration announced that it would stop seizing drugs, and Bush signed a bill allowing individuals to travel to Canada and purchase a 90-day supply of prescription drugs (Basler, 2006; Bloomberg, 2006; CBC, 2006).

When combined, resistance by the industry and friendly politicians did have some impact on the burgeoning reimportation industry. Some marginal operations were forced to close and profit margins shrank for the major companies (Lohn, 2006). Growth rates were halved, from 15 percent per year to 7 percent. It is impossible to tell which moves had the greatest impact, and none may have been as influential as the increasing value of the Canadian dollar compared to the currencies of the United States and other supplier nations (Macafee, 2006). However, it is clear that the actions forced reimporters to become more strategic and more proactive in their responses to industry–government alliances.

Interpretation, conclusion, and directions

We began this chapter with a position that is relatively new to health communication scholars. We suggested that, while both elites and nonelites have access to the same structural and rhetorical strategies in the construction and implementation of public health policy, their ability to use them to obtain desired outcomes is unequally distributed. Because elites have access to greater tangible resources and are more tightly networked with one another and with policy makers, they find it much easier to mold the structural configurations within which political action takes place, to act within those guidelines and constraints, and to modify the configurations when it is strategically advantageous to do so. Nonelites can engage in tactical action, which also can lead to changes in structural configurations, but are handicapped by limited resources, difficulty maintaining long-term network ties to policy makers, and by the need for structural stability within which they can devise and adjust their tactics. Our analysis of the drug reimportation issue both supports this model, and suggests two modifications.

The most important forms of strategic action by this elite industry involve the U.S. Congress and executive branch. In the legislative arena, public drug policy is privatized in plain sight. Extended patent protection and restrictions on generic drugs are overt parts of trade legislation.[28] But their meaning and importance is easily obscured by lumping together with other forms of "intellectual property rights." Other Congressional rules and procedures allow industry-friendly leaders to keep meaningful constraints from coming up for a vote, or to bury crucial changes in the private process of reconciling differences in bills passed by the U.S. House and Senate. Lobbying at both the federal and the state levels gives the industry disproportionate access to legislators, relative to consumer groups, and the ability to concentrate resources in the legislative chambers that constitute the greatest immediate threat to the industry. Policies that shift costs to taxpayers are especially easy to manage because the costs are borne by a group that is so diverse and disconnected that it is virtually impossible to mobilize.[29] Bills that "placate" the public, but have no effective enforcement provisions, are equally valuable. If legislative efforts fail, the court system, especially the federal courts, can be used to stop or water down state-level initiatives.[30] The industry can simultaneously move to weaken regulatory action.

New structures can be introduced to create seemingly objective "evidence" to support industry claims (Aune, 2001). Industry rhetors can legitimize their claims through the ethos of these "intellectual echo chambers" and/or regulatory agencies. Generalized "free market" and/or "miracle drug" rhetoric can be persuasive, especially as a way to frame critics' much more difficult-to-understand distinctions between "excessive" and "reasonable" profits, "miracle" and "new-but-not-improved and/or cost-beneficial" drugs, or "government price controls" and negotiated price ceilings. Dealing drugs on the border(s) clearly illustrates processes of outflanking.

However, our analysis of the drug reimportation case also suggests two modifications of the model. First, it clarifies the nature of the advantages available to organizational elites. As Anthony Giddens' analysis of globalization suggests (2000), today's multinational corporations have unprecedented "reach," both in terms of their ability to extend over time and space, and in terms of their capacity to insinuate themselves deeply into public policy making/enforcing bodies. Of course, not all corporate–government alliances are of equal importance—the "reach" of the U.S. government dwarfs all other possible alliances. On the surface, it appears that an alliance with the U.S. executive branch is most important—the use of trade agreements to undermine national sovereignty in the guise of protecting intellectual property, refusal to enforce legislation such as the Bayh–Dole act (repayment of federal R&D funds), or the use of the FDA to produce highly questionable rhetoric and policies (seizures of imports). However, the U.S. Congress has repeatedly acted in ways that ensure multinationals' continued policy monopolies, from continuing the "revolving door" of Congresspersons leaving the body to become industry lobbyists, to enacting industry-advantageous trade and consumer legislation, to funding the FDA in ways that encourage it to hasten the introduction of new drugs and delay the approval of generics, to enacting laws that the courts use to short-circuit state innovations. In short, although policy may be made in Washington, its impact is worldwide, and extended for decades into the future. Elites' ability to move seamlessly between public and private realms of action ensure the continuation of their privileged position.

The second extension involves the outflanking process itself. The drug reimportation experience highlights the dialectical nature of the outflanking–counteroutflanking process, and the relationship between social/political structures and rhetorical action. For example, it was action by state governments, spurred by grassroots activism, in response to the FDA's unbelievable safety claims that eventually led to changes in that organization's practices. Ironically, the agency's rhetoric has not changed, even though the active research efforts of state governments such as Illinois Governor Blagojevich's have completely undermined the credibility of its claims. Continued low-visibility civil disobedience by American customers "boldly crossing the line for cheaper drugs," to adopt the title of a related *New York Times* article, kept the issue on the public agenda and created a burgeoning market that was successfully exploited by Canadian and European entrepreneurs. As the U.S. industry–government coalition shifted its strategies and rhetoric, reimporters devised more sophisticated modes of operating. Eventually, grassroots pressure did lead to legislation at both the state and federal levels. New rhetoric leads to the creation of new structures, which created new rhetorical situations and opportunities while allowing the old ones to continue, in a complex and never-ending process.

Notes

1 The rapid increase from 1990 until 2003 was driven by increases in the number of prescriptions written (up 71 percent), increases in drug prices (which more than tripled the average annual inflation rate), and a shift toward expensive "new" drugs and away from older name-brand drugs and generics. The price moderation from 2003–2005 resulted from a reversal of these latter factors, primarily through increased uses of tiered copayment plans and varied cost-containment efforts among state Medicaid programs, all of which shifted spending toward older-but-comparably (or more) effective brand name drugs and generics (Gardner, 2007).

2 Tobin, 2007. Canada's economy is the tenth largest in the world, a bit larger than the state of California. The two have approximately the same population (*Houston Chronicle*, 2007). The nature and effectiveness of the Canadian system is routinely distorted in debates about U.S. health-care policy (Marmor, 1994, especially Chapter 12).

3 The Canadian Constitution explicitly declares that health care is a provincial, not a national, responsibility, with a few exceptions (e.g., the military and health care for indigenous peoples). As a result, Ottawa influences provincial systems primarily through financing arrangements. For excellent summaries of the development of the Canadian system, see Fuller (1998) and Rachlis and Kushner (1994). Over time, Ottawa's actual contribution to the Provinces' health-care costs has declined, reaching a low of 18 percent in 2004 (Ubelacker, 2004). It currently stands at just over 25 percent.

4 The act also increased the costs of generic drugs sold in Canada. Of the twenty-seven top-selling generic drugs sold in Canada during 2001, three-quarters could be purchased more cheaply in the United States (Neergaard, 2004).

5 Quebec's government seems relatively satisfied with its current plan, which covers a far larger percentage of residents than those of the other provinces and has frozen drug prices since 1994. However, reduced supplies of some drugs have led the province to consider allowing prices to rise, although it has made a commitment to absorb all increased costs (CBC, 2007). For more information on the "pharmacare" debate, see Canadian Press, 2005; Cordon, 2004; Perkel, 2004; and Ubelacker, 2004.

6 U.S. residents could save an additional 25–30 percent by purchasing prescriptions in the European Union. For example, a study conducted for the pbs series "Frontline" found that a group of four commonly prescribed drugs would cost $367 USD in the United States, $145 in Canada (39.5 percent of the U.S. price), and $103 in the EU (28 percent of the U.S. price and 71 percent of the Canadian price), Frontline, "The other drug war," 2003, transcript at www.pbs.org.

7 There also is a thriving reimportation system across the U.S.–Mexican border as a result of a 30–50 percent difference in costs. Most of this trade involves U.S. citizens physically crossing the border to shop in Mexican pharmacies, rather than internet mail orders. For example, *Houston Chronicle* personal finance columnist Scott Burns found that a month's supply of Zetia and Lipitor (which work together to control cholesterol) cost him a $30 copay thorough his company health plan, $93.03 at a pharmacy in Juarez, Mexico, and $181 at a Walgreens across the river in El Paso, TX. The dollar value of the trade is difficult to estimate (Bernstein, 2003; also see Harper, 2003).

8 For excellent summaries of industry rhetoric and critics' attacks and responses, see the materials available on the pbs.com website in conjunction with the Frontline episode, "The Other Drug War," and Abramson, 2004 and Angell, 2004. For the debate in Canada, see Rachlis (2004, ch. 10) and Fuller (1998, ch. 10). For an

excellent example of rhetorical criticism of pharmaceutical company rhetoric, see Quisenberry Stokes, this volume.

9   Dr. Taurel failed to mention that the seven countries that moved ahead of France also have some form of price control or government negotiation of prices.

10 For and extended analysis of this rhetoric, see Aune (2001). Ironically, PhRMa rhetors do not view protective tariffs, importation bans, government subsidies, or extended patent protections as governmental intrusions into the pharmaceutical "free market" (Antos, 2004).

11 The Bayh-Dole Act is a provision of the U.S. patent law that requires pharmaceutical firms that develop new drugs through research supported by federal funds to make those drugs available at a reasonable price. However, the law has never been enforced because the industry has successfully described it as an anti-competitive price control measure (Arno & Davis, 2002). Shifting federal funds to relatively rare conditions also could further reduce the need for massive profits on drugs with a larger market. Somewhat ironically, quasi-market forces are leading companies to shift more of their R&D activities to small-market drugs. Managed care plans and pharmaceutical middlemen are increasingly refusing to pay higher prices for "me too" drugs than for older drugs. As a result, firms have increased their own R&D spending (up an average of 6 percent in 2006) and focusing on niche conditions with small patient populations, and thus smaller clinical trial requirements (Agovino, 2006).

12 In the United States the most important free market think tanks are the Heritage Foundation and the Cato Institute; in Canada it is Vancouver's Fraser Institute. For an extended analysis of the role that these organizations play in free market rhetoric, see Aune (2001). Some political scientists take the somewhat counter-intuitive position that campaign contributions do not lead to favorable policy outcomes. For a critque of this position see Baumgartner and Leech (1998) and Clawson et al. (1998).

13 The strategies merged together somewhat, and regulatory capture was streamlined, on January 30, 2007 when the Bush administration announced that in the future all federal regulatory agencies must have a regulatory policy office run by a political appointee whose mandate will be to ensure that all regulatory actions be consistent with the President's priorities (Pear, 2007).

14 Dr. Frank is co-author, along with current Federal Reserve Chairman Ben Bernanke of *Principles of Economics*.

15 Mann defines classes in terms of economic power, not wealth or income: "that is, in persons' ability to control their own and others' life chances through control of economic resources—the means of production, distribution, and exchange" (1986, p. 216).

16 Keith Banting and Stan Corbett (2002) have persuasively argued that health policy making is distinctively complicated in federal systems like that of the United States and, to a lesser extent, Canada (see also Lammers & Liebig, 1990, and *Health Affairs*, 1998). The multiple levels of government created by a combined state/provincial and national system makes it less likely that major changes will be enacted or implemented. Federalism increases the number of "veto points" at which policy initiatives can be stymied, increases nonproductive inter-regional competition, and makes it more difficult for consumer or popular interest groups to influence policy making. Because they have fewer resources than the corporate lobby, they are less able to "cover" all of the sites where policy is being constructed. In short, a highly federal system provides a larger number of pressure points at which advocacy groups can attempt to stimulate policy change and for organizational actors to outflank those change agents. Immerschein et al. (1992)

trace state efforts to contain costs in the face of industry opposition during the 1980s and find very mixed results—in some states advocates are able to overcome elite dominance on some issues; in others they are not. For a similar analysis over a longer time period, see the essays in Leichtner (1997).

17   As far as we know, neither Mann nor de Certeau (1984) takes this position explicitly. In fact, Mann subsequently (1993) abandons the concept of "circuits of praxis," although Clegg (1989) expanded and refined it in his model of "circuits of power." We believe our extension is consistent with their overall arguments, but it is our extension of them.

18   Lobbyists who favor particular policy options establish ongoing relationships with policy makers and regulators and then introduce their pet "solutions" at opportune times through rhetoric that casts those options as viable solutions. For example, during the 1960s when it was politically viable to advocate expanding social service programs, advocates of Health Maintenance Organizations (HMOs) touted them as a means of increasing access to care by the poor. Later, when the Nixon administration focused on cost containment, HMO advocates argued that health-care cost increases were driven by the fee-for-service payment system and could be controlled by increased reliance on managed care. Still later, when the public health community sought to focus on preventive care, HMOs were touted as a solution to that problem as well (Stone, 1988).

19   Political scientists have studied policy monopolies in a variety of settings, and have used a number of different terms to describe them—*iron triangles, policy whirlpools,* and *subsystem politics* are the most common. The classic study of health-care policy-making triangles is Starr (1982, 1994).

20   Of course, organizations may want to initiate new policies as well as block policy initiatives. For example, there was substantial corporate support for President Bush's tax reform package during 2001. But, large corporations were so successful in enacting desired policies from 1975 through 2001 (Greider, 1992; Kuttner, 1997; Phillips, 2002) that their primary concern today is with blocking policy.

21   Somewhat ironically, the Harper administration's position is based on free market ideology—restricting reimporation would be an undue government intervention in the economic system.

22   Although all parties admit that there is some risk that internet operations masquerading as pharmacies in high-safety countries (Canada, Germany, Ireland, and Australia) could pose a safety risk, it is excessively high U.S. drug costs that drive any potential black-market. Consequently, if reimportation actually reduces prices in the United States, it would reduce safety risks (Barry, 2004).

23   Recent FDA actions have helped the industry in another way. In the early 1990s Congress passed the Prescription Drug Users Fee Act, which required companies to pay up to a $500,000 USD fee so that the agency could hire more reviewers in an effort to speed the approval of new drugs. Today more than half of the FDA's reviewers are paid with industry money. Critics argue that the new funding system compromises drug safety, a claim that the FDA's leadership denies. It is clear, however, that the system has had two favorable effects for the industry: it has cut approval time from more than two years to less than six months (*Frontline,* "Dangerous Prescription," p. 13) and has slowed the approval of generic drugs. While the number of generic drug applications doubled between 2001 and 2005, the backlog also has doubled (Harris, 2006). The act also allowed the industry to market drugs directly to consumers (only New Zealand and the United States do so), and it is that provision that is likely to dominate debate over the extension and/or expansion of the act during early 2007 (Freudenheim, 2007). The industry uses a number of tactics to delay the introduction of generic drugs (Bridges, 2007; Kaplan, 2007; Kaufman, 2006; Saul, 2006b, 2006c, 2006d).

24 Reimportation was not the only cost-control strategy utilized by the states. In Oregon, Governor John Kitzhaber, facing massive increases in the costs of Medicaid prescription drugs, focused on improving customer decision making by providing information on the relative costs and effectiveness of various drugs for common conditions. Again, lobbyists attacked, but the governor gained support from the business lobby whose members faced similar cost inflation. For a time, they were able to keep the bill bottled up in committee, but Kitzhabers's threat to veto the $1 billion USD Department of Human Services budget, and start a publicity campaign in which he argued that legislative leaders were denying consumers the information they needed to make effective decisions because of their financial ties to the industry. In addition, the bill was carefully designed to *not* substitute state regulations for individual judgment. It passed with a comfortable margin, and the list of preferred drugs, minus a large number of highly advertised and expensive, but no more effective, was made public (see *Frontline*, "Other War."). The states of West Virginia and Kentucky won similar battles over drugs included in their Medicaid formularies, while New York state legislature over-rode Governor Pataki's veto of a bill preventing the creation of a preferred-drug list for its Medicaid program (Harris, 2003).

25 Tennessee and Michigan are currently considering plans to use the program as well.

26 Though I-SaveRx still operates, most of those eligible to use the program have not done so. To date, it has processed approximately 16,200 orders in comparison to Illinois retail pharmacies, which filled 141 million prescriptions in 2003 alone (Landa, 2005). However, reports and polls indicate that safety does not appear to have caused its lack of use. Instead, the governor's office admits that it has not publicized the program well to Illinois residents eligible for the program and doctors, and many of those who have tried to use I-SaveRx found the website too confusing. Still others have not seen enough savings to find the program, money wise, worthwhile.

27 One bill, sponsored by Sen. Snowe (R-Maine) and Sen. Byron Dorgan (D-ND) also would prohibit drug companies from cutting off supplies to foreign pharmacies that participate in the program (Barry & Basler, 2004).

28 Accepting extended patent periods and other restrictions on generic drugs also have been used as requirements for a country entering the WTO (Rabinowitz, 2007).

29 The threat imposed by state-level initiatives led PhRMa to shift its attention to federal legislation. The eventual result was the creation of Medicare Plan D, generally considered to be the largest shift of taxpayer money to corporate coffers in U.S. history (Applebaum, 2003; Bartlett, 2006; Common Cause, 2004; Gilpin, 2003). Unfortunately, space limitations preclude any systematic analysis of the political and rhetorical processes that led to Plan D, or of its impact on drug reimportation. Congress continues to consider proposals designed to allow reimportation, continues to succumb to industry and Bush administration pressure, and Americans continue to import drugs from abroad (Gorham, 2007).

30 See, for example, Aune's (2001) analysis of the influence that free-market advocates have on the federal court system.

References

AARP Bulletin (2007). You can trim your prescription drug bill. May, p. 6.

Abramson, John (2004). *Overdosed America*. New York: HarperCollins.

Agovino, Theresa (2006). Drug makers re-evaluate approaches to research. *Houston Chronicle*, December 10, D9.

Angell, Marcia (2004). *The Truth About the Drug Companies*. New York: Random House.

Antos, Joseph (2004). *Private Discounts, Public Subsidies*. Washington, DC: AEI Press.

Applebaum, Anne (2003). Bipartisanship the worst kind of Medicare politics. *Houston Chronicle*, June 27, 35A.

Arno, P., & Davis, M. (2002). Drug pricing law never enforced. *Houston Chronicle*, April 17, 27A.

Aune, Jame Arnt (1994). *The Rhetoric of Marxism*. Boulder, CO: Westview Press.

Aune, James Arnt (2001). *Selling the Free Market*. New York: Guilford Press.

Bakan, Joel (2004). *The Corporation*. Boston: Free Press.

Banting, Keith, & Corbett, Stan (2002). *Health Policy and Federalism*. Kingston, Ontario, CA: Queens University Institute of Intergovernmente.

Barry, Patricia (2004). States defy FDA on drug reimportation. *AARP Bulletin*, October, pp. 10–12.

Barry, Patricia, & Basler, Barbara (2004). Battle lines drawn on Rx imports. *AARP Bulletin*, July–Aug, p. 2.

Bartlett, Bruce (2006). *Imposter*. New York: Doubleday.

Basler, Barbara (2006). Public favors Canada imports. *AARP Bulletin*, November, p. 8.

Baumgartner, Frank & Jones, Bryan (1993). *Agendas and Instability in American Politics*. Chicago: University of Chicago Press.

Baumgartner, Frank, & Leech, Beth (1998). *Basic Interests: The Importance of Interest Groups in Politics and Political Science*. Princeton: Princeton University Press.

Beauchamp, Donald (1996). *Health Care Reform and the Battle for the Body Politic*. Philadelphia: Temple University Press.

Bernstein, Alan (2003). Seniors flock to Mexico for savings. *Houston Chronicle*, June 8, 1A.

Bloomberg News (2006). U.S. steps back on drug confiscations. *NY Times on the Web*. October 4. Retrieved October 4, 2006.

Bridges, Andrew (2007). Settlements delay generic drugs, regulators argue. *Bryan-College Station Eagle.com*. January 18. Retrieved January 18, 2007.

Broder, John (2006). Amid scandals, states overhaul lobbying laws. *NY Times on the Web*. January 24. Retrieved January 26, 2006.

Burns, Scott (2005). Prescriptions become a pricey investment. *Houston Chronicle*, January 31, D3.

Canadian Press (2004). UN says U.S.-Peru trade pact could raise prices of essential drugs in Peru. www.canada.com. July 14. Retrieved July 14, 2004.

CBC (Canadian Broadcasting Corporation) (2006). Canada shouldn't be "medicine cabinet" for U.S., pharmacists warn. www.cbc.ca. October 5. Retrieved October 6, 2006.

CBC (Canadian Broadcasting Corporation) (2007). Quebec to end freeze on drug prices. January 18. www.cbc.ca. Retrieved January 18, 2007.

Center for Responsive Politics (2007). Pharmaceuticals/health products: long-term contribution trends. www.opensecrets.org/industries. Retrieved January 11, 2007.

Cheney, George, Christiansen, Lars, Conrad, Charles, and Lair, Daniel (2004). Organizational rhetoric as organizational discourse. In D. Grant, C. Hardy, C. Oswick, & L. Putnam, (eds), *The Handbook of Organizational Discourse*. Thousand Oaks, CA: Sage, pp. 79–104.

Choudhry, Niteesh K., & Detsky, Allan S. (2005). A perspective on US drug reimportation. *Journal of the American Medical Association, 293*(3): 358–362.

Clawson, Don, Neustadtl, Alan, & Weller, Mark (1998). *Dollars and Votes.* Philadelphia, PA: Temple University Press.

Clegg, Stewart (1989). *Frameworks of Power.* London: Sage.

Clegg, Stewart, Courpasson, David, & Phillips, Nelson (2006). *Power and Organizations.* London: Sage.

Cobb, R.W., & Ross, M.H. (eds) (1997). *Cultural Strategies of Agenda Denial.* Lawrence: University of Kansas Press.

Common Cause (2004). Democracy on drugs: The Medicare/Prescription drug bill, a study in how government shouldn't work. Washington, DC: Common Cause.

Connolly, Ceci. (2004). Industry backers have strong voice at public session. *Washington Post*, April 15, p. A3.

Conrad, Charles, & Abbott, Je'Anna (2007). Corporate social responsibility and public policymaking. In Steve May, George Cheney, & Juliet Roper (eds), *The Debate Over Corporate Social Responsibility.* New York: Oxford, pp. 413–437.

Cooper, M. (2006). New prescription pricing law faces repeal in Pataki budget. *NY Times on the Web.* January 20. Retrieved January 21, 2006.

Cordon, Sandra (2004). Pharmacare program too costly: Goodale. www.canada.com. August 19. Retrieved August 20, 2004.

Davey, Monica. (2003). Illinois to seek U.S. exemption to buy drugs from Canada. *New York Times*, December 22, p. A27.

de Certeau, Michel (1984). *The Practice of Everyday Life.* Berkeley: University of California Press.

Delong, Bradford (2004). Phony case against drug imports. *Houston Chronicle*, October 10, 1E.

Drabant, Steve M. (2003). Letters to the editor. *Chicago Sun-Times*, November 13, p. 46.

Frank, Robert (2006). State governments overreach in taking on problems best solved at the national level. www.nytimes.com. April 13. Retrieved April 13, 2006.

Freudenheim, Milt (2007). Showdown looms in Congress over drug advertising on tv. *NY Times on the Web.* January 22. Retrieved January 22, 2007.

Fuller, Colleen (1998). *Caring for Profit.* Vancouver: New Star Books.

Gardner, Amanda (2007). But out-of-pocket costs continue to rise, annual government report says. www.cbc.ca. January 9. Retrieved January 9, 2007.

Giddens, Anthony (1984). *The Constitution of Society.* Berkeley: University of California Press.

Giddens, Anthony (2000). *Runaway World.* New York: Routledge.

Gilpin, Kenneth (2003). The winners in the Medicare bill, and why. *NY Times on the web.* December 14. Retrieved December 14, 2003.

Girion, Lisa (2006). More medicines from abroad seized. www.latimes.com. February 11. Retrieved February 13, 2006.

Gorham, Beth (2007). U.S. Senate guts latest attempt to legalize bulk drug imports from Canada. May 7. www.cbc.ca. Retrieved May 8, 2007.

Gormley, M. (2006). Bid to cut pollution reports criticized. *Houston Chronicle*, January 22, A6.

Goverde, Henri, Cerny, Philip, Haugaard, Mark, & Lentner, Howard (2000). *Power in Contemporary Politics.* London: Sage.

Office of Gov. Rod Blagojevich. (2006). Press Release. October 5. www.illinois.gov/gov/.

Greider, William (1992). *Who Will Tell the People?* New York: Simon & Schuster.

Greider, K. (2004). Get drugmakers' attention with both carrot and stick. *Houston Chronicle*, October 23, B9.

Gross, D. (2003). *Prescription Drug Prices in Canada.* Washington, DC: AARP Policy Institute.

Hacker, Jacob (1997). *The Road to Nowhere: The Genesis of President Clinton's Plan for Health Security.* Princeton, NJ: Princeton University Press.

Hall, James, & Jones, Bryan (1997). Agenda denial and issue containment in the regulation of financial securities. In R.W. Cobb, & M.H. Ross, (eds), *Cultural Strategies of Agenda Denial.* Lawrence, KS: Kansas University Press, pp. 40–69.

Harper, Tim. (2003). Illinois wants Canadian drugs. *Toronto Star*, September 16, p. A1.

Harris, Gardiner (2003). States try to limit drugs in Medicaid, but makers resist. *NY Times on the Web.* December 18. Retrieved December 18, 2003.

Harris, Gardiner (2006). For generics, bumpy road to pharmacy. *NY Times on the Web.* February 23. Retrieved February 23, 2006.

Health Affairs (1998). Special issue on "states and the new federalism." *17*, 3.

Houston Chronicle (2003b). FDA takes its war on imported drugs to New England. December 17, 6A.

Houston Chronicle (2003c). FDA: Legalizing Canadian drugs too costly. December 24, 11A.

Houston Chronicle (2007). Just how big is that economy? January 16, D3.

Illinois Policy Institute (2003). Does the Blagojevich prescription drug reimportation proposal threaten public safety, fund terrorism? Springfield: Illinois Policy Institute.

Imershein, Allen, Rond, Philip, & Mathis, Mary (1992). Restructuring patterns of elite dominance and the formation of state policy in health care. *American Journal of Sociology*, 97: 970–993.

Iyengar, Shano (1993) *Is Anyone Responsible?* Chicago: University of Chicago Press.

Kain, J. (1974). Urban problems. In J. McKie (ed.), *Social Responsibility and the Business Predicament.* Washington, DC: Brookings Institution, pp. 217–246.

Kaiser Family Foundation (2007). Health care spending in the United States and OECD Countries. January. www.kff.org. Retrieved January 5, 2007.

Kaiser Family Foundation (2006). Prescription drug trends. www.kff.org. June. Retrieved July 1, 2006.

Kaplan, Peter (2007). Senate bill aims to end deals on generic drugs. www.washingtonpost.com. January 17. Retrieved January 19, 2007.

Kaufman, Marc (2006). Drug firms' deals allow exclusivity. www.washingtonpost.com. April 25. Retrieved November 26, 2006.

Kingdon, James (1984/1995). *Agendas, Alternatives and Public Policies.* Boston: Little Brown.

Krauss, Clifford (2005). Going global at a small-town Canadian drugstore. *NY Times on the Web.* March 5. Retrieved March 5, 2005.

Krauss, Clifford (2006). Kinks in the Canada drug pipeline. *N.Y. Times on the Web.* April 6. Retrieved April 6, 2006.

Kuttner, Robert (1997). *Everything for Sale.* New York: Alfred Knopf.

Lammers, William, & Liebig, Phoebe (1990). State health policies, federalism, and the elderly. *The Journal of Federalism*, 20: 131–148.

Landa, Amy Snow. (2005). Illinois drug import program falls flat with doctors. www. ama-assn.org. December 5. Retrieved January 25, 2007.

Leichter, Howard (1997). *Health Policy Reform in America: Innovations from the States.* Armonk, NY: M.E. Sharpe.

Lohn, Martiga (2006). Fewer American seniors are turning to Canada to fill prescriptions. www.canada.com. February 22. Retrieved February 22, 2006.

Lynx, Donald, & Salmon, J. Warren (2006). Confronting the denial of drugs to Americans in need. Working Paper. Chicago: University of Illinois at Chicago.

Macafee, Michelle (2006). Internet pharmacists await fallout from new U.S. drug benefit. www.canada.com. January 1. Retrieved January 1, 2006.

Mann, Michael (1986). *The Sources of Social Power*, Vol. 1. Cambridge: Cambridge University Press.

Mann, Michael (1993). *The Sources of Social Power*, Vol. 2. New York: Cambridge University Press.

Manheim, Jarol (2001). *The Death of a Thousand Cuts.* Mahwah, NJ: Lawrence Erlbaum.

Marmor, Theodore (1994). *Understanding Health Care Reform.* New Haven: Yale University Press.

May, Steve, Cheney, George, & Roper, Juliet (2007). *The Debate over Corporate Social Responsibility.* New York: Oxford.

McClelland, Colin (2005). Canada considers blocking internet drug sales. *Houston Chronicle*, January 6, A14.

McNeil, Kenneth (1978). Understanding organizational power. *Administrative Science Quarterly*, 23: 65–90.

Munro, Margaret (2006). Canada's prescription drug bill continues to skyrocket. www.canada.com. May 11. Retrieved May 11, 2006.

Neergaard, Lauran (2004). Study: U.S. generics cheaper than many Canadian drugs. *Houston Chronicle*, January 18, 9A.

Pear, Robert (2003). Drug companies increase spending to lobby Congress and government. *NY Times on the Web.* June 1. Retrieved June 1, 2003.

Pear, Robert (2006). Drug industry is on defensive as power shifts. *N.Y. Times on the Web.* November 24. Retrieved November 24, 2006.

Pear, Robert (2007). Bush directive increases sway on regulation. *NY Times on the web.* January 30. Retrieved January 30, 2007.

Perkel, Colin (2004). Premiers call on Martin to explain Liberal election promise on pharmacare. www.canada.com. September 2. Retrieved September 9, 2004.

Phillips, Kevin (2002). *Wealth and Democracy.* New York: Broadway Books.

Porter, Eduardo (2004). Importing less expensive drugs not seen as cure for U.S. woes. *NY Times on the Web.* October 16. Retrieved October 16, 2004.

Rabinowitz, Gavin (2007). Hundreds protest Swiss pharmaceutical giant's challenge to Indian patent law. www.cnc.ca. January 29. Retrived January 29, 2007.

Rachlis, Michael (2004). *Prescription for Excellence.* Toronto: Harper Collins.

Rachlis, Michael, & Kushner, Carol (1994). *Strong Medicine.* Toronto: Random House.

Redford, E.S. (1969). *Democracy in the Administrative State.* New York: Oxford University Press.

Saul, S. (2006a). In the newest war of the states, forget red and blue. *NY Times on the Web.* January 31. Retrieved January 31, 2006.

Saul, Stephanie (2006b). Marketers of Plavix outfoxed on a deal. *NY Times on the Web*. August 9. Retrieved January 19, 2007.

Saul, Stephanie (2006c). Generic of Plavix is blocked. *NY Times on the Web*. September 1. Retrieved September 9, 2006.

Saul, Stephanie (2006d). Plavix makers say a generic threatens research. *NY Times on the Web*. September 19. Retrieved September 19, 2006.

Schattschneider, E.E. (1935). *Politics, Pressures and the Tariff*. New York: Prentice Hall.

Skocpol, Theda (1996). *Boomerang*. New York: W.W. Norton.

Starr, Paul (1982). *The Social Transformation of American Medicine*. New York: Basic Books.

Starr, Paul (1994). *The Logic of Health Care Reform*. New York: Penguin.

Stone, Deborah (1988). *Policy Paradox*. Glenview, IL: Scott Foresman.

Tobin, Anne-Marie (2007). Study in new journal compares health outcomes in Canada and U.S. www.cbc.ca. April 17. Retrieved April 18, 2007.

Ubelacker, Sheryl (2004). Dosanjh still nixing pharmacare. www.canada.com. August 16. Retrieved August 17, 2004.

Vogel, David (1989). *Fluctuating Fortunes*. New York: Basic Books.

Wilson, James Q. (1973). *Political Organizations*. New York: Basic Books.

Wilson, J.Q. (1974). The politics of regulation. In J. McKie (ed.), *Social Responsibility and the Business Predicament*. Washington, DC: Brookings Institution, pp. 135–168.

Chapter 17

Technologies of neoliberal governmentality

The discursive influence of global economic policies on public health

Heather M. Zoller

In 1997 the World Health Organization (WHO) predicted that, "The interrelationship between global trade and industrialization, environmental sustainability and public health will become major public policy issues" (WHO, 1997, p. 4). Indeed, some argue that the locus of power in health policy making has shifted as the World Bank (WB) now outspends the WHO in health-related funding (Barris & McLeod, 2000). This chapter examines the significant influence of global economic and trade agreements on public health. The development and growth of neoliberal policies through organizations such as the World Bank, International Monetary Fund (IMF), World Trade Organization (WTO), and North American Free Trade Area (NAFTA) materially affect key structural predictors of health including income levels, education, access to basic resources, safety measures, and environmental quality (Millen & Holtz, 2000). At the same time, the neoliberal ideologies that undergird these policies actually impede health promoters' ability to address these problems by discursively privileging the private market and undermining the language of public investment and protection we associate with public health promotion. Thus, although economic policies may seem far from the purview of health communication, these policies represent vital communication issues for the field to address.

As Conrad and Jodlowski describe in this volume, policy negotiation, construction, and implementation are communicative processes that involve struggles over meaning among actors with different levels of access and power (see also Conrad & McIntush, 2003). Although the field of health communication works internationally and has given some attention to health policy, little research has considered the influence of global trade policy discourse on the social context of health and illness. Examining economic discourse may at first seem removed from the work of health communication, thus one goal of this chapter is to illustrate its centrality to understanding health in both its symbolic and material/biological dimensions. The chapter begins by describing how a critical, multisectoral approach to public health demonstrates the linkage by prioritizing the political, economic, and social roots of health inequality across social domains. I then present the concept of governmentality (Foucault, 1991; Rose & Miller, 1992) as an analytic framework. The chapter demonstrates the utility of this critical framework by interrogating three significant neoliberal policy mechanisms as governmental technology. These technologies include Structural Adjustment Policies (SAPs), Harmonization mechanisms, and Investor-to-State Lawsuits (ISLs).

The analysis illustrates how these policies, in privileging commercial interests, make it difficult to promote good health by raising standards of proof for health protection, disqualifying health as a counter-discourse, and discouraging democratic decision-making. The chapter ends with discussion of the ways that health communication scholars can address the problems of neoliberalism in our research, and support health activism that seeks to resist and transform economic policies in ways that serve rather than undermine public health.

Global trade and development discourse: economic governmentality and public health

First, I define some key terms related to globalization and public health. "Globalization" is a polysemic term that may be used to refer to growing interplay between multiple cultures, homogenization of cultures due to the growth of international media, and the growth of particular trade and economic relationships. This chapter is limited in its scope to the latter meaning, focused on the set of economic arrangements usually associated with the development of the post-World War II Bretton Woods economic institutions, including the WB, IMF, the General Agreement on Tariffs and Trade (GATT) that gave way to the WTO, and a host of multilateral trade agreements, including NAFTA and proposed Free Trade Area of the Americas (FTAA).

The WTO is a mechanism to manage the world trade system that allows member countries to make commitments to trade liberalization and hold one another accountable through dispute settlement. The WB facilitates multilateral development loans primarily to developing countries, originally for certain development projects (e.g. building a dam), and now for more broad-based structural support. The IMF is charged with coordinating global economic policy (monetary policy, inflation) for economic stability, and it imposes structural economic requirements on countries receiving development loans (Falk, 1999).

The WB and the IMF were originally designed to prevent economic crises (Gershman & Irwin, 2000), and it has been argued that members felt the goal of opening trade would be achieved through government support for social welfare. However, Western financial leaders adopted policies known as the "Washington Consensus," "free trade" and "neoliberalism" (Falk, 1999; Gershman & Irwin, 2000) in the face of the "debt crisis" of the 1970s and 1980s, as Western investors feared that heavily indebted "third world" countries would default on international loans due to global stagflation. Rose and Miller

(1992) describe neoliberalism as "A re-organization of political rationalities" (p. 199) that aims to decouple government, business, and welfare issues, while proliferating strategies for creating markets. In this system, development is equated with "economic growth, privatization, and minimal state interference" (Carpenter, 2000, p. 344). This market-based economic agenda directly influences health by affecting key predictors of health status. It also influences the ability to protect and promote health discursively by privileging market ethics over the normative foundation that supports public health efforts.

The discourse of public health

Trade policy is often discussed as a health issue in narrow terms, such as intellectual property and AIDS mediciation. Yet economic decisions guide the public investments and social protections that are at the heart of public health, which involves population-based efforts to prevent disease and promote health (Garrett, 2000; Petersen & Lupton, 1996) such as sanitation, epidemiology, vaccination, public safety regulations, health promotion campaigns, and medical care access. Unfortunately, dominant discourses of public health (and health communication) have helped to shield linkages between health and economic policy. Theories of health and disease causation act as discourses in the Foucaultian (1980) sense, as constructed sets of meaning that create and are created by power relations. Discourse as knowledge production mediates between the symbolic and material, as Fairclough (1995) notes: "Discourse contributes to the creation and constant recreation of the relations, subjects . . . and objects which populate the social world" (p. 73). Public health is guided by different theories about disease causation, and these discourses act politically to guide interventions.

"Germ Theories" of public health focus on micro-organisms (germs, viruses) and represent a prevailing rationale of health; they are popular efforts that seem to embody scientific progress. This discourse focuses public attention at the individual body first, lifestyle choices second, environmental issues third, and only lastly sociopolitical issues (Tesh, 1994). Another dominant approach to public health is the lifestyle theory of causation, which promotes the idea that good health can be achieved through better individual choice-making. This discourse operates similarly to maintain the political status quo by directing attention toward the individual and away from social and political contexts.

An alternative is the environmental theory of disease, which attempts to place more emphasis on ecological contexts of health. Yet Tesh (1994) argues that prevailing institutions tend to define the environment in discrete terms to include lifestyle choices over more comprehensive definitions that would attend to such issues as resource depletion or industrial practices. Similarly, the multicausal web approach to health promotion (exemplified by the U.S. *Healthy People* initiative) examines health as a multifactorial issue, but fails to prioritize structural and political issues, making discrete changes an easier choice for decision makers (e.g. asthma treatment over pollution reduction) (Zoller, 2005b).

Thus, only the critical approach to public health prioritizes interventions in sociopolitical power (including poverty, access to decision making, and capitalist production processes). Originators of radical approaches to public health include Virchow, Engels, and Allende (Tesh, 1994; Waitzkin, 1983). As early as 1840, Chadwick's publication of the *Inquiry into the Sanitary Conditions of the Labouring Population of Great Britain* connected poverty and environmental pollution with health and disease, and framed efforts to redress these problems as the common good. Engels documented the relationships among class structure (housing, work conditions), and infectious disease, nutrition, and alcoholism, and pointed for the need for fundamental change in class inequality (Waitzkin, 1983). This work influenced Virchow, one of the founders of social medicine, who focused on reforming resource availability as a key to good health (Waitzkin, 1983). Allende worked in the 1930s and 1940s to address the role of underdevelopment and imperialism in public health problems. Although the three point to different solutions (from revolution to reform), each prioritizes intervention in political, economic, and social inequities as the work of health promotion. Waitzkin also notes that each is "multisectoral," demonstrating that health policy must transcend the health sector alone to address political changes such as wages, housing, planning, occupational safety, and social safety nets. Critical scholars should also note that social disparities including gender, sexuality, ethnicity and nationality must be considered in understanding health inequality.

The discourse of the "new public health" makes reference to economic and political change using the language of empowerment, cooperation, and community participation (Petersen & Lupton, 1996); for instance, WHO's 1978 Alma Ata declaration of "Health for All by the Year 2000" links health to social and economic justice, political autonomy, and resistance to Western, biomedical definitions of health (Carpenter, 2000). Yet programs such as the WHO's "Healthy Communities" initiative continue to emphasize individual responsibility, localize what are often national and international problems, ignore power imbalances at the local level, and justify state rollbacks in health protection investments (Petersen & Lupton, 1996). Moreover, many argue that the rising power of market-based policies from the IMF and WB has encouraged the WHO to largely abandon any comprehensive approach to social change and adopt a reformist stance in order to survive, focusing on discrete campaigns such as vaccinations or health education (Banerji, 1999). Thus, there is an absence of critical, multisectoral public health discourse that prioritizes social change in the roots of inequality.

Public health and health communication

Scholars of health communication play an increasing role in promoting public health, both in the United States and globally. As they do so, researchers tend to operate within dominant discourses of public health focused on lifestyle theories and medical compliance, producing models and persuasive initiatives to alter individual behavior, with little attention to the social and political circumstances of target audiences (Dutta-Bergman, 2005). As a result, many projects take existing political and economic contexts as a given, such as research into vaccine information in the Philippines (McDivitt et al. 1997), Bolivian contraceptive promotion (Valente & Saba, 2001), radio programming in Nepal (Storey et al., 1999), nutrition communication in Sub-Saharan Africa (Pratt et al., 1997), and organizational factors in HIV/AIDS campaigns in Africa (Kiwanuka-Tondo & Snyder, 2002; Witte, 1998).

Yet health scholars are beginning to articulate linkages between communication theory and health-policy changes. Research examines policy construction as both a communicative process (Murphy, 2001; Sharf, 1999) and a power-laden activity (Conrad & McIntush, 2003; Dejong & Wallack, 1999; Zoller, 2003). A growing number of projects acknowledge the role of policy in influencing the cultural, political, and economic foundations of health in countries outside the United States, and their impact on risk communication and disease prevention (Airhihenbuwa et al., 2000; Melkote et al., 2000). For example, Chay-Nemeth (1998) links the growth of the sex industry, a risk for the spread of HIV/AIDS in Thailand, in part to unequal wealth distribution, poverty, and low educational levels of women. Such studies largely have focused on the decisions of individual governments. This chapter expands this research by critically examining international policies that transcend the specific domain of health. In the next section, I provide a framework for analyzing global trade as a governmental discourse to understand its communicative implications for health promotion.

Neoliberal governmentality

Neoliberalism, understood as a set of international trade, economic, and development arrangements, can be analyzed as a governmental effort. Drawing from Foucault (1991), *governmentality* is not necessarily linked with state authority, although the state may participate. Rather, Foucault describes governmentality as an ensemble of "institutions, procedures, analyses and reflections, the calculations and tactics" (p. 102) that facilitates the exercise of a form of power concerned with managing populations and addressing issues of political economy. Governmentality is constituted by and implemented through discourse.

Lupton (1995) provides an excellent discussion of governmentality in terms of the productive and coercive efforts of public health groups to establish "voluntary" social norms regarding the body and care for the self. Rather than examine public health as a governmental discourse, this chapter examines the governmental practices of neoliberal market economics as they shape public health efforts.

Rose and Miller's (Rose, 1996; Rose & Miller, 1992) discussion of governmentality can be read to provide a framework for analyzing governmental discourse. First, the authors argue that governmentality is primarily a problematizing activity: "it poses the obligations of rulers in terms of the problems they seek to address" (1992, p. 181). Programs of government develop around these defined problems, rendering them apparently governable through diagnosis, prescription, and intervention. Thus it is necessary to understand the problems a governmental system construes and the process through which they form intervention.

Second, Rose and Miller (1992) argue that the problematics of government can be analyzed "in terms of their political rationalities, the changing discursive fields within which the exercise of power is conceptualized" (p. 175), or "principles to which government should be directed" (p. 179). This involves explaining not just systems of thought but also "systems of action" (p. 177). Analysis should discern how tasks are divided among different social authorities (family, politics, spiritual, etc.).

Third, political rationalities also must be understood in terms of governmental technologies, "the complex of mundane programmes, techniques, apparatuses, documents, and procedures through which authorities seek to embody and give effect to governmental ambitions" (Rose & Miller, 1992, p. 175). Thus we can examine the systems created for executing goals. That these systems are understood as "technologies" is important. Peterson (1990) defines technological discourse as "language used to structure human action according to rules of closed systems" (p. 78). She notes that technological discourse can become problematic when experience that cannot be managed or utilized within a particular system is rejected or ignored. Technological discourse emphasizes efficiency, substituting procedure for creative invention. Thus, analyzing technological discourse can reveal "orthodoxies": the organizational sense making or public consciousness embedded in it (Vickery, 1990).

When looking at neoliberalism generally, we see that the problems to which neoliberalism addresses itself are state interference and economic inefficiency. Neoliberal institutions forward solutions to these problems based on the rationalities of privatization, deregulation, and trade liberalization, particularly among developing countries in the global south (Falk, 1999). In this system, what were previously thought to be issues of political governance are "to be transformed into commodified forms and regulated according to market principles" (Rose & Miller, 1992, p. 198). For example, services such as health care, water, and utilities should be privatized and delivered through the market. This chapter focuses on three specific trade mechanisms as neoliberal technologies to understand their material and symbolic influence on public health and its promotion. These mechanisms include structural adjustment, harmonization, and investor lawsuits. These three were chosen because they significantly influence the material/biological elements of health, but also because they have, somewhat quietly, altered the landscape for public health actors.

The discursive influence of neoliberal governmentality on health: three exemplars

For each of these mechanisms, I describe the problems the policy defines and addresses, the guiding political rationality, and technologies of implementation. In doing so, I trace the discursive implications of these policies for global public health promotion.

Structural Adjustment Package (SAP) loans: neoliberalism and public investment

Development loan policies are key governmental mechanisms that greatly influence the ability to promote health. Loans to "developing" nations require the approval of the IMF, which imposes a set of requirements on borrower nations. These "structural adjustment policies" reflect neoliberal rationality by demanding austerity measures (drastically reducing social expenditures) and privatization (selling state-owned facilities to for-profit groups) (Stiglitz, 2002). From a public health perspective, this orthodoxy prioritizes investment concerns, thereby failing to account for its material effects on health in individual countries, and disqualifying health as a substantive counterdiscourse.

IMF and WB discourse constructs the central problem around which they orient their actions in terms of the need for borrower countries to repay debts, which is thought to be impeded by inflation and closed markets (Stiglitz, 2002). The corresponding solutions have been to require that borrowing nations dramatically decrease spending to balance the budget and avoid inflation (austerity), privatize governmental services such as education, health care, and water systems to open markets for business, and deregulate markets to improve efficiency. Advocates believe open markets will push countries to develop a comparative advantage (Neumayer, 2001).

The political rationality of SAP programs transfers authority in social decision making from the nation-state and indigenous actors to global economic elites. For example, in developing nations, health care is often defined as public goods distributed by need, after SAPs, financial institutions redefine health care as a private commodity to be distributed by ability to pay. Policies direct governments to attempt cost-recovery through health measures.

Evidence suggests that these technologies, the programs and procedures used to implement SAPs, have become ends in themselves. For example, the interest paid to multilateral banks has exceeded the amount of money borrowed by many developing nations (Schoepf et al., 2000).[1] Although lowering interest rates was an original rationale for these policies, Stiglitz (2002) argues that eventually, "To the fund, a liberalized financial system was an end in itself" (p. 35). Thus, the technological discourse of the WB/IMF shows itself as a closed system as described by T. Peterson (1990) in at least two ways. First, economic advisors ignored contextual evidence that these policies did not lower interest rates.[2] They ignored data that showed that developing countries undergoing SAPs have experienced increased poverty and political instability, continuing to focus on a country's ability to repay debt in the short term to the detriment of building infrastructure that would create long-term social improvements (Gershman & Irwin, 2000). Second, alternate approaches were dismissed as "ideological," such as policies that would account for historic imperialism and income inequalities in producing poverty rates for countries such as Africa (Schoepf et al., 2000). In light of publicized failures and public pressure, the WB and IMF instituted "poverty reduction strategy paper" (PRSP) requirements in the late 1990s that emphasize poverty reduction, however, the economic calculus remains largely the same[3] (Craig & Porter, 2003).

The direct health influence of SAP discourse has been severe. Since the inception of neoliberal policies, the incidence of poverty has risen dramatically to an estimated 1.5 billion people (Carpenter, 2000). Although trade advocates argue that liberalization will result in a transfer of capital between developed and developing countries, between 1965 and 1995, GDP per capita fell by half in sub-Saharan Africa and by 30 percent in Latin America (Rowson, 2000). "Free trade" has resulted in negative income growth for the poorest 40 percent of the population. Mounting evidence documents the ensuing public health crises. As government spending declines, safety nets for the increasing number of poor have disappeared. In Nicaragua after structural adjustment, three out of four people live below the poverty line, and debt repayments exceed the entire social-sector budget (Gershman & Irwin, 2000). SAPs in Bolivia led to poverty as $400 million in taxes from the state-owned petroleum industry shrank to $80 million in taxes after privatization (Brubaker, 2001).

There are now more homeless and higher rates of disease and malnutrition throughout Africa. A longitudinal study by UNICEF in Brazzaville Congo, before and after SAPs, demonstrated that as adjustment policies took effect, there was a doubling in low-birth weight babies for children of the poor, and an increase in acute malnutrition and growth stunting (Schoepf et al., 2000). Privatization and subsidy cessation policies play a significant role in increasing hunger. In 1999, when Mexico eliminated some agricultural price controls and subsidies, the price of tortillas increased 350 percent, while wages increased only 10 percent that year (Brubaker, 2001). Privatization threatens global access to clean water, a major public health issue when more than a third of people living in developing countries lack access to clean water and sewers (Sidel, 2000). Following IMF requirements to privatize public holdings, the Bolivian government sold its publicly built and funded water system to Bechtel Corporation, which raised rates to what was for most people one third of their salary (Brubaker, 2001).

These direct health effects are particularly pernicious for health promoters because as disease rises, the re-definition of health care as a commodity under SAPs reduces access to health care. Thus the policies create discursive barriers to addressing the very problems they create. Studies in Zaire, Zimbabwe, and Nigeria show attendance rates for health-care services plummet when fees are charged (Millen et al., 2000). The WB itself found that in fifty-three countries under structural adjustment, health expenditures fell from 2.3 to 1.1 percent of their budget (Carpenter, 2000).

In 1988, O'Brien, chief economist of the WB, stated about structural adjustment policies in sub-Saharan Africa: "We did not think that the human costs of these adjustment programs could be so great, and economic gains so slow in coming" (cited in Bienefeld, 2000, p. 53). SAP policies suggest that global trade and economic institutions are forms of governing the global south on behalf of economically advanced countries. They represent the uneven application of neoliberal theories that disproportionately affect already poor countries. Developed countries such the United States and the European Union retain trade tariffs, monetary support for industry (such as steel, agriculture, and aviation), and public investment in education and health (Navarro, 1999) while continuing to require privatization and austerity measures in developing countries. The privileging of *privatization* and liberal markets is an inherent barrier to those who promote *public* health with its basic need for public expenditure and infrastructures.

Harmonization: neoliberal governance and the discourse of regulation

We have seen that "trade negotiations" extend beyond traditional concepts of trade such as tariffs to the domestic policies of individual states. Advocates refer to achieving standardization as "harmonization" whether bilaterally (e.g., European Union–United States), or multilaterally (e.g., the WTO). Harmonization agreements, whereby nation states and industries attempt to make uniform regulatory requirements for everything from car headlights to chemicals, now influence public health, environmental, and safety regulations. These policies fail to account for health effects, and impede health promotion by raising the discursive burden to create or maintain regulation as a means of protecting public health and safety.

The key problem for global capital, according to proponents, is that the burden to meet different regulatory requirements is cumbersome and deters trade (Green Cowles, 2001). Additionally, proponents note that domestic regulation may disguise protectionism for national industries (Cameron, 1999). Critical analysis suggests that harmonization discourse privileges the problem of market efficiency for goods producers over public health.

Examples of harmonization technologies include two discursive mechanisms, the Technical Barriers to Trade (TBT) and Sanitary and Phytosanitary (SPS) agreements of the WTO, which stipulate that members should "base their technical regulations, standards, and conformity assessment procedures on international standards, guides, and recommendations" (Motaal, 1999, p. 226). More specifically, these rules "require that technical regulations and health and safety laws are not more trade restrictive than necessary to achieve their legitimate objectives, and do not create unnecessary barriers to trade" (Martin, 2001, p. 114). WTO rules require that public health goals be achieved in the "least trade restrictive" manner possible.

This guiding political rationality transfers a good deal of public health authority to global trade institutions such as the WTO, NAFTA, where public health advocates play no formal role, and where business leaders have access to trade officials that public advocates do not (Greider, 2001; Zoller, 2004). This is particularly problematic because, from a communication perspective, establishing that laws are not "more trade restrictive than necessary" is a discursive process that involves definitional conflicts among competing interest groups. The use of scientific measures of risk adds to this conflict rather than ameliorates it, given that the negotiation of risk itself is ideological, involving value-laden choices that benefit some over others (Sass, 1999).

TBT and SPS agreements are technologies that protect investor rights, but discursively restrict public health protections. Although the clause requiring regulation to be implemented in the least trade restrictive way appears reasonable from an economic perspective, it also acts as a mechanism for industry to challenge domestic public health standards. Critics refer to harmonization as the "race to the bottom." In practice, we see Japan and the European Union claim that U.S. nutrition labeling requirements are too trade restrictive, and argue for voluntary labeling (Goldman & Wagner, 2000). Canada submitted a challenge to a French asbestos ban, arguing that "protective clothing and other measures that limit exposure would be less burdensome on trade than a ban" (Goldman & Wagner, 2000, p. 265). Milmo (2002) reported that the European Chemical Industry Council was openly optimistic that the EPA will assure that harmonization procedures match the United States' more lenient chemical testing program rather than the stricter policies of Europe.[4] As these examples suggest, industry uses harmonization mechanisms to promote lenient regulatory standards.

Harmonization technology makes public health protection more difficult as business interests attempt to establish standards of certainty over the precautionary approach to risk. Environmental and health advocates argue that WTO rulings should rely upon the Precautionary Principle (PP), which holds that in the face of incomplete or uncertain evidence of harm, decision makers will protect the public from potential harms rather than await total certainty. However, harmonization advocates frame the PP as an unfair trade barrier that keeps foreign products out of domestic markets (Martin, 2001). By calling for evidence of "statistical human assessments and certainties of harm" in order to establish regulation (Labonte et al. 1999, p. 27), industry leaders shift the burden of proof from producers proving a product or service safe to advocates establishing a certainty of harm to warrant regulation.

For example, the pharmaceutical "Expert Group" of the TABD, a business advisory group to the WTO states, "It is essential that regulatory decisions be made on the basis of sound scientific and medical risk assessment, with clear, reasoned, and unambiguous methodology. The so-called Precautionary Principle is neither necessary nor appropriate, especially with respect to the pharmaceutical sector" (p. 42). The United States and Canada used SPS measures before the WTO to protest the European Commission's import ban on beef from hormone treated cows, arguing that scientific certainty did not exist regarding the harms of hormone-treated animals on humans. The decision resulted in authorization to impose trade sanctions of 191.4 million dollars against the European Union.[5]

The concept of "sound scientific risk assessments" obscures the very uncertainty in establishing causation that the PP was designed to deal with. Appeals for resolute scientific findings are problematic because such data are rarely available in biological contexts, given multifactorial causation and an inability to use controls (Sass, 1999). Standards of certainty would have prevented passage of much existing regulation intended to prevent potential harms. For example, the U.S. Food Quality Protection Act of 1996 added protections for children against pesticides, based on the *lack* of epidemiological research that demonstrates safe levels of pesticide exposure for children (Goldman & Wagner, 2000).

Additionally, SPS and TBT mechanisms may alter the definition of the "status quo." If the burden of proof rests with those who want to change the unaltered environment, producers must provide evidence that what they produce is safe, whereas if it rests with those who want to alter existing production processes, public health and environmental groups must prove a substance harmful before it can be regulated (Cameron, 1999).

In sum, harmonization agreements that construct a burden to prove a substance harmful before it can be regulated discursively create a significant barrier to promoting health protections. Trade negotiators can use private, market-based mechanisms to undermine important public health protections. These technologies exclude open public processes, reducing the influence of public health advocates.

Investor-to-State Lawsuits: neoliberalism and the discourse of investment protection

Investor-to-State Lawsuits (ISLs) are global trade mechanisms in treaties such as the WTO and NAFTA that protect global corporate economic investments. However, these governance technologies also assert and expand the notion of a corporation's right to profits (Greider, 2001) by allowing corporate legal claims against governments for lost profits and potential profits due to domestic laws. By discursively defining regulation as expropriation, these obscure policies shift the locus of public health and environmental lawmaking from democratic localities to investor courts.

ISL mechanisms define and address the problem of protecting foreign investment from seizure or unfair competition. The solutions forwarded include those such as NAFTA Article 1110, which states that "governments must compensate foreign investors for measures that 'expropriate' their property or are 'tantamount to a direct or indirect expropriation'" (Public Citizen, 2002, p. 2). Also known as Chapter 11 lawsuits, NAFTA cases transfer governing authority to a private three-judge arbitration tribunal. Unless both sides agree otherwise, tribunal decisions are secret and never made available to the public (Greider, 2001).

In addressing these problems, the discourse of ISL treaties expands corporate rights through key re-definitions of property rights and regulation through the everyday terminology of "taking" and "tantamount."[6] The concept involves defining public regulation as "a government 'taking' of private property that requires compensation to the owners" (Greider, 2001, p. 22). This idea finds expression in the term "tantamount to expropriation." As a result of this re-definition, lawsuits are now filed against foreign governments for loss of *potential* profits due to regulation. Such suits involve large damage claims that could be very difficult to pay, particularly for impoverished countries.

Labonte et al. (1999) reported that under NAFTA and the WTO, every challenge to a resource conservation effort had succeeded. For example, the WTO ruled that the United States must allow gas products from Brazil and Venezuela to be sold in the United States despite being below U.S. environmental standards or pay $150 million a year in damages. Rather than pay the fine, the Clean Air Act was altered to allow this gasoline, damaging public respiratory health (Labonte et al., 1999, p. 30).

The rationale of ISLs is to protect a corporate right to profit, and it delegitimizes state action in protecting the public. Once the language of "taking" is legally instituted, public health and safety measures become potentially actionable offenses. The possibility of "regulatory chill," the weakening or removal of regulation in the face of lawsuits, creates a significant barrier for public health and environmental protection.

In 1997, Canada passed a law banning the import of MMT,[7] a manganese additive. Although the substance was already banned in the United States due to health concerns, Ethyl Corporation sued Canada for 250 million dollars in lost potential profits under NAFTA, citing the law as a Chapter 11 infraction as "measures undertaken tantamount to expropriation of its investment" (Neumayer, 2001, p. 80). Supporting the notion of regulatory chill, Public Citizen (2002, p. 4) reported that "After learning that the NAFTA tribunal was likely to rule against its position, the Canadian government revoked the ban, paid Ethyl $13 million in damages, and issued a public statement declaring there was no evidence that MMT posed health or environmental risks" (p. 4). Thus, the threat of such lawsuits encourages state self-discipline, potentially preventing health protection efforts even before rulings are made.

Methanex Corporation sued the U.S. government under NAFTA, seeking compensation for a March 1999 California-imposed phase-out and ban on MTBE (methyl tertiary butyl ether) a fuel additive (Neumayer, 2001). The U.S. Environmental Protection Agency views the product as a potential human carcinogen and groundwater contaminator. Methenex Corporation sued the US for $970 million for damage to future profits expected from its sale of methanol, an ingredient in MTBE (Greider, 2001). Neumayer argues that the company used the lawsuit to prevent other states from enacting similar legislation.

ISL lawsuits also may influence efforts to change health and safety claims by product manufacturers. For example, in 2002 Philip Morris announced their intent to sue Canada under NAFTA Chapter 11 for a proposed ban on the words "light" and "mild" from cigarette packaging. Philip Morris argued that the proposed health regulations would be "tantamount to expropriation" of its trademarks that involve those words (Public Citizen, 2002). It demanded compensation for money spent in developing brand loyalty around these terms if such rules went into effect. In this case, Canada imposed the ban and faced potential lawsuits.

This Canadian case illustrates that states maintain the ability to impose health regulations, when public attention is drawn to health threats, and resources are available. However, ISL mechanisms significantly shift the playing field for health advocates by privileging profit through a private court system versus the public mechanisms used to create health protections.

Implications: communication research and global health advocacy

Critical analysis of these three globalization policies demonstrates how these technologies of economic policy, normally thought to be outside the domain of health policy, materially and discursively impede global health promotion. Neoliberal discourse problematizes state intervention and public investment, which are key to protecting health, and forward the private market as a solution in ways that prioritize investment protections. Furthermore, the technological discourse of trade forms a closed system that closes off the context-sensitive decision making needed to promote public health.

Global financial rules remain in flux in the face of multiple negotiations among nations. Indeed, given the breakdown of consensus about the global economy and international cooperation (Saul, 2004), now may be an opportune moment to alter the rationality guiding trade and investment institutions, and to prevent the same rationality from re-emerging in other forms (as witnessed in the privatization of Iraq (Roy, 2004), CAFTA—the Central Americas Free Trade Agreement, and the continued promotion of the FTAA). The preceding analysis provides the basis for some specific courses of action to promote public health protections, whether incrementally or more transformatively.

First, countering structural adjustment/conditionality systems involves discursively redefining and prioritizing public investment and re-valuing health as a public good. A critical discourse of public health can challenge the dominant logic of privatization. These broad changes may be facilitated by a) by moving health decisions from the economic to the political realm, b) educating the public, governments, and trade participants that improved health and economic growth have occurred where nations protect vulnerable industries and retain state investments in health and education (Navarro, 1999), and c) framing health protection as capacity building rather than an opportunity for "aid." Additionally, economic remediation must go beyond debt forgiveness to remove harmful austerity and privatization requirements if developing countries are to escape poverty and disease. The contradiction between enforcement of these rules in developed and developing countries can be used to counter the assumption that such policies result solely from a value-free economic calculus.

Second, to effectively counter harmonization procedures and reduce or remove their influence on safety standards, health advocates must work to codify the precautionary principle, place the burden of proof for safety on industry,[8] and include health professionals in trade negotiations. Such work has been achieved in the United Nations, but its relative lack of authority in relation to the financial institutions means that more work remains to be done. Additionally, health communication scholars can publicize the effects of harmonization decisions on public health and democratic processes (which involves educating the public about the importance of seemingly technical, scientific procedures).

Third, protecting health regulations and preventing regulatory chill from ISLs requires redefining "expropriation" and "taking" to exempt existing health laws that are not designed to impede foreign investment. Health communicators may achieve such goals by insisting on a participatory role in trade agreements, or through democratic advocacy, activism, and lobbying. In order to fight Chapter 11 provisions, consumer advocates recommend the inclusion of "social development and environmental protective measures" in trade policies as a safeguard (Labonte et al., 1999, p. 25). More fundamentally, health advocates also must reject ISL mechanisms and contest the notion of a "right to profits" in order to move debate and decision-making into the public and democratic arenas, away from commercial-interest tribunals.

Health communication research and practice

The critical, multisectoral approach to public health guiding this chapter provides insight into the potential role of health communication research and practice to address neoliberal governmentality more broadly. The field needs to address some of its own practices, and it can also facilitate academic and public activism.

First, we must work to remove the field of health communication's complicity with the rationale of neoliberal governmentality. For example, health campaign efforts that emphasize behavior choices without attention to social contexts are problematic on several levels. Targeting behavioral choices such as dietary patterns, condom use, and drug abstinence, and focusing on compliance with biomedical authorities, ignores the political decision making that alters the infrastructure guiding personal agency, health knowledge, and risk decisions. It cruelly ignores the lived experience of populations around the world to emphasize only personal choice making when basics such as access to clean water are threatened by global agreements outside local control.

Individualistic communication research reinforces the rationale of individualism and personal responsibility that is a counterpart to market-based decision making. It is more difficult to argue for public investment in health protections when publics (particularly Western publics) define health as a matter of personal choices. Health communication scholars should see within its purview the job of helping to persuade the public that the individualistic approach does not adequately address the social foundations of health, including poverty, access to food, water, shelter, education, and health care, as well as health and environmental regulation. Furthermore, when health promoters ignore or treat as a given current economic arrangements, they facilitate the dominance of economic institutions in setting policies that influence health.

Thus, this analysis (along with other chapters in this book) demonstrates that challenging and constructing global policies is a communicative issue that must be considered alongside other domains of health communication research such as interpersonal interventions, health promotion campaigns, health organizations, and medical practice. Poverty rates, education levels, health investments, and protective legislation are at least in part the result of political decisions based on governance strategies that depend upon the negotiation of public meaning. The developing countries whose health status some communication researchers are working hard to improve (South Africa,

Bolivia, Nepal to mention a few) are some of those made most vulnerable by structural adjustment policies and investor protections.

With this recognition in place, health communication researchers can evaluate and promote strategies of public participation for challenging neoliberalism and develop positive alternatives. Strategies may include advocacy from health organizations and grassroots health activism (Zoller, 2005a). Examples of successful health advocacy include the Canadian Public Health Service (CPHS), which played a role in derailing the 1998 Multilateral Agreement on Investments by researching and sharing findings about the potential impact of such an agreement on public health (Pinder, 1998). This group also publicized the need for a formal role for public health in trade agreements, which became known as the "social clauses campaign" (p. 39).

It is important for us to investigate what communication strategies allow maximum policy-making input on the part of affected communities and populations. Insights from organizational studies and public relations give the field unique contributions to debates among health advocates about how to achieve change. For example, advocates disagree about whether to work within the WTO framework to create a global commitment to public health, debt forgiveness, and public participation (Carpenter, 2000), or to attempt to defeat these global trade institutions and replace them with alternate systems ("Fix it or nix it"). Debate exists about the role of transnational nongovernmental organizations (NGOs). For example, there are disagreements about whether to strengthen and reform WHO and its "Health for All" campaign (Carpenter, 2000) or to abandon it as an institution of social change (see for discussion Banerji, 1999). Communication researchers can also investigate strategies to build alternate sources of power. Rather than emphasize divisiveness by choosing a single way to proceed, research should focus on how multiple strategies might operate together to achieve public health improvements that are flexible and context-sensitive, rather than technological.

Also, health communication researchers can examine how health-related economic policies are experienced, resisted, and transformed by actual people acting locally, nationally, and transnationally. Grassroots health activism is an important area for growth in health communication scholarship (Zoller, 2005a). How are individual communities, cultures, or countries finding ways to promote health in the face of these policy conditions (see for example Dutta-Bergman, 2004)?

These questions place research and advocacy of the movement of "globalization from below" squarely within the purview of health communication research. Falk (1999) describes this movement as grassroots resistance aimed at altering social norms for social justice, sustainability, and compassion in contrast to the elite policy making of neoliberalism. Globalization from below focuses on re-asserting democracy, local control, and establishing economies that serve human interests rather than the reverse (Falk, 1999). Perhaps because health activists tend to focus on single issues or diseases (such as AIDS activism) rather than forge a common identity, the health focus of much of this grassroots resistance may be overlooked (Zoller, 2005a). This fragmentation also may prevent activists from using arguments about public health to their full advantage. Our field can address the role of these networked activists in challenging the market-based logics and rearticulating health equity as a social good. We also can play a role in fomenting an integrated public health movement.

Critical approaches to public health emphasize the economic, social and political roots of public health, and thereby prioritize fundamental, multi-sectoral changes that may be overlooked by health efforts that work within the status quo. The obdurate outcomes of increased death and disease particularly for poor and marginalized populations provide a potentially powerful basis to bring criticisms of neoliberal techniques to public consciousness. Inequality is a problem for everyone; the rich cannot exist in a healthy state alongside the poor and sick.

Acknowledgments

The author wishes to thank Mohan J. Dutta, Shiv Ganesh and Ed Schiappa for their review of drafts of this chapter, and Gail Fairhurst and Dennis Mumby for helpful comments on the chapter.

Notes

1   "In 1996, sub-Saharan Africa received $15 billion in loans but paid out $12 billion in debt service" (Schoepf et al., 2000, p. 121). Eighty percent of the loans to Africa in the 1970s are estimated to have stayed in Western hands, yet most African countries have been using 30–70 percent of their export revenues to pay debt (Schoepf et al., 2000).
2   When confronted with problems such as unemployment, IMF economists explain it away by holding that unemployment must be voluntary or caused by government or union intervention. For example, Argentina received an "A" rating in face of double-digit unemployment because its budget appeared balanced and inflation controlled.
3   In 1999, the WB and IMF responded to outcries about the effects of SAPs on poverty and democracy. They now require a Poverty Reduction Strategy Paper (PRSP) to be written as a condition for entry into the Heavily Indebted Poor Countries Initiative II. The paper assesses a country's ability to address poverty issues. However, critics argue that PRSPs are simply an extension of SAP policies (Bradshaw & Linneker, 2003). The WB claims that because participatory assessment occurs in each country, PRSPs demonstrate the absence of a formula for poverty reduction. Yet the organization continues to state that economic growth and macroeconomic stability are the keys to poverty reduction (Ellis et al., 2003), and features of SAPs remain in the strikingly similar plans for individual countries such as Honduras, Nicaragua, and Bolivia (Bradshaw & Linneker, 2003). Thus, Craig and Porter (2003) argue that PRSPs continue to favor technical procedures and a disciplinary approach over attention to contextual human needs related to political economy.

4 For example, the *Chemical Market Reporter* (Milmo, 2002) states: "The EPA's drive for greater compatibility in the way chemicals are controlled raises hopes that the European Union (EU) can be persuaded to adopt a more conciliatory approach to chemical regulations" (p. 4).

5 The WTO dismissed carcinogenicity findings from the "benchmark" International Agency on Research of Cancer (Cameron, 1999). The Appellate Body of the WTO ruled that "the precautionary principle cannot override our finding . . . namely that the EC import ban . . . is not based on risk assessment" (Cameron, 1999, p. 259). According to Neumayer (2001), the WTO appellate decision shows that "in tendency the appellate body seemed to side with those who dispute that the precautionary principle is internationally and widely accepted" (p. 129).

6 Treaty negotiators, who typically come from and return to private corporate law, have discussed alterations in the meaning of property and regulation in the U.S. Council for International Business since the mid-1980s (Greider, 2001).

7 Methylcyclopentadienyl manganese tricarbonyl.

8 The Precautionary Principle should be applied so that the burden of proof rests with those who want to alter the environment rather than those who want to alter existing production processes.

References

Airhihenbuwa, C., Makinwa, B., & Obregon, R. (2000). Towards a new communications framework for HIV/AIDS. *Journal of Health Communication*, 5(1), 101–111.

Banerji, D. (1999). A fundamental shift in the approach to international health by WHO, UNICEF, and the World Bank: Instances of "intellectual Fascism" and totalitarianism in some Asian countries. *International Journal of Health Services*, 29(2), 227–259.

Barris, E., & McLeod, K. (2000). Globalization and international trade in the twenty-first century: Opportunities for and threats to the health sector in the south. *International Journal of Health Services*, 30(1), 187–210.

Bienefeld, M. (2000). Globalization and social change: Drowning in the icy waters of commercial calculation. In J. Dragsbaek Schmidt & J. Hersh (eds), *Globalization and Social Change*. London: Routledge, pp. 46–66.

Bradshaw, S., & Linneker, B. (2003). Civil society responses to poverty reduction strategies in Nicaragua. *Progress in Development Studies*, 3(2), 147–169.

Brubaker, P.K. (2001). *Globalization at What Price? Economic Change and Daily Life*. Cleveland: The Pilgrim Press.

Cameron, J. (1999). The Precautionary Principle. In G.P. Sampson, & W.B. Chambers (eds), *Trade, Environment, and the Millennium*. New York: United Nations University Press, pp. 239–270.

Carpenter, M. (2000). Health for some: Global health and social development since Alma Ata. *Community Development Journal*, 35(4), 336–351.

Chay-Nemeth, C. (1998). Demystifying AIDS in Thailand: A dialectical analysis of the Thai sex industry. *Journal of Health Communication*, 3(3), 217–231.

Conrad, C., & McIntush, H.G. (2003). Organizational rhetoric and healthcare policymaking. In T.L. Thompson, A.M. Dorsey, K.I. Miller, & R. Parrott (eds), *Handbook of Health Communication*. Mahwah, NJ: Lawrence Erlbaum Associates, pp. 403–422.

Craig, D., & Porter, D. (2003). Poverty reduction strategy papers: A new convergence. *World Development, 31*(1), 53–70.

Dejong, W., & Wallack, L. (1999). A critical perspective on the Drug Czar's antidrug media campaign. *Journal of Health Communication, 4*(2), 155–160.

Dutta-Bergman, M. (2004). Poverty, structural barriers, and health: A Santali narrative of health communication. *Qualitative Health Research, 14*(8), 1107–1123.

Dutta-Bergman, M. (2005). Theory and practice in health communication campaigns: A critical interrogation. *Health Communication, 18*(2), 103–122.

Ellis, F., Kutengule, M., & Nyasulu, A. (2003). Livelihoods and rural poverty reduction in Malawi. *World Development, 31*(9), 1495–1511.

Fairclough, N. (1995). *Critical Discourse Analysis: The Critical Study of Language.* London: Longman.

Falk, R. (1999). *Predatory Globalization: A Critique.* Cambridge: Polity Press.

Foucault, M. (1980). *Power/knowledge: Selected Interviews and Other Writings 1972–1977* (C. Gordon, L. Marshall, J. Mepham, K. Soper, trans.). New York: Pantheon.

Foucault, M. (1991). Governmentality. In G. Burchell, & P. Miller (eds), *The Foucault Effect: Studies in Governmentality.* London: Harverster/Wheatsheaf, pp. 87–104.

Garrett, L. (2000). *Betrayal of Trust: The Collapse of Global Public Health.* New York: Hyperion.

Gershman, J., & Irwin, A. (2000). Getting a grip on the global economy. In J.Y. Kim, J.V. Millen, A. Irwin, & J. Gershman (eds), *Dying for Growth: Global Inequality and the Health of the Poor.* Monroe, Maine: Common Courage Press, pp. 11–43.

Goldman, P., & Wagner, J.M. (2000). Trading away public health: WTO obstacles to effective toxic controls. *Journal of Public Health Policy, 21*(3), 260–267.

Green Cowles, M. (2001). The transatlantic business dialogue: Transforming the new transatlantic dialogue. In M.A. Pollack, & G.C. Shaffer (eds), *Transatlantic Governance in the Global Economy.* Boulder: Rowman & Littlefield, pp. 213–264.

Greider, W. (2001). The right and US trade law: Invalidating the 20th century. *The Nation, 273*, 21–29.

Kiwanuka-Tondo, J., & Snyder, L.B. (2002). The influence of organizational characteristics and campaign design elements on communication campaign quality: Evidence from 91 Ugandan AIDS campaigns. *Journal of Health Communication, 7*(1), 59–77.

Labonte, R., International Union for Health Promotion and Education, & The Canadian Public Health Association. (1999). Brief to the World Trade Organization: World trade and population health. *Promotion & Education, VI*(4), 24–32.

Lupton, D. (1995). *The Imperative of Health: Public Health and the Regulated Body.* London: Sage.

Martin, C. (2001). The relationship between trade and environment regimes: What needs to change? In G.P. Sampson (ed.), *The Role of the World Trade Organization in Global Governance.* New York: The United Nations University Press, pp. 137–154.

McDivitt, J.A., Zimicki, S., & Hornik, R.C. (1997). Explaining the impact of a communication campaign to change vaccination knowledge and coverage in the Philippines. *Health Communication, 9*(2), 95–118.

Melkote, S., Muppidi, S., & Goswami, D. (2000). Social and economic factors in an integrated behavioral and societal approach to communications in HIV/AIDS. *Journal of Health Communication, 5*(3), 17–27.

Millen, J.V., & Holtz, T.H. (2000). Dying for growth, Part I: Transnational corporations and the health of the poor. In J.Y. Kim, J.V. Millen, A. Irwin, & J. Gershman (eds), *Dying for Growth: Global Inequality and the Health of the Poor.* Monroe, Maine: Common Courage Press, pp. 177–224.

Millen, J.V., Irwin, A., & Kim, J.Y. (2000). Introduction: What is growing? Who is dying? In J.V. Millen, A. Irwin, J.Y. Kim & J. Gershman (eds), *Dying for Growth: Global Inequality and the Health of the Poor.* Monroe, Maine: Common Courage Press, pp. 3–10.

Milmo, S. (2002). EPA and EU collaborate on chemicals regulations. *Chemical Market Reporter, 261,* 4–6.

Motaal, D.A. (1999). The Agreement on Technical Barriers to Trade, the Committee on Trade and Environment, and eco-labelling. In G.P. Sampson, & B. Chambers (eds), *Trade, Environment, and the Millennium.* New York: United Nations University Press, pp. 223–238.

Murphy, P. (2001). Framing the nicotine debate: A cultural approach to risk. *Health Communication, 13*(2), 119–140.

Navarro, V. (1999). Health and equity in the world in the era of "globalization". *International Journal of Health Services, 29*(2), 215–226.

Neumayer, E. (2001). *Greening Trade and Investment.* London: Earthscan Publications.

Petersen, A., & Lupton, D. (1996). *The New Public Health: Health and Self in the Age of Risk.* London: Sage.

Peterson, T.R. (1990). Structuring closure through technological discourse: The Mormon Priesthood Correlation Program. In M.J. Medhurst, A. Gonzalez, & T.R. Peterson (eds), *Communication & the culture of technology.* Pullman: Washington State University Press, pp. 77–94.

Pinder, L. (1998). Health promotion meets globalisation. *Promotion & Education,* V(3&4), 37–39.

Pratt, C.B., Silva-Barbeau, I., & Pratt, C.A. (1997). Toward a symmetrical and an integrated framework of norms for nutrition communication in Sub-Saharan Africa. *Journal of Health Communication, 2*(1), 43–58.

Public Citizen. (2002). NAFTA Investor-To-State cases. *Harmonization Alert, 2,* 1–4.

Rose, N. (1996). Governing "advanced" liberal societies. In A. Barry, T. Osborne, & N. Rose (eds), *Foucault and Political Reason: Liberalism, Neo-liberalism and Rationalities of Government.* Chicago: University of Chicago Press, pp. 37–64.

Rose, N., & Miller, P. (1992). Political power beyond the state: Problematics of government. *British Journal of Sociology, 43*(2), 173–205.

Rowson, M. (2000). Globalization and health—Some issues. *Medicine, Conflict, and Survival, 16*(2), 162–174.

Roy, A. (2004). The new American century. *The Nation, 278,* 11–14.

Sass, R. (1999). The unwritten story of women's role in the birth of occupational health and safety legislation. *International Journal of Health Services, 29*(1), 109–145.

Saul, J.R. (2004). The collapse of globalism and the rebirth of nationalism. *Harper's* (March).

Schoepf, B.G., Schoepf, C., & Millen, J.V. (2000). Theoretical therapies, remote remedies: SAPs and the political ecology of poverty and health in Africa. In J.Y. Kim, J.V. Millen, A. Irwin & J. Gershman (eds), *Dying for Growth: Global Inequality and the Health of the Poor.* Monroe, Maine: Common Courage Press, pp. 91–125.

Sharf, B.F. (1999). The present and future of Health Communication scholarship: Overlooked opportunities. *Health Communication, 11*(2), 195–199.

Sidel, V.W. (2000). Working together for health and human rights. *Medicine, Conflict, and Survival, 16*(4), 355–369.

Stiglitz, J.E. (2002). *Globalization and its Discontents.* New York: W.W. Norton and Company.

Storey, D., Boulay, M., Karki, Y., Heckert, K., & Karmacha, D. (1999). Impact of the Integrated Radio Communication Project in Nepal, 1994–1997. *Journal of Health Communication, 4*(4), 271–294.

Tesh, S. (1994). *Hidden Arguments: Politics, Ideology and Disease Prevention Policy.* New Brunswick: Rutgers University Press.

Valente, T.W., & Saba, W.P. (2001). Campaign exposure and interpersonal communication as factors in contraceptive use in Bolivia. *Journal of Health Communication, 6*(4), 303–322.

Vickery, M. (1990). Rhetorical maintenance of technological society: Commercial nuclear power and social orthodoxy. In M.J. Medhurst, A. Gonzalez & T.R. Peterson (eds), *Communication & The Culture of Technology.* Pullman: Washington State University Press, pp. 137–156.

Waitzkin, H. (1983). *The Second Sickness.* New York: The Free Press.

WHO. (1997). Trade and health. *Health for all in the 21st Century Newsletter, Winter* (97/98).

Witte, K. (1998). A theoretically based evaluation of HIV/AIDS prevention campaigns along the Trans-Africa Highway in Kenya. *Journal of Health Communication, 3*(4), 345–363.

Zoller, H.M. (2003). Health on the line: Identity and disciplinary control in employee occupational health and safety discourse. *Journal of Applied Communication Research, 31*(2), 118–139.

Zoller, H.M. (2004). Dialogue as global issue management: Legitimizing corporate influence in the Transatlantic Business Dialogue. *Management Communication Quarterly, 18*(2), 204–240.

Zoller, H.M. (2005a). Health activism: Communication theory and action for social change. *Communication Theory, 15*(4), 341–364.

Zoller, H.M. (2005b). Women caught in the multicausal web: a gendered analysis of Healthy People 2010. *Communication Studies, 56,* 175–192.

Chapter 18

The paradox of "fair trade"

The influence of neoliberal trade agreements on food security and health

Rebecca Desouza, Ambar Basu, Induk Kim, Iccha Basnyat, and Mohan J. Dutta

> Last year, it was the monsoon season. It rained every day. The rains kept coming. It was as if the rains would never end. I had to stay home. Could not go out to find work. Ten days I was out of work. I went and begged for job but did not find one. My children would wait at the door for me to return, their eyes were hungry. They wanted food.
>
> (Dutta-Bergman, 2004, p. 25)

One of the essential components of health is food. Food calls our urgent attention because it constitutes "the overriding human need, the very means of life, recognized in the charter of United Nations as a human right" (Madeley, 2000, p. 25). Food is a fundamental necessity in our lives. The Food Research Action Center (2005) notes a wide range of negative health outcomes due to hunger and malnutrition: hungry persons suffer from two to four times as many individual health problems, such as unwanted weight loss, fatigue, headaches, inability to concentrate and frequent colds; the mortality rate is closely related to inadequate quantity or quality of the diet; iron-deficiency anemia in children can lead to negative health effects such as developmental and behavioral disturbances that can affect children's ability to learn; pregnant women who are undernourished are more likely to have low-birthweight babies and these babies are more likely to suffer delays in their physical and cognitive development; in addition to having a detrimental effect on the cognitive development of children, malnourishment results in the loss of knowledge, brainpower, and productivity for the nation; hunger and malnutrition aggravate chronic and acute diseases and speed the onset of degenerative diseases among the elderly; finally, hunger and food insecurity have an emotional impact on children, their parents, and the communities. Hunger, therefore, has tremendous impact on people's health, quality of life, and the decisions made along the life path.

In spite of the basic role of food, much of the existing literature in health communication has typically ignored the question of access to food. In fact, state-sponsored programs such as population-control programs and immunization programs are often critiqued by the community because they do not seek to meet the basic needs, but instead focus on promoting behavior change. With respect to food, campaigns continue to target different aspects of healthy eating without paying much attention to the issue of access; this is often based on the assumption that individuals and communities are indeed capable of securing the healthy food they need. Health communication scholarship conducted in the marginalized sectors of the globe, however, is starting to draw our attention to the need for basic food capabilities in marginalized communities (Dutta-Bergman, 2004, 2005). In such communities, health is talked about in terms of the ability to secure enough resources to feed the family. In the absence of food, community members point out that it is impossible to think about other health resources, supplies, and behavior changes.

There is little research that interrogates macro-structural factors such as global politics and policy making, which impact a community's access to food. Historically, much of health communication scholarship has focused on individual factors (i.e., beliefs, attitudes and individual capabilities) affecting health, while environmental conditions within which health behaviors arise have been ignored. The distribution of health and life opportunities, however, are heavily influenced by the interaction of social, cultural, economic, and political factors (McLeroy et al., 1988; Minkler 1999). This makes it important to shift the focus of health research from the individual to the identification of factors within the environment collectively responsible for the condition of ill-health (Lupton, 1994). However, Sharf (1999) laments that health communication scholars have not always recognized opportunities available to them to influence public policy, and have not taken the initiative to bring communication knowledge to bear on public health practices. Interrogating macro-structures such as policy also enables advocacy processes. Lupton (1994) affirms that health communication has the role of assisting communities in the processes and skills of advocacy, and health advocacy provides an avenue by which structural elements of ill health can be challenged and changed. Zoller (2005) argues for health activism that focuses on issues of power and conflict, and that uses a multisectoral perspective to examine the broad spectrum of determinants (e.g., political and economic) that shape health.

Responding to the calls of health communication scholars for scholarship that looks at policy, the goal of this chapter is to set the stage for scholars to address the ways in which neoliberal trade policy shapes "food security" in marginalized communities. Food security is defined as "physical and economic access by all people at all times to sufficient, safe and nutritious food to maintain a healthy and active life" (World Bank, 1986). In Chapter 17 (this book), Heather Zoller analyses three neoliberal technologies—structural adjustment, harmonization, and investor lawsuits—from a critical, multi-sectoral perspective to demonstrate how economic policies usually thought to be outside the domain of health policy impede global health promotion. This chapter is yet another positive demonstration of how the multisectoral lens can serve to illuminate the causes and consequences of health inequities in the world. Here, we use descriptive case studies to illustrate how neoliberal trade agreements specifically influence food security in developing regions of the world and how such food shortages pose multiple threats to the health of these communities. The three major trade related policies and cases interrogated here are the General Agreement on Trade and Tariffs (GATT) and its impact on the banana trade in Latin America and the African-Caribbean regions; the Agreement on Agriculture (AoA) and its impact on sugar trade in the Pacific Islands, and the Agreement on Trade-Related Aspects of Intellectual Property Rights (TRIPS) and its impact on the rice trade in South Asia. Culture is pivotal to the understanding of health and its determinants, thus the chapter uses the culture-centered approach (Airhihenbuwa, 1995; Dutta-Bergman, 2004, 2005) as a starting point to theorize about the role of culture, structure, and communication in the context of trade agreements and food security.

This chapter begins with a brief description of the culture-centered approach, after which, each trade agreement and its corresponding case study is presented to illustrate the impact of the agreements on food security. The discussion explicates the linkages between health and hunger, and problematizes the role of culture and communication in health policy making.

Culture-centered approach to health communication

The significance of culture in the realm of health is manifold. First, culture is important because it affects every aspect of people's lives, including attitude toward illness, health status, and health-related behaviors. In the culture-centered approach, culture is deemed central to the planning, implementation, and evaluation of health communication and health promotion programs (Airhihenbuwa, 1995; Jack & Airhihenbuwa, 1993; Dutta-Bergman, 2005). Airhihenbuwa (2005) defines culture as "a collective sense of consciousness that is vocal enough to reveal its sense of history and language but quiet enough to render its structures, values, and beliefs neutral and common" (p. 17). Scholars (Airhihenbuwa & Obregon, 2000; Jack & Airhihenbuwa, 1993) emphasize that culture is always historically specific because it is based on shared memories and a sense of continuity between generations. In the context of neoliberal trade policies, the culture-centered approach is a useful lens because it enables us to ask questions pertaining to culture. For example, what cultures and communities are represented by the trade agreements? Whose attitudes, values, and beliefs do these policies articulate?

Secondly, the culture-centered approach is relevant to the interrogation of macro-policy, because it emphasizes the importance of structural realities in health decision-making. The focal point of the cultural approach is not just the individual, but also the individual's social network of communities, infrastructure, and institutions, and the legal, political, and economic realities that encompass his or her life (Dutta-Bergman, 2005). Structure defines, limits, shapes, and constrains the nature of communicative practices (Dutta-Bergman, 2004, 2005). According to Dutta-Bergman (2005), "Health decisions might be located in the capability of community members to gain access to some of the primary resources of life, such as food, clothing, and shelter. In the face of the absence of these basic resources, engaging in higher order health behaviors such as getting mammograms, not smoking cigarettes, or having safe sex might seem irrelevant" (p. 109). Using the culture-centered approach thus allows us to attend to the contextual nature of health, especially since health is not separable from social structure, economics, politics, and other features of human activity. More specifically, the culture-centered approach enables us to interrogate how structures such as neoliberal trade agreements marginalize communities by restricting their access to food.

Finally, the culture-centered approach is instructive to the current analysis because it underscores the importance of communication and "dialogue" in health decision making. The approach argues that members of the community or culture should be actively engaged in decision-making processes that shape their realities (Dutta-Bergman, 2004, 2005). The notion of "voice" and "reciprocal communication" are central to the approach; it is based on the rationale that if the voices of communities are allowed to emerge, more effective solutions will be put in place. The culture-centered approach locates communication at the center of theorizing about health solutions. The approach stresses that communication theories develop from within the culture or community, rather than from the outside (Airhihenbuwa, 1995; Dutta-Bergman, 2005; Jack & Airhihenbuwa, 1993). According to Dutta-Bergman (2005), "Explanations of phenomena and articulations of pragmatic solutions based on the nature of the phenomena emerge from within the culture or subculture being studied . . . the culture-centered approach becomes the conduit through which members of indigenous communities find ways to articulate their voices and participate in social change" (p. 116). The culture-centered approach thus allows us to address issues of communication and voice in the context of trade agreements. Whose "voice" is represented in the trade policies? What are the conduits and platforms available for communities to articulate themselves and participate in social change? Thus the culture-centered approach sets the stage for us as health communication scholars to ask questions pertaining to culture, structure, and "voice" in the context of neoliberal trade policies, and it provides us with a starting point to theorize about the role of communication in policies and political agreements.

Neoliberal trade agreements and food security

Neoliberal ideology manifest in the "new policy agenda" or "Washington Consensus" was first promoted by leading political ideologues Regan and Thatcher. The term neoliberal refers to a set of economic reforms or policies that usually include cutting tariffs and other trade barriers, reducing government intervention in the economy, cuts in social spending, reducing or eliminating subsidies that provide important benefits for the poor, privatizing public enterprises and services, and emphasizing exports as the engine of growth (Korten, 1995, 1999). The basic principle of the agenda is an assertion of the inherent superiority of economic liberalism including the design of an international economic order based on free markets, private property, individual incentive and a minimal role for the state (Labonte, 2001; Labonte & Torgerson, 2002). Neoliberal ideology is most evident in global trade policies and agreements. Scholars (Labonte, 2001; Labonte & Torgerson, 2002) argue that what distinguishes this globalizing era from previous ones is the scale of movement of financial capital and the establishment of binding rules through global institutions, such as the World Trade Organization or the World Bank and their trade policies.

Neoliberal trade agreements have been associated with negative health and dependency patterns in developing regions of the world. Clarkson (1999) concurs that nation-states today often find themselves locked into neoliberal principles by structural adjustment programs in the South and by international agreements and international institutions in the North. Scholars (Harris & Seid, 2004; McMichael & Beaglehole, 2000) argue that the principal promoters of the contemporary market-based economic system advocate development strategies that often impair population health in countries affected by the strategies and reforms. According to Labonte (2001; Labonte & Torgerson, 2002), globalizing influences such as enforceable trade agreements and various forms of international development affect the national context of health through effects on labor rights, food security, the provision of public goods and services, and environmental protection.

The next section of this chapter provides a brief description of three trade agreements (i.e., GATT, AoA, and TRIPS) and corresponding case studies to illustrate the impact of the agreement on food security of marginalized populations. We highlight the linkages among culture, structure, and communication in the context of trade policies, and then further explicate the linkages in the discussion section.

General Agreement on Trade and Tariffs (GATT)

The formation of the General Agreement on Tariffs and Trade in the postwar era was a major landmark in the history of trade liberalization. Immediately following the World Wars, the loss of colonies threatened the economies of European nations and the United States predicted significant deterioration in its international trade due to economic nationalism in the postwar environment (Hudec, 1987). There existed the consensus among developed countries that economic growth and reconstruction was essential to prevent further political unrest (Weiner, 1995). The rationale of trade liberalization was simple—if countries specialize in goods that they can produce efficiently, and exchanged these goods with other countries, the cost of production will be reduced at the global level, and every nation participating in free trade will benefit with economic growth (Madeley, 2000). Upon this consensus, twenty-three countries signed a contract with a code of rules for international trade called the General Agreement on Tariffs and Trade (GATT) in 1947. The GATT centered around three central principles (Dam, 1970; Hudec, 1987). First, all contracting parties (i.e., the signatory governments of the GATT) were required to eliminate many nontariff protectionist measures[1] affecting international trade; second, all tariff levels could not exceed the level of those at the time of the Agreement and all contracting parties would engage in negotiations to gradually decrease the levels of tariffs; and third, the most-favored-nation principle[2] required all participating governments to eradicate discriminatory trading practices and treat all other contracting parties equally (see United Nations, 1947).

Critics argue that the GATT was a symbol of the hegemonic leadership of the United States. The specific objectives of the United States in negotiating the GATT were twofold: a) to abolish nontariff barriers and to significantly reduce all tariffs to eradicate economic protectionism, and b) to put an end to the discriminatory trading practices originating from the colonial system (Dam, 1970; Hudec, 1987). The first objective was achieved in the subsequent decades. Seven rounds of GATT meetings were held between 1947 and 1979 to liberalize trade in manufactured goods, and this resulted in a significant reduction of trade barriers within the framework of GATT (Madeley, 2000). The second objective of removing discriminatory trading practices, however, was not realized. The promise of economic growth proved to be empty as importation and international debts increased in developing countries, and exportation remained insufficient (Hudec, 1987; Madeley, 2000). Developing countries struggled to protect their infant industries and to gain special status in the international trade market. There were some amendments made to the GATT in subsequent years, but developing countries soon realized that the modifications, aimed to assist the economic development of developing countries, were merely obligations with no legal binding (Hudec, 1987; Madeley, 2000).

The need for major trade reforms led to the formation of the World Trade Organization (WTO) on April 14, 1994, when trade ministers from more than 100 countries met in Marrakesh, Morocco to sign The Final Act Embodying the Results of the Uruguay Round of Multilateral Negotiations. The purpose of the WTO was to oversee a new and equitable multilateral trading system, and to administer the trade agreements negotiated during the 1986–1994 Uruguay Round of trade negotiations. A key feature added to the WTO was a considerably more effective procedure for the adjudication of legal disputes called the "dispute settlement" procedure (Hudec, 1987). Unlike the GATT dispute settlement procedure, the new GATT/WTO procedure gave governments automatic access to tribunals, made legal rulings by tribunals automatically binding, introduced appellate review, and made trade sanctions automatically available in cases of noncompliance. Currently, the GATT represents the umbrella agreement, which covers other agreements such as the Agreement on Agriculture and TRIPs, while the WTO stands as an independent international organization, which oversees and regulates its members' trade practices and disputes (Madeley, 2000).

Impact of GATT/WTO on ACP regions and Latin America: the case of bananas

The repercussions of the GATT/WTO can most clearly be seen in the case of the "banana war" involving Latin America, Africa and the Caribbean and Pacific (ACP),[3] and U.S. and European stakeholders. The ongoing banana trade war is a result of U.S. and Latin-American objections to the European Union's preferential treatment of banana exports received from ACP regions (Finley, 2003; Joseph, 2000).The origins of the banana dispute can be traced to the late 1950s when the European Community first established preferential trading arrangements with former European colonies in the ACP. Preferential treatment by the EU involved a) limiting Latin America's access to the European market, and b) allowing duty-free importation of ACP bananas in the European Union. According to the European Union, the purpose of the duty-free treatment was to make ACP bananas competitive with banana imports from Latin America. Latin-American countries have significantly cheaper production costs because several multinational corporations (e.g., Dole Food Company, Inc. and Chiquita Brands International, Inc.) have large capital investments in Latin America's banana industry. As a result, Latin-American banana plantations are larger and more efficient than ACP banana-production, which suffers from poor soil conditions, independent farmers, natural disasters, and more expensive shipping costs due to the absence of mass production mechanisms. For example, production and transport prices on the Windward Islands in the ACP are 1.5 to 2 times higher than in Latin America.

The dispute was taken to the WTO, which in its newly established role was in charge of overseeing trade-related disputes. In 1996, five countries (i.e., Honduras, Guatemala, Ecuador, Mexico, and the United States) lodged a complaint with the WTO against the banana regime, which they considered discriminatory to their interests. The United States became involved on behalf of the multinational companies because it was especially keen to increase its access to the European market. In 1997, the WTO ruled in favor of Latin American and U.S. interests; the WTO adjudicated that the European Union banana regime was discriminatory and ordered it to be amended. In 1999, the WTO, using a seemingly aggressive measure, authorized the United States to impose trade sanctions of $191 million against the European Union for not making satisfactory modifications, and finally, in 2001, the United States and the European Union after protracted negotiations agreed on a new European Union banana importation regime (Clark, 2002; Joseph, 2000). The new banana importation scheme was designed to abolish all individual country quotas and phase in a tariff-only system by 2006 (Clark, 2002; Joseph, 2000). In other words, the ACP regions could not have preferential access to European markets for much longer.

The new importation scheme, which denies preferential access of ACP bananas to the European Union markets, has already had devastating effects on the economy of ACP regions (Grossman, 1998). This is because a large proportion of the ACP population (i.e., 50 percent of St. Vincent and 30 percent of St. Lucia and Dominica) is engaged in banana production. The statement made by Jamaican Prime Minister Percival Patterson (as cited in Grossman, 1998), "Bananas are to us what cars are to Detroit," illustrates the extent to which ACP banana producers depend on access to the European market for their subsistence. A 1997 fact-finding mission by European parliamentarians argued that the loss of the banana trade with the European Union would lead to mass poverty and high levels of unemployment because small farmers in the ACP regions cannot compete on a "free market" (Bananalink, 2004). This has proved true; over the past years, the increased competition from Latin-American "dollar" bananas in the European Union has reduced the market share of Caribbean farmers, as a result, many small-scale marginal farmers in the ACP are abandoning their lands for the only other economic alternatives, which include the cultivation of illegal drugs, emigration, or poverty (Clark, 2002; Joseph, 2000).

Negative repercussions of the banana trade are witnessed in Latin America as well. Given that the WTO ruled in favor of Latin-American interests, one would imagine that it would bring about positive outcomes in the region. But this is far from the lived reality. According to Banana Link (2005), a nongovernmental organization, Latin-American plantation workers and producers do not benefit from changes to the European Union banana regime. In fact, increased social and environmental deregulation negatively affects their health, and further decreases their share of the benefits. Plantation workers in Latin America earn as little as 1 percent of the final price of a banana, workers in Nicaragua earn as little as $1 a day, and workers in Ecuador earn between $3 and $5 a day, these wages are often insufficient to meet basic needs of communities. Furthermore, the establishment of mass producing plantations results in the displacement of indigenous people; for example, indigenous populations such as the Cabecar and the Bribri peoples are seriously threatened by the colonization of vast tracks of land by banana companies, contamination of rivers, and pressure on their lands. The displaced people are either transformed into plantation workers or migratory labourers, who often have no official documents and thus cannot benefit from any medical or social facilities.

Central to the culture-centered approach is the structural capacity of community members to be healthy. The current policies are threatening the livelihood and health of both the farmers of Latin America and the ACP regions. In these regions, however, the falling economies, the environmental losses, and the displacement of workers threaten food security to the extent that community members lack both the economic means to buy food and the environmental resources to cultivate their own food. Furthermore, the "banana war" has resulted in developing countries losing their means of sustenance as they compete with other countries for access to markets in Europe and the United States. Thus, the WTO policies produce winners and losers, but the winners are generally large enterprises, such as transnational corporations, while the losers are poor farmers and rural laborers, whose livelihood and health is undermined by falling commodity prices and by the loss of rural employment.

Agreement on Agriculture (AoA)

The Agreement on Agriculture came into effect in 1994 as a result of the 1986–94 Uruguay Round of the GATT. The objective of the agreement was to amend the 1947 GATT to include fairer agricultural trade agreements and to establish a "significant first step towards order, fair competition and less distorted sector" (WTO, 2005). Prior to the Uruguay Round, agricultural commodities were largely exempt from the application of GATT requirements, thus developing countries taxed the agricultural sector in order to earn badly needed revenue, while industrialized countries used a number of techniques to promote agricultural production (e.g., export subsidies, import tariffs, import quotas, and other nontariff barriers). Moreover, under the pre-Uruguay GATT, the United States and the European Union adopted a variety of measures to protect and promote agricultural production, which conferred a big advantage on agricultural producers in industrialized countries compared to their competitors in developing countries. The AoA was significant because it represented for the first time since the creation of GATT that agricultural commodities were subject to the multilateral trading rules (Gonsalez, 2002). The Agreement obliged participating nations to provide market access to other nations and to significantly reduce traditionally allowed domestic supports and export subsidies to farmers (Wiener, 1995). Specifically, the AoA obligates WTO members to liberalize agricultural trade in three respects: the expansion of market access by requiring the conversion of all nontariff barriers to tariffs[4] (i.e., tariffication) and the binding and reduction of these tariffs; the reduction of both the volume of and expenditures on subsidized exports; and, the reduction of trade-distorting domestic subsidies.

It is important to note that while the agricultural trade negotiations were meant to remove trade inequities, the AoA was shaped by the intense rivalry between the United States and the European Union for world agricultural markets, and developing countries were almost entirely left out of the negotiating process. The United States called for a phase-out of agricultural export subsidies over a five-year period, while the European Union, seeking to protect its Common Agricultural Policy,[5] argued for a more modest subsidy reduction proposal designed to preserve status quo. Japan and South Korea, both net food-importing nations, placed great emphasis on the need to support domestic production in order to promote food security, South Korea argued for special and differential treatment for developing countries, including longer timeframes to remove import restrictions, and developing countries (led most often by India, Jamaica and Egypt) advocated the elimination of developed country protectionism, the importance of agricultural support for the economic development in nonindustrialized nations, and the prime importance of food security for developing countries (Gonsalez, 2002). In the end, however, the AoA only served to institutionalize the existing inequities between developed and developing countries by restricting policy options available to developing countries to promote food security; the agreement enabled developed countries to continue to subsidize and protect domestic producers while requiring developing countries to open up their markets to foreign competition.

Impact of Agreement on Agriculture in Pacific Islands: the case of sugar

The repercussions of the AoA can most clearly be seen in the case of sugar in the Pacific Islands. Pacific Island nations have long sustained their economy by keeping high tariff level and maintaining preferential measures from the previous colonial system. However, as the Islands joined the WTO and adopted the rules of trade liberalization, the economic, social, and political scapes of these Island countries are dramatically changing. Abiding by the rules in the AoA, the entrance to the WTO mandated the nations to significantly reduce tariffs and inhibited their traditional reliance on preferential relationship with few major trading partners. For example, the sugar industry, the Island nations' primary export sector and income source, was one of the hardest-hit by the trade liberalization rules. The Island nations' (see Kelsey, 2005, for the case of Fiji) sugar export to the European Union was interrupted by the AoA; this was because the goal of the AoA was to inhibit any preferential measures that disrupted free market trade. This resulted in the loss of market access from the part of the Island nations. At the same time, the application of the Most-Favored-Nation principle provided other WTO members with the access to the Island's economy. The tariff cuts, in the mean time, significantly decreased governmental revenues and increased reliance on imported foodstuffs, and deprived agricultural rural areas of workers (see Kelsey, 2005, for the case of Tonga). A 1999 study by the Food and Agriculture Organization (FAO) reported that agricultural trade liberalization has resulted in a concentration of landholding in a wide cross-section of countries, so while large, export-oriented agricultural enterprises reaped the benefits of trade liberalization, small farmers frequently lose title to their plots of land. Add to that, government cuts in agricultural input subsidies has increased the price of farm inputs thereby forcing farmers to pay more for agricultural inputs while receiving less for their output.

The application of the Agreement on Agriculture is also threatening communities' access to healthy food in the Pacific Islands. The AoA negatively impacts food security and the economic livelihood of small farmers by producing a flood of cheap food imports and restricting domestic food production in developing countries (Gonsalez, 2002; FAO, 2000). According to the FAO Report, the AoA resulted in an increase in food imports (e.g., meat and dairy products), which proved a threat to key agricultural sectors important for economic development, employment, food supply, and poverty alleviation. In addition, the AoA resulted in a decline in domestic food production in developing countries. Trade liberalization has led to an increased emphasis on export production, thus developing countries have begun to devote more land and resources to export crops, but due to declining world prices for many agricultural commodities, small farmers do not necessarily receive better prices for export commodities. In the Pacific Islands, cheap but unhealthy import foodstuffs (e.g., mutton flaps) are replacing healthier traditional diets, such as fish, organic chicken, and taro, because they cannot compete with cheap imports. For example, in the discussion of the Tongans' increased consumption of mutton flaps, Kelsey (2005) notes that "Tongan people made economically rational, but nutritionally detrimental, decisions to eat less healthy foods because they were cheap and available" (p. 22). Mutton flaps, a fatty waste product of sheep, is campaigned against in the developed nations for the negative health impacts but the same developed countries are selling the product at a cheap price in the Island nations. The result of unhealthy eating is that obesity and cardiovascular diseases are also becoming serious health problems in the Islands.

The lack of importance given to food security in the Agreement on Agriculture has had negative repercussions for small farmers. The application of the AoA has resulted in reduced access to economic resources, which significantly limits communities' access to healthy food. AoA creates structural nodes that limit practices related to health on the ground. This ties in well with the culture-centered approach to health communication, which situates structure at the center of health communication practices that a community engages in. The lack of healthy food and inadequate income to access the healthy food are structural nodes that inhibit an individual's and community's ability to partake in communication processes that promote health. Health communication practices are transformed from the realm of awareness to ability. Though a person or a community is aware of the need to remain healthy and ways to do so (i.e., by eating healthy food), she/he is not able to choose the healthy practice due to structural barriers (i.e., lack of income, lack of availability of healthy food).

Agreement on Trade-Related Aspects of Intellectual Property Rights (TRIPS)

The Agreement on Trade-Related Aspects of Intellectual Property Rights (TRIPS) came into effect in 1995 as a result of the 1986–94 Uruguay Round of the General Agreement on Trade and Tariffs (GATT). TRIPS was seen as a step toward applying basic principles of GATT—to foster seamless international trade, while protecting the rights of creative minds. The WTO describes intellectual property rights as "the rights given to people over the creations of their minds" (WTO, 1994). It is these creations of the mind that the trade regulating body seeks to protect through the Agreement (WTO, 1994). According to the WTO, governments need to ensure that innovators have the right to prevent others from using their innovations and the right to negotiate payment from others in return for using their innovations. However, since the extent of protection and enforcement of these rights varied widely across geographical boundaries causing much tension, the "new internationally agreed trade rules for intellectual property rights (i.e., TRIPS) were seen as a way to introduce more order and predictability, and for disputes to be settled more systematically" (WTO, 1994). The TRIPS Agreement covers the following areas of intellectual property: copyright and related rights (the rights of performers, producers of sound recordings and broadcasting organizations); trademarks; geographical indications including appellations of origin; industrial designs; patents including the protection of new varieties of plants; the layout-designs of integrated circuits; and undisclosed information (WTO, 1994). The agreement stresses on fair and equitable action against infringement of intellectual property rights, and the need to make redressal procedures less complicated, less costly and short in duration.

Impact of TRIPS in South Asia: the case of basmati

The repercussions of TRIPS can most clearly be seen in the case of basmati in South Asia. The TRIPS Agreement threatens food security by a) not recognizing indigenous communities' rights over their resources and b) by enabling biopiracy.[6] According to Woods (2002) and Bodekar (2003), the agreement inadequately protects indigenous knowledge. "The view under TRIPS is that if it is not patented it is not owned. If it is not owned, it represents knowledge that is part of a global commons available for exploitation by all who so wish" (Bodekar, 2003, p. 787). According to legal analysts such as Woods (2002) and Bodekar (2003), the TRIPS Agreement does not extend either patent or geographic protection to the traditional knowledge of indigenous people; for example, the patent laws under TRIPS do not adequately recognize traditional form of breeding as "prior art" (i.e., the entire body of knowledge available to the public before a given filing or priority date for any patent, utility model, or industrial design). This has thus led to multinational biotechnological corporations successfully seeking patents on food grains (Woods, 2002), which in turn negatively impacts local economies. In addition, TRIPS enables biopiracy to take place with relative ease especially in lesser-developed countries that are rich in genetic resources and low in technology. Access to technology in developed countries allows richer countries to harness and reproduce genetic material for patenting, thereby enabling the expropriation of local resources.

The attempt of RiceTec, a Texas-based company to patent basmati rice is a case in point. Basmati rice is traditional to India and Pakistan, and in 1997 comprised 4 percent of India's export earnings, receiving premium prices in the international market. In September 1997, RiceTec, a U.S. multinational agro-company, successfully applied for several patents on the basmati rice and grain lines. The Pakistani and Indian governments refuted the patents stating that the plant varieties and grains already exist as a staple in India, and that neither variety of rice can be grown in the United States. The United States Patent and Trademark Office rescinded fifteen of the twenty patents granted. However, the five remaining patents continue to permit RiceTec to exclude others from making, using and selling its patented basmati rice in the United States until September 2017. What this means is that the rice-producing nations in South Asia will have a smaller (and perhaps non-existent) international market in the coming years. In addition to marginalizing access that developing countries have to international markets, TRIPs also enables biopiracy. For example, the RiceTec's U.S. patent claimed the invention of "novel rice lines with plants that are semi-dwarf in stature, substantially photoperiod-insensitive and high-yielding, and that produce rice grains having characteristics similar or superior to those of good quality basmati rice grains produced in India and Pakistan." However, what the policy does not take into account is that the patent takes ownership of genetic material originally developed by South Asian farmers; the germplasm from these varieties were initially collected in the Indian subcontinent and later deposited and processed in the United States and other places. Add to that, TRIPS also allows the patent holder to usurp the "basmati" name, which itself could jeopardize the sale of basmati from South Asia due to confusion (TED, 2005).

The patenting of food grains can have major implications for the economy and food security in the least developed countries (LDC). In many of the LDCs, food grains such as rice form a vital part of people's diet. According to the Trade and Environment Database (TED, 2005), with the basmati patent rights, RiceTec will be able to not only call its aromatic rice basmati within the United States, but to also label it basmati for its exports. This means farmers that depend on basmati cultivation and export in India and Pakistan will not only lose out on the 45,000-tonne US import market, which forms 10 percent of the total basmati exports, but also its position in markets such as the European Union, the United Kingdom, Middle East, and West Asia. This would certainly hit the local economy in rice-growing regions of India and

Pakistan. As farmers lose markets for their crops, their incomes will be hit hard, leading to increased inability to spend on a basic necessity such as food. Thus, the very resources that are a part of the day-to-day life of indigenous groups have to be purchased at a price from the technologically advanced countries and from transnational corporations, creating the scenario for continuous exploitation.

This has a direct bearing on the health of the affected population and on the communicative practices that influence health. The culture-centered approach to health communication emphasizes the importance of structural factors in health decisions. Health decisions are situated in the ability of community members to gain access to basic resources of life, such as food, clothing, and shelter. In the case of basmati farmers in India and Pakistan, a decrease in their income structures their (in)ability to procure food for themselves and their families. Looking for ways and means to provide the needed food then overrides larger health concerns, and influences communicative patterns that emanate from these food-deprived cultural spaces. Day-to-day practices center around fighting hunger and the structures (such as TRIPS and other global trade policies) that create and reinforce it. Practicing and propagating healthy practices such as immunizing children and going for health check-ups becomes a second-order derivative of hunger and the need to fight it. As Madeley (2000) notes, agreements such as TRIPS establish private, monopolistic control over plant resources and lead to dislocation of farmers, loss of food security and ultimately denial of "the right to survive."

Discussion

There is no doubt that hunger and food security are the quintessential issues that necessitate the immediate attention of health communication scholarship. However, the dominant research frameworks for studying health issues (i.e., the individual behavior change model) fail to capture the complex nature of health inequality: the economic, political, and cultural contexts in which health is embedded. There is the need for a shift of paradigm that contextualizes health inequality and listens to the voices of marginalized communities in order to generate more culturally appropriate and empowering ways for social and health change. For example, without accounting for the structural issues surrounding health, researchers run the risk of obtaining a myopic picture of and yielding marginal explanations of the phenomenon. Consequently, the resulting solutions cannot be adequately applied to the context of health problems in marginalized communities. This chapter is a step toward the paradigm-shift. By using the framework of culture-centered approach (Dutta-Bergman, 2005), we examine neoliberal trade policies and their relevance to public health in the context of hunger and food security.

The culture-centered approach argues for the importance of basic structures (e.g. food) in the context of health. From the evaluation of policies and cases presented in this chapter, the conclusion drawn is that "hunger is not caused by lack of food in the world, but rather by the inability of hungry people to gain access to the plentiful food that exists" (Food First, 2005). The result of the strict imposition of neoliberal trade policies is that people who suffer from hunger lack the resources to either buy food or produce it themselves. The cumulative effects of trade liberalization and neoliberal policies are the reduction in food subsidies, higher food prices, and lower wages in rural poorer households. With their low incomes, lost jobs, and farmlands taken away, people in the marginalized sectors cannot afford to buy food, and thus suffer from hunger and malnutrition. At a global level, the exercise of trade liberalization rules have caused the governments of developing countries to undergo high levels of foreign indebtedness and severe cutbacks in the health-care funding (Madeley, 2000). A high level of indebtedness means that countries must shift money away from agriculture and other essentials so as to repay debts. Thus, more resources are allocated to debt repayment than health-care services and public supports crucial for the protection of people's rights to health.

It is important to point out that in addition to structural marginalization and food deprivation, neoliberal trade policies also facilitate cultural violation as seen in the case studies presented. For example, in the ACP regions and Latin America, community life revolves around the production of bananas; banana production is not just a means of livelihood, but central to the lives and well-being of communities. Displacement, the increase in crime, changes in the social environment, and devastation of the natural environment has disturbing effects on the culture and society of these communities. Thus, GATT has not just affected the economies of these regions, but also disrupted the ways in which communities in the ACP regions and in Latin America live. In the Pacific Islands, food habits, which are so inherent to the culture of communities, have also undergone changes for the worse. Cheap imported food has replaced healthier local food because indigenous production cannot compete with cheap imports legislated by the AoA. In South Asia, the patenting of basmati has negatively impacted the ways of livelihood of farmers who are dependent rice production. Furthermore, since TRIPS does not acknowledge or distinguish between indigenous knowledge and industry knowledge, it has enabled the expropriation of traditional and cultural knowledge of communities. The knowledge that indigenous people have nurtured, developed and passed on through generations is systematically expropriated by property rights agreements. Communities are not compensated for their cultural knowledge, but rather, the very resources that are a part of the day-to-day life of indigenous groups now have to be purchased at a premium from technologically advanced countries. Thus, it is important to note that the effects of neoliberal trade agreements are not confined to structural implications, but rather, the policies marginalize the very cultures of such communities through direct and indirect pathways.

As health communication scholars, we must locate such policy issues in the context of those communicative processes that limit and impede the possibility of achieving good health, thus the question we raise is whose "voice" is represented in the policies? Viewed through the lens of the culture-centered approach, neoliberal trade agreements clearly do not represent the "agreement" of *all* cultures and communities. Globalizing influences such as enforceable trade agreements negatively affecting the food security, economy, culture, and overall health of communities. Trade policies do not account for the voices of marginalized populations as is evident from the stunning paradox of food insecurity. The world has more than enough food to meet its needs because global food production has surpassed population growth in recent decades, but there are still more than 20,000 people that die of the effects of hunger everyday (Madeley, 2000). There is enough food available such that countries that do not produce all the food they want can import necessary food, but still millions of people do not share this security. Thus while international institutions believe that trade liberalization is the key to solving hunger, in fact, the "globalization of food markets is an instant strategy for creating hunger" (Madeley, 2000; Shiva, 2000; Labonte, 2001; Labonte & Torgerson, 2002; Harris & Seid, 2004; McMichael & Beaglehole, 2000).

The policies undoubtedly privilege those actors that have access to power. The voices of developed countries, multinational companies, and large agro-chemical industries are allowed to emerge in the public sphere, while poor communities silently endure the consequences of neoliberal practices and processes. Neoliberal agreements create a scenario for continual exploitation of the poor, and legitimate this exploitation under the rubric of "intellectual property rights" or "fair trade". For example, TRIPS which was formulated by the industrialized world clearly does not serve the interests of indigenous farmers and local communities. The analysis reveals that TRIPS serves the transnational empire by facilitating the exploitation of indigenous knowledge, and by opening up new markets for transnational corporations. In most instances, indigenous groups lack access to communicative platforms, legal structures, and civil society systems to contest such policies, thus making it easy for outsiders to exploit them. Furthermore, neoliberal agreements create a situation in which communities are so entrenched in fighting for their very survival that the very act of "staging a protest" as we know it becomes a rather far-fetched notion. Consider the statement, "Ten days I was out of work. I went and begged for job but did not find one. My children would wait at the door for me to return, their eyes were hungry. They wanted food" (Dutta-Bergman, 2004, p. 25). This *is* a protest, but unfortunately, this form of protest does not surface at the time when "fair trade" agreements are decided.

Thus, there is the recognition that advocacy is required as a means to improving health conditions. As health communication scholars, we should not limit ourselves to working within the policy frameworks that are handed down to us. According to Lupton (1994), "advocacy activities seek to change the political agenda, to direct the spotlight of public accountability away from individuals and toward vested interests in industry and government, to influence public policy, and to encourage the initiation and enforcement of regulation of industrial activities that perpetuate unhealthy environments and manufacture unhealthy products" (p. 63). The politicization of health communication allows for opening up alternative spaces that question the fundamental assumptions that drive the constructions of health and the communicative practices that emerge around it. As health communication scholars, we need to pay attention to public advocacy such that we can develop strategic communicative mechanisms for influencing policy makers. Zoller (Chapter 17, this book) suggests that health communication research should evaluate the potential of various communicative strategies to challenge neoliberalism and to develop positive alternatives that place public health on the global agenda. Specifically, macro policies need to be amended such that they take into account indigenous rights. Ghosh (2003) suggests that since there is no normative principle to assist decision makers when faced with conflicting alternatives, empowering traditionally subordinated groups should be the relevant norm for structuring rights involving local indigenous communities. Thus health advocates should emphasize the creation of dialogical platforms that listen to the voices of indigenous people and document the critical aspects of policy that further marginalize them. This creation of dialogical platforms provides the recipe for social change in a world replete with exploitative tendencies of those with power directed at further marginalization of the poor.

Notes

1   Any restriction imposed on the free flow of trade is a trade barrier. Trade barriers can either be tariff barriers (i.e., a levy of ordinary customs duties) or nontariff barriers (i.e., any trade barriers other than the tariff barriers, such as import policy barriers; standards, testing, labeling and certification requirements; and, anti-dumping and countervailing measures, services barriers etc.)

2   "Most-favored-nation-treatment" (MFN) requires parties to accord the most favorable tariff and regulatory treatment given to the product of any one contracting party for import or export to all "like products" of other contracting parties. For example, if contracting party A agrees with contracting party B to reduce the tariff on the product X to 5 percent, this same "tariff rate" must apply to all other contracting parties for products that are the same as X (i.e., like products). In other words, if a country gives most-favored-nation treatment to one country regarding a particular issue, it must handle all other countries equally regarding the same issue.

3   The ACP is comprised of seventy-eight nations of which the twelve traditional banana producing ACP countries are Cameroon, Cape Verde, Ivory Coast, Madagascar, Somalia, Jamaica, Belize, St. Lucia, St. Vincent, Grenada, Dominica, and Suriname.

4   One of the most important aspects of the Agreement on Agriculture is tariffication. This requires countries with nontariff measures, such as quantitative restrictions

and import licensing, to abolish them by transferring the nontariff measures to the tariff equivalents and adding these into fixed tariffs. The tariff equivalent was calculated based on average world market price of the product to which nontariff measures were applied traditionally.

5   The Common Agricultural Policy is a system of European Union agricultural subsidies that guarantees a minimum price to producers and provides direct payment of a subsidy for crops planted. The Common Agricultural Policy has been providing some economic certainty for European Union farmers and production of a certain quantity of agricultural goods.

6   Biopiracy refers to the appropriation of biological resources without the prior informed consent of the local people and/or of the competent authority of the respective state, for access and benefit sharing, under mutually agreed terms.

References

Airhihenbuwa, C. (1995). *Health and Culture: Beyond the Western Paradigm*. Thousand Oaks, CA: Sage.

Airhihenbuwa, C., & Obregon, R. (2000). A critical assessment of theories/models used in health communication for HIV/AIDS. *Journal of Health Communication, 5*, 5–15.

Banana Link Website (2004). Retrieved 5 May, 2004 from www.bananalink.org.uk/.

Bodekar, G. (2003). Traditional medical knowledge, intellectual property rights & benefit sharing. Symposium: Traditional knowledge, intellectual property, and indigenous culture. *Cardozo Journal of International and Comparative Law, 11/785.*

Clark, H. (2002). The WTO banana dispute settlement and its implications for trade relations between the United States and the European Union. *Cornell International Law Journal, 35*, 291.

Clarkson, S. (1999). The global-continental-national dynamic: some hypotheses on comparative continentalism. In S. Nagel (ed.), *Global Public Policy: Among and Within Nations*. New York: St. Martin's.

Dam, K.W. (1970). *The GATT: Law and the International Economic Organization*. Chicago, IL: University of Chicago Press.

Dutta-Bergman, M. (2005). Theory and practice in health communication campaigns: A critical interrogation. *Health Communication, 18*(2), 103–122.

Dutta-Bergman, M. (2004). The unheard voices of Santalis: Communicating about health from the margins of India. *Communication Theory, 14*(3), 237–263.

FAO. (2000). *Agriculture, Trade and Food Security Issues and Options in the WTO Negotiations from the Perspective of Developing Countries*. Geneva, Switzerland: Food and Agriculture Organization.

Finley, M. (2003). The bitter with the sweet: The impact of the World Trade Organization's settlement of the banana trade dispute on the human rights of Ecuadorian banana workers. *New York Law School Law Review, 48*, 815.

Food First (2005). Democratizing market. Retrieved April 12, 2006, from www. foodfirst.org/programs.

Food Research Action Center (2005). Health consequences of hunger. Retrieved April 12, 2006, from www.frac.org/html/hunger_in_the_us/health.html.

Ghosh, S. (2003). Reflections on the traditional knowledge debate. *Cardozo Journal of International and Comparative Law, 11*, 497–510.

Gonsalez, C. (2002). Institutionalizing Inequality: The WTO Agreement on Agriculture, Food Security, and Developing Countries. *Columbia Journal of Environmental Law, 27*(433).

Grossman, L.S. (1998) *The Political Ecology of Bananas: Contract Farming, Peasants, and Agrarian Change in the Eastern Caribbean.* Chapel Hill: The University of North Carolina Press.

Harris, R., & Seid, M. (2004). *Globalization and Health in the New Millennium.* Boston, MA: Brill.

Hudec, R.E. (1987). *Developing Countries in the GATT Legal System.* Aldershot, UK: Gower.

Jack, L., & Airhihenbuwa, C. (1993). Cancer among low-income African-Americans: Implications for culture and community-based health promotion. *Wellness Perspectives, 9*(4), 57–69.

Joseph, A.L. (2000). The banana split: Has the stalemate been broken in the WTO banana dispute? The global trade community's a-peel for justice. *Fordham International Law Journal, 24,* 744.

Kelsey, J. (2005). World trade and small nations in the South Pacific region. *Kansas Journal of Law and Public Policy, 14,* 247.

Korten, D. (1995). *When Corporations Ruled the World.* London: Earthscan.

Korten, D. (1999). *The Post-Corporate World.* San Francisco, CA: Kumarian.

Labonte, R. (2001). Globalization and reform of the World Trade Organization. *Canadian Journal of Public Health, 92*(4), 248–249.

Labonte, R., & Torgerson, R. (2002). *Frameworks for analyzing the links between globalization and health.* Saskatoon: University of Saskatchewan.

Lupton, D. (1994). Toward the development of critical health communication praxis. *Health Communication, 6*(1), 55–67.

Madeley, J. (2000). *Hungry for Trade: How the Poor Pay for Free Trade.* New York: Zed Books.

McLeroy K., Bibeau, D., Steckler, A., & Glanz, K. (1988). An ecological perspective on health promotion programs. *Health Education Quarterly, 15,* 351–377.

McMichael, A.J., & Beaglehole, R. (2000). The changing global context of public health. *Lancet, 356,* 495–499.

Minkler, M. (1999). Personal responsibility for health? A review of the arguments and the evidence at century's end. *Health Education & Behavior, 26* (1), 121–141.

Sharf, B. (1999). The present and future of health communication scholarship: Overlooked opportunities. *Health Communication, 11*(2), 195–200.

Shiva, V. (2000). The historic significance of Seattle. *Splice,* January/February 2000.

Trade and Environment Database (TED). Retrieved October 14, 2005 from www.american.edu/TED/basmati.htm.

United Nations. (1947). *General Agreement on Tariffs and Trade.*

Weiner, J. (1995). *Making Rules in the Uruguay Round of the GATT: A Study of International Leadership.* Aldershot, UK: Dartmouth.

Woods, M. (2002). Food for thought: the biopiracy of jasmine and basmati rice. *Albany Law Journal of Science & Technology, 13,* 123.

World Bank (1986) Poverty and hunger—Issues and options for food security in developing countries. Washington DC.

World Trade Organization (2005). *Understanding the WTO—Agriculture: Fairer markets for farmers.* Retrieved September 13, 2005, from the World Trade Organization website: www.wto.org.

World Trade Organization/WTO (1994). Intellectual property rights and the TRIPS Agreement. Retrieved March 14, 2004 from www.wto.org/english/tratop_e/trips_e/trips_e.htm#WhatAre.

Zoller, H.M. (2005). Health activism: Communication theory and action for social change. *Communication Theory, 15*(4), 341–364.

Chapter 19

Globalization, social justice movements, and the human genome diversity debates

A case study in health activism

*Rulon Wood, Damon M. Hall,
and Marouf Hasian, Jr.*

During the past two decades, there has been an increased interest in providing studies that recover the agency of the "other," the subalterns who were once considered the passive recipients of Western-oriented epistemologies. Authors such as Said (1978), Spivak (1988), and Bhabha (1992) are only some of the interdisciplinary writers who have provided provocative readings that invite us to rethink the ways that we write about disparate power relations, discursive social constructs, and effective postcolonial resistance. Whereas some writers believe that we need to give voice to the "other" through the study of alternative histories that come from those who might be engaged in activities such as peasant uprisings in India (Guha, 1983), other authors focus their attention on the contrapuntal readings of "colonial discourse" (Moore-Gilbert, 1997, p. 19). While many of these authors have disagreements about preferred methods of analysis or choice of artifacts that need deconstructing, they share the common goal of demonstrating the ways in which subalterns have some active social agency and control over their circumstances. The cumulative effect of introducing these postcolonial themes and methods is that scholars and researchers have a much more nuanced understanding of how "development" programs (Spivak, 1999) and other ostensibly neutral Western projects are tied to a host of ideological prefigurations, politicized histories, and polysemic international texts.

This growing awareness of the need to give voice to the national or international "other" has also potentially altered the ways that researchers think about the ontological and epistemic dimensions of health communication and medicinal public practices. For example, Airhihenbuwa et al. (2000) contend that the current health communication models are inadequate in addressing the needs of a variety of groups and cultures. These authors argue that "Western cultures, to varying degrees, tend to view the self as a production of the individual, whereas many other cultures view the self as a production of the family, community, and other environmental influences for which we do not have, or desire, total control" (pp. 106–107). The work of Airhihenbuwa et al. (2000) thus invites us to rethink the ways that we approach the creation, dissemination, and reception of various health communication systems that might be Eurocentric.

Even more recently, Dutta-Bergman (2004), has suggested that we need to supplement our traditional monological (purportedly neutral and generalizable) health communication models with more "culture-centered" approaches that encourage the polysemic and polyvalent study of health care. This "approach to health communication foregrounds the voices of marginalized people, in dialogue with the academic researcher or theorist, with the goals of developing mutual understanding and respect, as opposed to imposing the dominant worldview" (Dutta-Bergman, 2004, p. 241). This collaborative way of thinking about individual and communal health care means that we take seriously the possibility that nonWestern voices have something substantive to say about the co-production of health-care systems. In essence, the culture-centered approach to health communication foregrounds agency and context in the co-construction of meanings through subaltern participation.

In this chapter, we extend the work of Airhihenbuwa et al. (2000) and Dutta-Bergman (2004) and argue that communication critics who study genetic epistemes need to take seriously the possibility that researchers should attend to both the power of dominant texts and the heuristic value of alternative, subaltern, health commentaries. If postcolonial critics and other researchers are truly interested in finding more (co) productive health dialogues, then they need to constantly be self-reflexive about the ways that they write about the agency and voice of the subaltern—especially in situations where "development" projects are touted as modern, nonexploitative forms of progress (Spivak, 1999). As we argue below, we hope to show in our study of the controversial Human Genome Diversity Project (HGDP) that indigenous voices had much to say about the goals, timing, desirability, legality, and ethicality of these programs. Moreover, we argue that some of these critics did much more than simply "stall" or interfere with the trajectories or agendas of the scientists who touted the program—they may have helped alter the very way that we think about genomic knowledge or methods.

Zoller (2005) has recently averred that "health communication can benefit in the study of activism by adopting critical and multisectoral lenses" that focus in on issues of power, inequality, and "multiple social domains" (p. 342), and we are firmly convinced that a culture-centered study of the HGDP offers important insights into the ways in which traditional modes of scientific research have been informed and changed through a process of indigenous health activism. With this in mind, we have divided this chapter into four major sections. In the first, we provide some background information and explain how subaltern voices were excluded during initial planning stages of the HGDP. In the second section, we demonstrate how alliances of subaltern voices came together as a force for activism and change, primarily through the internet, engaging researchers in a new discursive space. Additionally, we identify the primary concerns voiced by this new collective. In the third section, we demonstrate the ways in which these marginalized voices were able to make a difference in both the formation and the implementation of the HGDP, and we illustrate how various subaltern commentaries may have influenced the direction of future genetic "diversity" research. Finally, in the concluding portions of the essay, we comment on how this study might help alter the ways that we think about genomic "development," the assumptions that are built into health communication paradigms that try to eliminate "misunderstanding," and the role that subalterns play in the co-production of genomic knowledges.

Background: an absence of the subaltern voice

In the late 1980s, U.S. officials had decided to spend billions of dollars on the mapping and sequencing of genetic material, and under the auspices of the Human Genome Project (HGP), these scientists were able to secure large amounts of federal funding (some 3 billion dollars). The renascent public and elite interest in genomic research seemed to open the possibilities that there might be other genomic projects that would build on the good will that had been created by promoters of the HGP.

Within a matter of a few years, a second group of scientists proposed a related project, one that would focus on genomic "diversity"—or the study of various genetic patterns so that scientists could understand genetic differences and similarities in and among various human populations. The popular HGP had indeed constructed a "map" of the human genome, but most of the samples that were used in making generalizations about larger populations had purportedly come from non"diverse" subjects. As one investigator (Jackson, 1998) would later remark, the HGP genomic baseline had been built on molecular taxonomies that were skewed toward "North Atlantic European lineages," and this lack of scientific representativeness militated against the possibility that this type of research might have broader health applications (pp. 155–170).

In 1991 a small group of geneticists—in an apparently innocuous article about the importance of "diversity"—first introduced to the world the idea that humanity needed to amply fund the newly forming Human Genome Diversity Project (HGDP). In theory, this project would supplement scientific understanding of "prehistoric migrations, natural selection, the social structure of populations, and the frequency and types of mutations [that] our species has experienced" (Cavalli-Sforza et al., 1991, p. 490). In addition, the architects of the HGDP also believed that it could help indigenous people cope with modern challenges that came from population growth, famine, war, transportation, and communication (p. 490); however, no specifics were mentioned on how these goals would be accomplished. At first glance the objectives of the project seemed fairly straightforward—the scientists planned to locate isolated, indigenous groups from around the globe, collect samples, and then from those samples, construct a map of genetic variation. Given this orientation, it is not surprising that there was very little discussion of the social agency or cultural beliefs of those "subjects" who would provide the diverse genetic material that would be stored in various international data banks.

Shortly after Cavalli-Sforza and his co-authors began writing about these early planning stages, the HGDP came under intense national and international scrutiny. Both scientists and lay publics were divided when they were asked about the efficacy or need for a project that required the genomic study of "disappearing" "tribes." Part of the problem lay in the way the project was initially framed—the promoters often simply assumed that these diverse cultures either wanted these genomic projects or would understand the humanitarian side-benefits that might come from a massively funded study of diversity. At the same time, the HGDP project was being touted when many humanists and social scientists were having extensive debates about the social construction of "race," the lines that divided genetics from eugenics, and the promise and perils of privileging Western-oriented views of medicine. In the words of Swedland (1993), the project was "21st century technology applied to 19th century biology" (quoted in Reardon, 2005, p. 92). Greely (2001a)—a Stanford law professor who was familiar with many of Cavalli-Sforza's initiatives—touched on one facet of this complex palimpsest when he claimed that the hostile reception of the HGDP may have been tied to the schism that existed within the field of Anthropology. Greely (2001a) elaborated by explaining that while "Physical anthropology is aligned with the natural sciences" much "of cultural anthropology seems to have adopted a post-modern critique of science," and this in turn meant that many of the essentializing categories that informed HGDP research were coming under attack. Alliances were being formed that brought together some subaltern critics and cultural anthropologists, and this created a situation where "even talk about 'human populations'" was taken as a "sign of dangerous naiveté" (p. 224).

The beleaguered architects of the HGDP aligned themselves with some physical anthropologists who shared their basic assumptions about the physical or genetic nature of racial or ethnic differences, and the usage of some nonculturally oriented approaches meant that the HGDP could be viewed as a desirable, neutral, scientific, and reasonable program. These early advocates of the HGDP had a difficult time understanding just why the enterprise was characterized as modern form of neocolonialism. For example, advocates of the project had to hear or read about "biocolonialism" (Marks, 2003, p. 2) or "bioprospecting." Many health-care activists and interdisciplinary scholars commented on the potential links that sutured together historical "Western exploitative practices" with contemporary "production of diversity as a site of informational and commercial value" (Reardon, 2001, p. 367). Spivak (1999) echoes this concern, specifically in the commercialization of DNA. She stated that "DNA patenting is the dead end road of the native informant as 'new proletarian,' owning nothing but his/her body" (p. 388). In short, these early critiques complained about the exploitation of the "other," and the fact that very few promoters of the HGDP seemed to care about the co-production of knowledge, the need to take into account culturally sensitive ways of thinking about genomic science, and the potential existence of contradictory genetic paradigms. In many ways, the defenders of the HGDP simply assumed that this early criticism was simply a matter of a potential public relations crisis, one that could be fixed by more active publicity and the reduction of scientific "misunderstanding." For example, Whitt (2000) demonstrates how early criticisms were diverted by focusing on the "value free" rhetoric of pure science. In this way, early complaints were contained at the "level of application" (p. 422).

One distinctive feature of these early debates is the absence of indigenous voices. No representatives were involved in any of the early planning stages, and it was simply assumed that the scientists would be the primary or exclusive social agents who would be involved in the collection, storage, interpretation, funding, and dissemination of "diverse" genetic information. This mirrors the problems identified by Dutta-Bergman (2004) and Airhihenbuwa et al. (2000) in the application of traditional health communication models. In this instance, it appears that there was very little consideration—at least in the initial planning stages of the project—of the possibility that the spread of genomic information might require the active participation of the "other," the "subjects" who carried the "diverse" genomic materials. As long as researchers were operating from modernist frameworks that focused on the need for individuated consent or assumed the desirability of collecting information from "vanishing tribes," then they could not help but view indigenous criticism as inherently nonscientific. The idea of looking for some interplay between diverse social/scientific epistemes was lost on HGDP advocates who were worrying about timelines and the elite formation of ethical protocols. This problem, however, was soon addressed as various subalterns formed new alliances, engaged in debates about the desirability and feasibility of the project, and asked for the formation of more culturally sensitive scientific communities.

The subalterns: collective voices and critical social activism

In many ways, the types of modernist arguments that were used in the early defenses of the HGDP created a situation that facilitated the formation of alliances between communities that were worried about the culture insensitivity of the promoters. At the same time that Marks (2003) and other scholars were complaining about the racial or ethnic taxonomies that formed the basic underpinnings of the HGDP, other lay persons or indigenous leaders were taking the debate into cyberspace, and list serves and blogs were used as forums for harsh critiques of the alleged cultural insensitivity of HGDP defenders. When defenders of the project talked about some specific selection protocols that would be used in the targeting of key "vanishing" tribes, they galvanized critics and inadvertently helped with the creation of new collective alliances. Critics and indigenous communities came together against a common foe. For example, "The Declaration of Indigenous Peoples of the Western Hemisphere Regarding the Human Genome Diversity Project" lists seventeen different groups who oppose the project. These groups range from the Kuna Indians of Panama to the En'owkin in British Columbia (Indigenous Peoples of the Western Hemisphere, 1996).

Given the framing of these debates as public relations concerns, perhaps we should not be surprised to find that some of the supporters of the project began to debate those representatives of the subalterns, and that the voice of the "other" could no longer be ignored. Blending together scientific, legal, and cultural commentaries about the project, some of the leaders of these indigenous communities engaged in forms of health activism that they hoped would alter the trajectory or scope of the HGDP. For example, Liddle, director of the Central Australian Aboriginal Congress, stated that:

> If the Vampire Project goes ahead and patents are put on genetic material from Aboriginal people, this would be legalized theft. Over the last 200 years, non-Aboriginal people have taken our land, language, culture and health—even our children. Now they want to take the genetic material which makes us Aboriginal people as well.
>
> (quoted in Nason, 1994, p. 3)

This general concern, which was raised by numerous critics, received a response from the director of the HGDP as well as its legal council. Greely and Cavalli-Sforza (1993) posted this response on Native-L, an electronic bulletin board hosted by Native.Net:

> The proposed HGD Project is not and will not be a commercial venture. The chance that this research will lead to the development of commercially valuable products is very remote. Our current planning anticipates that this unlikely event is not impossible and so we are seeking to ensure that, should the cell-lines have commercial value, the benefits will flow back to the sampled populations.
>
> (Greely & Cavalli-Sforza, 1993, paragraph 7)

Note here that no credit is being given to the activists who were complaining about genetic exploitation—it is the scientists who are characterized as the enlightened elites who will gratuitously try to protect the "sample populations." Moreover, note the tone and framing of this particular argument—this electronic response is framed as an argument that is meant to clarify the "true" goals of the project, which in turn assumes that critics simply misunderstood the goals of the project. Note the absence of any detailed discussion of how or when these benefits will flow back to the sampled populations, and little discussion of how subaltern leaders might aid in the dispensation of genomic knowledge.

It is important to note that we are not suggesting that the framers of the HGDP engaged in completely productive dialogue, nor are we suggesting that the response was adequate. But we do find it encouraging that the location of the debates (Native-L) indicates that rather than ignoring the voices of the subaltern, the researchers were at least paying some attention to those who have traditionally been silenced. The question of course, is whether this provides subalterns with some substantive social agency—were these cultural critics ever viewed as informed decision makers who might shape the nature, scope, or trajectory of the HGDP?

Many of the indigenous critics of the project certainly viewed themselves as equals who were engaged in social reformist efforts. In our analysis, we found that there were three primary concerns that were voiced by the indigenous participants, each of which we have outlined below. These concerns, although appearing at some time or another on the internet, also appeared in other media outlets. Although at times, the researchers appeared to have ambivalent feelings about these requests, they tried to address many of these cultural, political, or social queries. Unfortunately, the use of elite frameworks constrained the ways that some of the defenders of the HGDP could write about this social activism. For example, in a recent article, Cavalli-Sforza (2005) refers to those who questioned the project as "naïve" (p. 333).

What we believe our analysis demonstrates is that the subaltern voices could not be silenced, and in the final analysis, we believe that researchers must be keenly aware of a more culture-centered approach to health communication activities, including research design and implementation (Airhihenbuwa et al., 2000; Dutta-Bergman, 2004).

A second lesson that we hope that this study demonstrates is that the concerns voiced by the participants resulted in policy changes (Greely, 2001a). In other words, whether the vocal defenders of the HGDP liked it or not, the subalterns had some agency in defining the contours of the debates that took place over the very existence of the project, the sampling methods that would be used in the collection of blood and tissue samples, and the framing of the project as a "diversity" endeavor. Lexicons that were once filled with labels such as "vanishing tribes" were replaced with essays that mentioned targeted "populations" (Cavalli-Sforza, 2005). Fewer essayists wrote about genetic "goldmines" or the hourly rate of blood collection. Many of these critics were able to fight against a system that positioned them as subjects, and although the fight is not over, we will demonstrate how the three concerns listed below eventually resulted in some genomic reforms.

Scientific curiosities

One early complaint about the HGDP focused in on the idea that the indigenous communities were being treated as scientific curiosities rather than as partners in the research process. This is certainly understandable in light of several off-handed comments made by Dr. Luca Cavalli-Sforza, who is quoted as saying "one person can bleed 50 people and get on the airplane in one day" (cited in Harry, 1995, paragraph 4). Cavalli-Sforza's comments appear to reinforce Spivak's (1999) concerns noted earlier, where the collection of DNA created a situation where subaltern "proletariat" bodies "are nothing more than" commodities, conveyers of genetic code (p. 388).

As noted earlier in this chapter, some indigenous communities were also bothered by genomic discourses that treated various tribal people as "endangered species." This allegedly created the impression that these groups were historical anomalies that had members who were doomed for extinction. Publics could get the impression that these isolated communities were superfluous or on cultural peripheries, losers in the social-Darwinian battle for cultural survival.

The World Council of Indigenous Peoples (WCIP) spoke out against these assumptions, describing the HGDP's goal as one that focused on the gathering of "DNA samples from the living before they disappear forever, and so avoid the irreversible loss of precious genetic information" (Settee, 2001, p. 2). Another activist noted that this "assumption that indigenous people are doomed adds insult to the indignity of being used as human guinea pigs" (Burrows, 2001, p. 244). With such strong accusations as these being voiced against the HGDP, the scientists must have realized that totally ignoring these critiques might mean that they were endangering the life of their project.

Clashing epistemes

As Airhihenbuwa and Obregon (2000) suggest, scientific ways of knowing are often in conflict with other cultural epistemes (pp. 11–12). In these situations, scientists are often unwilling to acknowledge these differences— perhaps because of worries that these "pseudosciences" might infect more pristine scientific investigations. In the HGDP debates, the subaltern voices refused to privilege dominant scientific ideas about the genetic formation of cultures, genetic migrations, or genetic tales of human "origins." These counter-narratives highlighted the importance of alternative social knowledges, and these critics circulated a host of cultural or historical stories that had other explanations for human diasporas or community markers. For example, some indigenous people argue that they "already possess strong beliefs and knowledge regarding their creation and histories" (Harry, 1995, paragraph 12). These "cosmologies of indigenous people are environmentally and culturally specific and are not congruent with popular Western theories" (Harry, 1995 paragraph 13).

Debra Harry, the director of the Indigenous Peoples Council on Bio-colonialism (IPCB), argued that the search for new explanations of origins and migrations of indigenous populations does not consider the "impact of the findings" on indigenous communities. For example, she wonders—"will theories of migration be used to challenge aboriginal territorial claims or rights to land?" (Harry, 1995, paragraph 14). Marks (2003) pointed out to HGDP proponents what they seemed to have overlooked is that tribes are "likely to have different ideas about blood, human bodies, and heredity" and that these views should be considered when approaching, educating, and performing informed consent processes for genomic research (Wallace, 1998, p. 60).

In each of these arguments, opponents of the HGDP were able to successfully battle what many considered to be the neocolonialist ideology of the HGDP, and in turn, garner support for their cause. One of the issues that we still are grappling with is whether the consciousness-raising that is taking place actually influences the co-production of genomic knowledge.

Patenting of DNA

The confusing messages concerning how the knowledge generated by the HGDP would actually benefit the indigenous communities left some opponents thinking that the "real agenda is the future development of pharmaceuticals that will generate huge corporate profits, long after indigenous peoples have been left to disappear" (Burrows, 2001, p. 245). The ethics and morality of the commodification, selling, patenting, and ownership of indigenous genetics became a key component of the most prominent, long-lasting, and developed critiques of the HGDP.

The perceptual problematics of the HGDP were not helped by the fact that sometimes nonHGDP activities could be linked to the troubled project. While defenders of the project constantly reiterated the point that they were not interested in the patenting of human life, the ideas surrounding the HGDP were entering into the public consciousness at the same time that the World Trade Organization (WTO) Trade-Related Intellectual Property Rights Agreement (TRIPS) was commenting on the need for regulating the eventual patenting of genetic materials. In 1993, some scientists applied for a patent based on the genes of a 26-year-old Guaymi Indian woman from Panama (WO 9208784) ("1996 Biopiracy update," 1996). On March 14, 1995, a patent was awarded (patent, U.S. 5, 397,696) based on the discovery of cell lines from the Hagahai tribe in Papua New Guinea. This was considered among opponents as the "first" patent on indigenous genes. These, and other nonHGDP patenting activities, were used by HGDP critics to argue that the real beneficiaries of this project would be financial interests. Although the HGDP scientists adamantly denied that there were any concerns over monetary gain, some critics continued to worry.

These problems will not go away, and the only way to really address them is through a dialogue in which there is a true collaboration between researchers and participants—a dialogue in which traditional, scientific discourse does not silence the voice of any shareholder. In the following section, we demonstrate how the concerns voiced by the critics of the HGDP were able to transform scientific practices and policies.

The subaltern: a voice for meaningful genomic change

Although the reforms that we will address in this section are not perfect or complete, we wish to demonstrate the power of activist voices in the arena of genomic health. We have focused our analysis on three main areas: the model ethical protocol; greater participation in future genetic endeavors; and more specific designation of material benefits to the participants.

The model ethical protocol and informed consent

One of the major shifts that came about, in our estimation, through the HGDP debates, was a re-articulation of the concept of informed consent, and further, group consent. In many of the early genomic debates, defenders of the HGDP hoped that they could satisfy some of their critics when they promoted the ideas that researchers needed to be active in their pursuit of "individual" consent forms. Simply improving the process of writing these forms, or ensuring that potential subjects understood and signed these forms, could therefore be characterized as a major legal or ethical improvement that would help protect the rights of subalterns. In theory, researchers must inform their subjects of the potential risks and benefits of any project. For the individual, the task of obtaining consent is fairly simple because the subject of the study and the person providing consent are one and the same; however, when one addresses the risks and benefits of genetic/population research, suddenly, the "subject" becomes much larger. Suppose, for example, that a scientist sampled a small group of individuals from a given population, only to find that this population had a genetic predisposition toward alcoholism. Suddenly, the potential risks to the larger population from which the samples were taken become an issue, perhaps even resulting in loss of jobs and health insurance. In this case, it seems to make more sense to obtain the consent of the entire population before engaging in research. To date, some Native American and indigenous groups "require" group consent (Greely, 2001b, p. 790).

Other interesting problems also arise as one considers the ramifications of this concept. Who, for example, is the appropriate individual who can theoretically provide single or group consent—a religious leader, a political leader, or some other spokesperson? And furthermore, how does one even define a population? In the words of Greely (2001b), Stanford professor and the legal council for the HGDP,

> Is the relevant group a particular village in the Navajo Nation (the proper term for the Navajo Reservation)? Is it the entire Navajo Nation? Is it all Southwestern Native Americans who speak languages related to Navajo, thus encompassing the Apache? Is it all Native Americans who speak a language in the NaDene language family, from inland Alaska to the Southwest? Or is the relevant group all Native Americans?
>
> (p. 791)

Note the complexity of Professor Greely's analysis. He appears to have adopted some mix of both modernist and post-modern thinking, as he grapples with the complexities of the social construction of genomic knowledge. While he does not go so far as to acknowledge the constructive nature of "samples" or "populations," he at least helps us see some of the political or cultural assumptions that inform the way that we think about "group" designations.

Our argument here is that whether the defenders of the HGDP like it or not, the social commentators who have critiqued the project have helped provide the types of culture-centered arguments that can be appropriated in polysemic and polyvalent ways. For example, the legal authors who have written "model" genomic protocols might view themselves as independent or modernist reformists who have clarified the goals of the HGDP, but the wording of this document clearly provide with clues of how critics have helped co-produce some of the legal framing of these debates. Note, for example, how this 1996 model ethic protocol seems to answer some early indigenous concerns: It states,

> The HGDP requires that researchers participating in the HGDP show that they have obtained the informed consent of the population, through its culturally appropriate authorities where such authorities exist, before they begin sampling. If, for example, the Navajo Nation decided that it would not participate in the HGDP, the HGDP would not accept samples taken from members of that population.
>
> (quoted in Greely, 2001b, p. 790)

Of course, as is probably apparent, there are no easy solutions, and the model ethical protocol does not negate any of these complex issues, but we are encouraged by the fact that the issue has become part of the debate. We would argue that the researchers are writing in more complex ways, and that they are at least trying to answer some of the concerns of the indigenous communities. Rather than the modernist assumptions that appear to have a certain "taken for granted-ness" that bracket out certain social or political concerns, the researchers are considering cultural aspects of the problem, even in the adopted legal protocols of this project.

Greater participation/inclusion

A second way that we have noted that the general climate surrounding genetic research is changing is the way that the participants have been positioned. As noted in previous sections, one of the concerns of the indigenous groups was that they were seen more as curiosities and objects of study rather than partners in the research process. Although it is difficult to demonstrate all of the ways this is changing, we have noted that in a recent genetic project, one that is a kind of offshoot of the HGDP, care has been taken to avoid some of the pitfalls that haunted the HGDP. National Geographic has recently unveiled the Genographic project, a project with many of the same goals as the HGDP.

In many ways the promoters of the Genographic project differentiate themselves as educators who have learned from the troubles of the HGDP, and they distance themselves from their more trouble-laden precursor. On the surface, this rhetorical move bypasses many of the early HGDP critiques, and stresses the importance of co-participation in these types of projects. The Genographic website states:

> Ours is a true collaboration between indigenous populations and scientists. Helping communicate their stories and promoting preservation of their languages and cultures is integral. Before any fieldwork begins, we have been and will continue to seek advice and counsel from leaders and members of indigenous communities about their voluntary participation in the project.
> (*National Geographic*, 2005, "FAQ Questions," paragraph 3)

Again, we want to stress that we are not claiming that the Genographic project is truly collaborative or that their efforts are completely altruistic. What we are noting, however, is that there is an increased sensitivity—one that may result in reform. Notice the change in language from the way the HGDP was framed. Now, instead of talking about subjects in a more paternal way, the Genographic project frames them as equal partners, even from the initial design stages. We see this as a direct result of the activist efforts of the individuals and groups who critiqued the HGDP.

Monetary benefits funneled back to participants

As mentioned above, the commercialization and patenting of DNA has been a primary concern among indigenous populations. As we have seen, there is enormous potential for financial rewards for those who patent this material, particularly for future medical uses. This is troubling to indigenous groups because, as has happened in the past, colonizers have been prone to take indigenous resources and leave the colonized with nothing in return.

As with issues of group consent, due to the issues raised by those opposed to the HGDP, scientists have begun to grapple with these issues. According to

Greely (2001b), the Chinese government now requires profit sharing for any exported DNA (p. 796), resulting in monetary compensation for research participants. Additionally, the Canavan Foundation has sued a hospital that holds a patent on certain genes because researchers patented the genetic marker for Canavan disease without informing the parents of children affected with the malady (Greely, 2001b, p. 796). Moreover, many researchers fear that as profit sharing becomes more common, the promise of wealth may be used to coerce participants to take part in studies.

It is our contention that the subaltern critiques of power and economic disparities have helped raise consciousness about the material conditions of the "other," the subjects of many of these studies. According to Greely (2001b), "The HGDP, both in North America and worldwide, committed itself to providing a fair share of any financial benefits to the participating populations" (p. 796). Again, whether the HGDP's promise becomes a reality, or whether this is simply a way to placate the activists, remains to be seen. However, if we look to the Genographic project as an indication of the future of genetic research, the rhetoric is promising. Perhaps it is possible that future decision makers may be constrained by their own rhetorics, rhetorics that were in part created from the shards of commentaries from detractors. As National Geographic has recently stated,

> In addition to answering questions of scientific interest to indigenous populations and the general public, we feel it is imperative to give something tangible back to the participating communities through Genographic's legacy project, which will include educational activities and cultural preservation projects. Proceeds from the sale of the participation kits will help fund the legacy project.
>
> (National Geographic, 2005, "FAQ," paragraph 4)

While skeptics might argue that this may simply provide readers with one more example of public relations management, we believe that the existence of these texts might provide future critics with the strategically essential tools that they will need in many post-colonial debates about neocolonial exploitation.

Conclusions

From the onset of this chapter, we attempted to show that there is a very real need to consider genomic health activism within the field of health communication. In this, we take up the call of Zoller (2005), who has invited us to rethink the ways that we study the formation of various health epistemes. In our analysis of the Human Genome Diversity Project, we have argued that the indigenous critiques of research methods and protocols did more than simply react to the claims of empowered scientists and other promoters of the project. They engaged in culture-centered critiques of the HGDP that provided constructive forms of social activism. A loose collective of indigenous groups and activists came together to address what many saw as the neocolonialist agenda of the HGDP. We believe that these disenfranchised groups were able to make a difference. They have been able to at least shape some genetic policies, as decision makers grappled with such issues as the implementation of the model ethical protocol or the future practices of genetic research, as witnessed in National Geographic's Genographic project. Interestingly enough, we are even now hearing debates over whether these activist groups have stalemated the HGDP, or drastically altered the packaging of related genomic projects. To date, noted Greely in 2001, "the HGDP has generated more debate than samples" (2001b, p. 787). While Greely might be interpreting this "debate" as some impediment that stands in the way of the inexorable collection of genetic material from "diverse" sources, we applaud the advent of indigenous critiques that refuse to take at face value the valorizing claims of researchers who treat the HGDP as an unalloyed scientific or public good. The alliances that have been created have helped facilitate some unique forms of health activism. The subaltern voice has been heard.

In sum, we hope that we have extended the work of communication scholars who have called for more integrated collaboration. As Dutta-Bergman (2004) suggests, it is critical that we follow a health communication model that is culture centered, not only in the dissemination of medical aid, but also in research design and implementation. If not, as has been illustrated in the HGDP, researchers face an uphill battle, one that is riddled with implicit or explicit neocolonial ideologies. We believe that true collaborations will allow us to address these important issues in more productive ways, and hopefully they will provide us with the informed choices that come from greater cultural sensitivity and understanding.

References

1996 Biopiracy update. (1996). Retrieved December 14, 2005 from www.etcgroup.org/article.asp?newsid=197.

Airhihenbuwa, C., Makinwa, B., & Obregon, R. (2000). Toward a new communications framework for HIV/AIDS. *Journal of Health Communication*, 5, 101–111.

Airhihenbuwa, C., & Obregon, R. (2000). A critical assessment of theories/models used in health communication for HIV/AIDS. *Journal of Health Communication*, 5, 5–15.

Bhabha, H. (1992). *Postcolnial Criticism*. In S. Greenblatt, & G. Gunn (eds), *Redrawing the Boundaries: the Transformation of English and American Literary Studies*. New York: Modern Language Association of America.

Burrows, B. (2001). Patents, ethics, and spin. In B. Tokar (ed.), *Redesigning Life? The Worldwide Challenge to Genetic Engineering*. Montreal: McGill-Queen's University Press.

Cavalli-Sforza, L., Wilson, A., Cantor, C., Cook, D., & King, M.C. (1991). Call for a worldwide survey of human genetic diversity: A vanishing opportunity for the Human Genome Project. *Genomics*, 11(Summer), 490–491.

Cavalli-Sforza, L.L. (2005). The Human Genome Diversity Project: past, present and future. *Nature*, 6(4), 333–340.

Dutta-Bergman, Mohan. (2004). The unheard voices of Santalis: Communicating about health from the margins of India. *Communication Theory*, 14(3), 237–263.

Greely, Henry T., & Luca Cavalli-Sforza. (1993). Human Genome Diversity Project—Organizers' Response. Retrieved December 8, 2005 from www.native-net.org/archive/nl/9307/0046.html.

Greely, H. (2001a). Human genome diversity: What about the other human genome project? *Nature*, 2, 222–227.

Greely, H. (2001b). Informed consent and other ethical issues in human population genetics. *Annual Review of Genetics*, 35(1), 785–800.

Guha, R. (1983). *Elementary Aspects of Peasant Insurgency in Colonial India*. Delhi: Oxford University Press.

Harry, D. (1995). The human genome diversity project and its implications for indigenous peoples. *Information about Intellectual Property Rights*, 6. Retrieved December 15, 2005 www.ipcb.org/publications/briefing_papers/files/hgdp.html.

Indigenous Peoples of the Western Hemisphere. (1996). Declaration of Indigenous Peoples of the Western Hemisphere Regarding the Human Genome Diversity Project. Retrieved October 15, 2005 from www.indians.org/welker/genome.htm.

Jackson, F. (1998). Scientific limitations and ethical ramifications of non-representative Human Genome Project: African American Response. *Science and Engineering News*, 4, 155–170.

Marks, J. (2003). Human Genome Diversity Project: Impact on indigenous communities. *Encyclopedia of the Human Genome*, 1–4. Retrieved December 8, 2005 from www.ehgonline.net.

Moore-Gilbert, B. (1997). *Postcolonial Theory: Contexts, Practices, Politics*. New York: Verso.

Nason, D. (1994). Tickner Warns over aboriginal Gene Sampling. *The Australian*, January 25, p. 3.

National Geographic. (2005). How to participate. Retrieved December 17, 2005 from www3.nationalgeographic.com/genographic.

Reardon, J. (2001). The Human Genome Diversity Project: A case study in coproduction. *Social Studies of Science*, 31, 357–388.

Reardon, J. (2005). *Race to the Finish: Identity and Governance in an Age of Genomics*. Princeton, New Jersey: Princeton University Press.

Said, E. (1978). *Orientalism*. New York: Pantheon Books.

Settee, Priscilla. (2001). The human genome project and the issue of biodiversity. Working Group on Women, Health, and the New Genetics. Retrieved December 14, 2005 from www.cwhn.ca/groups/biotech/availdocs/23-settee.pdf.

Spivak, G. (1988). Can the subaltern speak? In C. Nelson, & L. Grossberg (eds), *Marxism and the Interpretation of Culture*. Urbana: University of Illinoise Press.

Spivak, G. (1999). *A Critique of Postcolonial Reason*. Cambridge, MA: Harvard University Press.

Wallace, R.W. (1998). Perspectives. *Molecular Medicine Today*, 4, 59–62.

Whitt, L.A. (2000). Value-bifurcation in bioscience: The rhetoric of research justi-fication. *Perspectives on Science, 7*, 413–446.

Zoller, H. (2005). Health activism: Communication theory and action for social change. *Communication Theory, 15*(4), 341–364.

Part V

Afterword

Emerging agendas in health communication and the challenge of multiple perspectives

Heather M. Zoller and Mohan J. Dutta

The chapters in this book and the literature that they reference illustrate that the emergence of interpretive, critical, and cultural perspectives in health communication has broadened the theoretical, methodological, and pragmatic repertoire of the field. In this concluding discussion, we talk about how the scholarship on meaning, culture, structure and power advanced in this book contributes to health communication theory and practice. Taking stock of the work in this edited volume, we describe how we can expand on these through our future research agendas. Finally, given the growth of these "alternative" perspectives in health communication, we talk about how the field can maintain productive dialogue that builds health communication theorizing across different philosophical and methodological commitments.

Emerging contributions to the literature

In this section, we outline the theoretical contributions of interpretive, critical, and cultural studies in health communication. We follow with a discussion of methodological and pragmatic contributions of these lines of research.

Theoretical contributions

The chapters in this book are excellent examples of how meaning-centered research can contribute to health communication theorizing. Of course, what counts as a theoretical contribution is understood differently here than it would be by post-positivist theorists, who identify theory in terms of prediction, control, and generalizability. In our discussion of the implications of these chapters, we draw from Zoller and Kline (2008), who articulate the theoretical contributions of interpretive, cultural, and critical research to include in part: uncovering everyday, contextualized experiences of health and illness, facilitating a wider range of voices, and deconstructing biases in dominant approaches to health communication.

The use of interpretive methodologies allows for in-depth understanding of how people construct and interpret meanings associated with health and illness in everyday contexts. Interpretive perspectives should help us to understand relationships between discourse-in-use (text, daily talk and interaction) and larger social discourses (knowledge formations). Emily Cripe, for example, describes how women talk about their experiences of breastfeeding in a support group, and how this discourse both reflects and challenges larger social discourses of medicalization and motherhood. Deborah Lupton, who in many ways blazed the path for interpretive, critical, and cultural research, here connects mothers' talk about their children's health and their experiences as mothers to dominant gender constructions about motherhood and neoliberal conceptions of responsibility for health and illness. Many interpretive methodologies show us *how* meaning and social interaction are accomplished in daily life. For example, Harter et al. demonstrate how health-care workers actively respond to the limited material circumstances of the mobile health clinic.

The chapter by Cecilia Bosticco and Teresa Thompson demonstrates how grounded, contextualized research builds theory inductively, in this case, through the systematic development of the narrative perspective (a grounded concept *and* a theoretical lens). Comprehensive reviews that draw out commonalities and differences across individual studies of narrative are crucial in linking localized research to communication theory.

Chapters in the book illustrate how both interpretive and critical–cultural perspectives can deconstruct biases in dominant approaches to health communication. For example, several contributors critique the dominance of the medical paradigm. Geist-Martin, Sharf, and Jeha's study shows us the elements of communication that are missing from standard biomedical interactions by investigating alternative models that address connections among the mind, body, environment, and soul. Notably, they attend to tactile bodily practices and other nonverbal messages. They also describe the structural and economic barriers to holistic care within the dominant biomedical system. Murphy et. al and Ellingson elucidate how physician authority, so often taken for granted as an inevitable part of medical interaction, can become a communication problem as it interferes with health-care workers' ability to address patients' needs and experiences. Uncovering these biases lays the groundwork for the alternative models that the authors suggest.

Several chapters also broaden the range of critique by illustrating the biases of social policies and exploring the ideologies of these policies. For instance, Srinivas R. Melkote, Pradeep Krishnatray, and Sangeeta Krishnatray deconstruct the biases of neoliberal development discourse for individual responsibility, technological top-down solutions, and debt-repayment versus capacity building. They link these biases to the linear transmission model of communication that is intertwined with neoliberal approaches, focusing on individual lifestyles and drawing attention away from the need to address structural inequities in health care. Importantly, they contrast this with a resistance and empowerment model of development that uses participatory communication approaches and aims for increased access to material and cultural resources for citizens. Thus, they situate the communication of individual health campaigns within broader political policies and overarching worldviews. Zoller and Desouza et al. deconstruct dominant ideas about what counts as health policy by investigating the multisectoral effects of neo-liberalism, and exploring the discursive constitutions of neoliberal discourse. They provide multiple ways of theorizing about the role of communication in policy construction, and they help us to begin expanding what counts as health promotion from a focus on behavior-change and education models to political advocacy and intervention. This kind of critique promotes reflexivity as it asks us to examine how the field's work reinforces or challenges neoliberal approaches, and offers opportunities for transformative politics.

Interpretive, critical, and cultural perspectives facilitate the inclusion of a wider array of voices in the discipline because of their explicit concern with addressing the marginalized. Villagran, Collins, and Garcia engage with the voices of Hispanic women (and men) living in the Colonias along the Texas–Mexico border, elucidating how their health beliefs and needs are influenced by their culture, the local context, and the experience of poverty. This sheds light on Hispanic populations, which have been underrepresented in U.S. research, and also the complexity of health experiences in border areas. Dutta and Basnyat's chapter about the Radio Communication Project in Nepal shows us what it means to theorize and form interventions around the needs and cultural beliefs of the people with whom we study. They contrast this with interventions that treat audiences as the targets of elite messages. As they describe, unless it is possible for focus group members to truly challenge the goals, methods, and substance of the campaign, the use of focus groups to target campaign messages is not adequate to create a culture-centered approach. They further question the co-optive nature of participatory processes when they are made to look participatory in order to serve the agendas of dominant social actors. Each chapter in the culturally based health promotion section shows us that health promotion cannot be achieved without complex understanding of cultural, economic, and political contexts from the perspective of marginalized groups themselves. Additionally, research into motherhood, breastfeeding, and even cancer experiences allows us to hear, in women's own words, how health discourse is always a gendered discourse—reflecting, reinforcing, and sometimes resisting dominant assumptions about gender and sex roles.

Methodological contributions

The chapters presented in this book take us beyond the limited array of methods available to us in the dominant framework of health communication that are primarily quantitative in nature. These methods draw our attention to the ways in which health communication scholars might engage in meaning making with individuals, groups, and communities, and suggest alternative criteria for measuring and evaluating health communication scholarship. The chapters demonstrate the ways in which health meanings might be gathered, interpreted, and represented through scholarship. The emphasis on health meanings moves us beyond the typically accepted criteria such as reliability and validity that have large-scale acknowledgment in the established body of health communication work. Instead, they suggest new ways for approaching the study of health communication, with an emphasis on the deconstruction and co-construction of health meanings, and on relationships between local contexts and broader social structures.

The rhetorical methods used in this chapter use theory and textual analysis to understand the strategic use of language to achieve social goals in, among other discourses, pharmaceutical sales, health policies, and scientific discourse. This emphasis on the situated language of persuasion is one of the unique contributions made by our field. Rhetorical perspectives promote a deconstructive turn in health communication by demonstrating the need to continually interrogate the taken-for-granted assumptions about what it means to be healthy, about what constitutes health, and about who gets to define health issues. Reflexivity is one of the key elements of deconstruction.

It is through this deconstructive emphasis that we learn to continually interrogate our own privilege as health communicators and the politics of knowledge within which health communication efforts get situated. Knowledge production is political, and communicators play a vital role in establishing, recirculating and erasing discourses around policies, and this political vitality of communication is particularly evident in the realm of health. This intersection of communication, knowledge, and politics is articulated by the Zoller and Desouza et al. chapters as they interrogate neoliberal discourses and the dominant hegemonic structures served by these discourses. Similarly, Dutta and Basnyat deconstruct the participatory rhetoric of a health communication program, foregrounding the hegemonic possibilities of participatory platforms as they get co-opted within the dominant structures of health.

The use of a greater array of methodologies such as in-depth interviews and ethnographies is an emerging trend in health communication. Interviews provide in-depth insight into how health discourses are interpreted, such as mothers' sense of their responsibility for children's health and breastfeeding. Ethnographic research helps us to understand issues of culture and meaning by focusing on everyday communication-in-use in emergency rooms, clinics, and community organizations. Ethnographic works in this volume are reflexive, as they clearly articulate the relationship between the authors and research participants, and the lenses adopted to interpret their findings. At the same time, chapters in the book illustrate how these methods, though necessarily localized, contribute to health communication theory as they move beyond simplistic thematic analysis to address linkages between local instantiations of meaning and larger cultural practices. Both Murphy et al. and Ellingson use ethnographic investigations to begin formulating new communication models, and to build relationships with caregivers that allow them to implement such changes.

Similarly, ethnographic approaches to culture-centered health promotion such as Auger et al. show that interpretive research not only informs the development of alternative models of health promotion, but also constitutes a significant component of culture-centered interventions. Participatory methodologies emerge in this book as one of the key trends in health communication methodology. Chapters discuss the creation and evaluation of participatory health promotion, as well as barriers and limits to participation in health communication processes. For instance, Melinda Villagran, Dorothy Collins, and Sara Garcia participate in co-constructive meaning making with Latina community members as these participants explore interpretations of health and illness around cancer. Similarly, Camacho, Yep, Gomez and Velez invoke the principles of participation to present the concepts of critical health communication praxis, "third-order" research, and collaborative community dialogue to describe the communicative strategies utilized by Proyecto ContraSIDA Por Vida (PCPV) that was created, implemented, and evaluated in Latino communities in San Francisco, California. By highlighting controversial models of health promotion such as harm reduction, participatory research demonstrates the limits of empiricism for engaging the political landscape.

Practical contributions

Clearly then, chapters in this volume are connected to health communication practice, from those that are explicitly dedicated to engaging with and empowering research participants, to those whose analysis provides the basis for the revision of existing communication interventions and the construction of alternate models of practice. Zoller and Kline (2008) describe applied contributions of "alternate" research in terms of altering definitions of effectiveness, developing context-sensitive models of health communication, and highlighting the potential for resistance and social change. Indeed, the works presented here continually question the very basis of terms such as effectiveness and competence that are standard terminologies in health communication scholarship. In doing so, they rupture approaches to praxis that take for granted the assumptions and values underlying issues of health. The chapters illustrate that health praxis must acknowledge the contestation and negotiation of meaning that may not be captured well when aiming for standardization and replication.

This book highlights the growth of alternative models of health promotion. The culture-centered approach articulated by Dutta and Airhihenbuwa alters the definition of effective health promotion from the achievement of elite goals to the empowerment of local people to improve their material and cultural circumstances through the interrogation of the structures within which health meanings are constituted. In this sense, the culture-centered approach shares much in common with participatory and empowerment models of health promotion as described by Auger and DeCoster, and Camacho et al. Running through these different models is an emphasis on community participation as an entry point for communicating about issues of health. Melkote et al. describe an empowerment model of development that uses participatory communication approaches and aims for increased access to material and cultural resources for citizens. The participatory strategies of care they describe significantly alter standard treatment by health workers, and encourage the reduction of stigma by building personal knowledge with those who are ill.

McDermott, Oetzel, and White contribute to practice by adding complexity to our understanding of alternative models of health promotion, and cautioning against romanticizing empowerment and participatory models. They note that such projects often fail because leaders underestimate the complexity and commitment involved in collaboration. The chapter describes how we as researchers can deal with tensions between models of partnership promoted in participatory research and the realities of differential access to knowledge and resources. By applying their theoretical discussion to their own research, the chapter provides guidance for actively managing these tensions.

By tying theory to lived experience and studying the agency of nondominant groups, interpretive, critical, and cultural research helps to uncover the potential for resistance and social change, particularly at the margins of society (Zoller & Kline, 2008). Critical and cultural research should not treat power and hegemony as monolithic, but rather as a complicated, negotiated relationship (Gramsci, 1971; Mumby, 1997). Ellingson shows us subtle forms of resistance among technicians, who both reinforce and challenge physician authority in their daily work. Similarly, we see somewhat hidden forms of everyday resistance to medicalization among breastfeeding women that might go unnoticed in survey research. Also, we certainly can understand the discourse of the alternative healers studied by Geist-Martin, Sharf, and Jeha as a form of resistance to the dominant medical paradigm.

Comacho et al.'s study describes a more overt form of contestation as Proyecto ContraSIDA Por Vida actively resists dominant prevention communication models and prevailing scripts about sexuality and culture. Wood et al.'s chapter about the development of social justice movements aimed at participating in and altering debates about genetic research is an excellent example of how culture-centered analysis highlights the potential for activism. This study builds understanding of relationships between the rhetoric of science and the rhetoric of social movements. The research highlights not only the barriers to participation, but the potential material and discursive resources for resistance that can be crafted and exploited by health activists and advocates.

Theoretically, Chapters 17 and 18 describe the potential for broadening our conception of health activism to the array of forces aligned against neoliberal economics and development associated with globalization. Significantly, Conrad and Jodlowski articulate the imbalances involved in policy making, cautioning against romanticizing resistance, but also note the possibilities of "outflanking" as a means of resisting elite control of health-policy processes.

Emerging issues

We have highlighted the volume's contributions to theory, methods, and practice. The authors in this volume also set the groundwork for additional theorizing about an array of important emerging social concerns. Some of the chapters address contemporary, unfolding social issues that require attention because of their social influence, and because of their potential to refigure existing health communication theory. These topics include participatory health-promotion models, cultural representations, economic and cultural globalization, the influence of business and marketing on health knowledge, communication technology, biotechnology including genetic research and practice, food politics, complementary healing systems, and more. By attending to these issues, the chapters suggest the relevance of re-thinking what we fundamentally come to understand as health and what would fall under the purview of health communication.

For instance, the emphasis on complementary healing systems helps to depose the unquestioned dominance of the biomedical model that is often taken for granted in mainstream health communication scholarship. As scholars and practitioners of health communication, we are not located outside the value systems that imbue our theorizing and methodologies, but rather are situated within those very value systems that guide us and direct/constrain the questions we ask.

Research in this volume demonstrates emerging interest in addressing the role of business and global economic policies as a part of health communication studies. Communicating about health is almost always an economic issue, and the chapters presented in this book draw our attention to the role of commerce in health communication processes. This work theorizes about the role of social structures, looking beyond the mandate of changing individual lifestyles that is often dictated to us by policy makers and funding agencies. So for example, we have to question the framing of cancer prevention in terms of promoting five servings of fruits and vegetables per day from an economic perspective. Such a simplistic promotion fails to consider class and racially based inequalities in access to affordable fruits and vegetables. Such a promotion also highlights individual lifestyles and ignores industrial sources of cancer in capitalist societies such as environmental pollution and toxic exposures in the workplace. In this book, Dutta and Basnyat demonstrate the ways in which seemingly innocuous entertainment education programming serves dominant economic interests of globalization. The chapter by Stokes links business and health communication technologies, investigating how business interests influence the construction of knowledge about health and illness in new communication platforms.

Health communication is not only situated within the realm of economics, but is also an inherently political process. For too long, few researchers have acknowledged, let alone investigated, the political nature of health communication. Yet the politics of health guide the formation of health agendas, including the definition of health problems and solutions, as well as the absence of issues and interests from those agendas, from interpersonal and organizational settings to local, state, national and global health care and governmental systems. For instance, the omission of the question of food security from much of the talk of health communication completely draws attention away from the pressing issues of hunger and malnutrition in certain sectors of the globe. Similarly, the "otherizing" of cultures in dominant health discourses serves a certain political economic configuration in maintaining the hegemonic structures of dominant global health systems, and furthering neocolonial agendas. Taken together, the chapters in this book represent the emerging importance of addressing connections between micro and macro-level politics. For example, the medical communication section links the micro-practices of power in emergency rooms and clinics with larger issues of power and control in the medical industry. We see the importance of understanding politics at the level of everyday experience, such as managing children's health, as well as at the legislative level, such as pharmaceutical reimportation debates.

Some of the topics in the book represent "new" social issues such as the use of the internet, genetic research, the use of medical technicians, and the rise of alternative healing. Others, such as globalization, harm reduction campaigns, and power and authority in medicine, are subjects that are not necessarily "new," but have received little attention from health communication scholars. We see rising interest in culture-centered health promotion models, when of course the need to address culture is certainly not new. So, the erasure of these issues in dominant health communication scholarship enunciates the power structures within which health communication scholarship is constituted and practiced. That the study of health communication is itself situated within structures of knowledge is a vital point that is reiterated throughout the chapters. Next, we turn to discuss these structures as we suggest some research agendas that emerge from this volume.

Emerging agendas

By highlighting the growth of interpretive, critical, and cultural research, we hope this book spurs additional development of these perspectives in the field. Lingering perceptions of health communication as a post-positivist domain may be discouraging some scholars from participating in the field despite the centrality of health and communication to their work. Contributions in this volume provide evidence of a significant core of meaning-centered research in the field. Of course, there is still a long way to go in establishing a body of interpretive, critical, and cultural theory and praxis. The chapters in the book help to set potential research agendas for health communication in terms of both the directions of research that they represent, and the perspectives and topics that are not included in this particular collection.

First, and this is probably true of the larger field of communication, we see more growth in interpretive research than we do of explicitly critical or critical–cultural perspectives. We would like to see the development of a significant body of critical research that addresses issues of power, culture, and meaning in health communication. Many of the authors in this volume draw from Foucauldian theories of power. Foucault's theories of discourse, discipline, surveillance, and governmentality are key concepts that deserve more attention. We are glad to see development of theorists such as de Certeau, Said, and Spivak as well. Additionally, there are a range of critical theorists whose work would expand health communication theorizing, such as Karl Marx, Antonio Gramsci, and Jurgen Habermas. There is a need for a broad range of feminist theorizing as well, both critical and postmodern theorizing such as Susan Bordo and Donna Haraway. Also, critical theorists in the domain of health, illness, and medicine such as Ivan Illich, Howard Stein, Susan Sontag, Paula Treichler, Vandana Shiva, and Ashis Nandy have developed theories of power, language, culture, and structure that can inform health communication scholarship. Works of postcolonial scholars such as Chandra Mohanty can guide health communication scholarship toward understanding the politics of colonialism, neocolonialism and modernity within which knowledge formations are articulated and points of praxis are envisioned. Furthermore, works of subaltern studies scholars such as John Beverly, Ranajit Guha, and Gyan Prakash can guide us toward questions of erasures and epistemic violence as narratives of knowledge about health are written over, above and on the bodies of subalternized spaces and subject positions. It is through the interrogation of these epistemic structures that possibilities are suggested for emancipatory politics that invite dialogue with subaltern voices.

We mentioned that this book brings attention to relationships between health and economics. This volume investigates pharmaceutical sales and policy as well as neoliberal development models. It also highlights problems associated with health care access in the United States. Future critically oriented research, whether from a critical–interpretive, cultural studies, or materialist perspective, can add to this literature on the business of health care and the influence of economic systems on public health. Our field is uniquely situated to understand relationships among economics, structures, and the communicative construction of knowledge, and to investigate their implications for exacerbating or reducing health inequalities. In the United States, there is a need to understand the continuing evolution of capitation (HMO-style) systems and their influence on access and care, along with debates about pharmaceutical marketing and pricing. Globally, we are witnessing the growing dominance of market-based models for both medical care and public health services (and resistance to that dominance). Economic systems both influence and are influenced by particular conceptions of relationships among citizens. We believe that the fundamentally social nature of health provides a foundation for the critique of economic theories that treat health as an individual commodity. Communication research can address these relationships at the levels of public discourse and personal experience, drawing together research in organizational communication, public relations, issue management, and other areas.

We pointed out above that interpretive, cultural, and critical approaches in this volume bring more voices into communication research. Clearly, there is more to do in this area, as we work toward a systematic understanding of the dynamic role of culture (along with structures and individual influences) in the experience of health communication. We were pleased to include work in this volume that addresses health and sexuality. Moving forward there is significant need for more work to address the health issues of gay, lesbian, and transgendered people beyond the study of HIV/AIDS. Likewise, we need more research focused on the concerns of ethnic minorities in the United States, including African Americans, Hispanics, Asians, and many other groups. Dominant assumptions about race, sexuality, gender, and class influence the experience of health communication in unique ways depending upon how we are situated within these dominant frameworks (and within discourses among marginalized groups themselves). Research in multiple countries, particularly those of the global south, would help to dampen the assumption that Western models can, with just a little tweaking for local culture, be applied almost universally.

This volume highlights the growth of context-sensitive models for health promotion and medical communication. We would like to see the continued development of these culturally based models of intervention in order to develop a systematic understanding of their impact. If efficacy is to be understood in much broader terms, we need to examine not only a broad array of health outcomes, but also outcomes related to voice. How we can create genuinely open systems of participation in intervention goals and methods? How can interventions promote the capacity for social participation among those with whom we study? We need to address the complexity of empowerment while avoiding its co-optation. Longitudinal studies, case studies, ethnographies, and quantitative methodologies are all needed to achieve these goals. Furthermore, taking the culture-centered approach seriously requires continuing reflexivity about the politics of health interventions, the challenges of dialogue, and the complexities of ethical communication. It calls for sustained reflexivity of the scholar as she/he participates in journeys of solidarity with communities that have traditionally been rendered voiceless through the impetus on creating interventions and imposing such interventions on them. It requires scholars to question the privilege that allows us as health communicators to "intervene," "study," "design," and "evaluate." Interrogating this privilege offers an opening for discursive and material shifts in the unequal social structures within which health agendas are situated.

Emerging meaning-centered, health communication research can contribute to health communication theorizing by investigating the possibilities of increased agency and social change, particularly among marginalized groups themselves. For instance, works in this volume illuminate processes of decision making within systems of medical authority. More micro-level studies of resistance among medical staff can add insight into how these systems are experienced and contested. Macro-level research can address the development of alternatives to the biomedical model, including insider strategies of altering the institutional assumptions and education of biomedical actors, as well as outsider strategies of building legitimacy for alternative models. Future research can work toward greater understanding of the complexities of health and resistance in multiple contexts. These complexities arise from acknowledgment that, for instance, the potential implications of resistance to the voices that tell us how to live may include greater autonomy and the potential for change, but also may reinforce existing forms of power. Resistance to dominant health messages may actually promote better health (such as refusing an unnecessary cesarean section), or may damage health (such as refusing to stop smoking).

More broadly, at the level of political and social structures, we can give greater attention to community empowerment, grassroots activism, and advocacy (Sharf, 1997). We would very much like to see research address the role of communication in facilitating and impeding the growth of an overarching public health social movement to address health inequities. There is also need to attend to multisectoral linkages with other social movements including environmentalists and global justice activists.

In sum, the potential for theoretical and practical contributions from interpretive, cultural, and critical researchers is exciting. We hope that the emergence of these perspectives and the development of coherent lines of research make the task less daunting than it may have seemed only a decade ago. In the next section, we highlight some of the challenges that arise with the growth in perspectives in health communication.

Diversity and the discipline

Like the larger field of communication, the growth of the "alternative paradigm" in health communication has moved to a point where "Worldview II" approaches are no longer alternative but have become more mainstream. The field is now characterized by a greater diversity of philosophical and theoretical perspectives, methodologies, topics of study, and even geographies. This research is also highly interdisciplinary. We strongly believe that this pluralism is a strength rather than a weakness in the discipline. However, in order to capitalize on that strength, we need to understand how to work together across these differences. We need to work on the ways that we *value*, and *evaluate*, different forms of research. We need to create and continue productive conversations that build on one another's research to develop systematic theories, critiques, and practical interventions. Moreover, we need to continually attend to our language and discursive practices such that we are speaking with each other rather than talking past each other.

These emerging conversations must be built on understanding of and respect toward multiple paradigms (which does not rule out serious debate, criticism, and conflict, by the way). In the introduction, we described how different theoretical and methodological orientations may be understood in some ways as complementary and in others as conflicting. The important comparisons are not between "qualitative" and "quantitative," because any study might use one or both methodologies, but between the theoretical commitments of the researcher to more grounded, local knowledge aimed at insight and/or social change versus hypothesis-oriented work aimed at generalization (Zoller & Kline, 2008). We can value both approaches. Doing so, however, does not mean that one can accept interpretive research but treat it as merely a hypothesis generator (pre-scientific) that cannot build theory. Zoller and Kline note that we can just as easily treat post-positivistic research as pre-interpretive (research question generators). Thus, mutual respect involves understanding the goals and purposes of meaning-centered versus predictive research. Of course, for some people, pluralism involves a great deal of change because taking such an approach means that 1) "science" cannot be treated as the only valid way of knowing and 2) the values inherent in and hidden by the scientific process must be addressed. At the same time, those on the "other side of the fence" cannot dismiss out of hand post-positivist research aimed at understanding cause–effect relationships either. Many of the issues and agendas identified in this project would do well to be complemented with post-positivistic research in order to influence health-care policies. More than simply tolerating each other, perhaps there is a necessity for the various paradigms of health communication scholarship to come together with the goal of influencing practice, particularly in the context of the projects of social change that seek to transform unhealthy structures.

Emerging conversations in the field also must address differences among scholars in their commitments toward social change (particularly between 'interpretive' versus 'critical' perspectives). Productive conversations can be had about building reflexivity in our research to understand how our values and social positions influence the questions we ask, what counts as data, and how that data are interpreted. We can talk about how health communication scholars can become more engaged with those they study in a number of different capacities. These conversations become much less productive when they devolve into arguments about whether scholars who orient toward a consensus understanding of society or those who focus on conflict are more "right," more "scholarly" more "unbiased," or even more "moral." Debates often center around the explicit value-orientation of critical research, with some interpretive scholars arguing that ideological approaches are biased to the researcher's values and unnecessarily critical, and some critical scholars arguing that descriptive approaches are simply not reflexive about their values orientation and relationship to systems of power. The chapters in this book are good examples of how conflict- and consensus-based work can act in complementary ways to build local knowledge and to situate that knowledge within broader contexts, in the face of tensions among their approaches.

Theoretical and methodological pluralism, then, involves working in and across tensions across "paradigms" and within them. Building a measure of coherence is necessary to develop common understandings, build larger explanations, and guide practice. This coherence does not need to come from similar methodologies or even worldviews. Instead, it can develop around systematic attention to continued dialogue about common issues, questions, and concerns. Therefore, there is a need for new research that speaks within and across paradigms, continually engaging in the dialogic journey that celebrates the creative potential of health communication scholarship and practice. It is only perhaps through such dialogue that new spaces and ways of imagining health care might be envisioned, realized, and celebrated.

In closing

We envisioned this book as a discursive space for articulating new work in health communication, particularly paying attention to the need to attend to scholarship in the discipline that has otherwise been omitted and/or backgrounded. In some ways, although we did begin with an intuitive sense of where we might be headed, we really did not have an understanding of the scope of the new and interesting work that was being done by health communicators across the United States, theoretically, empirically, and in practice. We received a large number of submissions in response to our call for chapters, and had to narrow down the number of contributions in order to make sure that we had enough space for the predominantly theoretical and qualitative manuscripts we received. What we learned through this process is that scholars in a variety of health-related contexts are starting to question the taken-for-granted assumptions in traditional health communication scholarship, and articulate new ways to approach and understand health communication processes and phenomena.

The chapters presented in this book draw our attention to the process-based nature of health communication. In other words, they suggest that communicating about health ought to be understood as a process beyond the emphasis on messages in traditional health communication scholarship. Although designing and delivering effective messages is indeed important, these chapters suggest the relevance of understanding meanings and the ways in which meanings of health come to be discursively constituted. An emphasis on meanings situates health communication in the realm of social structures, cultural contexts and relational spaces within which health is negotiated. Building on the contributions presented here, we envision new and exciting work in the discipline that attends to the communicative processes within which health is constituted.

Also, there is a consistent articulation of the sociostructural nature of health communication, suggesting the importance of looking at unhealthy structures rather than simply studying individual-level health choices. Although individual choices are important, these choices need to be understood in the context of the social structures that both constrain and enable possibilities of health (Dutta, 2007). We welcome the move toward health communication scholarship that underscores the roles of health policies in the realm of health outcomes, and creates openings for new work that looks at the discursive processes and spaces through which unhealthy local, state, national and global policies are challenged and transformed.

We also are excited about the increasing emphasis on culture, and the impetus to look at the cultural contexts of health. That these contexts are dynamic, contested, and continuously negotiated draws our attention to the transformative and regenerative capacities of culture in the realm of health care. The lens of culture on one hand creates an entry point for challenging the dominant West-centric approaches in health communication; on the other hand, they offer opportunities for imagining other ways of approaching health, disease, and illness. The question of culture also brings us face-to-face with the modernist politics of health and the ways in which this modernist politics does violence to alternative ways of knowing. And ultimately, it creates discursive openings for listening to those voices that have otherwise been silenced in mainstream discourses of health communication.

The chapters offer new insights regarding the storied nature of health communication. Health is communicated and narrated through stories; therefore, stories are essential and central to communicating about health (Harter et al., 2005). Attending to these stories not only offers frameworks for interpreting how health is constituted, but also takes us beyond the realm of the biomedical to the realms of the human dimensions of health and healing. That stories can heal and that they can offer new ways of imagining the interstices of the mind, body, and spirit ruptures our ontological and epistemological foundations and creates new openings.

We close this epilogue with the hope that the presence of diverse voices here serves as hope and encouragement for health communication scholars to open up creative possibilities in health communication, to imagine new ways of understanding health, and to explore new avenues for observing health communication phenomena. We also hope that this work creates an opening for questioning the methods that we traditionally apply, and for creatively envisioning other ways in which we can come to know about health communication processes and practices. We note that the voices presented here are predominantly United States-based, although we have made an attempt to present different voices from multiple contexts within the United States. We hope that this spurs dialogue with researchers working globally, across a variety of social and cultural contexts, especially in those contexts that have otherwise been silenced and marginalized. Ultimately, we hope that this edited book serves as a point of encouragement for those scholars who want to continually question the practices we engage in so better possibilities might be imagined!

References

Dutta, M.J. (2007). Communicating about culture and health: Theorizing culture-centered and cultural sensitivity approaches. *Communication Theory, 17,* 304–328.

Gramsci, A. (1971). *Selections from the Prison Notebooks* (Q. Hoare, & G.N. Smith, trans.). New York: International Publishers.

Harter, L.M., Japp, P.M., & Beck, C. (2005). *Narratives, Health, and Healing.* Mahwah, NJ: Lawrence Erlbaum Associates.

Mumby, D.K. (1997). The problem of hegemony: Rereading Gramsci for organizational communication studies. *Western Journal of Communication, 61,* 343–375.

Sharf, B.F. (1997). Communicating breast cancer on-line: support and empowerment on the Internet. *Women & Health, 26*(1), 65–84.

Zoller, H.M., & Kline, K.N. (2008). Theoretical contributions of interpretive and critical research in health communication. *Communication Yearbook, 32.*

Contributors

Susan J. Auger (MSW, University of North Carolina at Chapel Hill, 1997) is president and founder of Auger Communications, Inc., an organizational and educational consulting firm. She has consulted on health-related research projects funded by CDC, CSAP, NIAAA, RWJ Foundation, and WHO. Her interests include cultural competency, health literacy, empowerment education, behavior change, minority health, and innovation diffusion.

Iccha Basnyat is a PhD candidate in health communication at Purdue University. Her research interests are in the areas of health communication campaigns, international health, cultural issues in health communication, and reproductive health. Currently, she is working on women's reproductive health in Nepal.

Ambar Basu is a doctoral candidate and graduate lecturer in the Department of Communication at Purdue University. He received his BA, and MSc from Calcutta University in 1995 then worked as a journalist with leading newspapers in India, covering health beats. His research on culture-centered approaches to health communication has been published in journals such as *Health Communication and Qualitative Health Research*.

Cecilia Bosticco (MA University of Dayton) is a mother and community volunteer who came to study communication at midlife. Her research interest in communication and bereavement flows from her personal experience of the death of her youngest daughter. She has published in journals including *Omega* and *Journal of Family Communication* among other publications.

Heather J. Carmack (MA, Ohio University) is a doctoral student in the School of Communication Studies at Ohio University who anticipates completing her degree in 2008. Her research in health communication focuses on medical mistakes, apologia, issues of patient safety, health law, and death and dying.

Melida D. Colindres (MPH, University of North Carolina at Chapel Hill, 1987), president and founder of INTER-AM English & Spanish Communications, provides consultation services regarding Latino health issues and translates and adapts medical and health-related programs and materials. She is actively involved in community outreach and health education programs related to chronic diseases, nutrition, and physical activity.

Dorothy Collins is a PhD student in the Department of Communication Studies at Texas A&M University. Her areas of research focus on the interplay of risk, health, and organizational communication.

Charles Conrad is professor of communication and honors scholar/teacher at Texas A&M University. He teaches classes in organizational communication; organizational rhetoric; discourse and healthcare policy; and communication, power, and politics. His research focuses on the symbolic processes through which organizations influence popular attitudes and public policies. His research has been published in *Communication Monographs*, *The Journal of Applied Communication Research*, *The Quarterly Journal of Speech*, *Critical Studies in Media Communication*, and others. He is a past editor of *Management Communication Quarterly*.

Emily T. Cripe is a doctoral student in the Hugh Downs School of Human Communication at Arizona State University. She currently serves as the editorial assistant for the *Western Journal of Communication*. Her research interests in health communication include narrative ethnography, the intersections between organizational communication and health, particularly related to work-life issues, and feminist approaches to health issues. Emily anticipates completing her degree in 2009.

Karen Deardorff is a doctoral student in the School of Communication Studies at Ohio University. She is the assistant director of the Cutler Scholars Program. Karen anticipates completing her PhD in 2008. Her research interests include health communication (particularly women's health), narrative ethnography, counter-narratives, and feminist rhetorical theory.

Mary E. DeCoster (MPH, University of North Carolina at Chapel Hill, 2002) is the program manager for communicable disease & infant mortality prevention in the Division of Health Education at the Durham County Health Department, in North Carolina. She is an International Board Certified Lactation Consultant (IBCLC) and trained childbirth educator. She has managed child survival projects in Latin America, and has trained lay health educators, peer educators, and community health workers. Her interests include empowerment education, minority health, and elimination of health disparities.

Rebecca Desouza is an assistant professor at the University of Minnesota, Duluth. She received her MA and PhD from Purdue University. Rebecca's research interests include HIV/AIDS campaigns, nongovernmental organizations and communication strategies, culture-centered approaches, and media coverage of global health. She is the winner of the 2006 Billsland Dissertation Fellowship and has published her work in outlets such as *Health Communication* and *Journal of Health Communication*.

Mohan J. Dutta is associate professor of health communication, public relations and mass media and director of graduate studies in the Department of Communication at Purdue University. He received his B.Tech. (Honors) in agricultural and food engineering from the Indian Institute of Technology (IIT), Kharagpur, MA in mass communication from North Dakota State University and PhD in mass communication from the University of Minnesota. He joined Purdue University in 2001 and was tenured in 2005. Professor Dutta is the 2006 Lewis Donohew Outstanding Scholar in Health Communication and conducts research on the culture-centered approach to health communication, marginalization in health care, social inequality, and the role of technologies in addressing health-care disparities. His most recent work explores the role of performance in health communication.

Eric M. Eisenberg is professor of communication at the University of South Florida. Dr. Eisenberg twice received the NCA award for the outstanding research publication in organizational communication, the Burlington Foundation award for excellence in teaching, and the Ohio University Elizabeth Andersch Award. Dr. Eisenberg is the author of over seventy-five articles, chapters, and books. He is an internationally recognized researcher, teacher, and consultant specializing in the strategic use of communication to promote positive organizational change.

Laura L. Ellingson, PhD, is associate professor of communication at Santa Clara University. Her research focuses on feminist qualitative methodology, gender studies, and communication in health-care organizations, including interdisciplinary communication, teamwork, and provider–patient communication. She is the author of *Communicating in the Clinic: Negotiating Frontstage and Backstage Teamwork* (2005, Hampton Press) and of the forthcoming, *Qualitative Crystallization* (Sage Publications).

Sara Garcia received her Bachelor's degree in communication from the University of Texas at San Antonio in 2005.

Patricia Geist-Martin is a professor in the School of Communication at San Diego State University. Her research interests focus on narrative and negotiating identity, voice, ideology, and control in organizations, particularly in health and illness. She has published three books, *Communicating Health: Personal, Political, and Cultural Complexities* (2004) (with Eileen Berlin Ray and Barbara Sharf), *Courage of Conviction: Women's Words, Women's Wisdom* (1997) (with Linda A. M. Perry), and *Negotiating* *the Crisis: DRGs and the Transformation of Hospitals* (1992) (with Monica Hardesty). She has published over fifty articles and book chapters covering a wide range of topics.

Prado Y. Gomez has spent the last fifteen years working in organizations, whose focus ranges from theater to HIV prevention in San Francisco. Most recently, he was the Director of Proyecto ContraSIDA Por Vida, a health and wellness program serving the queer Latina/o community. An advocate of the harm-reduction philosophy and promoter of social responsibility, Prado provides presentations and is a consultant to a variety of organizations. He is currently working at PAWS (Pets Are Wonderful Support) providing essential support services to low-income people with AIDS, other disabling illnesses and seniors.

Damon M. Hall is a PhD candidate and Boone and Crockett Conservation and Wildlife Policy Fellow in the Department of Wildlife and Fisheries Sciences at Texas A&M University in College Station, Texas. His research program interrogates the cultural and rhetorical aspects of environmental policy trends that affect the health and quality of life of human and nonhuman residents of ecological systems. He is currently involved in grants research for the Texas A&M Institute of Renewable Natural Resources (http://irnr. tamu.edu).

Lynn M. Harter (PhD, University Nebraska) is an associate professor in the School of Communication Studies at Ohio University and senior editor of *Health Communication*. Her research and teaching focus on discourses of health and healing and organizing for social change.

Marouf Hasian, Jr. is a full professor in the Department of Communication at the University of Utah. His areas of interest include law and rhetoric, social justice movements, and postcolonial studies. He is the author of the *Rhetoric of Eugenics in Anglo-American Thought* (Athens: University of Georgia Press, 1996), and *In the Name of Necessity: Military Tribunals and the Loss of American Civil Liberties* (Tuscaloosa: University of Alabama Press, 2005). He is currently working on a book that investigates how visual rhetorics are used to document atrocities and genocides.

Natalie J. Jeha (MA, San Diego State University) is currently a clinical research coordinator in the Division of Hematology and Oncology at the University of California, San Francisco. Her research interests include marginalization in medicine, the impact of illness on identity, and end-of-life negotiation strategies. Natalie's creative writing explores the value of holistic healing, communication, and interpersonal relationships in health care.

Denise Jodlowski is a doctoral candidate in the Department of Communication at Texas A&M University. Her dissertation focuses on the rhetorical construction of autism. Denise's research interests include the rhetoric of medicine and disability.

Pamela J. Kenniston (MA, MHA, Ohio University) is practice manager at Diles Hearing Center, Athens, Ohio. Her interests include rural health issues, narratives of social support, and the impact of illness on partners and families.

Induk Kim is a doctoral candidate in health communication at Purdue University. Induk conducts research in the areas of health-care activism, food politics, culture-centered approach to health communication, and the discursive framing of uncertainty in health communication.

Dr. Pradeep Krishnatray, is president of the NGO, Centre for Research and Education (CREED) in Andhra Pradesh and Madhya Pradesh, India. He is the editor of *Journal of Creative Communications*). Pradeep has over twenty-five years of experience in development communication, especially health communication. He has managed national level projects in rural communication, and has conducted research and training of health personnel in HIV/AIDS, TB, leprosy, family planning and other issues for UNFPA, UNICEF, ORBIS, and DANIDA, and others. He has published books and articles on using communication for destigmatizing health conditions and community mobilization.

Sangeeta Krishnatray has worked as a communication consultant with DANIDA and is state coordinator (Madhya Pradesh, India) with the Centre for Research and Education (CREED). She holds a postgraduate degree in communication, social work and law. She was coordinator of *Mahila Samkhya*, which empowered village women. Currently based in Hyderabad, India, she manages CREED's research and training activities. She has published a book (along with others) in Hindi on the role of communication in de-stigmatization and has articles in *MICA Communications Review* and *Journal of Health Management*.

Deborah Lupton is professor of sociology and cultural studies at Charles Sturt University, Australia. Her latest books are *Medicine as Culture: Illness, Disease and the Body in Western Societies* (2nd edition, Sage, 2003), *Risk and Everyday Life* (with J. Tulloch, Sage, 2003), *Risk and Sociocultural Theory: New Directions and Perspectives* (editor, CUP, 1999) and *Risk* (Routledge, 1999).

Virginia M. McDermott, PhD, is an assistant professor of communication at the University of New Mexico. Her research examines how problematic events change the nature of relationships and conversations, how communication facilitates coping, and how communication campaigns can be used to address health disparities and social inequities. She has extensive experience in organizational training and specializes in seminars on how to develop a positive organizational environment.

Srinivas R. Melkote is professor in the School of Communication Studies at Bowling Green State University, Ohio. He has taught at universities in India and the United States during the last twenty-five years. He has published extensively on communication in development support, participatory communication, and the theory and practice of communication in the third world. His research and teaching interests include media effects, international communication, communication strategies for HIV/AIDS prevention, and the impact and role of satellite television in the developing world.

Alexandra (Lexa) G. Murphy, PhD is an associate professor of communication and director of community service studies at DePaul University in Chicago, Illinois. Her research has centered on organizational communication and culture, focusing on the communication of marginalized groups in organizational and community contexts such as airlines, hospital emergency rooms, and on public health issues such as HIV/AIDS. She teaches courses that focus on cultural and political issues within organizations and communities.

Ariana Ochoa Camacho (MA, San Francisco State University) is currently in a PhD program in American Studies at New York University. In San Francisco, she worked as a volunteer coach for Las Diablitas at Proyecto ContraSIDA Por Vida, and as a Program Fellow at the San Francisco Foundation focused on issues impacting the Latino community of the Mission and Greater Bay Area, particularly immigration and environmental justice.

John G. Oetzel (PhD, University of Iowa, 1995) is professor and chair in the Department of Communication and Journalism at the University of New Mexico. His research focuses on the impact of culture on conflict communication in work groups, organizations, and health settings. His work has appeared in journals such as *Human Communication Research, Communication Monographs, Communication Research,* among others. He is co-author (with Stella Ting-Toomey) of *Managing Intercultural Communication Effectively* (Sage, 2001) and co-edited *The Sage Handbook of Conflict Communication: Integrating Theory, Research, and Practice* (2006).

Shawna J. Perry, MD is associate professor, assistant chair, and director of clinical operations at the University of Florida Health Science Center, Jacksonville, Florida. She is a graduate of Stanford University, Case Western Reserve University School of Medicine, and is a practicing emergency physician. Her primary research interest is patient safety. Dr. Perry has authored numerous articles and chapters and is involved in collaborative work in communication, human factors, and industrial engineering.

Elizabeth Rattine-Flaherty is a doctoral student in health communication with a particular interest in the health issues faced by women and minorities. She attends the Scripps College of Communication at Ohio University.

Barbara F. Sharf (PhD, University of Minnesota) is a professor in the Department of Communication at Texas A&M University, where she teaches classes in health communication, interpretive methods, narrative inquiry, and culture and health. She co-authored *Communicating Health: Personal, Cultural, and Political Complexities* (with Patricia Geist-Martin and Eileen Berlin Ray), as well as *The Physician's Guide to Better Communication*. Recent projects focus on *promatoras* (community health workers) in the *colonias* of South Texas.

Ashli Quesinberry Stokes is an assistant professor in the Department of Communication Studies at the University of North Carolina Charlotte. Dr. Stokes' research focuses on rhetorical analysis of public relations, with special interest in international health issues and public relations. She is co-authoring a textbook about international public relations. She has published in *Public Relations Review*, the *Southern Communication Journal*, *Studies in Communication Sciences*, the *Encyclopedia of Public Relations*, among others.

Teresa L. Thompson (PhD, Temple University) is professor of communication at the University of Dayton and editor of the journal *Health Communication*. She has published more than fifty journal articles and book chapters and has written or edited six books on health communication. Her primary research focus is provider–patient interaction.

Elissa Velez is a writer, filmmaker and community organizer from San Francisco. She is the administrative assistant for Mobilization Against AIDS International and its programs, including EL-LA a program for transgender Latinas. She served as program assistant for Proyecto ContraSIDA Por Vida for five years where she coordinated and implemented programming for queer Latinas and queer youth.

Melinda Villagran (PhD, University of Oklahoma, 2001) is an associate professor of Communication at George Mason University and an affiliate faculty member with the Culture and Policy Institute in San Antonio, Texas. Her primary research program investigates the intersections among organizational communication and culture in health-care practice. Dr. Villagran's research has appeared in journals including *Communication Monographs*, *Health Communication*, *Journal of Applied Communication Research*, *Communication Research Reports*, and *Analysis of Social Issues and Public Policy*.

Robert L. Wears, MD, MS is an emergency physician who works on safety in complex sociotechnical systems such as health-care organizations. He is currently professor in the Department of Emergency Medicine at the University of Florida, and visiting professor in the Clinical Safety Research Unit at Imperial College London; his writing and research focuses on technical work studies, joint cognitive systems, and particularly the impact of information technology on safety and resilient performance.

Kalvin White is an educator with the Navajo Nation Division of Education.

Rulon Wood holds graduate degrees in English, Film, and Instructional Technology. He is currently an adjunct assistant professor in the Arts Technology Program at the University of Utah and a doctoral student in the University of Utah's Communication Program. His research focuses on issues of film (narrative and documentary), technology, and rhetoric.

Gust A. Yep (PhD, University of Southern California) is professor of Communication Studies and Human Sexuality Studies at San Francisco State University. He is the lead editor of *Queer Theory and Communication: From Disciplining Queers to Queering the Discipline(s)* (2003) and co-editor of *LGBT Studies and Queer Theory* (2006). He also co-authored *Privacy and Disclosure of HIV in Interpersonal Relationships*. Awards include the 2006 NCA Randy Majors Memorial Award for Outstanding Lesbian, Gay, Bisexual, and Transgender Scholarship. Dr. Yep is currently the editor of the NCA Non-Serial Publications Program.

Heather M. Zoller (PhD, Purdue University) is an associate professor in the Department of Communication at the University of Cincinnati. Her research focuses on the politics of public health, including corporate issue management and occupational health, community organizing/public participation, and health activism. Publications appear in journals such as *Communication Monographs*, *Communication Theory*, *Communication Yearbook*, *Health Communication*, *Journal of Applied Communication Research*, and *Management Communication Quarterly* among others. Dr. Zoller's community outreach includes acting as spokesperson for the *Coalition for a Humane Economy*, and as a member of the *Addyston, OH Environmental Task Force*.

Index

Note: 'n' after a page number refers to a note.

AARP Bulletin 366
Abbott, J. 371
Abma, T.A. 48
abortion discourses 68
Abramson, J. 335, 337, 369, 370
Abuse NIoD 183
acculturation 217–18
action-reflection 142, 159, 160
activism: *see* health activism
acupuncture 88, 89–90, 99, 105–6; case study
    101–2, 103
Adler, H.M. 88
Africa 360, 397–8
Africa and the Caribbean and the Pacific
    (ACP) 417–19, 425
agency: and culture-centered communication
    149, 204–5, 206, 248, 253, 263, 432; in
    shaping genetic policy 362, 437, 440–3;
    subaltern 232, 259, 431
Agovino, T. 369
Agreement on Agriculture (AoA) 419–21
Agreement on Trade-Related Aspects of
    Intellectual Property Rights (TRIPS)
    422–4, 425, 426, 439
Airhihenbuwa, C.O. 7, 8, 9, 17, 133, 148,
    156, 158, 159, 161, 168, 177, 182, 193,
    226, 227, 228, 243, 248, 255, 256, 360,
    394, 413, 414, 431, 432, 435, 437, 438
Ajzen, I. 263
Albrecht, G.A. 131
alcohol abuse narratives 50–1
All India Radio 249
Allen, B. 277
Allende, S. 393
Allport, G.W. 138
alternative and dominant frameworks
    comparison 138–42
alternative models of health promotion 6, 22,
    453–4, 459
Altman, D.G. 190, 195
Alvesson, M. 320, 330

American Indians 185–98, 440
Anderson, E. 278
Anderson, J.A. 12
Anderson, R.A. 306, 309
Andrews, L.B. 275
Androutsopoulou, A. 43
Angell, M. 369
Antshel, K.L. 167, 207, 208
Apple, R.D. 67
Arend, E.D. 224
Armstrong, D. 32
Arnold, M. 341
Arnold, R. 159, 177
Arnstein, P. 42
Arsenio, W.F. 50
artistic work, Latino 239–40
Arvay, M. 43
Ascroft, J. 135
Ashcraft, K.L. 317, 327
Ashton, C.M. 203, 206
Asian Development Bank (ADB) 251
asthma care study 359
Astin, J.A. 87, 88
Atkinson, P. 275, 294
Auerbach, K.G. 65
Aune, J. 379
autism 270
Ayres, L. 51
Ayurveda 98

Babrow, A.S. 2, 10, 45, 68
Bach, P.B. 205
Backett-Milburn, K. 116
Bakan, Joel 365
Baker, E.L. 156
Balber, P.G. 43
banana wars 417–19, 425
Bandura, A. 263
Banerji, D. 393, 405
Baquet, C.R. 208
Barge, J.K. 298

Barley, S.R. 303, 306
Barrett, B. 87, 88
Barris, E. 390
Barry, P. 375, 376, 378
Bartlett, A. 67, 68
Bascom, A. 86
Basler, B. 378
basmati rice 422–4, 425
Basnyat, I. 33, 34, 151, 253, 255
Basu, A. 1, 14, 15, 150
Bath, P.A. 216
Bauer, J.J. 44
Baumgartner, F. 373
Baumslag, N.M. 64
Baxter, L.A. 183, 184, 185, 197
Bayh-Dole Act 382n
Beaglehole, R. 360, 415, 426
Bearison, D.J. 45
Beauchamp, D. 373
Beck, A. 169
Beck, C.S. 10, 22, 45, 46, 217, 316
Beck-Gernsheim, E. 126
Beck, U. 126
Becker, C. 92
Beckett-Tharp, D. 294, 304
Behara, R. 275
behavior change, campaigns promoting 8–9,
    12, 404, 411–12
Belknap, R.A. 45
Bellg, A. 43
Berger, C. 11
Bergsma, L.J. 182
Berkowitz, S. 341
Bernhardt, J. 352
Bernstein, A. 378
Bertero, C. 46, 51
Bevan, C. 51
Bevan, M.T. 295, 296, 299, 300
Beverly, John 457
Bhabha, H. 431
Bienefeld, M. 398
Biesanz, M.H. 88
Biggins, N.A. 51
'biocolonialism' 434
biomedical model 12, 86, 308, 316;
    alternatives to 6, 272–3, 453–4, 459;
    difficulties in combining with holistic
    medicine 98–9, 107; economic incentives
    of 99; holistic challenges to 90;
    patient-provider relationships in 88–9;
    power of 293, 297
biopolitics 36, 124
Birth of the Clinic, The 30
Bista, D. 250
Bitter Medicine (ABC broadcast) 375
Blagojevich, Rod 376, 377, 378
Bloch-Poulsen, J. 229
Blum, L.M. 64, 69
Blumberg, C.J. 49

Bochner, A.P. 11, 13
Bodekar, G. 422
body, discourses of the 68–9, 124
Bolivia 397, 398
Bonanno, G.A. 44
Bordo, Susan 457
Bosk, C.L. 275
Bosticco, C. 42, 46
Bottorff, J. 17
Boulay, M. 247, 248, 252, 263
Bowen, S.A. 302
Bowker, J. 204, 215
Bradley, L.R. 336, 337
Brashers, D.E. 15, 42, 206
Brazil 401
Brazzaville Congo 397
breast pumps 73–4
breastfeeding 34–5, 63–81, 113, 114, 116;
    dialectical tensions 64–70; difficulties in
    establishing 121; discourses 64–70; in
    public 66, 69, 75–6; racial, ethnic and
    class disparities in 66–7, 81–2n; receiving
    advice on 74–5, 76–7; resisting medical
    expertise 74–5, 77–80; support group case
    study 70–81
Brewer, M.B. 138
Brockmeier, J. 39
Broder, J. 373
Broussard, B.B. 50
Brown, B. 46
Brown, D. 17
Brown, J. 268
Browne, A. 17
Broz, S.L. 8
Brubaker, P.K. 397, 398
Brugge, D. 183, 186
Bruner, Jerome 49, 315
Buchbinder, R. 88
Bunton, R. 124
Burgoon, M. 8
Burke, K. 314, 315, 316, 326, 330, 338
Burkholder, T.R. 341
Burns, S. 378
Burrows, B. 438, 439
Burton, B. 335
Bush, George W. 378
Butterfoss, F.D. 182
Buzzanell, P.M. 7, 16, 47, 204, 205, 212, 215,
    269

Callister, L.C. 45
Cameron, J. 399, 400
Campbell, K.K. 341
Canada: health advocacy in 405; health
    care spending 366–7, 368; and
    Investor-to-State Lawsuits 401–2;
    pressures to restrict drug reimportations to
    US 375–6; use of SPS measures 400
Canada Medicare Act 1966 367

Canadian Public Health Service (CPHS) 405
Canavan Foundation 443
cancer: alternative therapies 88; narratives
    49, 50, 359; reducing risk 12
cancer care case study, Latino 206–20;
    dialectical tensions 207–9, 214–19;
    Latino cultural values affecting 206–9,
    219–20; method 209–14; results
    214–19
Cangemi, L. 85
capitalism and health 7, 33–4, 393, 413
CAQDAS (Computer Aided Qualitative
    Data Analysis Software) 72–3
care providers' narratives 46, 51
Carl, W. 270
Carpenter, M. 392, 393, 397, 398, 405
Carter, P. 64
Carver, C.S. 50
case review conferences 306, 309
Caspi, O. 85, 87
Cassileth, B.R. 88
Catlett, D. 335
Cavalli-Sforza, L. 433, 436, 437, 438
CBC 368, 378
Ceci, C. 276, 277, 278, 282
Cegala, D.J. 8
Centers for Disease Control 157, 233, 241
Certeau, Michel de 371, 457
Chadwick, E. 393
Chafee, S. 11
Charland, M. 338
Charmaz, K. 12, 299
Charon, R. 52
Chavez, V. 188, 193
Chay-Nemeth, C. 360, 394
Cheney, G. 182, 183, 184, 185, 191, 193,
    197, 198, 316, 317, 337, 371
Chicago Sun-Times 377
children 113–26; causes of death in Nepal
    251; co-sleeping with babies 78; diet 114,
    116, 120; disclosing donor-assisted
    conception to 44; immunization 113–14,
    116; malnutrition in 411; mothers'
    responsibility for the health of 117–26;
    obesity in 120–1; public health
    promotions 113–15; risk discourse in
    relation to 124–5; sharing narratives 49;
    social and cultural contexts in the care of
    116–17; UNICEF study in Africa 397;
    vulnerability of 119–20; Western societies
    focus on 126
China 443
chiropractic 88
Choi, K.H. 231
Choudhry, N. 377
Christensen, P. 125
Christiansen, A. 18
chronic fatigue 270
Clarkson, S. 415, 418

Clatts, M. 31
Clegg, S, 371
Cloud, D. 317, 327
Coates, J.R. 87
Cobb, R.W. 373
Coker, E.M. 47
Collard, S. 159
Colon-Emeric, C.S. 306
commodification of health 352, 458
community: building narratives 45–6;
    creating a Latino space 237–40;
    empowerment in destigmatizing leprosy
    139, 142; exploitation of indigenous
    knowledge 425, 426; indigenous rights
    422, 427; involvement in making health
    decisions 150, 414, 424; social activism
    against HGDP 435–40
community-based participatory research
    (CBPR) 151–2, 182–99; drug prevention
    campaign 185–98; ethical paradoxes in
    185–98
community coalition building 183
Community Service Program (CSP) 315, 317,
    318
community workers 142–4
complementary/alternative medicine (CAM)
    85, 87, 455; integration in US hospitals
    88; see also acupuncture; holistic medicine
compliance 300, 308
Computer Aided Qualitative Data Analysis
    Software (CAQDAS) 72–3
Condit, C.M. 7, 338, 341, 352
condoms 32, 238
confidentiality 190, 326–9
Conger, J.A. 339, 351
Connelly, J.E. 46, 52
Connolly, C. 352, 377
Conrad, C. 7, 17, 359, 371, 390, 394
Conroy, R.M. 88
consent 440–1
contact hypothesis 138
control narratives 42–3
Cook, M. 352
Cook, R.J. 189
Cooper, M. 374
Copeland, L. 45
coping narratives 42–3, 48, 49
Cora-Bramble, D. 208, 214
Corazón 234
Corbett, J.R. 336
Cortazzi, M. 320
Courtial, J.P. 47
Craig, D. 397
Craig, G. 125
Craig, R.T. 10
critical approaches 6–7, 10, 12, 17, 22, 148,
    269, 360; combining with narrative
    approaches 52–3; community voices in
    150; critical health communication praxis

225–9; methodology 15–16; to public health 393, 403, 406; theory 13–14, 34, 457
cultural geographies 237–8
cultural sensitivity approach 148, 149–50, 151, 269
cultural-symbolic systems 133–4
culture-centered approaches 148–51, 157–61, 227–8, 247–8, 269, 360, 453–4; 432 149; and agency for marginalized populations 204–5, 206, 248, 253, 263, 432, 444; combining with narrative approaches 52–3; in the context of neoliberal trade policies 413–14, 419, 426; to health campaigns 33; model of health communication 248; structural factors 151, 228, 413–14, 419, 421, 424; theoretical perspectives 7–8, 10, 14–15, 16, 17
Cummings, D.M. 314
Cunningham-Burley, S. 116
Curanderos 218
Curtis, J. 306
Cut Your Coat According to Your Cloth 252–3, 261, 263

Daaleman, T.D. 90
Dam, K.W. 416
Dana-Farber Cancer Institute 88
Darwin, T.J. 90
Das, T.K. 186
Dasberg, H. 42
DasGupta, S. 52
data analysis software 72–3
data protection 190–1
Davey, M. 377
Davies, B. 43
Dayton, C. 17
de Koning, K. 182, 183
De Madre a Madre Prenatal Care Photonovel Series 160, 163
DeCoster, M.E. 155–6
Deetz, S.A. 11, 13, 14, 226, 271, 278, 338
Dejong, W. 359, 394
deliberate disruptions 287–9
DelVecchio Good, M.J. 46
DeSantis, A. 16
Detsky, A. 377
Devine, P.G. 133
Día de Los Muertos 239–40
diagnosis narratives 49–50
dialectical tensions 185–6, 197; in breastfeeding discourses 64–70; in emergency care 286–7, 288; of hegemony 7; in Latino communication about cancer 207–9, 214–19; of materiality/social construction 10–11, 14; outflanking/ counterflanking in drug reimportation 380; in providing holistic

treatment 106–8; of social change/ status quo 10, 11; of universal/specific 10, 11, 13
dialogic models 253, 272–3
dialysis case study 271, 293–310; health care hierarchies 298–9, 306, 307–8; patient-care technician communication 302–7; patient communication 299–302; suggestions for practice 308–9
Díaz, R.M. 224, 225
Dickens, B.M. 189
Dietrich, P.J. 43
diffusion of innovations (DOI) model: absence of subaltern agency in 133; criticism of 134–42
DiGallo, A. 42, 49
Dimaggio, G. 52
Dionisopoulos, G.N. 15, 359
direct to consumer (DTC) drug marketing 336–7, 344
discourses, health 18–19, 30–4, 36
discursive closure 271, 278, 288
disease-based models 231, 233
Dixon-Woods, M. 50
DNA patents 434–5, 439–40, 443
Doak, C. 172, 178
dominant ideology 46–7, 226
Donnelly, G.F. 87
donor-assisted conception 44
Dorsey, A.M. 225
Dossey, Larry 89, 91
Dow, B.J. 7
Downs, B. 40
Drabant, S. 377
Drager, N. 360
Dreyer, J. 6, 9, 268
Drotar, D. 49
drug-prevention campaign 185–98
DTC (direct to consumer) drug marketing 336–7, 344
du Pré, A. 88, 89
Duquette-Smith, C. 338
Duran, B. 182, 183
Dutta-Bergman, M.J. 1, 5, 7, 8, 11, 16, 17, 33, 133, 148, 149, 151, 157, 158, 182, 193, 203, 204, 206, 207, 209, 219, 220, 227, 228, 241, 247, 248, 252, 253, 255, 256, 260, 261, 262, 339, 360, 394, 405, 412, 413, 414, 432, 435, 437, 444
Dutta, M.J. 1, 12, 14, 15, 17, 33, 34, 148, 150, 151, 462
dynamic equilibrium 108

E-E: *see* entertainment education (E-E)
economic policies, global 360, 361, 390–407; courses of action to promote public health 403–4; economic governmentality and public health 391–2; harmonization agreements 398–400, 403; health

communication research and practice 404–6; Investor-to-State Lawsuits (ISLs) 401–2, 403–4; neoliberal governmentality 394–404; public health discourse 392–4, 403; Structural Adjustment Package (SAP) loans 396–8, 406n
Economist 352
Edgar, T. 1
eDTC (e-direct to consumer) drug marketing 337; *see also* Healthology
Egbert, N. 108
Ehman, J.W. 90
Ehrenreich, B. 293, 345
Eisenberg, D.M. 87
Eisenberg, E. 275, 276, 278, 284, 285, 325, 326
elite, a priori approaches 11, 12, 14
elites, economic 371–2, 374, 379, 380
Ellingson, L.L. 6, 7, 10, 15, 16, 47, 204, 205, 212, 215, 269, 270, 293, 294, 297, 298, 302, 305, 308, 316, 328
Elliott, J. 52
Ellis, M. 90
Elofsson, L.C. 50
Elwood, W. 17, 338
emergency care case study 271, 275–90; decision-making processes 281–8; deliberate disruptions 287–9; dialectical tensions 286–7, 288; discursive closure 271, 278, 288; medical knowledge and power 271, 275, 276–80, 288; narrative rationality subjugated to technical rationality 279; NHS targets in 277; suggested interventions 289–90
Emerson, J.P. 327
empowerment 155, 158–9, 161; of a community 139, 142–3; development communication theories 139–42; online health information boosting consumer 339–40; paradox of pharmaceutical empowerment rhetoric 341–2, 343, 344, 349, 351, 352; of patients 339–40, 349, 351, 352
Engels, M. 393
English, D. 293
entertainment education (E-E): and imposition of the sender's value system 254, 261; participatory communication in 249–50; Radio Communication Project (RCP) 247–64
environmental theory of disease 392–3
Espino, S.L.R. 198
ethnic health disparities 151, 183, 205–6
ethnography 15, 297–8, 329, 453
Ethyl Corporation 402
European Union and the banana wars 417–19
Evans, J.W. 43
Extended Parallel Process model 11

Faber, S. 295
Fabj, V. 18
Falk, R. 391, 395, 405
Fals-Borda, O. 143, 183
familismo 167, 168, 208, 216, 217, 219
family planning project in Nepal 247–64
fatalismo 207–8, 215, 219–20
Feldman, P.J. 169
Filc, D. 86
financial barriers to health care 218, 220, 228, 398
Finley, M. 417
Fins, J.J. 43, 51
first-order research 227
Fishback, S.J. 159
Fishbein, M. 263
Fisher, Walter 41
Fletcher, P.N. 42
Flores, G. 207
Flower, L. 50
Food and Drug Administration (FDA) 336, 337, 345, 375, 376, 377, 378, 380
food imports 420, 421
food patents 423–4, 425
Food Research Action Center (2005) 411
food security 411–28, 456; access to food 411–12; banana wars 417–19; basmati rice trade 422–4; and hunger 412, 424, 425, 426; impact of neoliberal trade agreements on 412, 414–15, 424–7; paradox of 426; sugar in the Pacific Islands 420–1
Ford, L.A. 224, 226, 314, 331
Forey, J. 88
Fosgarde, M. 51
Foster-Fishman, P.G. 184
Foucault, Michel 7, 14, 30, 31, 32, 33, 65, 124, 125, 226, 270, 276–7, 293, 296–7, 300, 302, 308, 394, 457
Foulks, E.F. 198
Fox, S. 337
France 368
Frank, A.W. 48, 298, 316
Frank, R. 370
Frankfurt School 7, 14
Franks, H. 204, 215
Freidson, E. 31, 131
Freimuth, Vicky 8, 16, 32, 358
Freire, P. 142, 159, 183
Frey, L.R. 49
Friedman, E.A. 295, 300, 301, 308
Friends 47
Frist, Bill 378
Fuqua, J. 350, 351, 352
Furnham, A. 88
Fusco, C. 231

Galtry, J. 66
Galvin, K. 190, 195
Gardner, A. 366

Garrett, L. 392
Gates, L. 70
GATT (General Agreement on Trade and
    Tariffs) 415–19, 425
Gattuso, S. 51
Gaudet, T.W. 85, 87
Gaydos, E.L. 45
Geertz, C. 13
Geist-Martin, P. 10, 293, 304
Geist, P. 6, 9, 70, 268, 270
Gendall, P. 352
gender 7, 159, 451, 458
gender appropriate approaches 159
General Agreement on Trade and Tariffs
    (GATT) 415–19, 425
Genographic project 442, 443
genomic health reforms 440–3; see also
    Human Genome Diversity Project
    (HGDP)
German, K. 337
Gershman, J. 391, 397
Gevitz, N. 85
Gewirtz, A. 42
Ghaanti Heri Haad Nilaun 252
Ghosh, S. 427
Giacchino, F. 296
Gibbs, R.W. 204, 215
Gibson, T. 276
Giddens, A. 279, 371, 374
Gillespie, S.R. 7, 359
Gillotti, C. 268
Gilmour, J.A. 276, 277
Girion, L. 376, 378
Glaser, B.G. 319
globalization, economic 365, 380, 391
'globalization from below' 405
Gobé, M. 345, 348, 352
Goffman, E. 131, 270, 316, 328
Goldbeck-Wood, S. 88
Goldenberg, R.L. 169
Goldhammer, P. 337
Goldstein, L.S. 182
Gonsalez, C. 419, 420
Gonzalez, M.C. 89
Gordon, C. 125
Gorham, B. 373
Gormley, M. 372
Gossart-Walker, S. 42
Gould, A. 88
Goverde, H. 365
government relationships with multinational
    corporations 365, 370, 371–80
governmentality: see neoliberal
    governmentality
Graber, D.A. 342
Grace, V.M. 67
Graigie, F. 90
Gramsci, Antonio 7, 454, 457
Grassley, Charles 378

Gray, R.E. 46
Greely, H. 434, 436, 437, 440, 441, 443, 444
Greene, K. 224
Greider, K. 369
Greider, W. 399, 401
Grenier, L.M. 216
grieving process narratives 41, 42, 44
Griffith, D. 352
Grof, C. 103
Grof, S. 103
Gross, D. 367
Grossman, L.S. 418
Guajardo, M. 210
Guarnaccia, P.J. 216
Gudykunst, W.B. 216
Guha, Ranajit 431, 457
Gullickson, T. 43
Guttman, N. 67

Habermas, Jurgen 271, 457
Hacker, J. 373
Hadley, S.W. 89
Hahn, Steve 377
Hale, C.L. 45
Hales, C.P. 342
Hall, J. 373
Hall, S. 231
Hallberg, I.R. 43
Hancock, L. 184, 191, 192, 195
Handbook of Health Communication 2, 41
Hanson, J. 18
Haraway, Donna 457
Harden, J. 46
Hargraves, J.L. 218
harmonization agreements 398–400, 403
Harper, T. 377
Harré, R. 39
Harris, G. 375
Harris, R. 415, 426
Harry, Debra 438, 439
Hart, R. 341
Harter, L.M. 6, 10, 17, 18, 47, 53, 316, 462
Hartling, J.M. 161
Hatch-Woodruff, M.L. 43
Hauck, Y.L. 67, 69
Hausman, B. 67, 68
Hawkins, S.C. 46
Hawpe, L. 40
Hayes, V.E. 43
healing: definitions of 96–7; and narrative
    therapy 49–51
health activism 18, 340, 405–6, 412, 432,
    454; power in the genomic health arena
    440–4
health advocacy 402–4, 405, 412, 426–7
Health Belief Model 11
health campaigns: contributing to
    marginalization 7; culture-centered
    approach 33; methodologies in studying

15; participatory approaches 138; promoting behavior change 8–9, 12, 404, 411–12; promoting children's health 113–15; resistance to 459

health care workers: and eradicating leprosy 142–4; experiences using TWS methods 173–4, 178; narratives of 48; paraprofessionals 296, 303, 306; patient-care technicians 302–7; role of 139; *see also* hierarchies in the medical system

Health Communication 2, 3, 4

health communication as a discipline 1–5

health communication theories 1–18; contributions to 16–18, 449–51; defining 10–15; emerging agendas 456–9; emerging issues 455–6; historical development 8–10; interdisciplinary conversations 459–60; methodological issues 15–16, 22; theoretical perspectives 5–8

health disparities 7, 242, 262, 330, 331, 359, 360, 424; in the availability of services 314; empowerment-based strategies to improve 155; ethnic 151, 183, 205–6; and financial barriers 218, 220, 228; racial 148, 151, 157, 183, 205–6, 269; role of communication in producing 203; in treatment for HIV/AIDS 224–5

health literacy 177–8

health policy 17–18, 335, 358–60, 379, 394; inequalities in access to 371–4, 379; locus of power 390

Healthology 336, 337, 338, 340–53; analyzing pharmaceutically supported websites 342–50; paradox of empowerment rhetoric 341–2, 343, 344, 349, 351, 352

healthy eating campaigns 12, 412

Healthy People 63, 66–7, 183, 359, 392

Heartfield, M. 276, 277

hegemony 7, 226, 293

Hellstrom, O. 43

Helman, C. 31

Hemphill, L. 52

Henderson, A. 276

Henwood, F. 340, 344

Herman, K. 89

Herzenstein, M. 344

Hess, J.D. 46

Hiemstra, R. 158

hierarchies in the medical system 282, 289, 298–9, 306, 307–8

Hindu epistemology 95–6

Hines, S.C. 295, 296

Hirmani, A.B. 130

Hirt, E.R. 133

History of Sexuality, The 30

HIV/AIDS: access to online health information 340; in Asia and Africa 360, 394; disparities in treatment 224–5; in the Latino community 224–5, 241–2; mobile health clinics 314; narratives 42; Reagan's rhetorical management of 359; stigmatization 129; *see also* Proyecto ContraSIDA Por Vida

HIV Prevention Council 233

Hobbs, R. 90

Hoek, J. 352

Hoffman, J.R. 337

Hoffman, M. 203

holistic medicine 35, 85–109; case study methodology 91–2; case study results 92–106; communication 88–9, 105–6; defining 86–7; dialectical tensions 106–8; difficulties combining with biomedicine 98–9, 107; future research 108–9; the history of 87–91; modifying the script to help the patient 107; restrictions of licensing regulations 99, 107; spirituality in 89, 90–1, 108, 176

Holmer, A.F. 336

Holtz, T.H. 390

Honos-Webb, L. 48

Horn, A. 49

Horrigan, J.B. 337

Horvath, A.O. 89

Hospital Insurance and Diagnosis Services Act (HIDS) 1957 366

House, J.S. 224

Houston Chronicle 376

Howard, K.I. 89

Hubbard, R.S. 157

Huberman, A.M. 73

Hudec, R.E. 415, 416

Huggins, C.E. 87

Hughey, J. 142

Human Genome Diversity Project (HGDP) 432–5; critical social activism 435–40; DNA patenting concerns 434–5, 439–40, 443; genomic health reforms 440–3; online debate 435–6, 437

Human Genome Project (HGP) 433

Humlog 249

hunger 411, 424, 425, 426

Hunter, C.P. 208

Hunter, K.M. 316

Huntington, A.D. 276, 277

Hyder, A.A. 183

Ickovics, J. 155

identity 17; in constant formation 231–2; Latino 216–19; pharmaceutical public relations' impact on 337–8, 340, 351; in Proyecto's work 231–2, 235, 238–9; transforming narratives 43–5, 49; and understanding of health communication 17

ideology, dominant 46–7, 226

Illich, Ivan 31, 457

illness narratives 50
illness, taking control of 351
IMF (International Monetary Fund) 365, 390, 391, 393, 396, 397, 398
immunization 113–14, 116
Imperative of Health, The 9
India: basmati rice trade 423–4; *see also* leprosy, destigmatizing
Indigenous Peoples Council on Biocolonialism (IPCB) 439
infant formula 66, 74, 78, 80, 82n
infertility discourse, age-related 17, 47, 53
information avoidance 216, 220
Institute of Medicine (IOM) 88, 155, 156, 158, 177
Institutional Review Boards (IRBs) 186
integrative medicine 87
intellectual property rights 422–4, 425, 426, 439
International Monetary Fund (IMF) 365, 390, 391, 393, 396, 397, 398
interpretive approach 6, 10, 16–17, 22; advancing patient-centered theories 269; community voices in 150; methodology 15; theory building 12–13
intervention narratives 50–1
Investor-to-State Lawsuits (ISLs) 401–2, 403–4
Irurita, V.F. 67, 69
Irwin, A. 391, 397
Israel, B.A. 183, 184, 187
Iyengar, S. 374

Jack, A. 352
Jack, L. 413, 414
Jackson, F. 433
Jacobson, T.L. 248, 249, 250, 252, 253, 262
Jain, N. 88
Janani 250
Japan 420
Japp, D. 270
Japp, P.M. 10, 45, 46, 270
Jasinski, J. 338
Jaye, C. 51
Jennings, Peter 375
Jensen, P.S. 187
Johns Hopkins University/Center for Communication Programs (JHU/CCP) 248, 251, 252, 255, 256, 257, 260
Johnson, J.L. 17, 31, 41, 51, 269, 330
Johnston Lloyd 155
Johnstone, S. 295
Jones, B. 373
Jones, C.P. 187
Jones, D.W. 43
Jordan, J. 159
Jordan, N. 88
Jordens, C.L. 46
Joseph, A.L. 417, 418

Journal of Applied Communication Research 3
Journal of Health Communication 3, 4
Jovchelovitch, S. 339
Juanillo, N.K. 8

Kain, J. 365
Kaiser Family Foundation 366
Kakai, H. 208
Kalischuk, R.G. 43
Kameny, R.R. 45
Kanugo, R.N. 339, 351
Kaptain, D.C. 49
Kaufert, J. 52
Kaye, G. 142
Keeley, M.P. 49, 215
Kegler, M.C. 182
Kelsey, J. 420–1
Keranen, L. 49
Kerik, Bernard 377
Keyton, J. 299
Kierans, C.M. 295
Kim, J.Y. 360
King, G. 270
Kingdon, J. 373
Kirkcaldy, B. 88
Kirkman, M. 44, 47
Kirkwood, W.G. 17
Kirsi, T. 51
Kiwanuka-Tondo, J. 394
Klein, K. 49
Kliewer, S. 90, 91
Kline, K.N. 3, 10, 15, 16, 32, 33, 460
knowledge: discourse, and social practices 30, 31; exploitation of indigenous 425, 426; physicians' power and 272, 298, 302, 303–4, 307; and power in medical care 271, 275, 276–80, 288, 296–7, 308–9; power of 371; suppression of nurses' power and 277–8, 282–3, 302
Knowles, M. 158, 161
Koch, T. 52
Koenig Kellas, J. 49
Kole, A. 183, 186
Korten, D. 415
Krauss, C. 375, 376
Kreps, G. 203, 205
Kreuter, M.W. 184, 189
Krieshok, T.S. 49
Krishnatray, P. 129, 132, 137
Kristiansen, M. 229
Kroesen, K. 88
Kuipers, J. 275
Kushner, K. 52
Kuttner, R. 370
Kvale, S. 71

La Leche League 64
Labonte, R. 43, 400, 401, 404, 415, 426
Lakoff, G. 31

Lammers, J.C. 270
language barriers to health care 207, 218–19; overcoming 238
Lani, J.A. 48
Lara, M. 217
Larson, D.B. 91
Latin American banana wars 417–19, 425
Latino(s): cultural values and norms 166–8, 176–7, 206–9; health disparities 157, 205–6; living with HIV/AIDS 224–5, 241–2; physicians 218–19; relationships with practitioners 176, 208; *see also* cancer care case study, Latino; prenatal education case study; Proyecto ContraSIDA Por Vida (PCPV or Proyecto)
Lax, W. 190, 195
Leape, L.L. 275
LeDreff, G. 47
Leibovitz, Z. 295
Lenzin, N.L. 189
leprosy, destigmatizing 36, 129–44; criticism of dominant diffusion of innovation approach 134–42; empowerment of the local community 139, 142; participatory approaches to communication and cure 134–44; role of health/community workers in eradicating 142–4; stigma of 130–1
Levy, J.A. 131
Lewin, K. 183
Leydon, G.M. 216
Li, R. 64
licensing regulations in the US 99, 107
Lichtenthal, W.G. 43
Liebman, J. 314
lifestyle theory of causation of disease 9, 11, 392, 404
Lindlof, T.R. 6, 71, 297
Lindsay, E. 302
listening 88–9, 105
loans, developmental 396–8
lobbyists, professional 372–3, 375, 379
'local, emergent' approaches 11, 14
Loftus, L.A. 51
Loghman-Adham, M. 295
Lohn, M. 378
Lowenberg, J.S. 89
Lu, L. 207
Luborsky, L. 89
Ludwig, M.J. 226
Lule, J. 40
Lundin, A.P. 308
Lupton, D. 7, 8, 9, 12, 13, 14, 16, 30, 31, 32, 65, 68, 69, 113, 114, 115, 124, 125, 148, 205, 225, 226, 337, 338, 392, 393, 412
Lurier, A.C. 43
Lynch, J. 276, 277
Lynx, D. 367
Lysaker, P.H. 49, 50

Macafee, M. 378
Macaulay, A.C. 190
machismo 208
MacPherson, H. 88
Madeley, J. 411, 416, 417, 425, 426
Madness and Civilization 30
Maduro, R. 215, 218
Mahera, J.M. 51
Maine reimportation program 375, 376
Makoul, G. 5
Manheim, J. 371
Manias, E. 276, 277
Mann, Michael 371
March of Dimes 157
Marchand, L. 52
marginalized groups: access to online health information 273, 351–2; agency 149, 203–4, 206, 253, 263, 432, 444; and health communication campaigns 7; in health communication theory 7, 17; health policy and 359–60; mobile health clinics reaching 272, 273, 321–2, 330; *see also* food security
marianismo 208, 216, 219
Marks, J. 434, 435, 439
Markus, H. 340
Martin, C. 399, 400
Martin, J.N. 209, 214
Martin, M. 182, 183, 185, 198
Martins, A.J. 46
Marx, Karl 457
Marxism 14
Masi, C.M. 339, 340
Masilela, S. 135
Massad, S. 88
Massey, D. 315
Massey, Z. 155, 169
materiality/social construction dialectic 10–11, 14
Mattson, M. 2, 10, 68
May, S. 371
May, T. 278
Maynooth, N.U.I. 295
McAdams, D.P. 40
McClelland, C. 375
McCormick, S,. 340–1
McCreight, B.S. 42
McDaniel, Jr., R.R. 332
McDivitt, J.A. 394
McDowell, J. 51
McGillion, M. 46
McGorry, S.Y. 207
McIntush, H.G. 7, 18, 359, 390, 394
McKinley, A. 314
McKnight, J. 7, 9
McLeod, K. 390
McLeroy, K. 412
McMichael, A.J. 415, 426
McNeil, K. 365

M.D. Anderson Cancer Center 88
media 8, 33, 247–50, 373
media studies, interpretive 16
medicalization of women 65–8, 73
Meeker, M.A. 51
Mehl, M.R. 49
Melkote, S. 7, 18, 129, 132, 137, 360, 394
Mercer, S.W. 88
metaphors 31
Methanex Corporation 402
Mexico 378, 381n, 397; *colonias* on the border
    with Texas 210–11; ideculture and the
    medical system 216–19
Meyer, B. 50
Meyer, I.H. 42
Meyrowitz, J. 352
Michels, D.L. 64
Mickey, T. 338
Miles, M.B. 73
military discourse in health 31, 34
Millen, J.V. 390, 395
Miller, D. 116, 126
Miller, J.B. 159, 161
Miller, K. 325, 332
Miller, N. 138
Miller, P. 391
Miller, W.R. 91
Milton, C.L. 46
Mindt, T. 49
Minkler, M. 183, 184, 185, 187, 188, 193,
    224, 412
mobile health clinic case study 313–32;
    difficulties of maintaining privacy 326–9;
    improvisation 321–6; marginalized
    patients 271, 272, 321–2, 330; providing
    continuity of care 321–6; research
    practices 318–20
Mobilization Against AIDS International 230
modernization framework 138–42
Mohanty, Chandra 232, 457
Mokros, H.B. 13, 226
Monk, G. 43
Montello, M. 51, 52
Moore-Gilbert, B. 431
Morgan-Witte, J. 45, 46, 300, 316, 328
Mori, M. 336
Morris, D.B. 316
Moss, A.H. 295
Most Favored Nation principle 420
Motaal, D.A. 399
mothers: case study on responsibility for their
    children's health 35–6, 117–26; class and
    cultural differences in attitudes to the care
    of children 116, 123; concerns over
    childhood obesity 120–1; concerns over
    children's diet 116, 120; feelings of
    disempowerment 123–4; feelings of guilt
    and inadequacy 121–3; pressure from
    other mothers to conform 122–3, 126;

previous research 115–17; responsible
    motherhood discourses 36, 124; *see also*
    breastfeeding
multinational corporations and relationships
    with government 365, 371–80
Mumby, D.K. 7, 317, 327, 454
Munro, M. 367
Murdoch, R.O. 45
Murphy, P. 359, 394
Murphy, S.A. 41
Murray-Johnson, L. 6, 15
Murray, M. 46
Mutchler, K. 31
Myers, G.E. 48

Nadesan, M.H. 17, 66, 69, 270
Nairn, S. 46
Nakayama, T.K. 185
Nama, N. 182, 186
Nandy, Ashis 457
narrative competence 51–2
narrative perspectives 6
narrative theory 39, 320
narrative therapy 49
narratives 6, 34, 39–53, 315–17, 320, 462;
    discourses as 31–2; functions of 41–7;
    health and healing 49–51; influencing
    health policy 359; local health decision
    150; patient 48, 279, 285, 298; structure
    of 48; women's 159, 296
*Narratives, Health and Healing: Communication
    Theory, Research and Practice* 6
Nason, D. 436
National Geographic 442, 443
National Health Service 277
Native Americans 185–98, 440
Navarro, V. 360, 398, 403
Nease, D.E. 90
Neff, J.A. 208
Neimeyer, R.A. 42
Nelson, S. 46, 50
neoliberal governmentality 124, 394–6;
    discursive influence on global public
    health promotion 396–402; economic
    governmentality and public health 391–2
neoliberal trade agreements: *see* trade
    agreements, neoliberal global
neoliberalism 390–2, 402, 405
Nepal 250–1; Radio Communication Project
    (RCP) 247–64
Neumayer, E. 396, 402
New Scientist 352
Nicaragua 397
Nigeria 398
Nilsson, M. 44
Nochi, M. 42
Noland, C. 270
non-compliance 300, 301, 308
nonverbal communication 105–6

Norberg, A. 51
North American Free Trade Agreement
(NAFTA) 210, 390, 399, 401, 402
Nurius, P. 340
nurses: changing role 303; nurse-patient
relationship 295–6; nurse-physician
relationship 302–3; nursing rounds 289;
suppression of knowledge and power of
277–8, 282–3, 302
NVivo qualitative data analysis software 72

Obregon, R. 228, 413, 438
O'Brien, M. 43
O'Callaghan, F.V. 88
Office of Ministry of Health (OMH) 203,
205
Ogle, K. 42
O'Hair, D. 204
Ohlen, J. 50
Olbrechts Tyteca, L. 342
Olesen, F. 49
Olofsson, B. 51
online health information 273, 337, 339–40,
351–2; see also Healthology
Opie, A. 302, 308, 309
Orbe, M. 270
organizational effectiveness 142
organizational paradoxes 185–6, 197–8
organizational rhetoric 371–4, 379
Orlinsky, D.F. 89
Other Drug War, The (PBS Frontline) 375,
381n
othering 269, 431, 456

Pacanowsky, M. 339, 347, 349
Pacific Islands 420–1, 425
Pakistan 423–4
Palmer, G. 66
Pals, J.L. 44
Papa, M. 249
paradoxes in comparison to dialectics 185–6
Pargament, K.I. 216
Park, C.L. 49
Parrott, R. 89, 108
participation, paradox of 191–5
participatory approaches 134–8, 140–1,
157–60, 227, 249–50, 454; see also
community-based participatory research
(CBPR)
Patai, D. 143
Pataki, George 374
Patankar, P. 131, 137
Patented Medicines Price Review Board 367
patient-care technicians 302–7
patient case reviews 306, 309
patient-centered approach 70, 155, 156,
157–8, 269, 308–9
patient-practitioner relationships: with
dialysis nurses 295–6; in holistic medicine

89, 105–6; Latino 176, 208; listening in
88–9, 105; researching 15; see also
physician-patient relationships
patients: case study in a dialysis centre
299–302; empowered 339–40, 349, 351,
352; issues of compliance/noncompliance
300, 301, 308; as members of the care
team 308–9; narratives 48, 279, 285, 298
Patton, M.Q. 13
Payne, J.G. 192
PCPV: see Proyecto ContraSIDA Por Vida
Pear, R. 341, 370
pedagogy 158, 161
Pennebaker, J.W. 49
Penson, R.T. 42
Perelman, C. 342
Perez, T.L. 15, 359
personal responsibility 7, 12, 404; objectives
in the RCP program 258–60; for poverty
258, 259, 260
personalismo 167, 208
Petersen, A. 113, 115, 124, 125, 392, 393
Peterson, T.R. 395, 397
Petoskey, E.L. 182
pharmaceutical advertising 335
pharmaceutical health public relations:
constitutive theoretical approaches 337–8,
350–1; empowering patients 339–40, 349,
351, 352; impact on consumer identities
337–8, 340, 351; pharmaceutical
promotion 336–7; vested interests of 352;
see also Healthology
pharmaceutical reimportation 365–80; drug
costs for seniors 374, 375; economics of
366–8; FDA drug seizures 378; media
events 375; New York consumer price
comparison website 374; political
contributions 370; pressures on the
Canadian government 375–6; the pricing
rhetoric 368–70; rhetoric and outflanking
in 371–8, 379, 380; safety rhetoric 376,
377–8; strategic action 361, 379; US state
reimportation programs 375, 376–8, 384n
Philip Morris 402
photonovels 156–7, 163
physician-nurse relationship 302–3
physician-patient relationships 8, 9, 11,
268–9, 275; and authority 176–7, 208,
283; bounded/unbounded 294; context of
social policy and patients' lives 359–60;
cultural sensitivity approach 149; in
dialysis treatment 294, 295–6;
disempowerment in 337; importance of
listening 88–9; research methods 15
physicians: knowledge and power 272, 298,
302, 303–4, 307; Latino 218–19; rounds
289
Pinder, L. 405
Pingree, Chellie 375

Pires, G. 339, 340
Plan, Do, Study, Act (PDSA) Cycle 163, 164–5
Polaschek, N. 296, 298, 299, 301, 302, 303, 308
Policastro, M. 39
policy: *see* health policy
political contributions of the pharmaceutical industry 370
Poltorak, M. 116
polymorphism 204, 207
Poole, M.S. 270
population control 251–2, 262
Porter, D. 397
Porter, E. 375
Porter, L.G. 46
post-positivistic approach 5, 8–9, 22; methodology 15; theory building 11–12, 449; voices of local communities 150
postcolonial theory 7, 432, 457
postmodern theory 7, 14, 457
poststructuralism 32, 269
poverty: blaming individuals for their 258, 259, 260; increases under SAPs 397, 406n; interventions in 393
Poverty Reduction Strategy Paper (PRSP) 406n
power 7, 14, 16, 32, 198, 226, 272, 454; challenging assumptions of 308–9; and culture in medical practice 269; health discourses in relationships of power 34; and knowledge in medical care 271, 275, 276–80, 288, 296–7, 308–9; paradox of 186–91; physicians' knowledge and 272, 298, 302, 303–4, 307; *power to* and *power over* 158; and the relationship with identities 231; structure in the US health system 293–4
Power, B.M. 157
Prakash, Gyan 457
Pratt, C.B. 394
praxis 4, 14
Precautionary Principle (PP) 400
pregnancy: narratives 47; social support in 169; women's behaviors in 114
prenatal education case study 151, 160–79; discussion 176–8; empowerment 158–9; gender appropriate approaches 159; method 161–3; participatory and culture-centered approaches 157–61; results 163–76; Teach-With-Stories (TWS) Method 151, 166–8
Prescott, P.A. 302
Prescription Drug Users Fee Act 383n
Price, P. 160, 208
privacy, maintaining 190, 326–9
privatization 397–8, 403
Prochaska, J.O. 161
professionalism 304–5

professionalization discourse 31
Prohaska, T.R. 225
promotional corporate discourse 338
Proyecto ContraSIDA Por Vida (PCPV or Proyecto) 152–3, 225, 229–43; critical health communication praxis 225–9; funding 232–3, 241; identities 231–2, 235, 238–9; Las Diablitas soccer team 232, 239, 240; RICCA model of 'living theory' 233–41; work with sex workers 236
Pryor, J.B. 129
psychotherapy 52
psychotherapy narratives 48
Public Citizen 401
public health: courses of action to promote global 403–4; critical approaches to 393, 403, 406; discourse 392–4, 403; discursive influence of neoliberal economic policy on 396–402; economic governmentality and 391–2; influence of health policy on 358–60
public opinion 335, 373

quest narratives 48
Quinn, S.C. 198

Rabin, S. 51
Rachlis, M. 367
racial health disparities 148, 151, 157, 183, 205–6, 269; in breastfeeding 66–7, 81–2n
racism, impacting on CBPR processes 187
Radio Communication Project (RCP) 153, 247–64; context 250–3; interrogating the participatory claims 253–61; participatory communication in E-E 249–50
radio dramas 249–50, 252
Ragan, S.L. 49, 51
Rainie, L. 337
Ramos-Marcuse, F. 50
Ramser, P. 43
Randall-David, E. 167
Rappaport, J. 183
Rawlins, W.K. 46, 316
Ray, E.B. 9, 10, 226
Reagan, Ronald 359
Real, K. 270
Reardon, J. 434
Reason, P. 188
Redford, E.S. 373
Reeder, G.D. 129
Rees, C.E. 216
Reeves, P. 340
reflexivity 432, 452
Regenstein, M. 157
Reilly, D. 88
Reinharz, S. 298
relational-cultural theory 158
religious beliefs 108; and Latino attitudes to cancer 207, 215–16, 220

resistance 102, 308, 315, 317-20, 454; to
    health messages 459; to medical expertise
    in breastfeeding mothers 74–5, 77–80;
    non-compliance of dialysis patients 300,
    301, 308; and the path to holistic healing
    102–3
respeto 208
RICCA model 233–41, 242
Rice, R.L. 169
RiceTec 423
Rich, M. 43, 192
Richard, A. 17
Rickheim, P.L. 169
Ricouer, P. 315
Riessman, C. 45
Riley, R. 276, 277
Rimal, R.N. 339
Rirodan, J. 65
Rising, S.S. 155
risk behaviors 182, 228, 239
risk discourses 124–5
Rissel, C.E. 182
Ritenbaugh, C.K. 89
Robert, S.A. 224
Roberts, K. 339, 352
Robinson, J.A. 40
Rodríguez, J.M. 230, 233
Rogers, E.M. 8, 9, 247, 249
Román, David 224, 243
Romyn, D.M. 46
Roosevelt, Franklin 47
Roque Ramírez, H.N. 224, 230, 233, 238
Rose, N. 391, 395
Ross, C.E. 208
Ross, M.H. 373
Roth, N.L. 50
Rouse, D.J. 169
Rowell, A. 335
Rowson, M. 397
Roy, A. 403
Ryan, K.M. 67
Rybarczyk, B. 43

Saba, W.P. 394
Sabogal, F. 217
Sadur, C.N. 169
Said, E. 431, 457
Sakalys, J.A. 47
Salmon, J.W. 367
Sanchez-Merki, V. 182
Sanitary and Phytosanitary (SPS) agreements
    399, 400
Santiago-Valles, W.F. 227
Sass, R. 399, 400
Saul, J.R. 403
Saul, S. 373
Saunders, J.M. 51
Scambler, G. 125, 131
Schatell, D. 294, 304

Schattschneider, E.E. 373
Schell, R. 314
Schenkel, S. 276
Scherer, C.W. 8
Scherman, M.H. 44
Schmied, V. 65, 68, 69
Schoepf, B.G. 397
Schrank, R.C. 40–1
Schulte, S.K. 192
Schwartz, L. 49
scientific discourses 11–12, 90, 433–5, 438–44
second-order research 227
Sedney, M.A. 40
Seid, M. 415, 426
self, cultural concepts of 431
self-regulation 124–5
Senge, P. 288
sense making narratives 41–2
Sensky, T. 302
Settee, P. 438
sex workers 228, 236
Shaffir, W.B. 73
Shah, Aparna and Suresh 93–4
Shapin, S. 278
Sharf, Barbara 6, 7, 9, 10, 15, 16, 32, 41, 43,
    45, 48, 268, 269, 273, 314, 358, 359, 394,
    412, 459
Shealy, C. Norman 89, 90
Shiro, M. 52
Shiva, V. 426, 457
Sholle, D.J. 337, 341
Siahpush, M. 88
Sibinga, E.M.S. 88
Sidel, V.W. 398
Siegel, K. 42
Singhal, A. 46, 247, 249
skepticism and the path to healing 101–2
Skinsnes, O.K. 129, 130
Skocpol, T. 373
Skoldberg, K. 320, 330
Skorshammer, M. 51
Skovdahl, K. 51
Skultans, V. 47
Slater, C.J. 169
Sleath, B. 88
Sloan, R.P. 90
Smedley, B.D. 205
Smith, S.L. 314
smoking narratives 50–1
Smyth, J. 49
Snyder, L.B. 394
Sobnosky, M.J. 18
social activism 437, 444
social change/status quo dialectic 10, 11
Solis, H.L. 205
Solomon, M. 15
Sontag, Susan 31, 34, 457
Sophia (holistic healer) 94–5
Sorlie, V. 46, 51

Sotirin, P. 17, 66, 69
Souter, K.T. 51
South Korea 420
Speer, P.W. 142
Speroff, T. 163
spiral model 142, 159, 160, 163
spirituality 89, 90–1, 108, 176
Spivak, G.C. 7, 232, 307, 431, 432, 434, 438, 457
Squier, S.M. 41, 42
Stacey, R.D. 332
stages-of-change theory 161
Stake, R.E. 71
Stalker, J. 159
Stearns, C.A. 69
Stein, Howard 268, 457
Stein, N.L. 31, 39
Stein, S. 338
Stern, S. 48
Stevens, E. 208
Stiglitz, J.E. 396
stigma: of AIDS 129; of leprosy 130–1
Stiles, W.B. 48
Stoecker, R. 194
Stohl, C. 182, 183, 184, 185, 191, 193, 197, 198
Stokes, A.Q. 337
Stone, D. 373
Stoner, M.H. 295
Storey, D. 247, 248, 249, 250, 251, 253, 262, 263, 394
Stormer, N. 68
strategic action 361, 379
Strauss, A.L. 319
Strayhorn, C.K. 210–11
Street, R.L. 15
Structural Adjustment Package (SAP) loans 396–8, 406n
structure: and culture 151, 228, 413–14, 419, 421, 424; and power 7, 14; unhealthy 462
Strupp, H.H. 89
substance abuse 9, 182; American Indian drug-prevention campaign 185–98
sugar 420–1
Sullivan, M.C. 216
Sunwolf 45, 49
Survey-Education-Treatment (SET) model 131–2
Sutherland, E.G. 89
Sutherland, L.R. 86, 87
Svedlund, M. 51
Swartz, L. 182, 186
Swartzman, L.C. 88
Symonds, B.D. 89

Tannen, D. 40
Tardy, R.W. 45
Taru 249–50

Taurel, Sidney 368
Taylor, B.C. 6, 71, 297
Taylor, J.A. 169
Teach-With-Stories (TWS) Method 151, 166–8
teacher-centered approach 157–8, 161
Technical Barriers to Trade (TBT) agreements 399, 400
technological discourse 395, 397, 402–3
Teinowitz, I. 337
Teng, B.S. 186
Tesh, S. 393
Tessaro, I.A. 314
theory: see health communication theories
Theory of Reasoned Action 11
'third-order' research 225, 227, 242
Thirtysomething 16, 32–3
Thomas-MacLean, R. 48
Thomas, S.B. 198, 205
Thompson, T.L. 2, 4, 42, 46, 358
Thorne, S.E. 299, 308
Tinkha Tinkha Sukh 249
Tonga 420, 421
Torgerson, R. 415, 426
Tracy, S.J. 197
trade agreements, neoliberal global 411–27; Agreement on Agriculture (AoA) 419–21; Agreement on Trade-Related Aspects of Intellectual Property Rights (TRIPS) 422–4, 425, 426, 439; General Agreement on Trade and Tariffs (GATT) 415–19, 425; impact on food security 412, 414–15, 424–7
transmission communication model 135
Transtheoretical Model of Change 161
traumatic narratives 49
Treichler, Paula 457
Trethewey, A. 70
Trevino, F. 208
Trickett, E.J. 192, 198
Trinh, C. 314
TRIPS 422–4, 425, 426, 439
True, N. 49
Trumbull, D.J. 71
Trummer, U.F. 155
Tudiver, F. 314
Tulloch, J. 115
Turner, B. 124
Turner, R.N. 85, 86
Turquist, C. 340
Tuskegee experiments 198

Ungar, M. 43
UNICEF 397
United States Agency for International Development (USAID) 251, 252
universal/specific tension 10, 11, 13
Urwin, C. 126
US Civil Rights Act 207

US Department of Health and Human Services (USDHHS) 63, 66
US Food Quality Protection Act 400

Valente, S.M. 51
Valente, T.W. 394
Vanderford, Marsha 6, 41, 45, 70, 269
Vegni, E. 51
Venezuela 401
Verhoef, M.J. 86, 87
Vibbert, S. 337
Vickers, A. 87
Vickery, M. 395
Video Intervention/Prevention Assessment 43
Villagran, M. 203
Villalobos, Alice 224
Virchow, R. 393
Vitri, N. 295
Vogel, D. 372

Waitzkin, H. 7, 13, 14, 16, 33, 268, 393
Walker, V.G. 131
Wall, G. 64, 66, 68
Wallace, R.W. 439
Wallack, L. 359, 394
Wallerstein, N. 182, 183, 185
Walters, A.S. 43
Ward, J.D. 64
Warren, S.L. 50
Washington Post 377
water, access to clean 397–8
Watsu 94, 105
weaning 78
Wear, D. 51, 293, 296, 298, 303
Weaver, A.J. 90
Weick, K. 40, 71, 279, 282
Weil, J. 87
Weiner, J. 415, 419
Welles-Nystrom, B. 116
Wendt, R.F. 183, 185
Whitt, L.A. 435
Whyte, W.F. 183
Widdershovern, G.A.M. 91
Wiegand, S. 352
Wilkes, M. 337

Wilkie, M.S. 344
Williams, L. 43, 208, 214
Wilson, H. 51
Wilson, J.Q. 370, 373
Wilson, R.H. 210
Wing, S. 186
Witte, K. 6, 8, 9, 15, 182, 394
Wittenberg-Lyles, E. 49
Wolff, T. 183, 184
women: behaviors in pregnancy 114; medicalization of 65–8, 73; narratives of 159, 269
Wood, M.L. 208
Woods, M. 422, 423
Workman, T. 46, 51
workplace: health discourses in the 33–4; participation in the 182–3
World Bank (WB) 390, 391, 393, 396, 397, 412, 415
World Council of Indigenous Peoples (WCIP) 438
World Health Organization (WHO) 87, 89, 129, 390, 393, 405
World Trade Organization (WTO) 365, 391, 399, 400, 401, 405, 415, 419, 420, 422; formation of 416–17
Wright, L. 340
www.I-SaveRx.com 377, 384n
Wynia, M.K. 88

Yamada, S. 52
Yep, G.A. 7, 17, 224, 226, 314, 331
Young, A. 50

Zabos, G.P. 314
Zaire 398
Zerwekh, J.V. 51
Zimbabwe 398
Zimmerman, D.R. 67
Zito, J.M. 336, 337
Zola, I. 31
Zoller, H.M. 3, 7, 15, 16, 17, 18, 188, 191, 229, 314, 339, 358, 359, 394, 399, 405, 406, 412, 426, 432, 443, 460
Zollman, C. 87
Zook, E.G. 9